EVANSTON HOSPITAL CORPORATION
EMERGENCY DEPARTMENT

DECISION MAKING IN
Trauma Management

A Multidisciplinary Approach

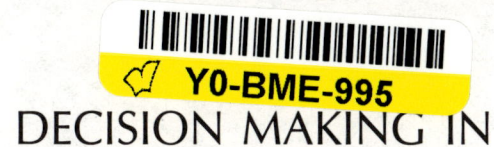

Medical Titles in the Clinical Decision Making™ Series

Consulting Editor
Ben Eiseman, M.D.

Balduini, Torg, Lehman, Gecha, Vegso:
   Decision Making in Sports Medicine
Berman:
   Pediatric Decision Making
Brain:
   Decision Making in Hematology
Bready, Smith:
   Decision Making in Anesthesiology
Callaham, Barton, Schumaker:
   Decision Making in Emergency Medicine
DeCherney, Polan, Lee, Boyers:
   Decision Making in Infertility
Don:
   Decision Making in Critical Care
Dubovsky, Feiger, Eiseman:
   Psychiatric Decision Making
Dunn, Epstein:
   Decision Making in Child Neurology
Friedman, Acker, Sachs:
   Obstetrical Decision Making
Friedman, Borten, Chapin:
   Gynecological Decision Making

Karlinsky, Goldstein, Lau:
   Decision Making in Pulmonary Medicine
Kohler, Jordan:
   Decision Making in Endocrinology and Metabolism
Korones:
   Neonatal Decision Making
Levine:
   Decision Making in Gastroenterology
Montgomery, Atkins:
   Decision Making in Emergency Cardiology
Nichols, Hyslop, Bartlett:
   Decision Making in Surgical Sepsis
Schein:
   Decision Making in Oncology
Shapiro, Chan:
   Decision Making in Nephrology
van Heuven, Zwaan:
   Decision Making in Ophthalmology
Weisberg, Strub, Garcia:
   Decision Making in Adult Neurology

Decision Making in Clinical Nursing™ Series

Baird:
   Decision Making in Oncology Nursing
Baumann, Johnston, Antai-Otong:
   Decision Making in Psychiatric and Psychosocial Nursing
Drain:
   Decision Making in Postanesthesia Nursing
Gorzeman, Bowdoin:
   Decision Making in Medical-Surgical Nursing
Knor:
   Decision Making in Obstetrical Nursing
Mancini:
   Decision Making in Emergency Nursing
Murphy:
   Decision Making in Pediatric Nursing
Wells:
   Decision Making in Perioperative Nursing
Williams:
   Decision Making in Critical Care Nursing

DECISION MAKING IN
Trauma Management
A Multidisciplinary Approach

Mary E. Mancini, RN, MSN, CNA

Vice-President
Nursing Administration
Parkland Memorial Hospital
Dallas, Texas

Jorie Klein, RN

Trauma Coordinator
Parkland Memorial Hospital
Dallas, Texas

B.C. Decker Inc. • Philadelphia

Publisher	B.C. Decker Inc
	320 Walnut Street
	Suite 400
	Philadelphia, Pennsylvania 19106

Sales and Distribution

United States and Puerto Rico
Mosby-Year Book Inc.
11830 Westline Industrial Drive
Saint Louis, Missouri 63146

Canada
Mosby-Year Book Limited
5240 Finch Avenue E., Unit 1
Scarborough, Ontario M1S 5A2

Australia
McGraw-Hill Book Company Australia Pty. Ltd.
4 Barcoo Street
Roseville East 2069
New South Wales, Australia

Brazil
Editora McGraw-Hill do Brasil, Ltda.
rua Tabapua, 1.105, Itaim-Bibi
Sao Paulo, S.P. Brasil

Colombia
Interamericana/McGraw-Hill de Colombia, S.A.
Carrera 17, No. 33-71
(Apartado Postal, A.A., 6131)
Bogota, D.E., Colombia

Europe, United Kingdom, Middle East and Africa
Wolfe Publishing Limited
Brook House
2-16 Torrington Place
London WC1E 7LT England

Hong Kong and China
McGraw-Hill Book Company
Suite 618, Ocean Centre
5 Canton Road
Tsimshatsui, Kowloon
Hong Kong

India
Tata McGraw-Hill Publishing Company, Ltd.
12/4 Asaf Ali Road, 3rd Floor
New Delhi 110002, India

Indonesia
Mr. Wong Fin Fah
P.O. Box 122/JAT
Jakarta, 1300 Indonesia

Japan
Igaku-Shoin Ltd.
Tokyo International P.O. Box 5063
1-28-36 Hongo, Bunkyo-ku,
Tokyo 113, Japan

Korea
Mr. Don-Gap Choi
C.P.O. Box 10583
Seoul, Korea

Malaysia
Mr. Lim Tao Slong
No. 8 Jalan SS 7/6B
Kelana Jaya
47301 Petaling Jaya
Selangor, Malaysia

Mexico
Interamericana/McGraw-Hill de Mexico, S.A. de C.V.
Cedro 512, Colonia Atlampa
(Apartado Postal 26370)
06450 Mexico, D.F., Mexico

New Zealand
McGraw-Hill Book Co. New Zealand Ltd.
5 Joval Place, Wiri
Manukau City, New Zealand

Portugal
Editora McGraw-Hill de Portugal, Ltda.
Rua Rosa Damasceno 11A-B
1900 Lisboa, Portugal

South Africa
Libriger Book Distributors
Warehouse Number 8
"Die Ou Looiery"
Tannery Road
Hamilton, Bloemfontein 9300

Singapore and Southeast Asia
McGraw-Hill Book Co.
21 Neythal Road
Jurong, Singapore 2262

Spain
McGraw-Hill/Interamericana de Espana, S.A.
Manuel Ferrero, 13
28020 Madrid, Spain

Taiwan
Mr. George Lim
P.O. Box 87-601
Taipei, Taiwan

Thailand
Mr. Vitit Lim
632/5 Phaholyothin Road
Sapan Kwai
Bangkok 10400
Thailand

Venezuela
Editorial Interamericana de Venezuela, C.A.
2da. calle Bello Monte
Local G-2
Caracas, Venezuela

NOTICE

The authors and publisher have made every effort to ensure that the patient care recommended herein, including choice of drugs and drug dosages, is in accord with the accepted standards and practice at the time of publication. However, since research and regulation constantly change clinical standards, the reader is urged to check the product information sheet included in the package of each drug, which includes recommended doses, warnings, and contraindications. This is particularly important with new or infrequently used drugs.

Decision Making in Trauma Management: A Multidisciplinary Approach   ISBN 1-55664-227-X

© 1991 by B.C. Decker Incorporated under the International Copyright Union. All rights reserved. No part of this publication may be reused or republished in any form without written permission of the publisher.

Library of Congress catalog card number: 90-83573   10 9 8 7 6 5 4 3 2 1

CONTRIBUTORS

EVANSTON HOSPITAL CORPORATION EMERGENCY DEPARTMENT

JAN AUERBACH, RN, MSN, EMTP

Paramedic Instructor, University of Texas Southwestern Medical Center at Dallas, Dallas, Texas

SUZY BAULCH, RN, BSN, CEN

Trauma Nurse Coordinator, NT Enloe Memorial Hospital, Chico, California

DAVID BARBA, MD

Assistant Professor of Neurosurgery, University of California San Diego School of Medicine, San Diego, California

JAN BEAR, MD

Chief Resident, Department of Orthopaedics and Rehabilitation, University of New Mexico Hospital, Albuquerque, New Mexico

BARBARA A. BIELAWSKI, RN, MS, CEN, TNCC

Quality Management Coordinator, Evanston Hospital Corporation, Evanston, Illinois

MELANIE DAETWEILER BOONE, BS

Surgical Critical Care Liaison, Parkland Memorial Hospital, Dallas, Texas

NANCY G. BROWN, RN, BSN

Assistant Trauma Coordinator, University of California Davis Medical Center, Sacramento, California

J. KENNETH BURKUS, MD

Assistant Clinical Professor, Department of Orthopedic Surgery, University of California Davis School of Medicine, Davis, California

DEBRA CASON, RN, MS, EMT-P

Assistant Professor, University of Texas Southwestern Medical Center at Dallas Southwestern Medical School; Emergency Medical Services Program Director, University of Texas Southwestern Medical Center at Dallas, Dallas, Texas

DONNA KAY CAUSBY, BS, PT

Chief Physical Therapist, Parkland Memorial Hospital, Dallas, Texas

BETTY M. CLARK, RN, MPA, CCRN

Nurse Manager, Surgical Intensive Care Unit, University of California Davis Medical Center, Sacramento, California

NATHAN COATES, MD

Assistant Instructor and Surgeon, University of Texas Health Science Center at Dallas Southwestern Medical School, Dallas, Texas

BRIAN COPELAND, MD, FACS

Staff, Division of Neurosurgery, Scripps Clinic and Research Foundation, Childrens Hospital and Health Center, San Diego, California

JANE CURRAN, RN, BSN

Staff Nurse, Emergency Services, Parkland Memorial Hospital, Dallas, Texas

KIMBERLY L. DAVIES, RN, BSN, CEN, EMT-P

Flight Nurse, Careflite Dallas, Helicopter Ambulance Service of North Texas, Plano, Texas

THOMAS DRURY, RN, BSN, BBA, CCRN, CEN

Assistant Trauma Coordinator, Trauma Department, Parkland Memorial Hospital, Dallas, Texas

KENDRA ELLIS, RN, BSN, CCRN, CEN

Critical Care Educator—Surgery, Parkland Memorial Hospital, Dallas, Texas

PATRICIA C. EPIFANIO, RN, MS, CEN

Emergency Nurse Coordinator, Maryland Institute of Emergency Medical Systems, Lutherville, Maryland

SHEENA M. FERGUSON, MSN, RN, CCRN, TNS

Student, University of Texas–Austin; Staff, Brackenridge Hospital, Austin, Texas

MAUREEN E. FLANAGAN, MS

Former Writer/Editor, Trauma Research Department, Washington Hospital Center, Washington, DC

TERI GALE, RN, BSN

Biotel Coordinator, Parkland Memorial Hospital, Dallas, Texas

GHALI E. GHALI, DDS

Chief Resident, Oral and Maxillofacial Surgery, University of Texas Southwestern Medical Center at Dallas Southwestern Medical School, Dallas, Texas

CAROL GOODYKOONTZ, RN, MS, EMT-P

Assistant Professor, University of Texas Southwestern Medical Center at Dallas Southwestern Medical School; Emergency Medical Services Assistant Program Director, University of Texas Southwestern Medical Center at Dallas, Dallas, Texas

ANITA L. GRUDDA, MOT, OTR

Staff, Department of Physical Medicine and Rehabilitation, Parkland Memorial Hospital, Dallas, Texas

GWEN J. HALL, MB

Forensic Pathologist, Oroville, California

MARINA G. HALL, BS, PT

Senior Staff Physical Therapist, Parkland Memorial Hospital, Dallas, Texas

LOUISE HAUBNER, RN, BSN, CEN, MICN

Base Hospital Nurse Coordinator/Disaster Coordinator, Sharp Memorial Hospital, San Diego, California

THOMAS S. HELPENSTELL, MD

Orthopaedic Surgeon, University of New Mexico Hospital and School of Medicine, Albuquerque, New Mexico

PEGGY HOLLINGSWORTH-FRIDLUND, RN, BSN

Trauma Coordinator, University of California San Diego Medical Center, San Diego, California

DAVID B. HOYT, MD

Associate Professor of Surgery, University of California San Diego School of Medicine; Director, Trauma Division, University of California San Diego Medical Center, San Diego, California

ANN HUDGINS, RN, BSN, EMT-P

Paramedic Instructor, Emergency Medicine Educators, University of Texas Southwestern Medical Center at Dallas

JOHN L. HUNT, MD

Professor of Surgery, University of Texas Southwestern Medical Center at Dallas Southwestern Medical School; Co-Director, Burn Unit, Parkland Memorial Hospital, Dallas, Texas

LISA B. JONES, RN, BSN, CEN

Former Head Nurse, Surgical Emergency Services, Parkland Memorial Hospital, Dallas, Texas

REBECCA P. JONES, BS, PT

Senior Staff Physical Therapist, Parkland Memorial Hospital, Dallas, Texas

LOUANN KITCHEN, RN, MS

Faculty, San Diego State University; Former Trauma Program Manager, Childrens Hospital and Health Center, San Diego, California

JORIE KLEIN, RN

Trauma Coordinator, Parkland Memorial Hospital, Dallas, Texas

KEVIN W. KLEIN, MD

Assistant Professor of Anesthesiology, University of Texas Southwestern Medical Center at Dallas Southwestern Medical School; Director of Anesthesiology, Zale-Lipshy University Hospital, Dallas, Texas

SALLY A. KNAUER, MD

Orthopedic Surgeon, Poudre Valley Hospital, Fort Collins, Colorado

VINETTE LANGFORD, RN, MSN, CEN

Co-Director of Critical Care Services, Louisiana State University Medical Center, Shreveport, Louisiana

MARY M. LAWNICK, RN, BSN

Nurse Research Assistant and MTOS Nurse Coordinator, Washington Hospital Center, Washington, DC

JEFFREY M. LOBOSKY, MD

Clinical Instructor, Department of Neurological Surgery, University of California Davis School of Medicine, Davis; Medical Director, Neurosurgical ICU, NT Enloe Memorial Hospital, Chico, California

MIGUEL A. LOPEZ-VIEGO, MD

Chief Surgical Resident, University of Texas Southwestern Medical Center and Parkland Memorial Hospital, Dallas, Texas

JODI LUKE, RN

Emergency Services Nurse, Parkland Memorial Hospital, Dallas, Texas

FRANK P. LYNCH, MD, FACS, FAAP

Clinical Professor of Surgery and Chief of Pediatric Surgery, University of California San Diego School of Medicine; Director of Trauma Services, Childrens Hospital and Health Center, San Diego, California

MARY E. MANCINI, RN, MSN, CNA

Vice-President, Nursing Administration, Parkland Memorial Hospital, Dallas, Texas

CONNIE MATTICE, RN, MSN

Trauma Nurse Coordinator, Butterworth Hospital, Grand Rapids Michigan

MARY C. McCARTHY, MD, FACS

Clinical Associate Professor of Surgery, Indiana University School of Medicine, Indianapolis, Indiana

EILEEN McMENEMY, RN

Homeless Outreach Medical Services Coordinator, Parkland Memorial Hospital, Dallas, Texas

BOB McMULLEN, PA-C, EMT-P

Assistant Instructor and EMT Training Coordinator, University of Texas Southwestern Medical Center at Dallas, Dallas, Texas

SHARON V. MOREL, RN, MSN, CRRN

Arthritis Care Center Manager, Saint Joseph Hospital, Ft. Worth, Texas

STEVEN L. MOULTON, MD

Senior Surgical Resident, University of California San Diego School of Medicine, San Diego, California

JANET NEFF, RN, MN

Trauma Coordinator and Base Station Coordinator, Stanford University Hospital, Stanford, California

ROBERT J. O'MALLEY, RN

Manager, Life Flight, University of California at Davis Medical Center, Davis, California

JOSEPH P. OSTERKAMP, MD

Chief Resident, Department of Anesthesia, University of California at Davis Medical Center, Davis, California

CONSTANCE D. PARRY, BS, PT

Senior Staff Physical Therapist, Parkland Memorial Hospital, Dallas, Texas

BRADLEY PETERSON, MD, FACA, FAAP, FCCM

Associate Clinical Professor of Pediatrics and Anesthesia, University of California San Diego School of Medicine; Director, Pediatric Intensive Care Unit, and Associate Director of Trauma, Childrens Hospital and Health Center, San Diego, California

EDWARD W. POTTMEYER, MD

Assistant Clinical Professor, Department of Surgery, University of California Davis School of Medicine, Davis; Staff Surgeon, Trauma Service, University of California Davis Medical Center, Sacramento, California

GARY F. PURDUE, MD

Associate Professor of Surgery, University of Texas Southwestern Medical Center at Dallas Southwestern Medical School; Co-Director, Burn Unit, Parkland Memorial Hospital, Dallas, Texas

WILLIAM GARY REED, MD

Professor, Department of Internal Medicine, University of Texas Southwestern Medical Center at Dallas Southwestern Medical School, Dallas, Texas

JOHN D. S. REID, MD

Clinical Assistant Professor, University of British Columbia Faculty of Medicine; Active Staff, St. Paul's Hospital, Vancouver, British Columbia, Canada

DOREEN REYNOLDS, RN

Director of Nurses, Operating Suite, Parkland Memorial Hospital, Dallas, Texas

MARY K. ROBERTS, BA, RN, MSN, CCRN

Critical Care Instructor and Critical Care and Trauma Nurse, Parkland Memorial Hospital, Dallas, Texas

R. BERNARD ROCHON, MD

Assistant Instructor, Department of Surgery, University of Texas Southwestern Medical Center at Dallas Southwestern Medical School; Trauma/Critical Care Fellow, Parkland Memorial Hospital, Dallas, Texas

MOLLY A. SEAMAN, RN, MSN, CEN

Quality Assurance/Risk Management Coordinator, Metroplex Emergency Physicians, P.A., Farmer's Branch, Texas

KATHLEEN C. SOLOTKIN, RN

Trauma Nurse Coordinator, Indiana University Critical Care and Trauma Center, Indianapolis, Indiana

JOHNESE SPISSO, RN, MPA, CCRN, CEN

Manager, Trauma Program, University of California Davis Medical Center, Sacramento, California

GREGORY G. STANFORD, MD

Assistant Professor, University of Texas Southwestern Medical Center at Dallas Southwestern Medical School; Staff Physician, Trauma/Critical Care Section, Parkland Memorial Hospital, Dallas, Texas

WILLIAM I. STERETT, MD

Professor of Orthopedic Surgery, University of California Davis School of Medicine; Staff, Department of Orthopedic Surgery, University of California Davis Medical Center, Davis, California

DENISE L. STEWART, RN, CEN

Staff Nurse, Emergency Services, Methodist Medical Center, Dallas, Texas

PATTI SUTTON-DIETRICH, RN, BSN, CCRN

Head Nurse, Pedi-Trauma Intensive Care Unit, Parkland Memorial Hospital, Dallas, Texas

PAULA TANABE, RN, MSN, CEN, TNS

Practitioner-Teacher, Emergency Department, Rush–Presbyterian–St. Luke's Medical Center, Chicago, Illinois

ERWIN R. THAL, MD

Professor, University of Texas Southwestern Medical Center at Dallas Southwestern Medical School; Medical Director, Surgical Emergency Room, Parkland Memorial Hospital, Dallas, Texas

JOHN TOMPKINS, MD

Clinical Instructor, University of Oklahoma College of Medicine; Chief, Orthopedic Surgery, Veterans Administration Medical Center, Oklahoma City, Oklahoma

ROBERT V. WALKER, DDS, FFDRCS(Ire), FDSRCS(Eng)

Professor and Past Chairman, Division of Oral and Maxillofacial Surgery, University of Texas Medical Center at Dallas Southwestern Medical School, Dallas, Texas

JOHN A. WEIGELT, MD, FACS

Professor of Surgery, University of Texas Southwestern Medical Center at Dallas Southwestern Medical School; Medical Director, Trauma/Surgical Intensive Care, Parkland Memorial Hospital, Dallas, Texas

PATTI WILLIS, RN, BSN

Head Nurse, Surgical Emergency Services Department, Parkland Memorial Hospital, Dallas, Texas

LINDA L. WILSON, RT

Staff, Department of Radiology, Parkland Memorial Hospital, Dallas, Texas

ROBERT P. WINTER, MD

Attending Surgeon and Vascular Specialist of Central Florida, Orlando Regional Medical Center, Orlando, Florida

DAVID H. WISNER, MD

Assistant Professor of Surgery, University of California Davis School of Medicine, Davis, California

PREFACE

Trauma care as a specialty has grown from infancy in the eighties to a specialized area of care and expertise as it enters the nineties. Health care professionals are faced daily with the challenge of providing care to the trauma patient population. Trauma continues to be the leading cause of death for children and adults under the age of 45. Each hour in the United States, 40 victims die from trauma injuries and approximately 1000 are injured and require medical treatment.

The purpose of *Decision Making in Trauma Management: A Multidisciplinary Approach* is to present the process of trauma management during the pre-hospital, resuscitation, stabilization, supportive, and rehabilitation phases in decision tree format. This format will be beneficial to everyone involved in trauma care from community hospitals to Level I Trauma Centers. The goal of the algorithm is to construct a format that is easy to follow and clearly demonstrates decision management. The narrative information is keyed to the decision points to provide further information and supportive references.

The contributors were targeted to provide a multidisciplinary group of authors. The contributors are established clinicians from different areas in the United States and Canada, which will provide the reader with a national perspective of trauma management. The reader will find chapters on specialty areas of trauma care, such as Pediatric Trauma, Trauma in the Elderly, and Trauma in the Homeless. The supportive care chapters cover the progression of the traumatic insult and the common complications that ensue. Procedures used in the initial evaluation and management and hospital course are included in the procedure chapters. The Rehabilitation section includes chapters on Spinal Cord Injury and Traumatic Brain Injury and other areas of rehabilitation expertise. Topics such as Trauma Scoring and Evidence Collection are also covered. We hope all clinicians involved in trauma care find the algorithms informative and useful in the daily setting of trauma management.

Thanks to all contributors who shared their clinical expertise and enthusiasm in producing this book. Thanks to Ms. Louann Kitchen for coordinating and being first editor of the Pediatric Trauma Section. Thanks to Brian Decker and Ellen Thomas for their help and support. Special thanks to Mr. Tom Drury, Ms. Tammy Morgan, Mrs. Jan Coder, and the Word Processing Department at Parkland Memorial Hospital for making this endeavor possible.

Jorie Klein
Beth Mancini

To

David, Laura and Carla

Mary E. Mancini

To

All health care professionals who give their time,
knowledge and expertise to provide
quality trauma care throughout our nation

Jorie Klein

CONTENTS

Mechanism of Injury 1
John A. Weigelt
Jorie Klein

PRE-HOSPITAL CARE

Dispatch 6
Debra Cason

Scene Management/Patient Evaluation 8
Carol Goodykoontz

Pre-Hospital Management 12
Debra Cason

EMT/Paramedic and Physician Communication ... 14
Jan Auerbach

Field Triage 16
Ann Hudgins

RESUSCITATION/STABILIZATION

Initial Assessment 20
Erwin R. Thal
Jorie Klein

Secondary Assessment 26
Erwin R. Thal
Jorie Klein

SHOCK MANAGEMENT

Hypovolemic Shock 36
Mary K. Roberts

Blood Administration 40
Thomas Drury

Fluid Warming 44
Thomas Drury

HEAD TRAUMA

Blunt Head Trauma 48
Gregory G. Stanford

Penetrating Head Trauma 52
Gregory G. Stanford

Skull Fracture 54
Jorie Klein

FACIAL TRAUMA

Maxillofacial Soft Tissue Trauma 58
Kimberly L. Davies

Nasal Trauma 60
Kimberly L. Davies

Dental Trauma 62
Kimberly L. Davies

Ear Trauma 64
Kimberly L. Davies

Eye Trauma 66
Patricia C. Epifanio

Maxillofacial Fractures: Airway Management 68
Robert V. Walker
Ghali E. Ghali

Maxillofacial Fractures: Treatment 70
Robert V. Walker
Ghali E. Ghali

NECK TRAUMA

Blunt Neck Trauma 76
   Kimberly L. Davies

Penetrating Neck Trauma 80
   Miguel A. Lopez-Viego

THORACIC TRAUMA: LIFE THREATENING INJURIES

Airway Obstruction 86
   Kimberly L. Davies

Tension Pneumothorax 88
   Lisa B. Jones

Massive Hemothorax 92
   Gregory G. Stanford

Open Sucking Chest Wound 94
   Jane Curran

Flail Chest 96
   Jane Curran

Cardiac Tamponade 98
   Lisa B. Jones

Emergency Thoracotomy 102
   John D. S. Reid

THORACIC TRAUMA: POTENTIALLY LIFE THREATENING INJURIES

Myocardial Contusion 106
   Johnese Spisso
   Edward W. Pottmeyer

Pulmonary Contusion 108
   Lisa B. Jones

Aortic Trauma 112
   Lisa B. Jones

Laryngotracheal Trauma 114
   Gregory G. Stanford

Traumatic Diaphragmatic Hernia 116
   Jorie Klein
   Thomas Drury

Esophageal Trauma 118
   Johnese Spisso
   Edward W. Pottmeyer

CHEST TRAUMA: OTHER MANIFESTATIONS

Simple Hemothorax or Pneumothorax 122
   Lisa B. Jones

Subcutaneous Emphysema 124
   Jane Curran
   Thomas Drury

Rib Fractures 126
   Jane Curran
   Thomas Drury

ABDOMINAL TRAUMA

Blunt Abdominal Trauma 130
   Thomas Drury

Penetrating Abdominal Trauma 134
   Thomas Drury

Trauma to the Pelvis 136
   Connie Mattice
   Nathan Coates

SPINAL TRAUMA

Cervical Spinal Trauma 146
   Suzy Baulch
   Jeffrey M. Lobosky

Thoracolumbar Spinal Trauma 150
   Jorie Klein

UPPER EXTREMITY TRAUMA

Shoulder and Clavicle Trauma 156
Johnese Spisso

Humeral Head, Elbow, Upper Arm, Forearm,
and Wrist Trauma 158
Johnese Spisso

Hand Trauma 160
Johnese Spisso

LOWER EXTREMITY TRAUMA

Acetabular, Hip, and Femur Trauma 164
William I. Sterett
J. Kenneth Burkus

Knee Trauma 166
William I. Sterett
J. Kenneth Burkus

Lower Leg, Ankle, and Foot Trauma 168
William I. Sterett
J. Kenneth Burkus

Mangled or Amputated Extremity 172
Patricia C. Epifanio

PERIPHERAL NERVE TRAUMA

Peripheral Nerve Trauma 178
Jan Bear

VASCULAR TRAUMA

Carotid Artery Trauma 184
Robert P. Winter

Subclavian, Axillary, and Brachial
Artery Trauma 186
Robert P. Winter

Iliofemoral Vascular Trauma 188
Robert P. Winter

Popliteal and Tibial Vascular Trauma 190
David H. Wisner

ENVIRONMENTAL TRAUMA

Thermal Burn 194
Gary F. Purdue
John L. Hunt

Electrical Burn 198
Gary F. Purdue
John L. Hunt

Chemical Burn 200
Gary F. Purdue
John L. Hunt

Hypothermia and Frostbite 202
Gary F. Purdue
John L. Hunt

Escharotomy and Fasciotomy 204
Gary F. Purdue
John L. Hunt

Smoke Inhalation 206
Gary F. Purdue
John L. Hunt

PEDIATRIC TRAUMA
Louann Kitchen, section editor

Pediatric Trauma Triage 210
Louise Haubner
Louann Kitchen

Resuscitation of the Pediatric Trauma Victim 214
Steven L. Moulton
Frank P. Lynch
Bradley Peterson

Pediatric Head Trauma 220
David Barba
Louann Kitchen
Brian Copeland

Pediatric Thoracic Trauma 224
    Steven L. Moulton
    Frank P. Lynch
    Louann Kitchen

Pediatric Abdominal Trauma 230
    Steven L. Moulton
    Frank P. Lynch
    Louann Kitchen

Pediatric Extremity Trauma 236
    Sally A. Knauer
    John Tompkins

Pediatric Burn Trauma 238
    Gary F. Purdue
    John L. Hunt

Child Abuse 240
    Gary F. Purdue
    John L. Hunt

SPECIAL CONSIDERATIONS IN EVALUATION OF TRAUMA PATIENTS

Dog Bite 244
    John A. Weigelt

Animal Bite 246
    John A. Weigelt

Spider Bite 248
    John A. Weigelt

Snake Bite 250
    John A. Weigelt

Alleged Criminal Assault 252
    Patti Willis

Trauma in Pregnancy 256
    Patti Willis

Trauma in the Elderly 260
    Denise L. Stewart
    Thomas Drury

Trauma in the Homeless 262
    Eileen McMenemy

Drowning and Near Drowning 264
    William Gary Reed

Evidence Collection 266
    Suzy Baulch
    Gwen J. Hall

TRAUMA SCORING

Data Collection for Trauma Patients 272
    Mary M. Lawnick
    Maureen E. Flanagan

E Codes 274
    Mary M. Lawnick
    Maureen E. Flanagan

CRAMS Score 276
    Mary M. Lawnick
    Maureen E. Flanagan

Trauma Score and Revised Trauma Score 278
    Mary M. Lawnick
    Maureen E. Flanagan

Injury Severity Score 282
    Mary M. Lawnick
    Maureen E. Flanagan

STABILIZATION/SUPPORTIVE CARE

Anesthesia for the Trauma Patient 286
    Kevin W. Klein

Nutritional Support 288
    Jodi Luke

Fluid, Electrolyte, and Acid-Base Imbalance 290
    Molly A. Seaman

Operating Room Management 292
    Doreen Reynolds

Management of Open Wounds 296
Janet Neff

Coagulation Problems 300
R. Bernard Rochon

Febrile Syndromes 302
Janet Neff

Acute Renal Failure 304
Molly A. Seaman

Gas Gangrene Infection 306
Sheena M. Ferguson

Hepatic Failure 308
Nathan Coates

Respiratory Failure 310
Joseph P. Osterkamp

Mechanical Ventilation 312
Joseph P. Osterkamp

Cardiogenic Shock 316
Barbara A. Bielawski
Paula Tanabe

Neurogenic Shock 318
Barbara A. Bielawski
Paula Tanabe

Septic Shock 320
Barbara A. Bielawski
Paula Tanabe

Multiple Organ Failure 322
Kathleen C. Solotkin
Mary C. McCarthy

Stress Gastritis 324
John A. Weigelt

Pulmonary Embolism 326
Jodi Luke

Deep Vein Thrombosis 328
Thomas S. Helpenstell

Therapy for Infectious Processes 330
Kathleen C. Solotkin
Mary C. McCarthy

Organ Procurement 332
Jodi Luke

Crisis Intervention 334
Melanie Daetweiler Boone

Helicopter and Fixed-Wing Transportation 336
Robert J. O'Malley

REHABILITATION

Rehabilitation of the Head-Injured Patient 338
Sharon V. Morel

Rehabilitation of the Spinal Cord–Injured
Patient 342
Sharon V. Morel

Rehabilitation After Upper Extremity
Amputation 346
Anita L. Grudda

Rehabilitation After Lower Extremity
Amputation 348
Marina G. Hall
Rebecca P. Jones

Rehabilitation of the Burn-Injured Patient 352
Donna Kay Causby
Constance D. Parry

PROCEDURES: AIRWAY/VENTILATION MANAGEMENT

Intubation 358
Kevin W. Klein

Cricothyroidotomy 360
Jorie Klein
Teri Gale

Tracheostomy 362
Teri Gale

Thoracentesis 364
Lisa B. Jones

Tube Thoracostomy 366
Jorie Klein

Arterial Blood Sampling 368
Janet Neff

PROCEDURES: VENOUS/CIRCULATORY ACCESS

Military Anti-Shock Trousers 372
Erwin R. Thal
Jorie Klein

Peripheral Intravenous Access Exchange 374
Jorie Klein

Intraosseous Line 376
Patti Sutton-Dietrich

DIAGNOSTIC PROCEDURES

Arteriogram/Aortogram 378
Lisa B. Jones

Computed Tomography Scan 379
Molly A. Seaman

Diagnostic Peritoneal Lavage 380
Jorie Klein
Gregory G. Stanford

Local Exploration 382
John D. S. Reid

Magnetic Resonance Imaging 383
Linda L. Wilson

Pericardiocentesis 384
Lisa B. Jones

Paracentesis 386
Lisa B. Jones

MONITORING

Arterial Line Insertion 388
Nancy G. Brown

Intracranial Pressure Monitoring 389
Kendra Ellis

Pulse Oximetry 390
Betty M. Clark

Pulmonary Artery Catheter Insertion 391
Johnese Spisso

THERAPEUTIC PROCEDURES

Pneumatic Pressure Device 394
Connie Mattice

Temporary Access for Catheter Hemodialysis . . . 396
R. Bernard Rochon

Cervical Spine Traction/Stabilization 397
Molly A. Seaman

Temperature Control Units 399
Janet Neff

Wound Dressing 401
Janet Neff

Steinmann Pin 403
Lisa B. Jones

Thomas/Hare Traction Splint 404
Kimberly L. Davies

Closed Reduction 407
Vinette Langford

Cast Care 408
Vinette Langford

Contact Lens Removal 409
Kimberly L. Davies

Eye Irrigation 411
Janet Neff

Helmet Removal 413
Bob McMullen

Corset-Type Extraction Devices 415
Bob McMullen

RESUSCITATION CRITIQUE

Trauma Resuscitation Videotaping 418
Peggy Hollingsworth-Fridlund
David B. Hoyt

AMERICAN HEART ASSOCIATION THERAPEUTIC MODALITIES

Asystole 422
Mary E. Mancini

Electromechanical Dissociation 424
Mary E. Mancini

Ventricular Fibrillation 426
Mary E. Mancini

Sustained Ventricular Tachycardia 430
Mary E. Mancini

INDEX 433

MECHANISM OF INJURY

John A. Weigelt
Jorie Klein

A. The mechanism of injury includes both the action of forces and their effects on the human body. Injury occurs when the force deforms tissue beyond its limits. The injury force can be penetrating or nonpenetrating. The resultant injury is dependent on the energy delivered and the area of contact, which can create anatomic (skeletal fractures) and physiologic (cardiac contusion) damage. Understanding the mechanism of injury and the forces involved alerts the evaluating team to the potential type of injury and helps them to predict eventual outcome and identify common injury patterns, thereby improving management of the trauma victim.

B. Factors that determine the amount of injury are the velocity of collision, the object shape, and tissue rigidity. Body tissue has inertial resistance as well as tensile, elastic, and compressive strength. Tensile strength equals the amount of tension a tissue can withstand and its ability to resist stretching forces. Elasticity is the ability of tissue to resume its original shape and size after being stretched. Compressive strength refers to the tissue's ability to resist squeezing forces or inward pressure.

C. Force is a physical factor that changes the motion of a body either at rest or already in motion. The more slowly a force is applied, the more slowly energy is released. If the force is dissipated over a large surface area, the tissue disruption is further reduced. The most common forces that produce injury are acceleration, deceleration, shearing, and compression. Acceleration is a change in the rate of velocity of a moving object. Deceleration is a decrease in the velocity of a moving object. Shearing forces occur across a plane with structures slipping relative to each other. Compression force is the ability of an object or structure to resist squeezing forces in an upward pressure.

D. Tissue or structure deformation can be measured according to strain, i.e., the change in shape, commonly defined as a change in length divided by the initial length. Two major types of strain are tensile and shear. A third type of strain is compression, which is less common and is responsible for crush injuries. An example of tissue strain is the stretching of an artery along its longitudinal axis. Shear strain occurs when the movement of tissue in opposite directions exceeds recoverable limits. Femur fractures and rib fractures are examples of tensile strain. Shear strain injuries include hepatic vein laceration from differential movement of hepatic lobes and brain injury from movement of the brain within the skull. Deceleration injury occurs as the chest wall has stopped, causing shear forces to be focused on the aorta at its point of attachment to the posterior chest wall. When the forces exceed tissue strength, an aortic laceration occurs.

E. Blunt injuries are caused by a combination of forces, as follows: deceleration, acceleration, shearing, crushing, and compression. Blunt trauma commonly produces multiple injuries to organs and tissue. The forces of blunt trauma set stable structures and organs into motion on impact. Blunt trauma is often more life threatening than penetrating trauma because the extent of injury is less obvious and diagnosis may be difficult and prolonged. Mechanisms of injury that produce blunt trauma include motor vehicle accidents, such as automobile, motorcycle, and motor vehicle related accidents (i.e., pedestrian or cyclist hit by a car), falls, and aggravated assaults.

Motor vehicle accidents account for approximately 50 percent of blunt trauma. Prehospital personnel should quickly survey the scene, making mental note of the appearance of the vehicle and damage sustained to the passenger compartment. The evaluating team should elicit a complete history of the accident from the prehospital personnel, police officers, and victim. It is important to know the rate of velocity, point of impact, type of impact (i.e., single vehicle, T-intersection collision), structure hit, amount of vehicle damage, and amount of compartment intrusion. The team also needs to know whether the patient was the driver or the passenger, whether restraints were used, and where the victim was found. Death of an occupant in the vehicle should alert the evaluating team that other passengers have a high likelihood of injury. The surviving victims have a high morbidity and mortality rate and warrant a thorough trauma evaluation. The team should assess the patient for potential deceleration injuries. A sudden stop of a vehicle traveling at approximately 30 mph or greater, with no brakes applied and no skid marks found, can produce deceleration injuries.

Frontal impact collisions with an identified bent steering wheel or column, knee imprints into the dashboard, and a broken windshield are associated with head injuries, hemopneumothorax, injuries to the spleen or liver, dislocated patella, femur fractures, and posterior fracture-dislocation of the hip. Deceleration injury to the aorta must be ruled out in many cases. Side impact collisions can produce contralateral neck sprain or cervical fracture, head injury, lacerations to the ear, lateral rib fractures or flail chest, pneumothorax, fractured spleen or liver (depending on the side of impact), and a fractured pelvis or acetabulum. Rear impact collisions can result in neck injuries. Usually there will be frontal impact complications as well because the occupant rebounds onto the steering wheel. Ejection from a vehicle produces a multitude of injuries and a 50 percent mortality rate. Deceleration injury must be ruled out. This victim may also suffer a penetrating impalement wound or road burn injuries as he or she lands. Head injuries and cervical spine fractures are possible. The risk of injury is increased by 300 percent when the occupant is ejected from the vehicle.

Motorcycle accidents comprise single or multiple vehicle accidents. Questions to be answered include the following: Was the motorcycle hit *by* another vehicle or did *it* hit another vehicle? Was control lost before im-

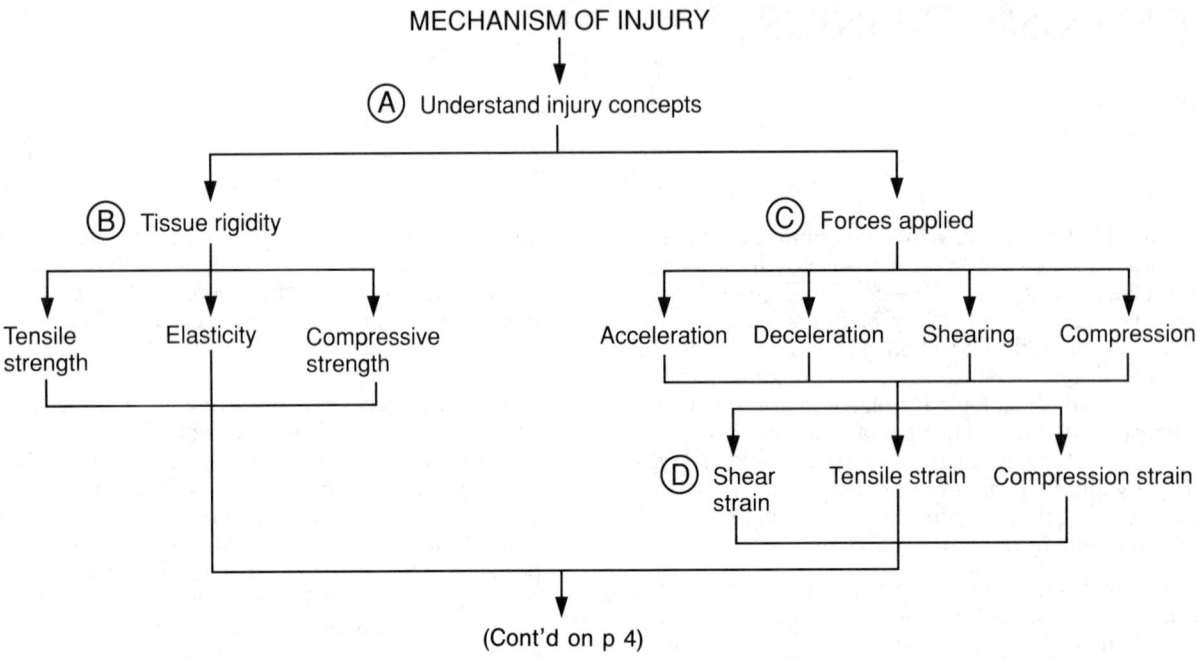

pact or was the driver able to "lay down" the cycle before impact? Was a helmet worn? Where was the victim found in relation to the motorcycle?

Pedestrians hit by vehicles suffer a magnitude of injuries. The prehospital provider should try to estimate how fast the vehicle was traveling, point of impact, and whether the victim was thrown or dragged. Waddell's triad, as follows, commonly occurs when a child is hit by a car: (1) the bumper and hood impact on the femur and chest, (2) the victim is thrown on impact, and (3) the contralateral skull is injured by the force of impact. Adult pedestrians receive a lateral impact from contact with the bumper and hood. Adults often try to protect themselves by turning sideways, which causes an injury to the ligaments in the other leg; this injury is often missed in the initial evaluation.

Falls are the second leading cause of death due to trauma in the United States. Important points for mechanism include the height of the fall, the victim's point of impact, and the surface on which the victim landed. It is important to determine whether the victim broke the fall. Falls of greater than 15 ft show impact injuries that include compression, stretching, and shearing, all of which can occur singly or in combination. Skeletal injuries, especially of the lower extremities, are likely consequences of fall. Wedge or compression fractures of vertebral bodies with fracture-dislocation of the spine occur secondary to flexion-compression and rotational injury forces. Torsion injury is also common and results from the force being transmitted to the feet and up the legs to the pelvis.

Aggravated assaults often present to the emergency department by private vehicle. The evaluating physician should determine the nature of the assaulting weapon. All body regions are to be evaluated for reddened areas, whelps, bruising, contusions, and lacerations that may indicate underlying occult injuries. The history of the incident is useful in determining potential injury. The evaluating team should evaluate the circumstances if a child is involved and be suspicious of potential child abuse. Women may often be the victims of battered wife syndrome.

F. Penetrating trauma refers to an injury produced when a foreign object passes through the tissue. The energy is dissipated through the tissue, thereby producing injury. The injuries caused by penetrating trauma are more predictable than those from blunt trauma. Organ and tissue disruption can generally be diagnosed as the trajectory of the instrument is traced. The most commonly involved organs are intestines, liver, vascular structures, and the spleen. The most common mechanisms of injury for penetrating trauma are stabbings and shootings associated with accidents, assaults, and other criminal activities.

Gunshot wounds can produce a variety of injury. High velocity gunshot wounds may involve gross tissue destruction with associated contamination and large gaping wounds and may produce profuse bleeding. Low velocity gunshot wounds may be small, clean, nonbleeding, and punctuate. Most civilian gunshot wounds are low velocity, whereas military injuries are high velocity. High velocity bullets travel at speeds greater than 3,000 ft per second. Damage from high velocity missiles is dependent on the three following factors: density and compressibility of the tissue, missile velocity, and the primary missile's fragmentation. High velocity bullets compress and accelerate tissue away from the bullet, thereby producing a cavity. The negative pressure created behind the missile contaminates the wound with foreign material. Tissue yaw may increase tissue destruction. Yawing is the deviation or deflection of the nose of the bullet from a straight path. Tumbling is the action of forward rotation around the center of the mass. Yawing and tumbling increase the area of the missile as it hits the tissue, which increases the amount of energy released and produces more damage. Low velocity missiles travel at speeds less than 1,000 ft per second or 305 m per second. Low velocity bullets cause little cavitation and blast effect; they essentially push the tissue aside.

Shotguns are short range, low velocity weapons with multiple lead pellets encased in a larger shell. Each pellet is considered a missile. There can be nine to 200 small pellets, depending on the size of pellet and the gauge of gun. The shell contains pellets, gun powder, and a plastic or paper wad separating the pellets from the gun powder. Gauge designates the bore of the gun. Common gauges include 10, 12, 16, 20, 28, and 410. Common shot sizes range from size 2 through 9 and have a respective pellet diameter of 0.15 to 0.08 inches. Larger shot sizes include buckshot and BBs. The shot pattern is of clinical importance. Most significant wounds occur between 0 and 15 yards. Wounding capacity is the function of mass and projectile velocity.

Stab wounds and impalements are low velocity wounds. Stab wounds may be inflicted by such instruments as knives, scissors, pencils, glass bottles, screwdrivers, and ice picks. Impalement can occur with motor vehicle accidents, motorcycle accidents, falls, and other forceful collisions. These wounds are usually obvious, but the patient must be totally undressed and inspected for all injuries. If the offending agent remains in place, its trajectory can be traced and underlying trauma predicted. The object should be left in place and secured to decrease further injury until definitive surgical therapy is available. If the object has been removed, the size, shape, and length of the object should be identified. It is also important to determine the trajectory of the instrument. Information regarding the gender of the assailant may be helpful in tracking the wound; men tend to stab upward and women downward. Injuries involving the upper abdomen may penetrate abdominal and thoracic structures. It is estimated that one out of every four patients who sustain a penetrating injury to the abdomen has an associated chest injury.

G. Explosive blasts are the result of detonated explosives that have been converted to large volumes of gas. Explosive devices inflict damage by several mechanisms. The pressure ruptures the explosive casing and resultant fragments become high velocity projectiles. The explosion center causes superficial burns to exposed areas, usually the hands, face, and neck. The rapidly expanding sphere of compressed gas molecules gives rise to a shock pressure wave, which expands outward in a radial direction. The blast's shockwave velocity is as high as 3000 m per second. The positive pressure phase is the maximum pressure reached by the blast wave and is greatest next to the actual explosion. The negative phase follows immediately and lasts 10 times as long. An equal volume of air is displaced along with the expanding gas and travels behind the blast. The rapid mass movement of air produces disruption of tissue, traumatic amputations, and evisceration. Patients may have combined penetrating trauma, impalement trauma, blunt trauma, and burn trauma. The type of explosion can also determine the severity and types of injury produced. Explosions in water are more severe than those in air; the blast wave travels farther and more rapidly in water because water is 800 times as dense as air. The positive pressure wave for an immersion blast peaks in 1 or 2 msec and then rapidly decays. Immersion blast produces intra-abdominal bleeding, bowel perforation, and lung injuries. Victims close to the explosion site may suffer avulsion of tissue and extremities, fractures, and severe internal injuries, and entry of the compressed air may produce tissue emphysema and symptomatic air emboli. Explosions in closed areas have a potential for being more severe because of toxic gases and smoke inhalation. Injury occurs most often at the tissue-air interfaces. Lung injury in the alveolar wall produces hemorrhage and edema. The abdominal organs show damage to the visceral wall and may produce perforation. The ear is the most sensitive organ to explosions.

H. Burn trauma is the third most common cause of accidental death in the United States and constitutes a major cause of morbidity and traumatized patients. Burn trauma includes thermal burns, scald burns, chemical burns, electrical burns, and frostbite injury. Burn injury not only destroys viable cutaneous elements but also elicits pathophysiologic alterations in other organ systems. Prehospital providers should stop the burning process: Clothes should be removed, chemical agents should be washed away, and contact with electrical current must be carefully interrupted. Once these activities are accomplished, the injured patient is managed like any trauma patient. The evaluating team should elicit a complete history, identifying the initial mechanism of injury, how long the patient was exposed, and whether the victim was in a closed space. Burn trauma may be compounded with blunt trauma from explosions, motor vehicle accidents, or jumping to escape further injury. The team should be alert for indications of attempted homicide, suicide, and child abuse.

Smoke inhalation is a direct insult to the alveolar level secondary to chemical fumes or the inhalation of smoke. The injury results from direct chemical irritation to the lung tissues. Nasopharyngeal burns and hoarseness may be present. Scald burns are treated and managed the same as heat or flame burns. The burning process should be stopped and the injury pattern quickly evaluated. A discrepancy in the injury pattern and history should alert the team to potential child abuse. Electrical burns account for less than 2 percent of the admission to burn facilities. Major electrical trauma occurs almost exclusively in men who work with electricity or in farm workers who move irrigation pipe. Toddlers occasionally suffer electrical shock from chewing on electrical cords. Voltage and type of current and the length of contact determine the amount of injury produced. These patients frequently have associated injuries from falls. Chemical burns occur when tissue components react with acids or alkalis to release thermal injury. The alkali burns are generally more serious than acid burns because alkalis penetrate tissue more deeply. The concentration of the chemical and the quantity of the agent determine the extent of injury. Frostbite or cold injuries are rarely the direct result of extreme weather conditions. Weather may be an associated contributing factor. The high risk population for cold injuries includes alcoholics, drug addicts, the mentally ill, the elderly, patients with decreased sensory perception, small children, and the homeless. Elderly people, infants, and young children are particularly susceptible to cold because of lack of adequate body insulation tissue. The patient most

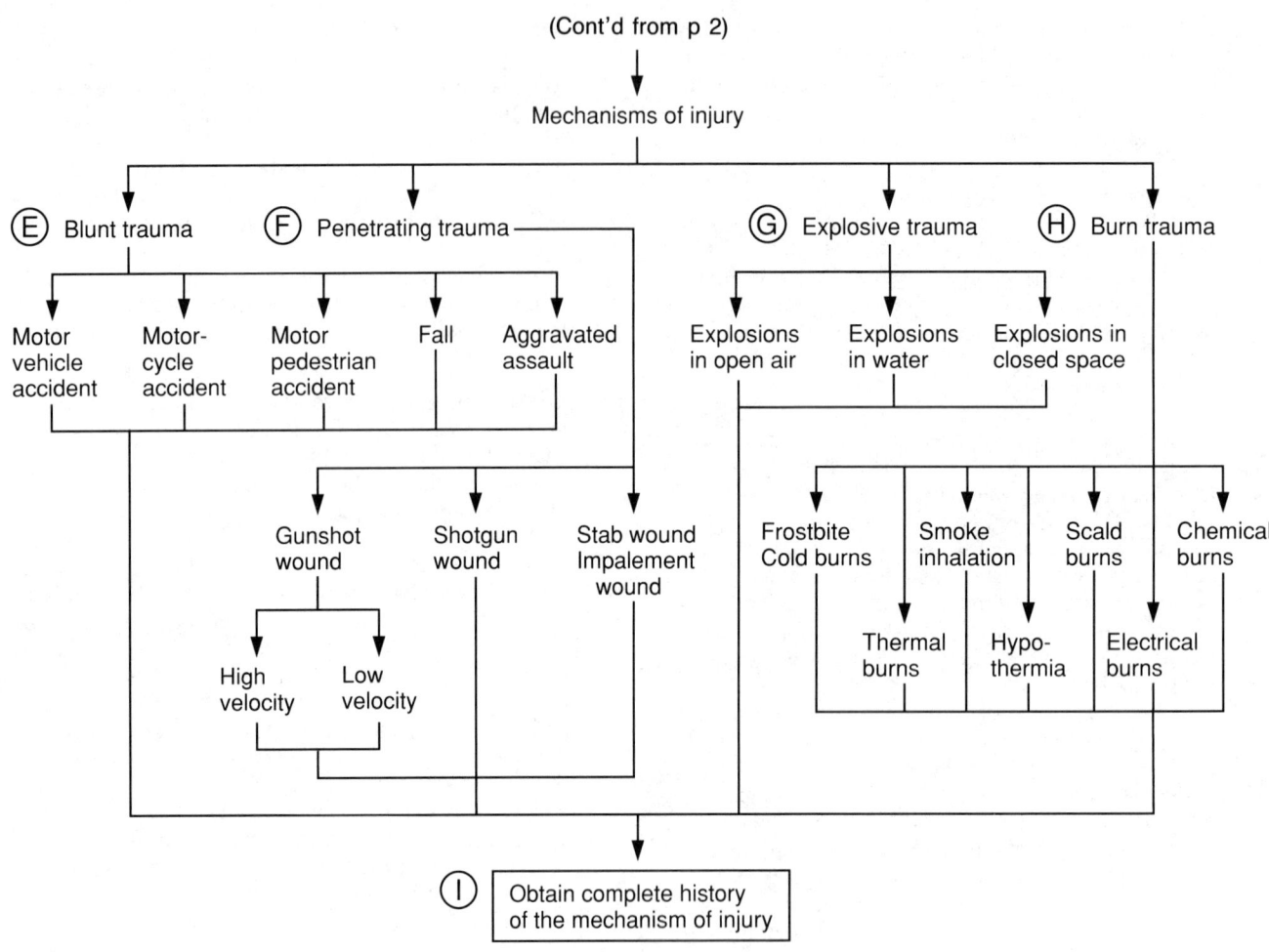

commonly presents to the emergency department days after the initial injury. Hypothermia is described as systemic trauma that occurs when the core body temperature drops below 35° C. Hypothermia is divided into two major categories: dry and immersion. Persons experiencing cold water immersion accidents are at greater risk for developing hypothermia resulting from evaporative heat loss. In addition, those persons not wearing flotation devices must use energy to stay afloat, which increases the rate of heat loss.

I. The prehospital provider must obtain as much information regarding the mechanism of injury as possible. This information should be given to the evaluating team. The team should obtain a complete history of the incident from the patient, family, and investigating officers. This combined information assists the team in creating an "index of suspicion" for potential injuries, which further aids in evaluating the patient and setting priorities.

References

American College of Surgeons. Advanced trauma life support course. Chicago: American College of Surgeons, 1989:20–24.

Baker JP, O'Neill B, Karpf RS. The injury fact book. Lexington, MA: Lexington Books, 1984.

Nahum AM, Melvin J. The biomechanics of trauma. Norwalk, CT: Appleton-Century-Crofts, 1985:1–30.

Weigelt A, McCormack A. Mechanism of injury. In: Cardona V, Huin PD, Mason PJ, Scanlon-Schilpp AM, Veise-Berry SW, eds. Resuscitation through rehabilitation. Philadelphia: WB Saunders, 1988:105–125.

Weiner SL, Barrett J. Explosions and explosion device-related injuries: trauma management. Philadelphia: WB Saunders, 1986:13–24.

PRE–HOSPITAL CARE

Dispatch
Scene Management/Patient Evaluation
Pre-Hospital Management
EMT/Paramedic and Physician Communication
Field Triage

DISPATCH

Debra Cason

A. In most areas, help for an emergency is obtained by calling 911. This number can be dialed on coin operated phones without inserting coins. Many trauma emergencies are observed by a third person who may not know the injured parties.

B. The emergency medical service (EMS) dispatcher collects pertinent information from the caller to dispatch the appropriate resources to the exact location. Necessary information to be obtained about the location includes the exact address, building name or number if applicable, and cross street. The telephone number being called from is important in case the emergency units are unable to find the patient. In "enhanced 911" systems, the telephone number of the calling phone is displayed on the dispatcher's monitor. Typically the caller is able to provide the dispatcher with information about the nature of the traumatic event or the cause of injury, which determines the resources to be dispatched. The precise body location and the severity of the patient's injury help the dispatcher provide pre-arrival instructions to the caller.

C. Appropriate resources to be dispatched depend on the caller's information. A motor vehicle accident (MVA) demands the police and fire equipment, in addition to EMS personnel. If victims are trapped in a vehicle, heavy rescue equipment such as a Hurst tool should be dispatched with the personnel. An aggravated assault would necessitate police dispatch as would a gunshot wound (GSW) and a stab wound. An industrial machinery accident may involve a victim's extremity caught in the equipment; consequently rescue resources and possibly a surgical team are required at the location.

D. Pre-arrival instructions to the caller are becoming a standard of care in EMS. Further injury to the trauma victim can be minimized by instructions such as "Don't move the victim" or "Apply direct pressure to the bleeding." Instructions for cardiopulmonary resuscitation (CPR) may also be given, even to untrained individuals.

References

Clawson JJ, Dernocoeur KB. Principles of emergency medical dispatch. Englewood Cliffs, NJ: Prentice Hall, 1988.

Eisenberg MS, Hallstrom AP, Carter WB, Cummins RO, Bergner L, Pierce J. Emergency CPR instruction via telephone. Am J Public Health 1985; 75:47–50.

National Association of EMS Physicians. EMS medical director's handbook. St. Louis: CV Mosby, 1989:66–67.

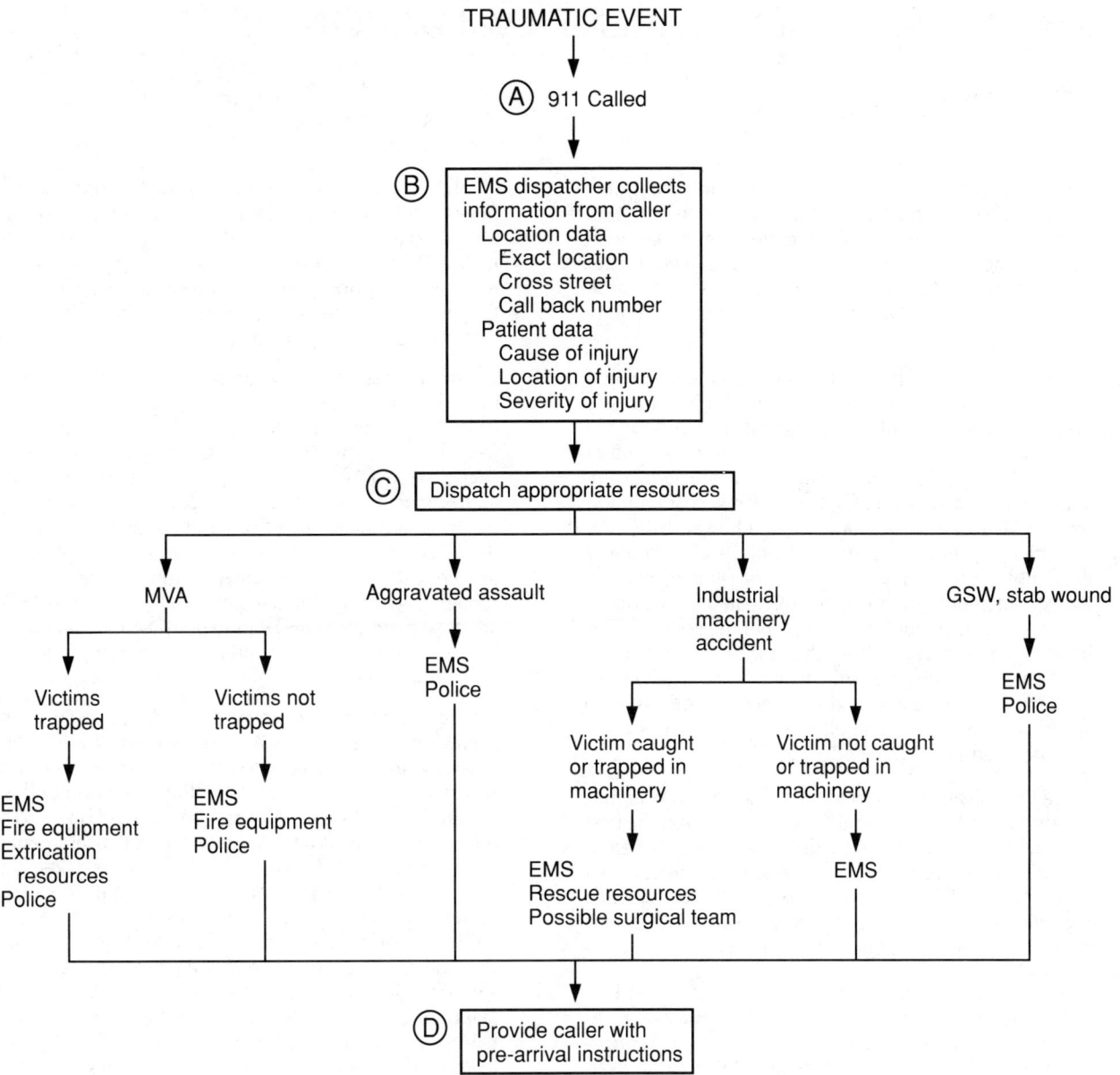

SCENE MANAGEMENT/PATIENT EVALUATION

Carol Goodykoontz

A. When the call for assistance is received, it is extremely important to obtain several vital pieces of information as follows: exact location of the patient, exact nature of the call, and call back number. Mental preparedness for the incident can be enhanced by having as much information as possible as well as having the necessary equipment available.

B. The scene survey is the quick, yet observant, evaluation of potential hazards and mechanism of injury that are provided by the patient's environment. The presence of environmental hazards, such as a downed powerline or busy highway traffic, should be quickly evaluated. Evaluation of the mechanism of injury is also key. Such information enables the paramedic, and eventually the physician, to anticipate potential injuries, particularly those not readily apparent. In a motor vehicle accident (MVA), different injuries can be anticipated for the driver and passengers depending on whether the collision was head on, broadside, or from the rear. A cracked windshield may lead the paramedic to anticipate head, chest, or abdominal injuries. Sudden deceleration, vehicle speed, and whether seatbelts were worn can also be helpful information.

C. Once the unit arrives on location, scene control becomes important. This takes special expertise, and even the best paramedics encounter many different situations before this skill is mastered. Control of the scene involves crowd control and gaining access to the patient. Any hazards identified in the initial scene survey are attended to, and police assistance is requested if indicated.

D. Quickly assess the number of victims involved and request additional units if indicated. It is crucial for the EMT/paramedic to have a sound understanding of treatment priorities in the case of a multi-victim incident. Various triage systems may be employed, but a standard one involves categorization as follows: first priority, second priority, low priority, and dead. Once the victims are identified and tagged, immediate treatment may be initiated. Be careful to assess, resuscitate, and package patients using a priority system. The key aspect in effective triage is to evaluate all victims quickly, then remain and direct others as help arrives.

E. The intactness of airway, breathing, and circulation is pivotal in this process. If the airway is obstructed or compromised, immediate attention is given to that problem. Several injuries may produce life threatening situations, such as tension pneumothorax, flail chest, fractured larynx, sucking chest wound, exsanguinating hemorrhage, or the presence of profound shock. Any hemorrhage is controlled by direct pressure, and shock is treated with two large bore intravenous lines (IVs) of Ringer's lactate. Pneumatic antishock garments (PASGs) are used if indicated and if time permits. Transport to the nearest trauma facility is indicated following stabilization of the patient.

F. Careful attention is given to the cervical spine as the survey continues. An MVA or fall victim should be removed with the use of a corset type extrication device and stabilized with a cervical collar, head immobilizer or head immobilizing device, and a backboard. The secondary survey is a brief but systematic assessment of all of the patient's injuries. Vital signs are taken and recorded, with any abnormalities noted. A history of the current incident is taken as well as any pertinent past medical history. Assessment of alcohol or drug use should be noted. The head-to-toe survey is begun with a neurologic evaluation of the patient. The AVPU (Alert, responds to Verbal stimuli, responds to Painful stimuli, Unresponsive) system should be employed to describe the patient's level of consciousness. This baseline information should be assessed and documented.

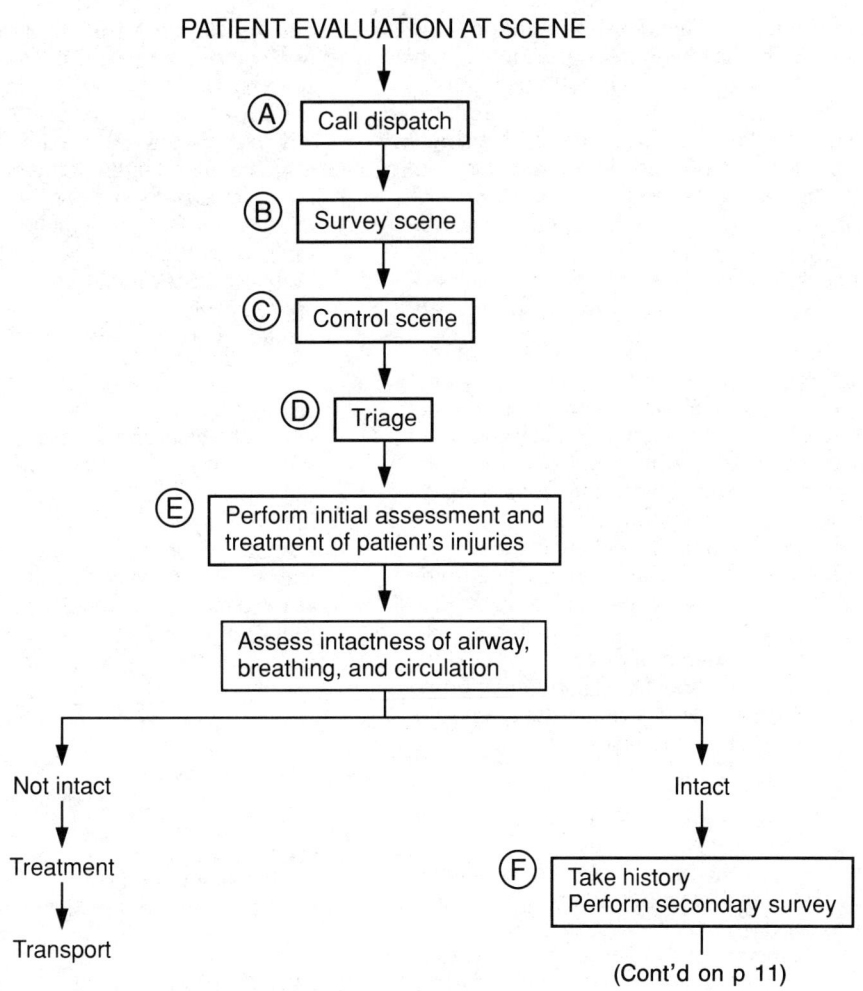

G. The head is examined for any depression in the scalp or obvious injury. The head and neck are immediately immobilized if indicated. The face is examined for edema, bruising, wounds, asymmetry, or bleeding from the nose or ears. The mouth is examined for loose teeth, dentures, injury, or other forms of possible obstruction. An obvious obstruction should be removed from the patient's mouth and bleeding controlled. The pupils can provide important clues for the paramedic and should be examined. The neck is checked for tracheal deviation, neck vein distention, subcutaneous emphysema, or other abnormality.

H. The examination of the chest and back is the next step in the secondary survey that yields important information about the respiratory and cardiovascular systems. In the trauma patient inspection of the chest includes noting any rib retractions, abdominal breathing, or paradoxical chest wall movement. Palpation of the chest may indicate rib fractures, pneumothorax, or subcutaneous emphysema. Auscultation of the lungs helps determine absent or diminished breath sounds and aids in evaluating pulmonary status prior to the administration of large amounts of IV fluids sometimes required for trauma patients. Any patient with suspected chest injury should have an IV started and an ECG reading done. Specific management of a tension pneumothorax, rib fracture, or flail chest should be done if indicated.

I. The abdomen and pelvic area should be evaluated. Inspection reveals any bruising, scars, swelling, or obvious deformity. A distended abdomen that is also tender may indicate intra-abdominal bleeding or an accumulation of fluid in the peritoneum. The iliac crests should be simultaneously palpated for the presence of pelvic instability. The genitourinary system is discreetly inspected for any obvious trauma, bleeding, evidence of incontinence, or priapism. IV fluids with Ringer's lactate are administered if indicated.

J. The last step in the head to toe survey is the examination of the extremities. The musculoskeletal system is inspected for deformity, swelling, or discoloration. Pain, pallor, paresthesia, paralysis, peripheral pulses, and capillary refill should be assessed in any injured extremity to evaluate the integrity of the peripheral vascular system. Neurologic status of the extremities is evaluated by testing for strength, movement, range of motion, and sensation. Throughout the examination a comparison of both sides is essential. Any fracture is treated with the appropriate immobilization device, such as board splints, a traction splint, or pillows and blankets.

K. Radio communication of patient data in the prehospital setting should provide a clear visual image of the patient to the physician and the receiving hospital. Data are communicated in a standard orderly format. Treatment requiring a physician's orders should then be instituted. If an EMS system has standing orders, treatment may be instituted prior to communication with base station medical control. A hospital destination should be established as the patient is prepared for transport. The priority (condition) of the patient and code (mode of travel) is then communicated to the receiving hospital.

References

Campbell JH. Basic trauma life support. 2nd ed. Englewood Cliffs, NJ: Prentice Hall, 1988.

Caroline NL. Emergency care in the streets. 3rd ed. Boston: Little, Brown, 1987.

Caroline NL. Emergency medical treatment: a text for EMT-A's and EMT intermediates. 2nd ed. Boston: Little, Brown, 1987.

Cason D, Goodykoontz C. Patient assessment: general principles and skills. In: Introduction to paramedic practice: theory and intervention. (Publication pending)

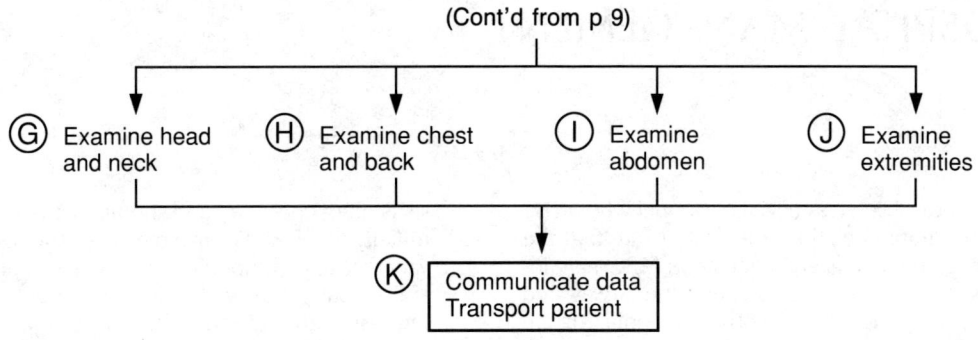

PRE–HOSPITAL MANAGEMENT

Debra Cason

A. Emergency medical services (EMS) personnel who arrive at the site of a trauma victim must first ensure that the patient's airway, breathing, and circulation (ABCs) are intact. This is done initially by assessing the airway and ventilatory status while simultaneously immobilizing the cervical spine. The patient who responds verbally to questioning has a patent airway and is ventilating. In the patient who does not respond verbally and consequently has an altered sensorium, the airway is opened with the chin lift or modified jaw thrust method (Fig. 1). These methods do not alter cervical spine alignment. If the patient is not breathing, ventilation is attempted with mouth-to-mouth or a bag-valve-mask. When manpower is available, the circulation is assessed simultaneously with ventilation.

B. Immediate intervention is required if the rescuer is unable to establish or maintain an airway with the chin lift or modified jaw thrust method or if spontaneous ventilation is absent. Oral or nasal airway devices may help maintain the airway. If necessary, endotracheal intubation (without cervical spine manipulation), nasotracheal intubation, or use of the esophageal obturator airway may secure the airway. Needle cricothyroidotomy with jet ventilation is necessary when the obstruction is below the level of the cords. This obstruction rarely occurs, and the procedure should be attempted only by personnel fully trained in this technique. Suctioning of blood and emesis is often necessary and should be available even if not initially required. Positive pressure ventilation with a bag-valve-mask and supplemental oxygen is provided for the apneic patient as well as for the patient who is breathing less than eight to 10 times per minute.

C. Once the airway is secured and ventilation is adequate, attention moves to the assessment of circulation. If the patient cannot be ventilated, paramedics must immediately transport and repeat attempts enroute to the hospital.

D. Circulation is assessed first by checking for the presence of a carotid pulse. If the pulse is absent, cardiopulmonary resuscitation (CPR) must be commenced and advanced cardiac life support (ACLS) procedures done enroute to the hospital. The presence of a strong, regular pulse with a rate between 60 and 100 likely indicates adequate circulation at that time. Such a patient would need an intravenous (IV) line of Ringer's lactate at a slow or keep open rate. Circulation is further assessed with the capillary refill test and evaluation of skin temperature and moisture. Active bleeding is treated with direct pressure. The patient with inadequate circulation requires one or two IVs of Ringer's lactate. The use of the pneumatic antishock garment (PASG) is considered also. Transport time to a trauma care facility is a consideration in the use of the antishock garment. No more than two attempts to start an IV are made prior to transporting.

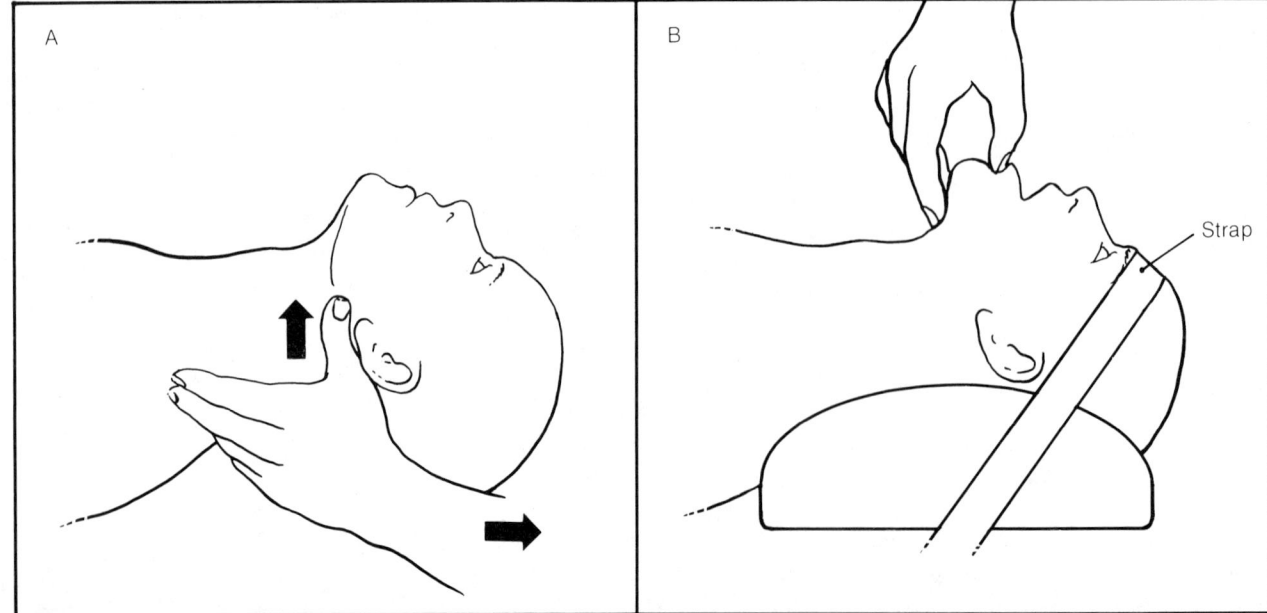

Figure 1 *A*, Modified jaw thrust; *B*, chin lift. (Redrawn after Campbell JE. Basic trauma life support. Englewood Cliffs, NJ: Prentice Hall, 1988:54.)

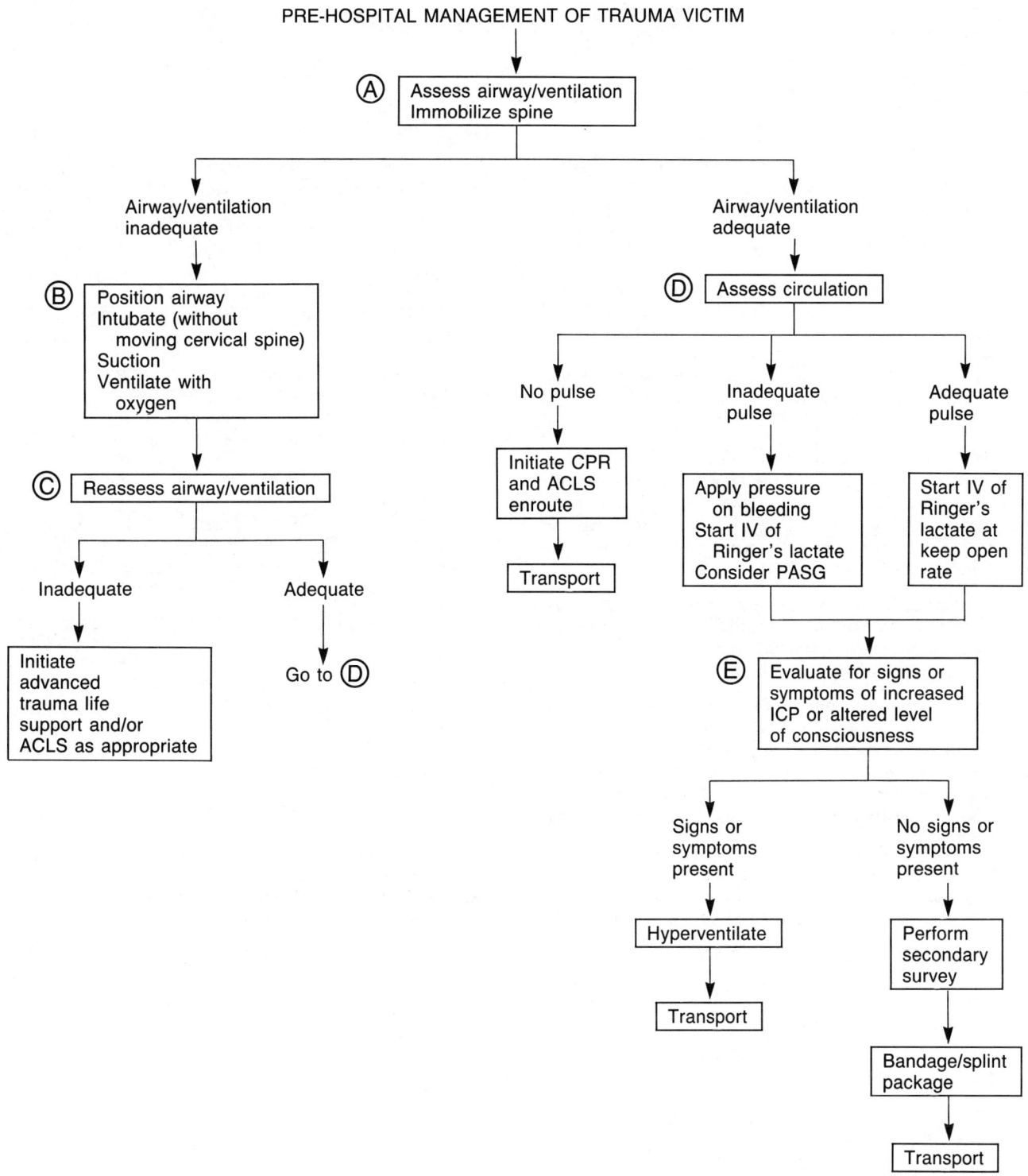

E. Signs and symptoms of altered level of consciousness or increasing intracranial pressure (ICP) indicate the need for hyperventilation and immediate transportation. In the absence of such symptoms, a secondary survey should commence with appropriate stabilization.

References

American College of Surgeons Committee on Trauma. Advanced trauma life support. Chicago: American College of Surgeons, 1989:33–38; 59–72.

Campbell JE. Basic trauma life support. Englewood Cliffs, NJ: Prentice Hall, 1988:21–90; 107–119.

The California EMSC Project. Prehospital care of pediatric emergencies. Los Angeles: Pediatric Society California, 1987:43–71.

EMT/PARAMEDIC AND PHYSICIAN COMMUNICATION

Jan Auerbach

A. When the EMT/paramedic in the field attempts to establish radio communication with the base station, he or she should identify which emergency medical service (EMS) is calling and the unit's level of function and its identification number.

B. The base station should respond by first identifying the facility. To minimize confusion when multiple units are involved in a single receiving facility, the base station should ask the EMS unit to repeat its identification information. Finally, it is important that the hospital based operator identify his or her title because the initial response is usually not by a physician.

C. After the EMT/paramedic has reidentified the EMS service and unit number, the on scene report should begin with patient's level of consciousness, age, complaint, and/or mechanism of injury. This provides the physician with a mental picture of the patient and an idea of the type of emergency involved.

D. Life saving therapy or emergency maneuvers performed during the primary survey should be reported next. If a finger-stick glucose result has been obtained on a comatose patient, it too should be reported at this time.

E. In an unstable patient, problems identified during the primary survey with the patient's airway, breathing, and/or cardiovascular stability should be reported next, along with vital signs. Additional history, physical findings, and medication usage should be reported at this time only if pertinent in obtaining treatment for the patient.

F. In a stable patient with a normal primary survey, vital signs and pertinent secondary survey findings are reported next. Secondary survey includes an elaboration of the chief complaint, past medical history, medications, and physical examination findings.

G. The EMT/paramedic should now inform the base station of established protocols that have been carried out and request or stand by for any additional orders from the physician. The EMT/paramedic should also state the estimated time of arrival (ETA) from the scene to the hospital.

H. The physician now proceeds with patient management by providing additional orders, if any, at this time. The physician may ask for additional information regarding the patient's condition before making treatment decisions.

I. The EMT/paramedic should now repeat any orders given by the physician for confirmation. If the EMT/paramedic needs more complete orders or disagrees with the orders given by the base station physician, additional patient history may be needed or an order requested again.

J. The sign off phase ends communication between the EMS unit and base station. The EMT/paramedic should now inform the base station that he or she is ending communication by signing off, using a common phrase. The base station should end communication by using the same phrase.

References

Caroline NL. Emergency care in the streets. 3rd ed. Boston: Little, Brown, 1987:563–574.

Slovis CM. In: Campbell JE, ed. Basic trauma life support. 2nd ed. Englewood Cliffs, NJ: Prentice Hall, 1988:355–360.

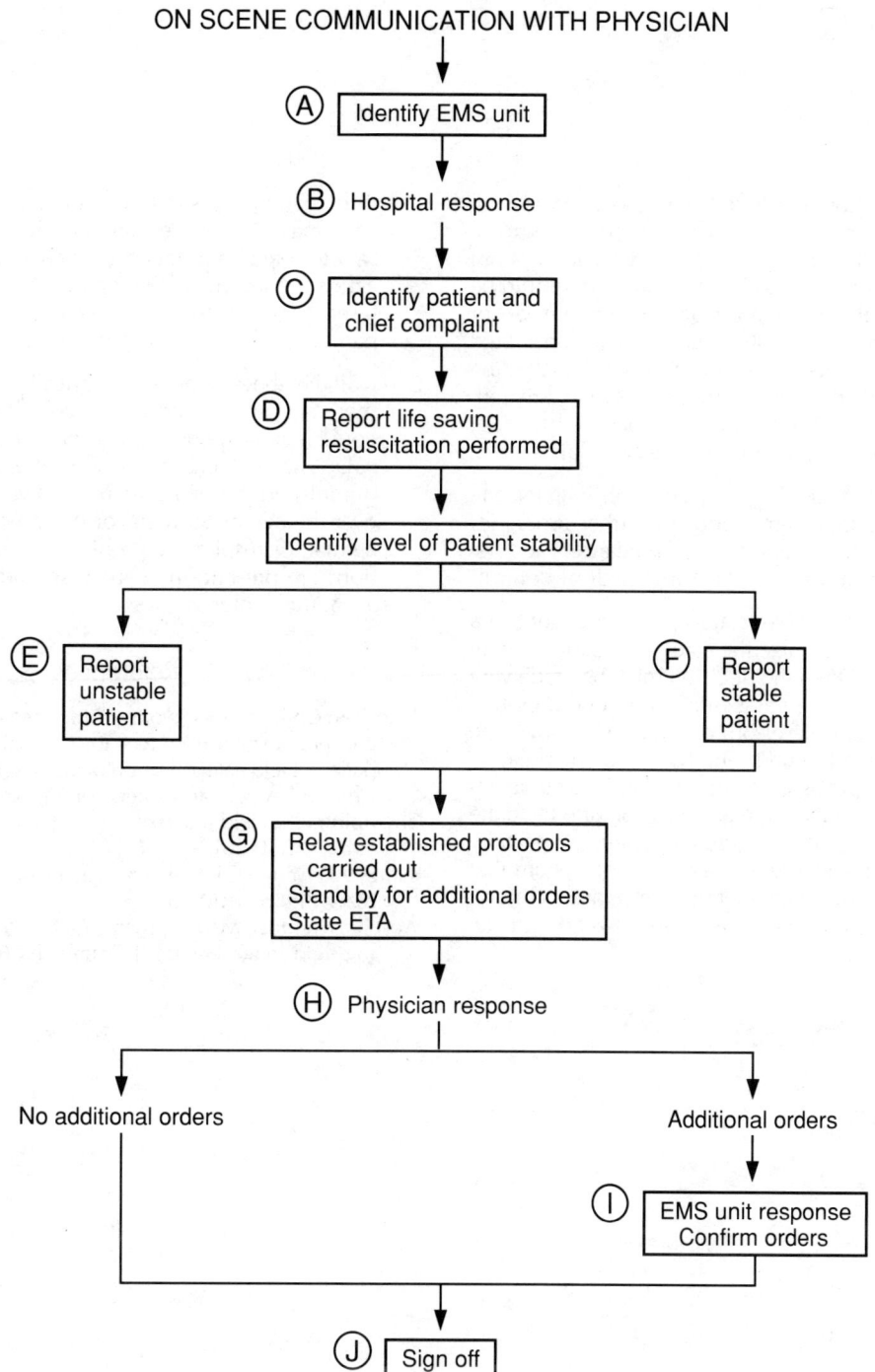

FIELD TRIAGE

Ann Hudgins

A. Scene response should include initial assessment of vital signs and a determination of baseline level of consciousness. Extricate the patient from the vehicle or from entrapment as soon as possible. Stabilization should be done to protect the patient from any further damages or to minimize current disability. Initial resuscitation should also be started and treatment given as permitted by the system's medical control. Any immediately life threatening conditions or injuries should be corrected without delaying transport to the appropriate hospital.

B. Medical control should be contacted after initial scene management or treatment to obtain further orders for treatment, medications, or additional guidance. Each system has its own procedure for using medical control.

C. A decision must be made to transport the patient to a hospital that can maximize the care needed for the traumatized patient. Often the decision must be made very quickly; therefore, rapid assessment of blood pressure, respiratory rate, and level of consciousness should be done to minimize the on scene time and any delay in transport. This rapid assessment can give an accurate indication of the severity of the patient's condition and the necessity of transport to a trauma center or specialty center. Many systems use a trauma scoring system that evaluates physiologic and anatomic response to injury; this scoring system facilitates field prioritization, triage, and transportation.

D. If the patient does not meet the criteria for transport to a trauma center or specialty center at this time, it is necessary to evaluate further the mechanism of injury and to assess the severity of the injuries. Normal vital signs and level of consciousness at the scene do not mean that the patient could not have potentially critical injuries.

E. If all the above steps reveal basically noncritical findings, there are other criteria to be considered that, if found, could make a moderately severe injury potentially critical. These include those patients with possibly diminished resources, such as the very young and those over the age of 55 years, or those patients with known cardiac or respiratory problems. If any of these conditions are present, the patient should be transported to a trauma center.

References

American College of Surgeons. Committee on trauma: Hospital and pre-hospital resources for optimal care of the injured patient. Field categorization of trauma patients (field triage). Chicago: American College of Surgeons, 1987.

Champion HR. Field triage of trauma patients. Ann Emerg Med 1982; 11:160–161.

Ramzy AI, Warren GT. Prehospital assessment and scoring. Trauma Q 1986; 3(1):1–13.

West JG, Murdock MA, Baldwin LC, et al. A method for evaluating field triage criteria. J Trauma 1986; 26:655–659.

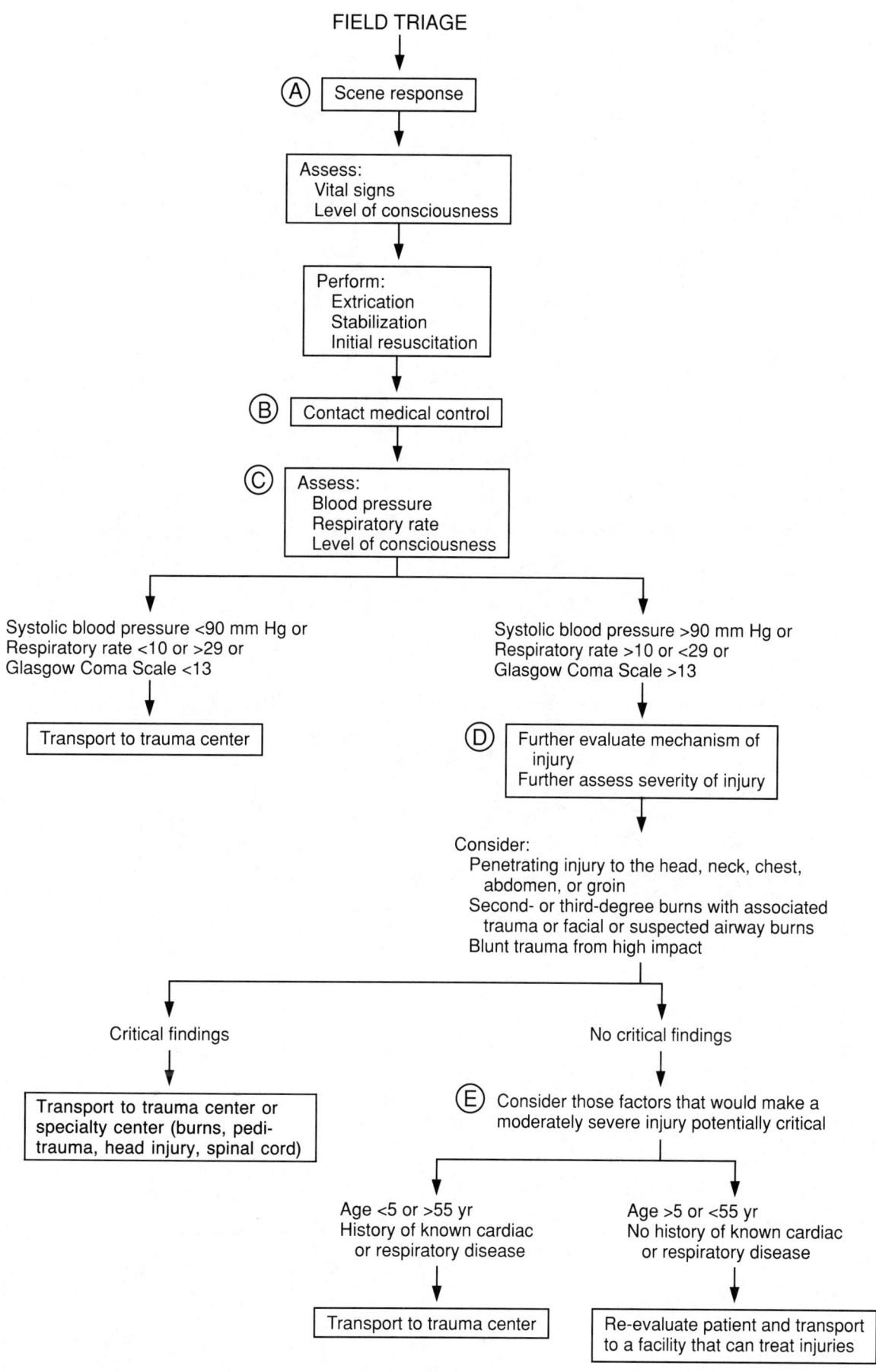

RESUSCITATION/ STABILIZATION

Initial Assessment
Secondary Assessment

INITIAL ASSESSMENT

Erwin R. Thal
Jorie Klein

A. Upon arrival in the hospital, the injured patient should be met by a qualified trauma team. This team should include a qualified physician with the American College of Surgeons Advanced Trauma Life Support (ATLS) training, an experienced trauma nursing team, a respiratory therapist, and a radiology technician.

B. A complete history of the mechanism of injury and prehospital care should be obtained. All preceding events should be taken into account to create a high index of suspicion for traumatic injury. The primary survey consists of an evaluation of the airway, breathing, circulation, and neurologic function. The patient is then classified according to severity of injury into one of the three following categories: (1) life threatening injury with interruption of vital physiologic function, (2) serious injury likely to require close observation or definitive surgical care, or (3) minor injury that may require extended observation or outpatient follow-up.

C. Management of the airway takes precedence over all other activity. Hypoxia generally occurs because of the patient's lack of ability to oxygenate the blood properly. This may be caused by mechanical problems or lack of oxygen exchange at the alveolar arterial interface. Hypoxia may be clinically manifested by an uncooperative, anxious, combative, and/or restless patient. These findings should not be confused with the alcoholic or drug abuser. Patients who present to the hospital with spontaneous respirations should be continuously reassessed. The airway should be protected and maintained.

D. The upper airway should be assessed for patency. Initial attempts to establish a patient's airway include the chin lift or jaw thrust maneuver and suctioning to remove foreign debris. The cervical spine should be stabilized in the neutral position to prevent injury. Excessive movement of the cervical spine can convert a fracture with no neurologic damage into a fracture-dislocation with neurologic injury.

E. Patients who have an upper or lower airway obstruction manifested by poor air exchange, slow or rapid respirations, or depressed central nervous system should be rapidly intubated. If time permits, lateral cervical films should be obtained. A normal lateral cervical spine film visualizing C7 and the top of T1 allows for oral endotracheal intubation with midline stabilization of the head and neck. One must remember that a normal lateral cervical spine film does not absolutely rule out a cervical spine injury. Spinal stabilization and immobilization must be maintained until a cervical fracture has been ruled out. If no cervical fractures are noted, oral endotracheal intubation is the procedure of choice. If a fracture is suspected, nasotracheal intubation may be performed according to clinical judgment. Intubation should be preceded by a period of pre-oxygenation with a bag mask device to help alleviate hypoxia.

F. Prior to attempted intubation the patient should be assessed for laryngeal injury, edema of the glottis, or severe oropharyngeal hemorrhage associated with facial trauma. Inability to intubate the trachea is the only indication for a surgical airway. A needle or surgical cricothyroidotomy is the preferable choice. (Surgical cricothyroidotomy is not recommended for children under 12 years of age.) If a fractured larynx is identified, a tracheostomy is indicated. An emergency tracheostomy may be difficult to perform and is best done in the operating room under more elective conditions.

G. Patients who arrive at the hospital already intubated must be evaluated for proper tube placement. The tube may have been inserted into a mainstem bronchus or dislodged enroute to the hospital. Placement can be checked quickly by listening for bilateral equal breath sounds and by listening over the stomach for improper placement. The tube must be repositioned if mainstem bronchus intubation has occurred and breath sounds then reassessed.

H. Once the tube is in place, regardless of the method selected, both lung fields must be auscultated to be certain the right mainstem bronchus has not been canulated. A chest film should be obtained to confirm proper placement.

I. The chest should be exposed to assess adequate ventilatory exchange. The team should note the rate, rhythm, and symmetry of the chest wall movement. One should look for distended neck veins, open wounds, lacerations, bruising, and abrasions that may indicate underlying injury. Adequate oxygenation and ventilation must be assured. Despite clear bilateral breath sounds, patients should be frequently reassessed. Oxygen should be administered to maintain a PaO_2 greater than 60 torr on room air or 100 torr on 40 percent O_2. Arterial blood gases should be obtained frequently.

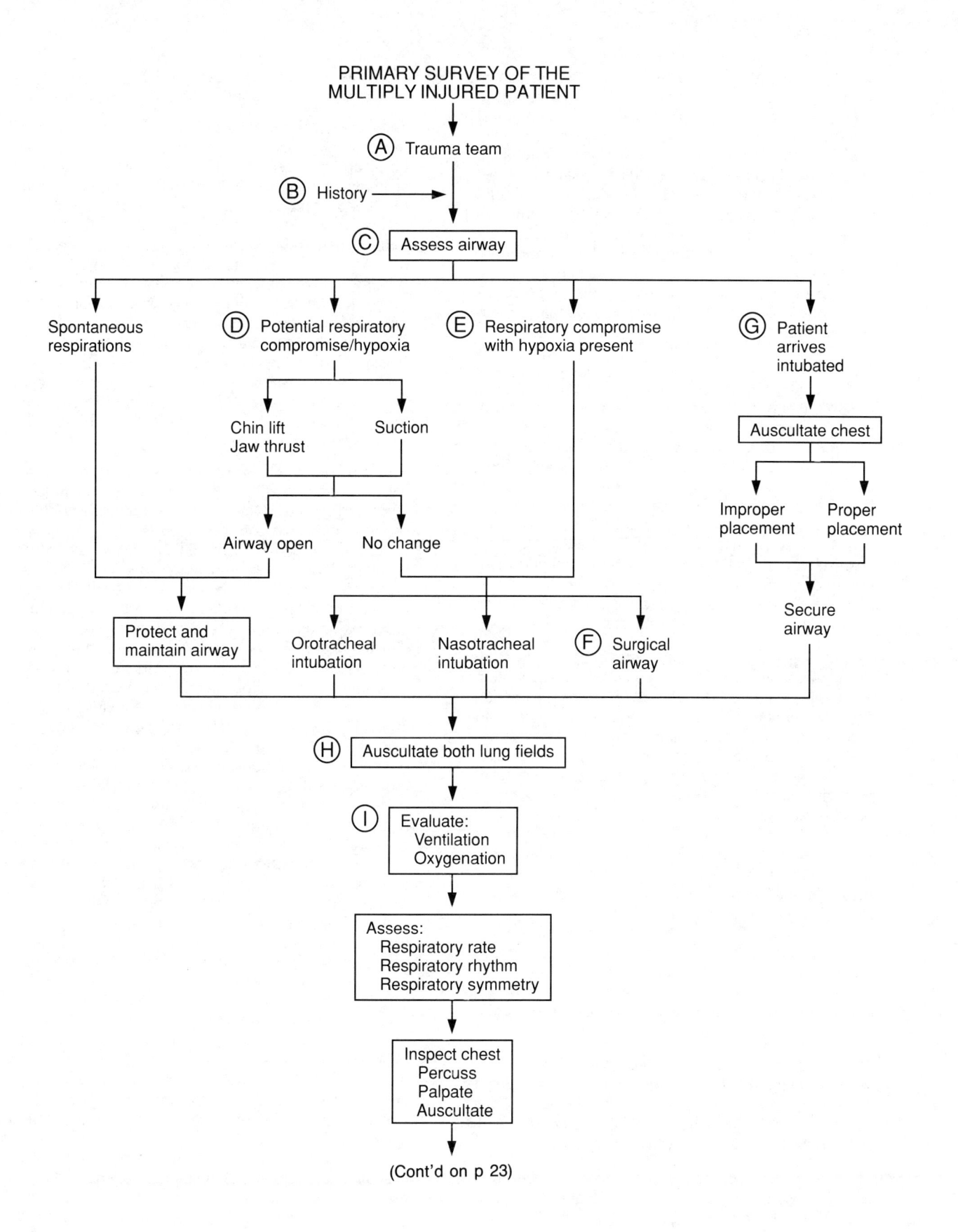

PRIMARY SURVEY OF THE MULTIPLY INJURED PATIENT

- (A) Trauma team
- (B) History
- (C) Assess airway
  - Spontaneous respirations
  - (D) Potential respiratory compromise/hypoxia
    - Chin lift / Jaw thrust
    - Suction
    - Airway open
    - No change
  - (E) Respiratory compromise with hypoxia present
  - (G) Patient arrives intubated
    - Auscultate chest
      - Improper placement
      - Proper placement
    - Secure airway

- Protect and maintain airway
- Orotracheal intubation
- Nasotracheal intubation
- (F) Surgical airway

- (H) Auscultate both lung fields
- (I) Evaluate:
  - Ventilation
  - Oxygenation
- Assess:
  - Respiratory rate
  - Respiratory rhythm
  - Respiratory symmetry
- Inspect chest
  - Percuss
  - Palpate
  - Auscultate

(Cont'd on p 23)

J. Simultaneously the chest must be assessed for mechanical factors that compromise the ventilatory process. Loss of chest wall stability, as seen in flail chest, mechanical compression due to a tension pneumothorax, an open pneumothorax, a massive hemothorax, or the encroachment of the chest cavity as seen with herniation of visceral contents secondary to a ruptured diaphragm should be carefully ruled out. Many patients may vomit and aspirate prior to arrival, thereby impairing adequate ventilation. Other less common entities that compromise breathing and ventilation are the exaggerated Trendelenburg position, the inflated military antishock trousers (MAST), and chest wall compression secondary to circumferential burns.

K. All life threatening injuries must be quickly treated. Rapid decompression by needle thoracentesis or chest tube insertion is essential in the patient with a tension pneumothorax. Evacuation of blood from the chest and re-expansion of the lung by closed tube thoracostomy controls most parenchymal bleeding. A sucking chest wound should be quickly sealed using a three corner flap dressing followed by closed tube thoracostomy. A large flail segment is splinted and, if it is contributing to inadequate ventilation, best treated by intubation and positive pressure breathing. The primary goal of ventilation is to achieve maximum cellular oxygenation. Chest films should be obtained as indicated but should not precede or delay life saving procedures.

L. Hemorrhage is one of the early causes of postinjury death that is amenable to effective treatment. Rapid assessment of the injured patient's hemodynamic status is essential. The key components to circulatory assessment are heart rate, skin color and temperature, and state of consciousness. The presence of a femoral or carotid pulse signifies coordinated cardiac action and at least 50 percent of residual blood volume. Rapid thready pulses are a sign of hypovolemia. An irregular heart rate is usually a warning of cardiac impairment. The patient's skin color should be evaluated; the ashen, gray skin of the face and pale white skin of the extremities are ominous signs of hypovolemia. When blood volume is lost, cerebral perfusion is impaired, and unconsciousness may result. Circulatory collapse in the trauma patient most commonly occurs as a result of hypovolemia secondary to hemorrhage. Compensatory mechanisms will frequently mask the magnitude of bleeding. A blood loss of 30 to 35 percent of the total blood volume can occur before significant changes are noted in the blood pressure.

M. The patient must be rapidly assessed for external, exsanguinating hemorrhage during the primary survey. Direct pressure to the wound is applied to control rapid ongoing blood loss. Tourniquets should not be used unless bleeding cannot be controlled by other means.

N. The severely injured patient who arrives with a normal blood pressure should be rapidly evaluated for occult injuries. Two large bore (16 gauge or greater) intravenous precautionary lines should be established and Ringer's lactate solution infused. Blood should be obtained for a complete blood cell count (CBC), type and crossmatch, and other routine trauma laboratory studies.

O. Three interrelated physiologic functions must be assessed in hypotensive patients, as follows: (1) the heart, (2) the blood and extracellular fluid volume, and (3) the arterial and venous resistance. Pump failure may occur as the result of primary cardiac disease, myocardial contusion, or mechanical problems such as cardiac tamponade. Volume deficits are most commonly associated with hemorrhage but may result from crush injuries, third spacing, or redistribution. Cardiac output may be diminished because of inadequate venous return as seen with tension pneumothorax. Vascular resistance may be altered by injury to the spinal cord, drugs, and sepsis. Regardless of the mechanism, circulatory collapse results in the low flow state and inadequately perfused cells. Normal aerobic metabolism is converted to anaerobic metabolism and, if untreated, leads to metabolic acidosis and eventual cell death.

P. Four types of shock are commonly recognized, as follows: (1) hemorrhagic or hypovolemic, (2) neurogenic, (3) cardiogenic, and (4) vasogenic. Although hemorrhagic shock is the most common type seen in the trauma patient, it is possible for more than one source to contribute to the patient's hypotension. Compensatory mechanisms may preclude a measurable fall in systolic pressure until the patient has lost up to 30 percent of blood volume; therefore, specific attention should be directed to the heart rate, respiratory rate, skin perfusion, and pulse pressure. A narrowed pulse pressure is one of the earliest signs of hypovolemia. The heart rate is a sensitive indicator but may be normally high in children or artificially low in the elderly. Older patients may have a limited cardiac response to catecholamine stimulation or may be taking medication such as beta blockers. The more common signs of hypovolemic shock, such as diaphoresis, cool clammy skin, decreased venous pressures, decreased urine output, thirst, and an altered state of consciousness, are easily recognized by the trauma team.

Neurogenic shock symptoms are much different than those of hypovolemic shock. The patient will have a motor and sensory deficit associated with dry skin, normal or slow heart rate, normal mentation, and normal urine output. Because of its infrequency, the diagnosis of neurogenic shock is often missed and patients inappropriately treated with large fluid volumes. (It is emphasized that neurogenic shock refers to spinal cord injury and not to head injury).

Cardiogenic shock caused by myocardial infarction or arrhythmias is often determined by history and should be confirmed by ECG monitoring. Myocardial dysfunction may occur from tension pneumothorax, myocardial contusion, cardiac tamponade, or an air embolus from the patient's associated injuries.

Cardiac contusion is not uncommon in rapid deceleration blunt trauma to the thorax. Patients with blunt thoracic trauma may need constant ECG monitoring to detect dysrhythmias. Any patient suspected of having cardiogenic shock should have careful monitoring of fluid resuscitation.

(Cont'd from p 21)

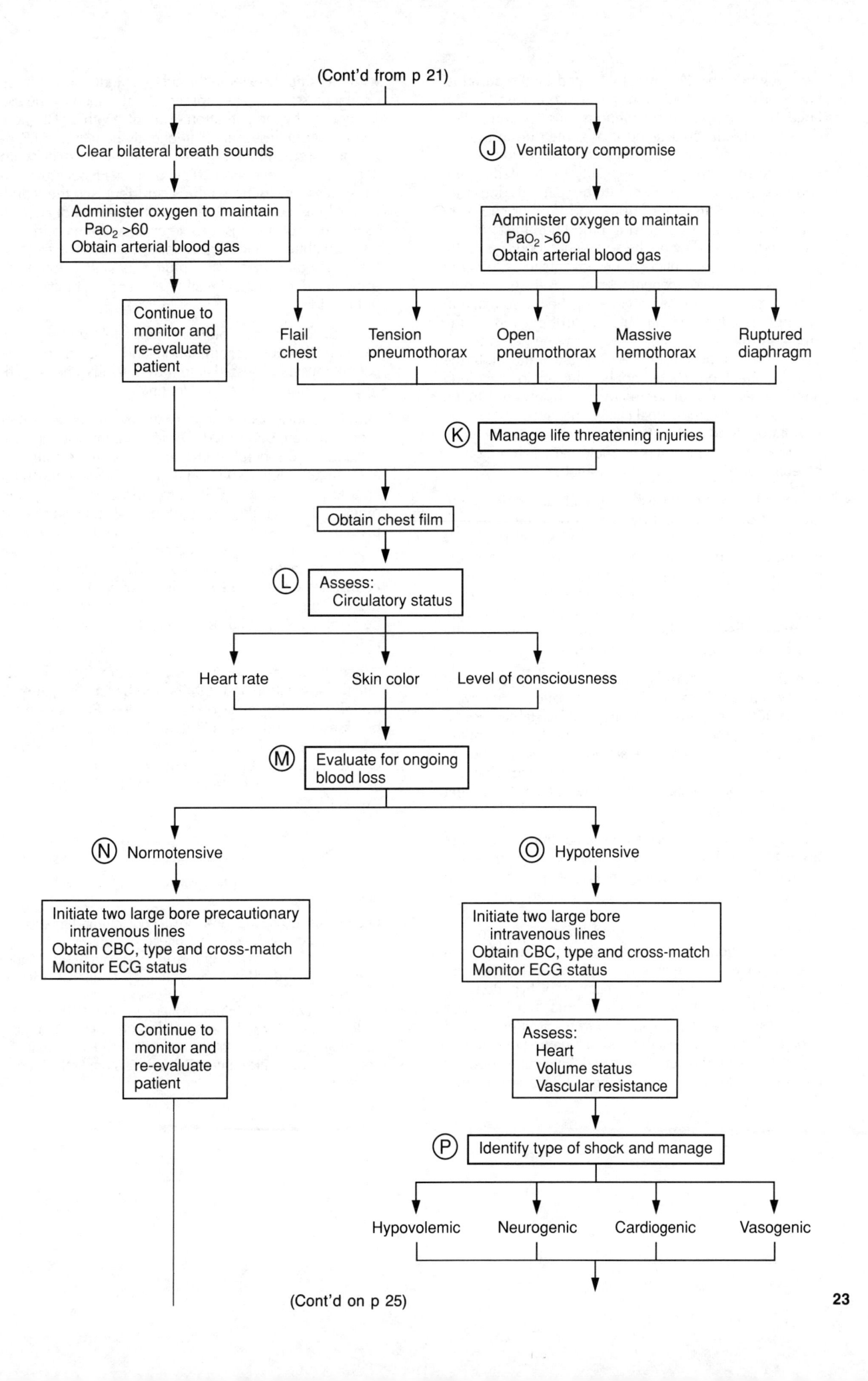

Clear bilateral breath sounds

Administer oxygen to maintain Pao₂ >60
Obtain arterial blood gas

Continue to monitor and re-evaluate patient

(J) Ventilatory compromise

Administer oxygen to maintain Pao₂ >60
Obtain arterial blood gas

- Flail chest
- Tension pneumothorax
- Open pneumothorax
- Massive hemothorax
- Ruptured diaphragm

(K) Manage life threatening injuries

Obtain chest film

(L) Assess: Circulatory status
- Heart rate
- Skin color
- Level of consciousness

(M) Evaluate for ongoing blood loss

(N) Normotensive

Initiate two large bore precautionary intravenous lines
Obtain CBC, type and cross-match
Monitor ECG status

Continue to monitor and re-evaluate patient

(O) Hypotensive

Initiate two large bore intravenous lines
Obtain CBC, type and cross-match
Monitor ECG status

Assess:
 Heart
 Volume status
 Vascular resistance

(P) Identify type of shock and manage
- Hypovolemic
- Neurogenic
- Cardiogenic
- Vasogenic

(Cont'd on p 25)

Q. Hypovolemic shock is initially treated by the administration of crystalloid solutions given through established large bore peripheral intravenous lines. Central line catheters should be avoided if possible during the initial resuscitation. Complications from the central venous route are more frequent, especially in the flailing uncooperative trauma patient. If the patient does not respond to the first 2 L of fluid, and if other causes of hypotension can be ruled out, blood administration is indicated. Depending on the source of blood loss, autologous replacement offers many advantages. Owing to the emphasis on component therapy, it is likely that only packed red cells will be provided by the blood bank. In urgent cases, type-specific blood can be given. In the emergent life threatening case, it may be necessary to use a universal donor such as O-negative blood. In the trauma patient, one should not be reluctant to give blood if there is evidence of hemodynamic instability. On the other hand, if the individual can be managed just as safely without blood administration, that should be the goal, provided that the patient is asymptomatic and no longer bleeding and blood is readily available.

R. As part of the primary survey, a brief neurologic examination is performed and baseline observations recorded. The Glasgow Coma Scale is used to help quantify the extent of neurologic injury. Patients with a coma score of less than 9 are classified as having severe injuries; 9 to 12, moderate injuries; and 13 to 15, minor injuries. Lateralizing neurologic signs generally indicate localized pressure phenomena in the brain usually caused by a subdural or epidural bleed.

S. The diagnosis of neurologic injury is best made on clinical evaluation. There are many diagnostic studies available, but the injured patient may not be stable enough to allow a time consuming work-up. The computed tomography (CT) scan is the single most useful study to obtain and, with proper planning, can frequently be performed without causing delay in the initial management of the trauma patient.

T. Increased intracranial pressure is a common sequela of blunt trauma. Evidence points to more favorable outcomes if the intracranial pressure can be quickly reduced and the duration of hypoxia kept to an absolute minimum. Cerebral ischemia or hypoxia results in insufficient substrate delivery to the injured brain. The principal metabolic requirements of the brain are oxygen and glucose, both used at extremely high rates. Elevated intracranial pressure is often accompanied by hypertension, temperature elevation, and bradycardia, but it may be masked in patients who are hypovolemic. Recognized hypotension cannot be attributed to bleeding in the head unless the patient is very young and the sutures have not closed or unless there is evidence of an open fracture with measurable external blood loss. Reduction of intracranial pressure can be rapidly accomplished by the use of modest hyperventilation. Patients with a Glasgow coma score of less than 11 frequently benefit if the Pco_2 can be lowered to 25 torr, which will usually occur with a respiratory rate around 20 per minute. Hypocarbia will cause vasoconstriction, which contributes to the reduction of brain edema. Diuretics such as mannitol are also used, but caution must be exercised and their administration withheld in the hypovolemic patient. The hypovolemic hypotensive head injured patient should be resuscitated in the usual manner, with no attempt to withhold fluids.

U. The trauma patient should be completely undressed to facilitate thorough examination and assessment. The patient must be assessed anteriorly, laterally, and posteriorly. All injuries must be identified.

V. Simultaneously, as the primary survey progresses, other procedures are performed. Oxygen is administered, two large bore peripheral intravenous lines are established, and Ringer's lactate solution is given. Blood is drawn for an arterial blood gas, CBC, type and cross-match, and other studies as indicated. A nasogastric tube should be placed in the stomach, and the contents evacuated. (Nasogastric tube placement is contraindicated if a cribriform plate fracture is suspected.) A Foley catheter should be inserted unless there is evidence of blood at the meatus or unless there is a scrotal hematoma, perineal hemorrhage, or a high riding prostate on rectal examination.

W. When the primary survey has been completed and the initial resuscitation and stabilization begun, the patient's overall condition must be re-evaluated. Priorities must be assessed, and the patient taken immediately to the operating room if indicated. It is essential that a single physician, preferably the general or trauma surgeon, assume the leadership and coordinate all the consultative activities.

References

American College of Surgeons. Advanced trauma life support course. Chicago: American College of Surgeons, 1989:11.

Levison M, Trunkey D. The multiply injured patient. In: Moore E, ed. Critical decisions in trauma. St. Louis: CV Mosby, 1984:44.

Shires G. Initial care of the injured patient. In: Shires GT, ed. Principles of trauma care. New York: McGraw-Hill, 1985:105.

Thal E. Initial management of the critically injured patient. In: Shires GT, ed. Surgical intensive care. Boston: Little, Brown, in press.

(Cont'd from p 23) Ⓠ Administer blood if indicated

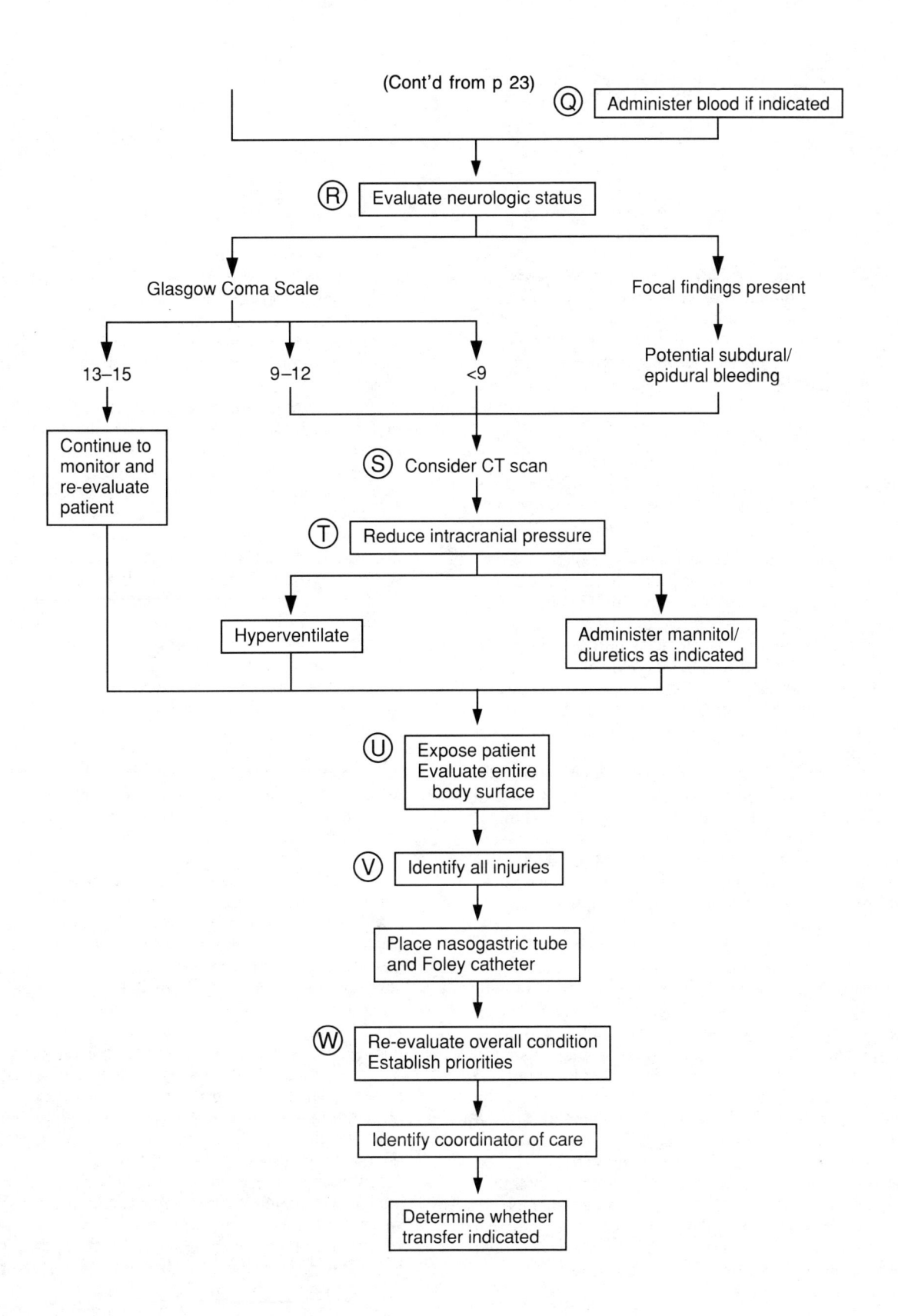

Ⓡ Evaluate neurologic status

Glasgow Coma Scale → 13–15, 9–12, <9

Focal findings present → Potential subdural/epidural bleeding

13–15 → Continue to monitor and re-evaluate patient

9–12 and <9 → Ⓢ Consider CT scan

Ⓣ Reduce intracranial pressure
- Hyperventilate
- Administer mannitol/diuretics as indicated

Ⓤ Expose patient. Evaluate entire body surface

Ⓥ Identify all injuries

Place nasogastric tube and Foley catheter

Ⓦ Re-evaluate overall condition. Establish priorities

Identify coordinator of care

Determine whether transfer indicated

25

SECONDARY ASSESSMENT

Erwin R. Thal
Jorie Klein

A. The secondary survey does not begin until the primary survey (i.e., airway, breathing, and circulation assessment) has been completed and until the resuscitation phase and management of all life threatening conditions have been initiated. The secondary survey consists of a complete head-to-toe physical examination. Following the secondary survey, the patient is again re-evaluated and priorities of care and diagnostic evaluation assessed.

B. The in-depth evaluation employs the look, listen, and feel techniques, which assess each body region. All body regions must be inspected, percussed, palpated, and auscultated. All vital signs are frequently monitored, i.e., blood pressure, pulse, respiration, and temperature.

C. Airway obstruction is the most serious problem to recognize and correct when assessing the head and face. Airway obstruction usually originates from uncontrolled secretions, bleeding, swelling, or mechanical causes associated with severe maxillofacial injuries. Scalp lacerations can produce significant blood loss that is sufficient to cause hypotension. The scalp must be palpated carefully to identify all lacerations, potential fractures, and changes in integrity. All penetrating wounds should be carefully identified. Some facial fractures are readily apparent, whereas others require special roentgenographic views to be identified. Bleeding associated with nasal fractures often requires anterior or posterior packing to achieve adequate hemostasis. Malocclusion may be the only finding present in mandibular fractures. Definitive treatment of maxillofacial injuries is often delayed until the initial swelling subsides. Ocular injuries must be assessed with the recognition that visual disturbances may occur as a direct result of trauma to the eye or because of a central source associated with brain injury. Assessment of pupillary function is important; a difference in pupil diameters of more than 1 mm is abnormal. It is important to perform a thorough funduscopic examination in all patients. Mydriatic solutions should not be used. The ears should be inspected for injury and hemotympanum. The presence of ecchymosis over the mastoid process (Battle's sign), hemotympanum, and otorrhea and/or rhinorrhea may be present in patients with a basilar skull fracture. The mouth should also be carefully inspected and palpated to identify potential fractures. Loose or broken teeth that may obstruct the airway should be identified. Any injuries to the tongue that may progress and potentially obstruct the airway should be assessed. All injuries should be noted.

D. The cervical region contains a greater variety and concentration of anatomic structures than any other area of the body relative to its size. The airway, vessels, thoracic duct, pharynx, esophagus, spinal cord, spinal column, thyroid gland, parathyroid glands, lower cranial nerves, brachial plexus, muscle, and soft tissue are all at risk for injury. The neck should be visually inspected to identify potential injury, lacerations, abrasions, and penetrating wounds. The examiner should note any deviation of the trachea, distention of the neck veins, palpable injury to the larynx, and subcutaneous emphysema. Injury to the airway is suspected in patients who have subcutaneous emphysema, hemoptysis, difficulty with phonation, or stridor.

Laryngeal trauma may be manifested by a fracture of the thyroid cartilage, subluxation of the arytenoid cartilage, or dislocation of the cricothyroid joint. Patients who sustain blunt trauma, are unconscious, or complain of neck pain must have the neck immobilized in a neutral position until a fracture has been ruled out. The cervical collar can be briefly removed to complete the physical examination. The cervical vertebral column should be palpated carefully with the neck stabilized in the neutral position. Any irregularities, step-off, or pain on palpation should be considered to be an injury until further diagnostic procedures can either identify the extent of injury or rule out injury. Lateral cervical films must include the seventh cervical vertebrae and the C7–T1 interspace. If additional films are needed to rule out injury, a complete radiologic survey can be obtained when all injuries are identified and prioritized. The hypopharynx and cervical esophagus are fairly well protected from injury by surrounding structures.

Endoscopy and contrast radiography are used to assess the aerodigestive tract. The zones of the neck associated with penetrating neck trauma must be evaluated to assist in diagnosis and in planning operative intervention. Zone I injuries occur at the thoracic outlet extending superiorly to 1 cm above the clavicles (approximately the level of the cricoid cartilage). Zone II injuries encompass that area from the cricoid cartilage to the angle of the mandible and Zone III from the angle of the mandible to the base of the skull. Patients who have injuries in Zone I are at greatest risk because they may have damage to major arterial structures in the root of the neck or upper mediastinum. These patients, when stable, benefit from preoperative arteriography. Patients with penetrating injuries in Zone II do not routinely require arteriography. Penetrating injuries in Zone III may be very difficult to manage if the internal carotid artery is injured. Arteriography is recommended to help define appropriate management. Unstable patients with indications for surgery, such as shock, expanding hematomas, or uncontrollable bleeding, are taken directly to the operating room (OR). Additional diagnostic studies such as arteriography, endoscopy, contrast radiography, and computed tomography (CT) may be obtained in the stable patient if the diagnosis is in question or if information is sought to plan an operative procedure.

E. Injuries to the thorax account for approximately 25 percent of the deaths attributable to trauma. Fifteen percent require operative intervention. Hypoxia may occur as a

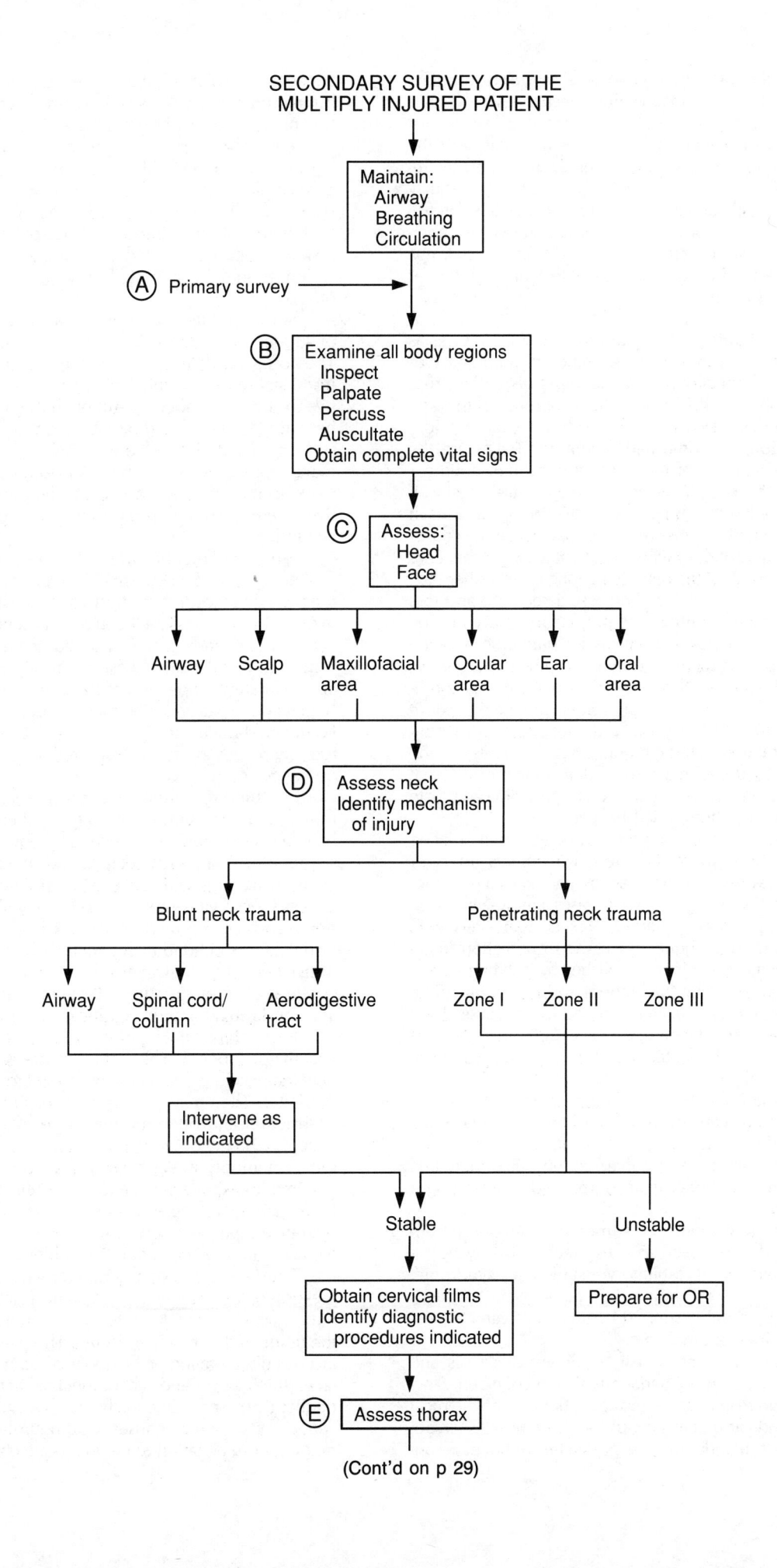

SECONDARY SURVEY OF THE MULTIPLY INJURED PATIENT

```
                    Maintain:
                     Airway
                     Breathing
                     Circulation
                          │
   (A) Primary survey ────┘
                          ▼
   (B)  Examine all body regions
          Inspect
          Palpate
          Percuss
          Auscultate
        Obtain complete vital signs
                          │
                          ▼
                     (C) Assess:
                          Head
                          Face
          ┌──────┬──────┬──┴───┬──────┬──────┐
          ▼      ▼      ▼      ▼      ▼      ▼
       Airway  Scalp  Maxillo- Ocular  Ear   Oral
                      facial   area          area
                      area
                          │
                          ▼
                   (D) Assess neck
                       Identify mechanism
                       of injury
              ┌───────────┴───────────┐
              ▼                       ▼
       Blunt neck trauma       Penetrating neck trauma
        ┌────┬─────┐              ┌────┬────┐
        ▼    ▼     ▼              ▼    ▼    ▼
     Airway Spinal Aerodigestive Zone I Zone II Zone III
            cord/  tract
            column
              │
              ▼
         Intervene as
          indicated
              │
              ▼                 ▼           ▼
            Stable                       Unstable
              │                              │
              ▼                              ▼
        Obtain cervical films         Prepare for OR
        Identify diagnostic
        procedures indicated
              │
              ▼
        (E) Assess thorax

          (Cont'd on p 29)
```

result of diminished blood volume, failure to ventilate the lungs, direct pulmonary injury, or changes in the pressure relationship in the pleural space that lead to displacement of mediastinal structures or collapse of the lung. During the secondary survey the chest is re-evaluated and any resuscitative procedures previously performed are again assessed. The chest wall is carefully inspected for evidence of external trauma, i.e., abrasions, contusions, crepitation, and frank instability. Injuries generally occur as a result of either blunt or penetrating trauma.

F. Blunt chest trauma is likely to produce such injuries as flail chest, hemothorax, pneumothorax, pulmonary or myocardial contusion, traumatic aortic disruption, ruptured diaphragm, rib fractures, tracheobronchial injuries, and on rare occasion traumatic asphyxia. Compression, deceleration, shearing, and barometric forces are the usual mechanisms of injury seen with blunt trauma.

Flail chest occurs when a segment of the chest wall loses its continuity with the rest of the rib cage as a result of multiple rib fractures. The chest wall instability causes paradoxical motion. Hypoxia associated with this condition is a result of the underlying lung injury rather than of the mechanical defect. The associated pain and loss of compliance resulting from pulmonary injury may be the cause of hypoxia. Crepitus on palpation and the presence of asymmetrical movement with inspiratory and expiratory effort are the classic findings with this condition. Chest films may initially underestimate the extent of lung injury and may fail to demonstrate costochondral separations. Arterial blood gases help to assess the degree of hypoxia. Treatment of flail chest is directed at correcting the underlying hypoxia by providing adequate ventilation and humidified oxygen.

Hemothorax is commonly associated with a lacerated lung or injury to the internal mammary artery or intercostal vessels. It may be accompanied by a pneumothorax, and bleeding generally ceases after re-expansion of the lung. Massive hemothorax is associated with hypovolemia and requires aggressive resuscitation. Treatment of hemothorax is accomplished by inserting a chest tube and quantifying the amount and rate of bleeding. A thoracotomy is indicated if blood loss exceeds 2000 ml or if the hourly rate is in excess of 200 ml. In the case of massive blood loss, the use of the autotransfuser may be beneficial.

A pneumothorax occurs when air enters the pleural space, thereby causing collapse of the ipsilateral lung. A ventilation perfusion defect occurs when the blood passes the nonventilated collapsed lung. Treatment of a simple pneumothorax is accomplished by inserting a chest tube.

Pulmonary contusion is the most common potentially lethal injury seen in chest trauma. It may be associated with adult respiratory insufficiency syndrome, which occurs over time rather than instantaneously. Vigorous pulmonary support beginning as early as possible provides optimal care.

Myocardial contusion is a difficult diagnosis and probably occurs more frequently than recognized. Electrocardiogram changes are variable but may be the most reliable indicator of this condition. Commonly seen abnormalities include multiple premature ventricular contractions, unexplained sinus tachycardia, atrial fibrillation, bundle branch block, and ST segment changes. Elevation of the creatine phosphokinase CPK-MB band isoenzyme level greater than 5 percent of the total CPK suggests a myocardial contusion. Two-dimensional echocardiography is a useful and reliable adjunctive study that should be obtained if the ECG is abnormal or if there is strong clinical evidence of myocardial contusion. Patients suspected of having a myocardial contusion should be admitted to a monitored bed and observed.

Aortic rupture is one of the most common causes of sudden death following rapid deceleration injuries. The aorta is usually torn at the ligamentum arteriosum just distal to the left subclavian artery at a point of relative fixation and mobility. Although the wall is torn, the hematoma is contained by the adventitia in those who survive. Knowledge of the mechanism of injury should make one suspect this injury. An aggressive diagnostic work-up that includes thoracic angiography is imperative. Definitive care requires urgent operative intervention.

A ruptured diaphragm is a less frequent injury and is often difficult to recognize. When present it may cause pressure changes in the chest cavity and contribute to hypoxia by compressing the lung. Auscultation might reveal bowel sounds in the chest, but these are often absent with small tears. Chest films fail to demonstrate approximately 30 percent of these injuries. A previously placed nasogastric tube may be seen on chest films. Peritoneal lavage and CT scans are notoriously poor in identifying this injury. The ruptured diaphragm requires operative intervention.

Fractured ribs are the most common thoracic cage injury and may compromise the patient's ability to handle tracheobronchial secretions adequately. This condition often leads to atelectasis and pneumonia, especially in patients with pre-existing pulmonary disease. Unless special views are obtained, many rib fractures are not seen on routine chest films. It is often difficult to visualize costochondral separations and anterior fractures; therefore, physical examination may be just as accurate as a radiologic survey. Local injection or epidural anesthesia may provide significant pain relief.

Tracheobronchial injuries involve the larynx, trachea, and major bronchi. These injuries are seen with both penetrating and blunt trauma but are more common with the latter. They may cause partial or complete airway obstruction and often are the cause of sudden death. Patients with major bronchial injuries present with a history of hemoptysis, subcutaneous emphysema, tension pneumothorax, or a persistent air leak after thoracostomy. Management of these injuries is individualized, and operative repair is reserved for those injuries in which airway maintenance cannot be achieved.

Traumatic asphyxia is a rare injury caused by compression of the chest that results in obstruction of venous return, which in turn leads to extravasation of blood into the tissue and to massive edema. The patient has a violaceous discoloration of the upper chest, neck, arms, and face. Bulging eyes and subconjunctival hemorrhages are frequently present. Cerebral hemorrhage may result from venous stasis, which causes focal neurologic problems ranging from agitation to death. Tissue changes resolve

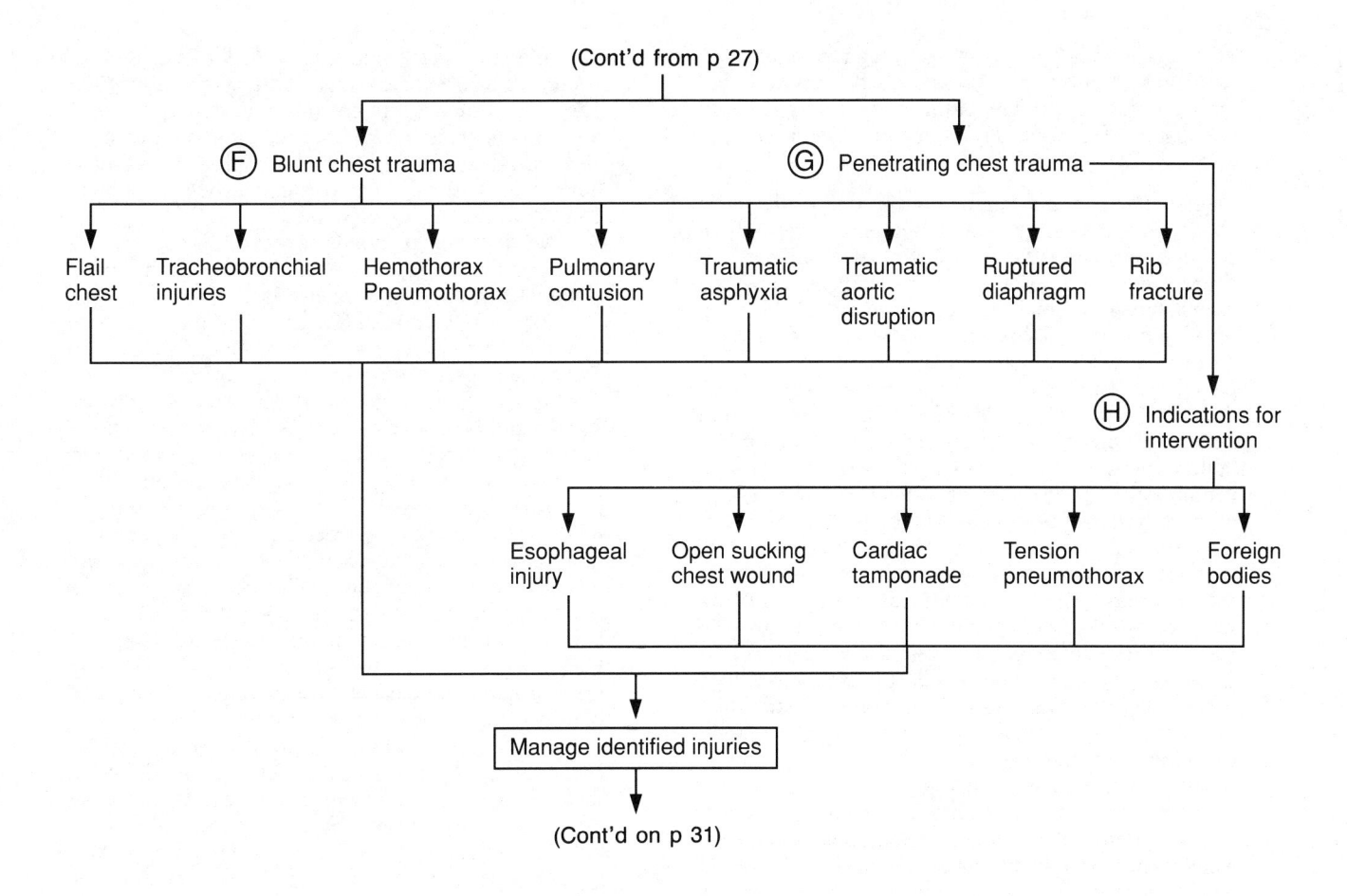

```
                        (Cont'd from p 27)
                    ┌───────────┴───────────┐
                    ▼                       ▼
              Ⓕ Blunt chest trauma    Ⓖ Penetrating chest trauma
```

- Flail chest
- Tracheobronchial injuries
- Hemothorax Pneumothorax
- Pulmonary contusion
- Traumatic asphyxia
- Traumatic aortic disruption
- Ruptured diaphragm
- Rib fracture

Ⓗ Indications for intervention

- Esophageal injury
- Open sucking chest wound
- Cardiac tamponade
- Tension pneumothorax
- Foreign bodies

Manage identified injuries

(Cont'd on p 31)

spontaneously, but attention must be directed to alleviation of the underlying injuries.

G. Penetrating chest trauma is more likely to cause tension pneumothorax, cardiac tamponade, open sucking chest wounds, esophageal trauma, and abdominal injuries. Anatomic landmarks are helpful in predicting potential problems. One cannot assume a bullet travels in a straight line; in reality, the missile trajectory is unpredictable because the bullet may ricochet, tumble, fragment, or embolize. Concern for abdominal injuries should exist any time a bullet enters, exits, or is located below the fourth to fifth intercostal space anteriorly, the fifth and sixth intercostal space laterally, or the sixth or seventh intercostal space posteriorly. These landmarks serve as indicators for celiotomy in patients with gunshot wounds to the chest.

H. Any patient who sustains a gunshot wound that enters the chest and transverses the mediastinum warrants a thoracotomy or, at minimum, a subxiphoid exploration in the OR. Any penetrating injury in the "box" outlined by the clavicles superiorly, the midclavicular lines laterally, and the xiphoid process inferiorly is an indication for a subxiphoid exploration.

Tension pneumothorax is a life threatening injury that involves clinical rather than radiologic diagnosis. This condition may be confused with cardiac tamponade; some of the signs, such as distended neck veins and cyanosis, are similar. The absence of breath sounds and hypertympanitic percussion on the ipsilateral side are diagnostic of this condition. Rapid decompress by either needle aspiration or chest tube insertion should be immediate.

Cardiac tamponade is most frequently seen in patients with penetrating trauma but must be considered in blunt trauma as well. This is a life threatening injury that warrants immediate intervention. Pericardiocentesis may be a diagnostic and life saving procedure, whereas thoracotomy is the definitive treatment.

Open sucking chest wounds occur when penetrating wounds fail to seal. If the wound is greater than two-thirds the diameter of the trachea, air will pass through the defect with each respiratory effort, taking the path of least resistance. This is a life threatening injury and leads to ineffective ventilation and ultimate hypoxia. These patients need a three-corner occlusive dressing put in place and a thoracostomy for the underlying pneumothorax. Definitive care includes primary closure of the chest wall.

Unrecognized esophageal injury that is left untreated is potentially lethal. Seen more commonly with penetrating trauma, it is suspected in patients with a left hemothorax or pneumothorax without rib fracture. Other signs and symptoms include pain, shock disproportional to the injury, particulate matter in the chest drainage, or mediastinal air usually seen on the left. Contrast radiography and/or endoscopy confirms the diagnosis, which demands prompt operative drainage and repair.

Foreign bodies are occasionally seen in conjunction with chest injuries. These should not be removed until the patient has been fully evaluated by a surgeon who is capable of treating any injury or ensuing complications.

I. Assessing abdominal trauma can be one of the most challenging tasks for the trauma surgeon. Unresponsive and uncooperative patients, lack of physical findings, and delayed symptom onset add to the challenge. Physical examination is one of the most accurate and reliable diagnostic modalities, although it can be misleading 10 to 15 percent of the time even in an alert, cooperative patient. The two major concerns in the evaluation of abdominal injuries are uncontrollable bleeding and peritoneal contamination secondary to perforation of a hollow viscus. Bleeding is best assessed by hemodynamic monitoring. The contamination from a hollow viscus injury is evaluated by repeated clinical evaluation in conjunction with adjunctive diagnostic studies.

The abdomen is divided into the three following major areas: (1) the peritoneal cavity; (2) the retroperitoneal space; and (3) the intrathoracic portion. Each of these areas requires special consideration for prompt injury recognition. The history and knowledge of the mechanism of injury are important. Many injuries within the peritoneal cavity cause enough irritation to be easily recognized. An exception is the presence of blood, which may or may not produce abdominal tenderness on physical examination. The degree to which it causes peritoneal irritation is unpredictable, and hence, a patient may have significant abdominal blood loss and a relatively benign appearing abdomen. It is not important to identify the specific organ injured, but rather to recognize the need and proper timing for operative intervention. Retroperitoneal injuries present more of a challenge because the lack of peritoneal irritation may allow the patient to be relatively asymptomatic in the early postinjury period. Intrathoracic injuries are suspected with penetrating injuries below the landmarks described under chest injuries (see *H*).

J. Abdominal trauma is divided into two major types, blunt and penetrating, each requiring a different philosophic and diagnostic approach. The process of careful monitoring and re-evaluation indicates the extent of the diagnostic work-up required. Patients with hemodynamic instability or positive evidence of an acute surgical abdomen, which suggests visceral injury, should be taken to the OR as quickly as possible following initial attempts at stabilization. Patients who sustain blunt trauma may require a variety of diagnostic procedures in the absence of obvious indication for celiotomy. These studies may include conventional radiography, laboratory determinations, diagnostic peritoneal lavage, CT scan, sonography, urologic survey, arteriography, and a variety of special procedures.

Conventional radiography usually consists of a chest film and an abdominal series consisting of a kidney, ureters, and bladder (KUB) and anterior-posterior (AP) view of the pelvis. These films help identify skeletal injuries. On rare occasions, they may demonstrate air under the diaphragm, which indicates a visceral perforation, or perirenal air on the right which suggests a retroperitoneal duodenal injury.

Laboratory determinations, with the exception of blood for a type and cross-match, play a relatively minor role in the evaluation of patients with abdominal trauma. All patients with an abnormally elevated amylase level should be admitted to the hospital for observation. A urinalysis is valuable in determining whether additional urologic studies are warranted.

The diagnostic peritoneal lavage (DPL) continues to be an excellent adjunctive procedure. Its use has been challenged by the recent interest in CT scans; however, when compared with the CT scan, the DPL appears to be the more sensitive test. It is extremely accurate in predicting injuries within the peritoneal cavity but less sensitive with retroperitoneal and diaphragmatic injuries. There is still lack of agreement as to what constitutes a positive study: most authors use 100,000 red blood cells per millimeter and 500 white blood cells per millimeter as their criteria. These numbers seem most reasonable in limiting the number of procedures in which minimal injury is found and identifying those patients who will benefit from early operation. DPL is particularly useful as a screening study in an unstable patient or in a patient with an altered state of consciousness. Other analyses, such as amylase level, presence of bile, liver function studies, and bacterial stains, are used, although there is no consensus regarding their efficacy.

The CT scan is rapidly becoming the most popular diagnostic study for assessing abdominal injuries in stable cooperative patients. To ensure a satisfactory study, it is necessary to use both intravenous and oral contrast material. Obtaining the scan is time-consuming and expensive but provides a good assessment of the retroperitoneal area, which is advantageous over the DPL.

Sonography has not been used frequently in the United States but is popular in Europe. The results have been excellent; however, the procedure requires further evaluation.

Special procedures, such as oral contrast studies, arteriography, magnetic resonance imaging, laparoscopy, and isotope scans, have all been described but infrequently used. The role of magnetic resonance imaging is as yet undetermined in the initial evaluation period; it may be an excellent modality to follow patients who are managed nonoperatively. Arteriography may be useful to assess a potential renal artery injury or to embolize pelvic vessels to control hemorrhage associated with pelvic fractures. Intravenous pyelography and cystography are obtained in patients with suspected urologic injury as evidenced by flank injury or microscopic or gross hematuria. A urethrogram is obtained prior to inserting a Foley catheter in those patients suspected of urethral injury.

Upon completion of the diagnostic process in patients with blunt abdominal trauma, a management decision must be made. Selective nonoperative therapy is now employed with more frequency. Conservative management must be carefully monitored, and until long-term outcome data verify its safety, surgery should remain a strong viable option.

K. Patients with penetrating abdominal injuries present different problems to the trauma team. Eighty to 90 percent of the patients who have penetration of the peri-

(Cont'd from p 29)

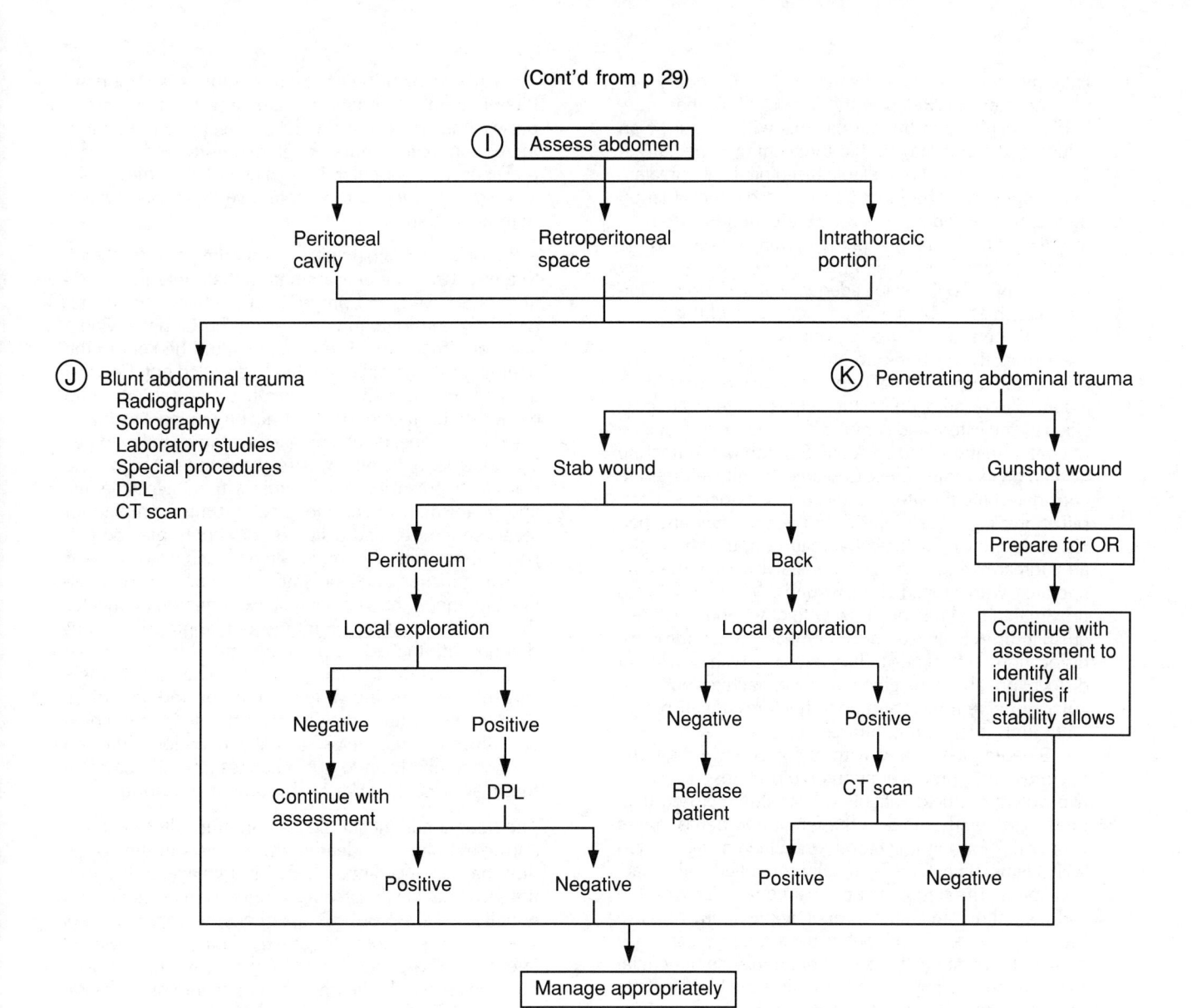

- Ⓘ Assess abdomen
  - Peritoneal cavity
  - Retroperitoneal space
  - Intrathoracic portion

- Ⓙ Blunt abdominal trauma
  - Radiography
  - Sonography
  - Laboratory studies
  - Special procedures
  - DPL
  - CT scan

- Ⓚ Penetrating abdominal trauma
  - Stab wound
    - Peritoneum → Local exploration
      - Negative → Continue with assessment
      - Positive → DPL
        - Positive
        - Negative
    - Back → Local exploration
      - Negative → Release patient
      - Positive → CT scan
        - Positive
        - Negative
  - Gunshot wound → Prepare for OR → Continue with assessment to identify all injuries if stability allows

Manage appropriately

(Cont'd on p 33)

---

toneum by a missile sustain visceral injury. Therefore, an aggressive approach is recommended, and essentially all patients with gunshot wounds to the lower chest, abdomen, flank, and back are taken to the operating room. Patients who sustain stab wounds are managed less aggressively. If there is no indication for celiotomy, the abdominal wound is locally explored. If the end of the tract is clearly seen and does not penetrate the peritoneal cavity, the wound is closed and evaluation for other injuries continued. However, if the end of the tract is not seen or if the peritoneum is violated, and if the patient remains asymptomatic, a DPL is performed and the patient managed accordingly. Local exploration is not recommended for lower chest wounds. DPL is not recommended for stab wounds of the back, but CT scans may be beneficial.

L. Extremity injuries are addressed in the secondary survey and have a lower priority of care. More than one-half of hospitalized trauma patients will have such an injury, and some may be life threatening, especially if accompanied by uncontrollable bleeding. Limb threatening injuries must be identified in the early evaluation period and treated aggressively. Evaluation of extremity injuries is an integral part of the overall approach to the trauma patient. The extremities are examined by paying close attention to the color, adequacy of perfusion, deformities such as angulation or shortening, swelling, bruising, and the status of open wounds.

Clinically, fractures are either closed or open. Any obvious or suspected fracture near a wound should be assumed to be an open fracture. Open fractures are classified by the extent and complexity of the wound, degree of contamination, and the configuration of the fracture as seen on extremity films. Certain extremity injuries are considered life threatening because of associated complications, e.g., crush injuries to the abdomen and pelvis; major pelvic fractures; traumatic amputations of the arm, forearm, thigh, or leg; and massive open long-bone fractures with ragged dirty wounds. Vascular injuries proximal to the knee or elbow with or without fractures; crush injuries to an extremity; compartment syndromes; dislocations of the knee or hip; fractures, with or without dislocation, about the elbow or knee; fractures with vascular or nerve injury; and open fractures are all potentially limb threatening injuries.

Bleeding associated with major closed long-bone fractures may produce enough blood loss to cause hypovolemic shock. Patients with multiple closed fractures, particularly those of the femur and pelvis, are at greater risk for ongoing blood loss. Bleeding associated with a femoral fracture is generally controlled with a traction splint. The trauma team must be familiar with the various splints and their proper application. Massive bleeding may occur with pelvic fractures. In the absence of urgent indications for operation, it may be beneficial to obtain an arteriogram and embolize the bleeding site as part of the initial therapy. External fixators and military antishock trousers (MAST) are two other modalities that may help control bleeding from pelvic injuries.

The signs and symptoms of a compartmental syndrome are pain, decreased sensation, tense swelling, and weakness or paralysis of the involved extremity. Intracompartmental pressure measurements may help diagnose a suspected compartment syndrome. The syndrome usually develops over a period of time and is associated with crush injuries, fractures, sustained compression of an extremity, reperfusion of a previously ischemic extremity, and electrical injuries. MAST may cause a compartment syndrome, particularly if left inflated for prolonged periods of time.

Under ideal circumstances, amputated extremities may be replanted. These procedures are performed at specialized centers. The evaluating physician should consult the surgeon at the definitive care facility to determine whether the patient is a candidate for replantation. If the patient qualifies, the amputated part should be carefully preserved and rapidly transported with the patient to the replantation center.

Early recognition of vascular injuries is important. Bleeding, an expanding hematoma, a bruit, abnormal pulses, impaired distal circulation, decreased sensation, increasing pain, and a cool extremity indicate the presence of a vascular injury. Doppler studies make assessment easier, but the definitive diagnosis is made with angiography.

M. A thorough neurologic evaluation completes the head-to-toe survey. Careful examination that looks for lacerations, CSF leaks, and presence of fractures and assessment of neurologic function using the Glasgow Coma Scale are important. The patient should be kept in the neutral position until injury has been ruled out. Cervical injuries are suspected in unconscious patients who demonstrate flaccid areflexia accompanied by diminished rectal tone, diaphragmatic breathing, ability to flex but not extend the elbow, pain above but not below the clavicle, hypotension, bradycardia without hypovolemia, and priapism. The conscious patient may complain of local tenderness, and a step-off deformity may be palpated. Examination for motor strength and weakness and sensory function and assessment of autonomic dysfunction are important. The physical examination delineates the precise location of injury, but appropriate films demonstrate the extent of injury and allow for proper planning and management. The CT scan is extremely valuable in assessing vertebral injuries and should be used liberally. Fluid administration should be monitored carefully. Continued reassessment of neurologic function allows the physician to note changes from the baseline that may necessitate re-establishment of priorities.

N. The trauma patient should be continuously monitored and re-evaluated to identify any changes in the condition that may warrant a change in management priorities. As initial life threatening injuries are managed, other equally serious problems may become apparent. Less severe injuries or underlying medical problems may need attention. The patient's pertinent past medical history must be assessed. The physician in charge must decide whether transfer is necessary and, if so, initiate the transfer process. If a patient needs to be transferred to a higher level facility, little time should be spent obtaining diagnostic procedures. Only those studies that will expedite resuscitation and stabilization should be obtained. Time is of the essence and the quicker the patient arrives at the appropriate definitive care center, the better are the chances for a successful outcome.

References

American College of Surgeons. Advanced trauma life support course. Chicago: American College of Surgeons, 1989:11–24.

Levison M, Trunkey D. The multiply injured patient. In: Moore E, ed. Critical decisions in trauma. St. Louis: CV Mosby, 1984:44–49.

Shires GT. Initial care of the injured patient. In: Shires GT, ed. Principles of trauma care. New York: McGraw-Hill, 1985:105–109.

Thal E. Initial management of the critically injured patient. In: Shires GT, ed. Surgical intensive care. Boston: Little, Brown, in press.

(Cont'd from p 31)

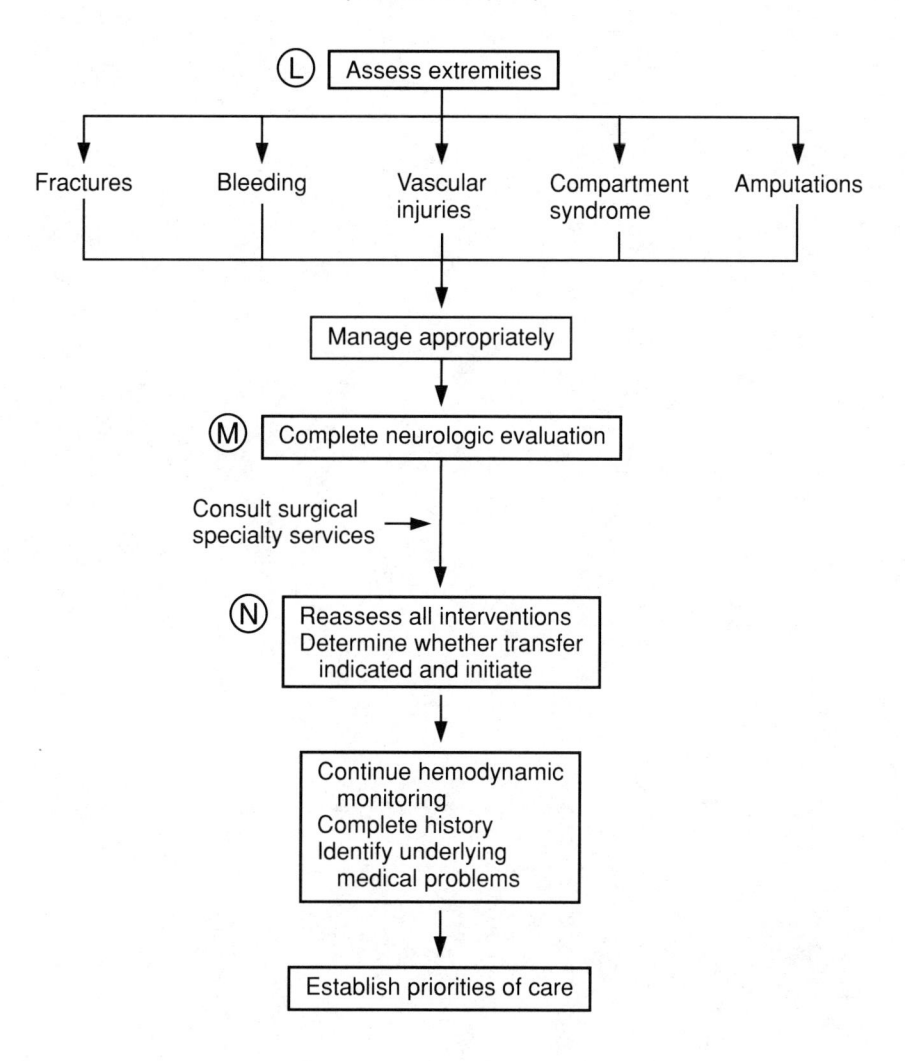

Ⓛ Assess extremities
- Fractures
- Bleeding
- Vascular injuries
- Compartment syndrome
- Amputations

↓

Manage appropriately

↓

Ⓜ Complete neurologic evaluation

Consult surgical specialty services →

↓

Ⓝ Reassess all interventions
Determine whether transfer indicated and initiate

↓

Continue hemodynamic monitoring
Complete history
Identify underlying medical problems

↓

Establish priorities of care

SHOCK MANAGEMENT

Hypovolemic Shock
Blood Administration
Fluid Warming

HYPOVOLEMIC SHOCK

Mary K. Roberts

A. A medical history is vital to determine the etiology of the shock. This can be quickly accomplished by an AMPLE history, as follows: A, allergies; M, medication currently being taken; P, past illnesses; L, last meal; E, preceding events.

B. Establishing and maintaining a patent airway with adequate ventilatory exchange is the first priority. If spontaneous ventilation is compromised, endotracheal intubation may be required to optimize oxygenation. In all cases, supplemental oxygen should be administered to improve oxygen transport to the tissues.

C. Cardiac monitoring should be initiated to determine whether shock induced arrhythmias are present.

D. Pulse, blood pressure, and respiratory rate should be immediately recorded and monitored every 5 to 15 minutes during the resuscitation phase. The degrees to which the pulse and respiratory rate are increased and the systolic blood pressure decreased are valuable indicators of the severity of the shock state and the progress made toward restoring tissue perfusion and tissue oxygenation. Hypothermia has been implicated in contributing to coagulopathies; therefore, temperature should also be closely monitored.

E. Direct manual pressure should be applied over any obvious external bleeding site. A pressure dressing can then be applied to the wound as bleeding slows. Elevation of a bleeding extremity above the patient's heart may also help control visible hemorrhage.

F. Blood should be obtained and laboratory samples sent for a complete blood count; arterial blood gas; electrolytes including serum glucose, blood urea nitrogen, and creatinine; coagulation profile; and typing and crossmatching. A baseline spun hematocrit level should also be obtained in the emergency department. This value may be misleading after acute hemorrhage because of hemoconcentration. The degree of blood loss may not be reflected in the hematocrit level for 4 to 6 hours after the patient has been resuscitated. Subsequent serial determinations are more valuable than this initial value. A urine sample should also be sent for urinalysis to determine the presence or absence of red blood cells.

G. Urine output is a reliable indicator of volume loss and of the adequacy of volume restitution and tissue perfusion. A Foley catheter must be inserted as soon as possible. A minimal adequate urine volume is 0.5 ml/kg per hour.

H. The term hypovolemic shock implies a condition in which there is a decrease in intravascular volume, resulting in inadequate tissue perfusion and insufficient cellular oxygenation. The classification system assists in determining the severity of shock and includes four simplified stages based on the amount of acute blood loss. For each stage the findings for each clinical indicator of tissue perfusion are predicted. Assessment assists in establishing the stability of the patient and determining the classification of shock. It also serves as a baseline from which to evaluate the patient's status during resuscitation. Indicators of tissue perfusion include patient's skin color, temperature, and moisture; capillary blanch test; neurologic status; and determination of the pulse pressure.

I. Because of compensatory mechanisms, the volume loss is minimized and the Class I patient exhibits few clinical symptoms.

J. In the absence of hypothermia, paleness and coolness of skin as well as a delay greater than 2 seconds in capillary refill are valuable indicators of a Class II patient. In addition, an increased diastolic pressure will decrease pulse pressure, and the patient may exhibit anxiety and restlessness.

K. The Class III patient manifests symptoms of shock in all clinical parameters. The compensatory mechanisms are inadequate, thereby resulting in a progressive decline in tissue perfusion and tissue oxygenation. Prompt treatment with crystalloids and blood products must be implemented with frequent reassessment of the clinical manifestations of shock to prevent further deterioration and to ensure adequate resuscitation.

L. Symptoms of profound shock include severe hypotension; irregular pulse with rate at 140 or greater; cold, cyanotic skin with no observable capillary refill; hyperventilation with shallow, irregular respirations; extreme alteration in level of consciousness; and oliguria.

M. If hypovolemic shock is not caused by overt hemorrhage, it is important to identify the etiology to help control fluid loss and to guide the subsequent medical treatment. Blood loss can be concealed in the thorax, abdomen, and fracture sites. Possible related causes for hypovolemic shock include burns, ascites, pancreatitis, bowel obstruction, diabetes insipidus, uncontrolled diabetes mellitus, and diuretic therapy.

N. If the patient is severely hypotensive and/or hemorrhage cannot be controlled, the pneumatic antishock garment might be considered as a supportive measure until adequate fluid volume has been restored.

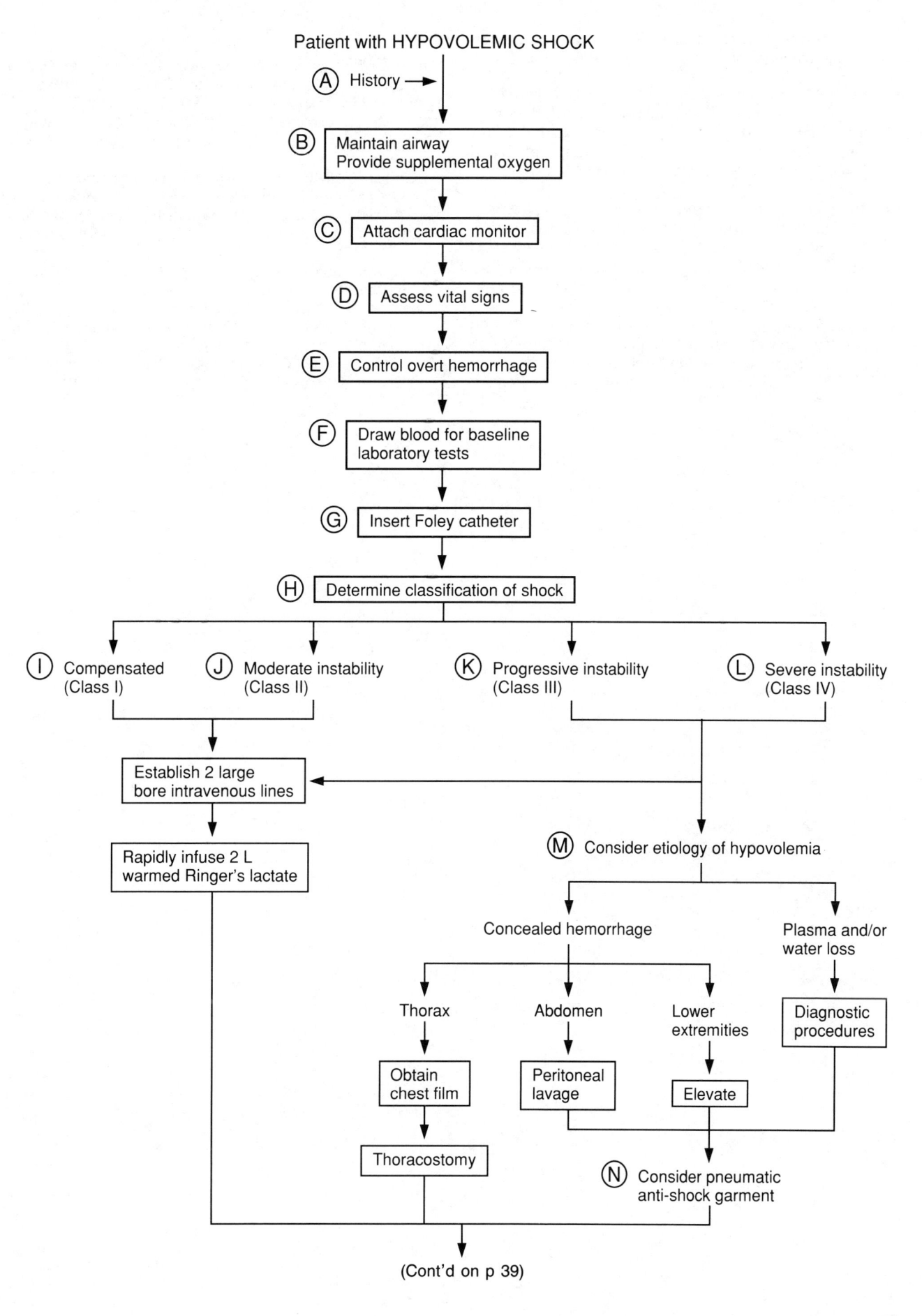

```
Patient with HYPOVOLEMIC SHOCK
              │
        (A) History ──→│
                       ↓
              (B) ┌─────────────────────────┐
                  │ Maintain airway         │
                  │ Provide supplemental oxygen │
                  └─────────────────────────┘
                       ↓
              (C) ┌─────────────────────────┐
                  │ Attach cardiac monitor  │
                  └─────────────────────────┘
                       ↓
              (D) ┌─────────────────────────┐
                  │ Assess vital signs      │
                  └─────────────────────────┘
                       ↓
              (E) ┌─────────────────────────┐
                  │ Control overt hemorrhage │
                  └─────────────────────────┘
                       ↓
              (F) ┌─────────────────────────┐
                  │ Draw blood for baseline │
                  │ laboratory tests        │
                  └─────────────────────────┘
                       ↓
              (G) ┌─────────────────────────┐
                  │ Insert Foley catheter   │
                  └─────────────────────────┘
                       ↓
              (H) ┌─────────────────────────┐
                  │ Determine classification of shock │
                  └─────────────────────────┘
```

(I) Compensated (Class I)
(J) Moderate instability (Class II)
(K) Progressive instability (Class III)
(L) Severe instability (Class IV)

Establish 2 large bore intravenous lines

Rapidly infuse 2 L warmed Ringer's lactate

(M) Consider etiology of hypovolemia

Concealed hemorrhage: Thorax, Abdomen, Lower extremities

Plasma and/or water loss: Diagnostic procedures

- Thorax → Obtain chest film → Thoracostomy
- Abdomen → Peritoneal lavage
- Lower extremities → Elevate

(N) Consider pneumatic anti-shock garment

(Cont'd on p 39)

37

O. Patients who present in progressive or severe shock states require blood transfusions during the resuscitation phase.

P. Central venous pressure (CVP) monitoring is helpful in ongoing evaluation of volume status. A CVP less than 5 mm Hg is strongly indicative of hypovolemia. This intravenous line is not used for primary resuscitation and should not be inserted on an emergency basis.

Q. The trauma patient who has been successfully resuscitated is usually anxious and requires verbal reassurance. Explanations of what has happened should be given as well as of the need for hospitalization. The patient should also be advised of when family will be allowed to visit.

R. Surgical intervention is required when shock cannot be corrected in the emergency department with fluid and blood administration. If shock recurs after initial correction, the need for definitive surgery is also evident.

References

American College of Surgeons. Advanced trauma life support course. Chicago: American College of Surgeons, 1984:175–190.

Casey MF. Hypovolemic shock. In: Sommers MS, ed. Difficult diagnoses in critical care nursing. Rockville, MD: Aspen, 1989:1–25.

McQuillan KA, Wiles CE. Initial management of traumatic shock. In: Cardona VC, Hurn PD, Mason PJ, Scanlon-Schilpp AM, Veise-Berry SW, eds. Trauma nursing: from resuscitation through rehabilitation. Philadelphia: WB Saunders, 1988:160–173.

Roberts MK. Fluid resuscitation in the adult trauma patient. Orthopaed Nursing 1989; 8(6):41–47.

Roberts MK. Hypovolemic shock. In: Mims BC, ed. Case studies in critical care nursing. Baltimore: Williams & Wilkins, 1990:85.

Trunkey D, Lewis FR. Current therapy of trauma–2. Toronto: BC Decker, 1986:60–69.

(Cont'd from p 37)

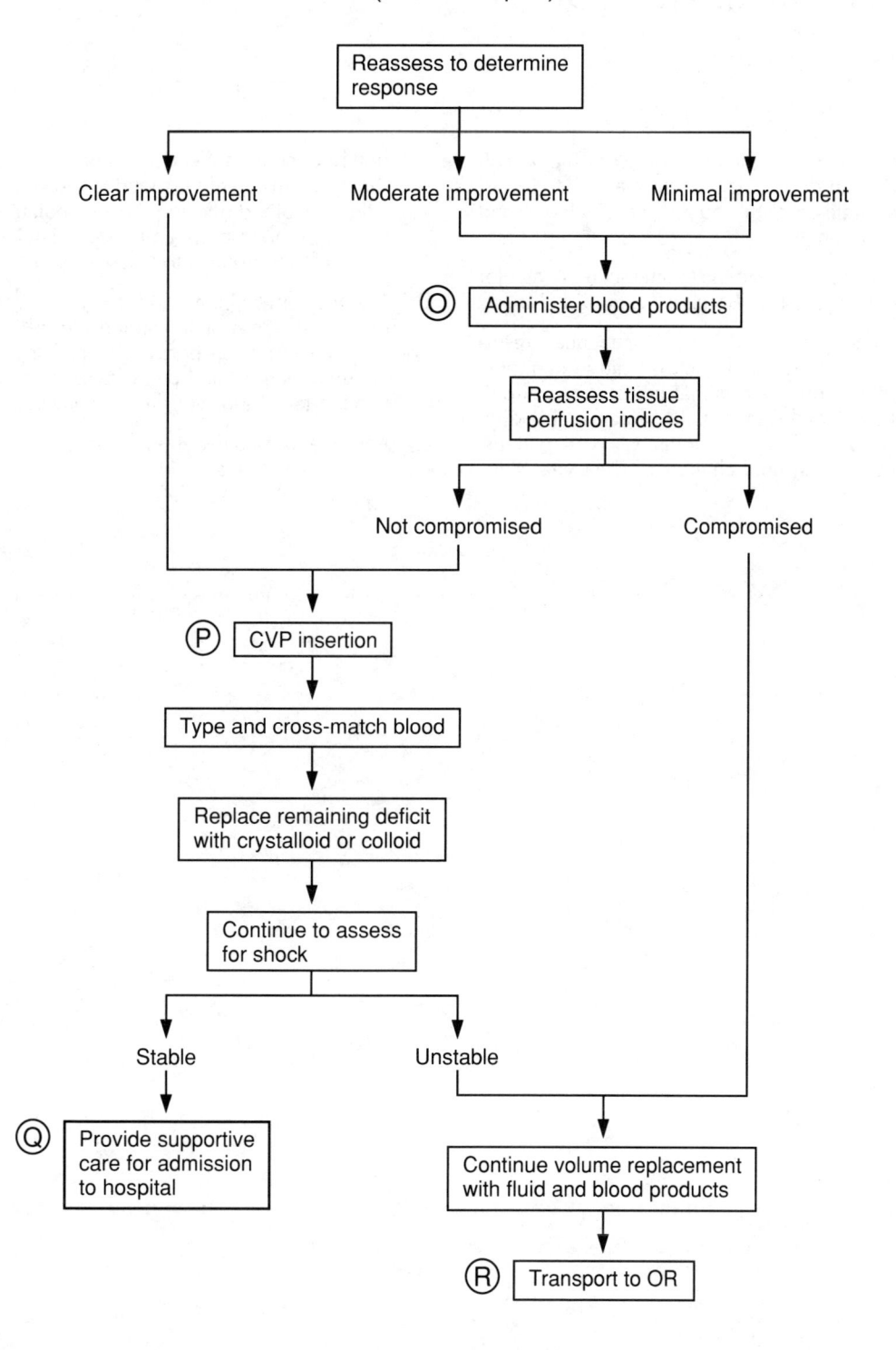

```
                    ┌─────────────────────┐
                    │ Reassess to determine│
                    │ response            │
                    └─────────────────────┘
           ┌───────────────┼───────────────┐
           ▼               ▼               ▼
    Clear improvement  Moderate improvement  Minimal improvement
           │               └───────┬───────┘
           │                       ▼
           │           ⓞ ┌─────────────────────┐
           │             │ Administer blood products│
           │             └─────────────────────┘
           │                       ▼
           │             ┌─────────────────────┐
           │             │ Reassess tissue     │
           │             │ perfusion indices   │
           │             └─────────────────────┘
           │                 ┌─────┴─────┐
           │                 ▼           ▼
           │          Not compromised  Compromised
           └─────────────────┤           │
                             ▼           │
                  ⓟ ┌──────────────┐     │
                    │ CVP insertion│     │
                    └──────────────┘     │
                             ▼           │
                    ┌──────────────────┐ │
                    │ Type and cross-  │ │
                    │ match blood      │ │
                    └──────────────────┘ │
                             ▼           │
                    ┌──────────────────┐ │
                    │ Replace remaining│ │
                    │ deficit with     │ │
                    │ crystalloid or   │ │
                    │ colloid          │ │
                    └──────────────────┘ │
                             ▼           │
                    ┌──────────────────┐ │
                    │ Continue to      │ │
                    │ assess for shock │ │
                    └──────────────────┘ │
                       ┌─────┴─────┐     │
                       ▼           ▼     │
                     Stable     Unstable │
                       │           └──┬──┘
                       ▼              ▼
          ⓠ ┌──────────────┐  ┌─────────────────────┐
            │ Provide      │  │ Continue volume     │
            │ supportive   │  │ replacement with    │
            │ care for     │  │ fluid and blood     │
            │ admission    │  │ products            │
            │ to hospital  │  └─────────────────────┘
            └──────────────┘           ▼
                              ⓡ ┌──────────────┐
                                │ Transport to OR│
                                └──────────────┘
```

BLOOD ADMINISTRATION

Thomas Drury

A. Laboratory tests should include complete blood cell count (CBC) with differential, serum electrolyte levels, coagulation studies, alcohol and drug toxicity levels, and a type and cross-match.

B. In addition to vital signs and the trauma score, skin color and temperature assist in the classification of shock.

C. The amount and type of fluid needed for adequate resuscitation are determined by the classification of shock. Class I patients require a minimal bolus of crystalloid. Class II patients' vital signs usually remain stable after the initial 1 to 2 L bolus of fluids. Class III patients respond to the initial fluid challenge. Their vital signs slowly decline, a clear indication for blood. Class IV shock victims do not respond to resuscitation with crystalloid or blood and require immediate surgical intervention. If not rapidly and appropriately treated, Class III shock deteriorates to Class IV shock (p 36).

D. The necessity of intravenous (IV) access is dependent on the classification of shock and the resuscitation needs of the patient. Large bore exchange kits (7 French), large "trauma tubing," and pressure bags can all be used to provide large and rapid resuscitation (p 36).

E. A warmer is used in delivering both crystalloid and blood to trauma patients (p 44).

BLOOD ADMINISTRATION

- **A** Obtain baseline blood studies
- **B** Assess: Vital signs, Trauma score
- **C** Determine classification of shock

Class I (15% blood loss) / **Class II** (20–25% blood loss):
- Provide 40% oxygen
- **D** Insert 2 large bore intravenous lines
- **E** Give 1–2 L warmed Ringer's lactate
- Patient stabilizes
  - Class I
  - Class II: May require type and cross-matched blood
- To operating room as needed
- Continue to assess and reassess for shock

Class III (30–35% blood loss):
- Provide 100% oxygen
- **D** Insert 2 large bore intravenous lines
- Consider additional venous access
- Consider #7 French exchange catheter
- **E** Begin with 1–2 L warmed Ringer's lactate

Class IV (40–50% blood loss):
- Provide 100% oxygen
- **D** Insert 2 large bore intravenous lines
- Obtain additional venous access
- Use #7 French exchange catheter
- **E** Obtain blood warmer. Begin rapid infusion of blood

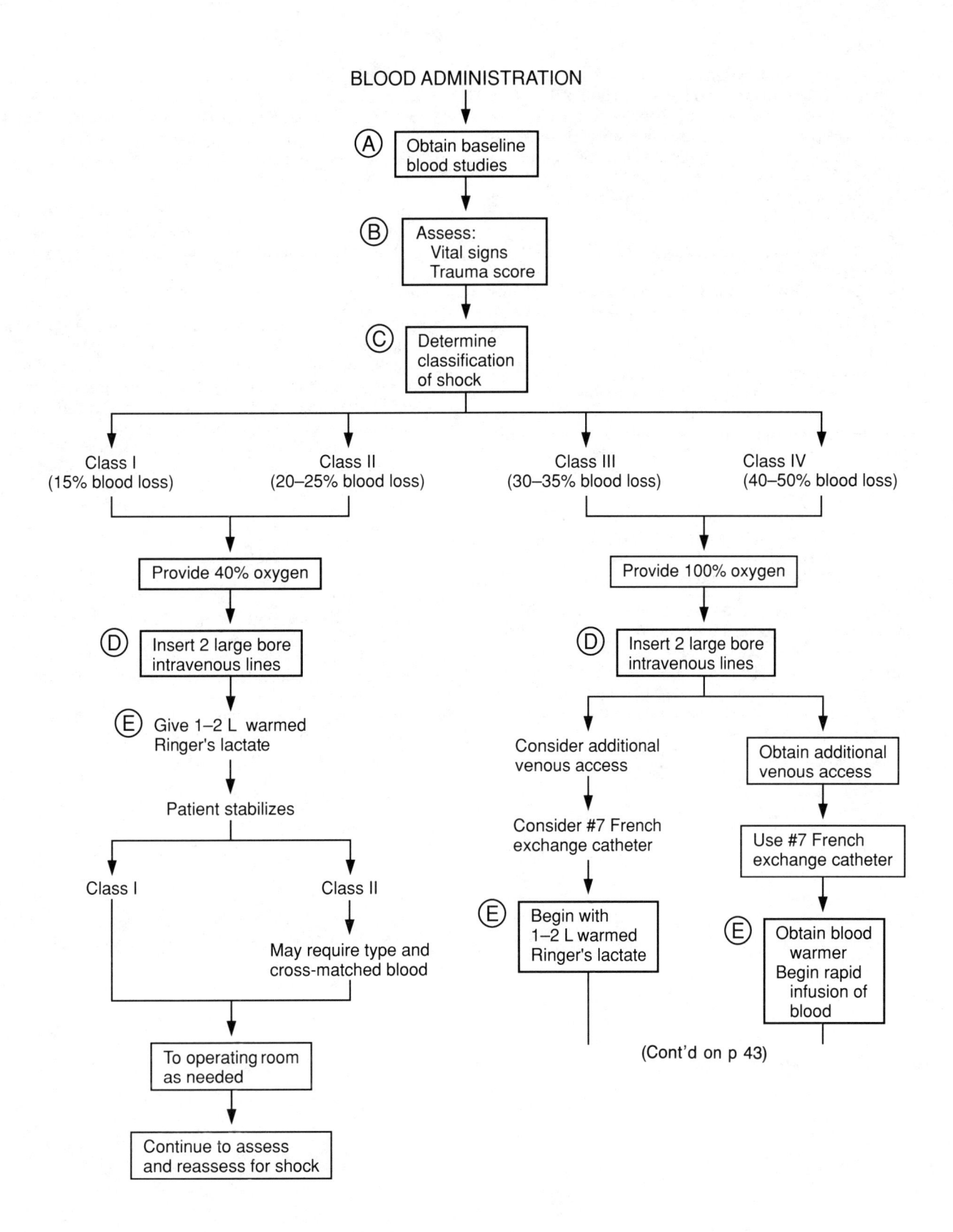

(Cont'd on p 43)

F. An autotransfusion system provides the patient with immediate type-specific and cross-matched blood. This provides clotting factors and platelets and avoids the chance of communicable disease transmission. A maximum of 4 hours may pass between collection and reinfusion. Care must be taken to ensure that fecal material is not present in reinfused blood if a lower chest wound is involved.

G. There are three types of packed red blood cells for the trauma patient, as follows:
1. Type O universal should be administered for patients in Class IV shock and those in late stages of Class III shock, i.e., if the hematocrit level is less than 30 and/or if blood pressure is less than 90 and fails to respond to resuscitation. Rh negative cells are preferred, especially in female patients.
2. Type specific can be ready in 10 to 20 minutes depending on blood bank facilities. It is compatible with ABO and Rh blood types and should be administered to patients in late stages of Class II shock and in Class III shock.
3. Type and cross-matched blood is always preferable. The process requires approximately 1 to 1.5 hours in most blood banks. Those patients in Class I and Class II shock should receive this blood.

There exists a controversy over the use of whole blood or packed cells in resuscitation. Advocates of whole blood use believe it best replaces the volume loss. Supporters of packed cell use believe whole blood use wastes components and increases chance of reaction. If coagulation times change, the depleted component can be administered.

H. Platelets, fresh frozen plasma, and cryoprecipitate are administered as needed. The partial thromboplastin time, prothrombin time, fibrinogen level, and platelet count are obtained to assess coagulation status. This is not usually a problem during resuscitation; however, a baseline level must be obtained.

I. The patient should be evaluated for hypocalcemia, caused by citrate in the stored blood, by monitoring the calcium blood level and by ECG monitoring. Hypocalcemia is not a problem during the early stages of resuscitation.

J. The patient must be monitored for a reaction. A urticarial eruption can be treated with antihistamine. If fever, chills, flank pain, chest pain, and urine positive for hemoglobin develops, the blood administration should be stopped and blood and urine samples obtained and sent to the laboratory with the blood bag. Treatment for a reaction includes administration of a large amount of fluid and diuretics (furosemide) to protect against renal failure.

References

American College of Surgeons. Advanced trauma life support course. Chicago: American College of Surgeons, 1988:57–89.

Gridley J Jr. Blood component therapy. Trauma Q 1986; 2:45–53.

Woolard RH. Venous access techniques: rapid volume administration. Trauma Q 1986; 2:74–79.

Zorko M, Polsky S. Rapid warming and infusion of packed red blood cells. Ann Emerg Med 1986; 79–82.

(Cont'd from p 41)

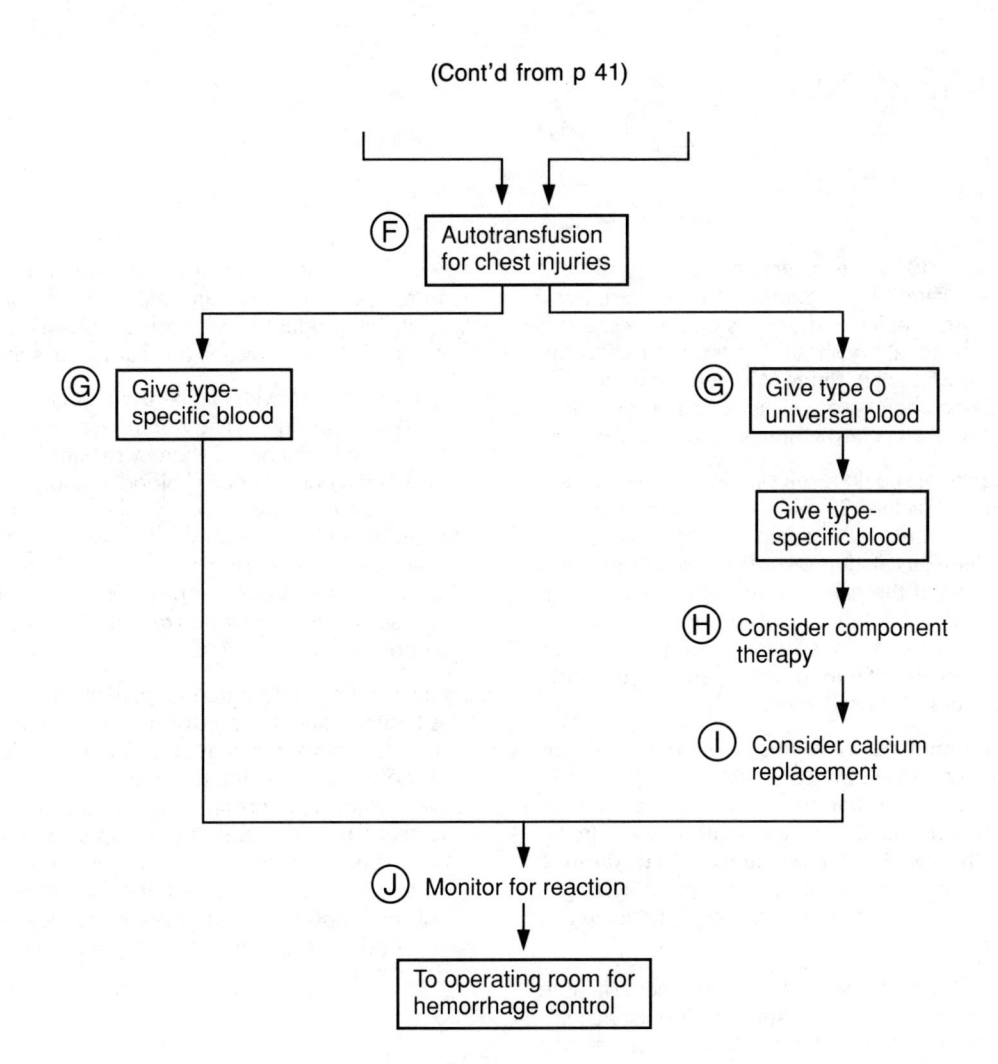

- Ⓕ Autotransfusion for chest injuries
  - Ⓖ Give type-specific blood
  - Ⓖ Give type O universal blood
    - Give type-specific blood
    - Ⓗ Consider component therapy
    - Ⓘ Consider calcium replacement
- Ⓙ Monitor for reaction
- To operating room for hemorrhage control

FLUID WARMING

Thomas Drury

A. Two large bore (16 gauge or greater) intravenous (IV) catheters are inserted in all trauma patients. Peripheral access is the first choice and venous cutdown second. During the resuscitation phase, the trauma patient requires large volumes of IV fluids. Warmed fluids are used to avoid further compromise such as decreased myocardial contractility, cardiac arrhythmias, and hypothermia.

B. The trauma patient should receive an initial 1 to 2 L fluid bolus of Ringer's lactate (20 ml/kg in pediatric patients). A careful reassessment of the patient's response is needed to avoid under-resuscitation or over-resuscitation. After the initial bolus, if the patient's vital signs remain stable, the crystalloid solution will continue to be administered. However, if the patient's vital signs do not stabilize or if they continue to drift to an unacceptable level, the patient will need blood.

C. A portable warming device is most frequently used during resuscitation. It is easily connected to IV poles and has disposable administration sets that can be rapidly changed between patients. These devices have electronic thermostats that regulate temperature, a rapid warming time, and flow rates of 150 ml per minute. When pressure bags are placed on the solutions, rapid infusion can be accomplished.

D. A warmed 37°C (98.6°F) water bath is another available method of fluid warming. Administration is accomplished via a coil submerged in the bath. There are also electronic devices that, in conjunction with a thermostat, maintain a uniform temperature. However, this latter method requires a large period of time for operational warming and is therefore not used during the resuscitation period.

E. A warming cabinet device is useful for crystalloid solution; however, it is not appropriate for blood. These systems allow large quantities of solution to be warmed for both parenteral and lavage purposes. The temperature can be easily set and frequently checked. However, unless fluids are rapidly used, the solutions are sensitive to temperature exposure and to length of exposure to heat. The product information can provide specific length of time of warming for the particular solutions used.

F. The microwave oven can be used for crystalloids but not for blood products. The microwave oven does not uniformly warm the blood, thereby causing hemolysis in one area and a pocket of cold blood in another. It works efficiently and effectively for crystalloid and allows for rapid warming of large amounts of IV solutions for parenteral and lavage fluids. Time and heating settings for microwave ovens vary among products, and therefore a particular oven must be tested to determine the settings used to obtain fluids of 37°C.

G. Any fluid given to a trauma patient should be warmed. A trauma patient is predisposed to hypothermia; therefore, failure to give warmed blood or fluid can further compromise the trauma patient's condition. Once warmed crystalloids are initiated, the patient should be re-evaluated constantly for a response to the resuscitation. Blood administration may be considered after an initial 1 to 2 L administration of crystalloid. Once warmed blood is begun, the patient must be monitored for a possible reaction (p 40).

References

American College of Surgeons. Advanced trauma life support course. Chicago: American College of Surgeons, 1988:57–89.

Leaman P, Martyak G. Microwave warming of resuscitation fluids. Ann Emerg Med 1985; 14:83–87.

Stamoulis C, Sawtelle S. Blood and fluid warming techniques. Trauma Q 1986; 2:1–6.

Zorko M, Polsky S. Rapid warming and infusion of packed red blood cells. Ann Emerg Med 1986; 79–83.

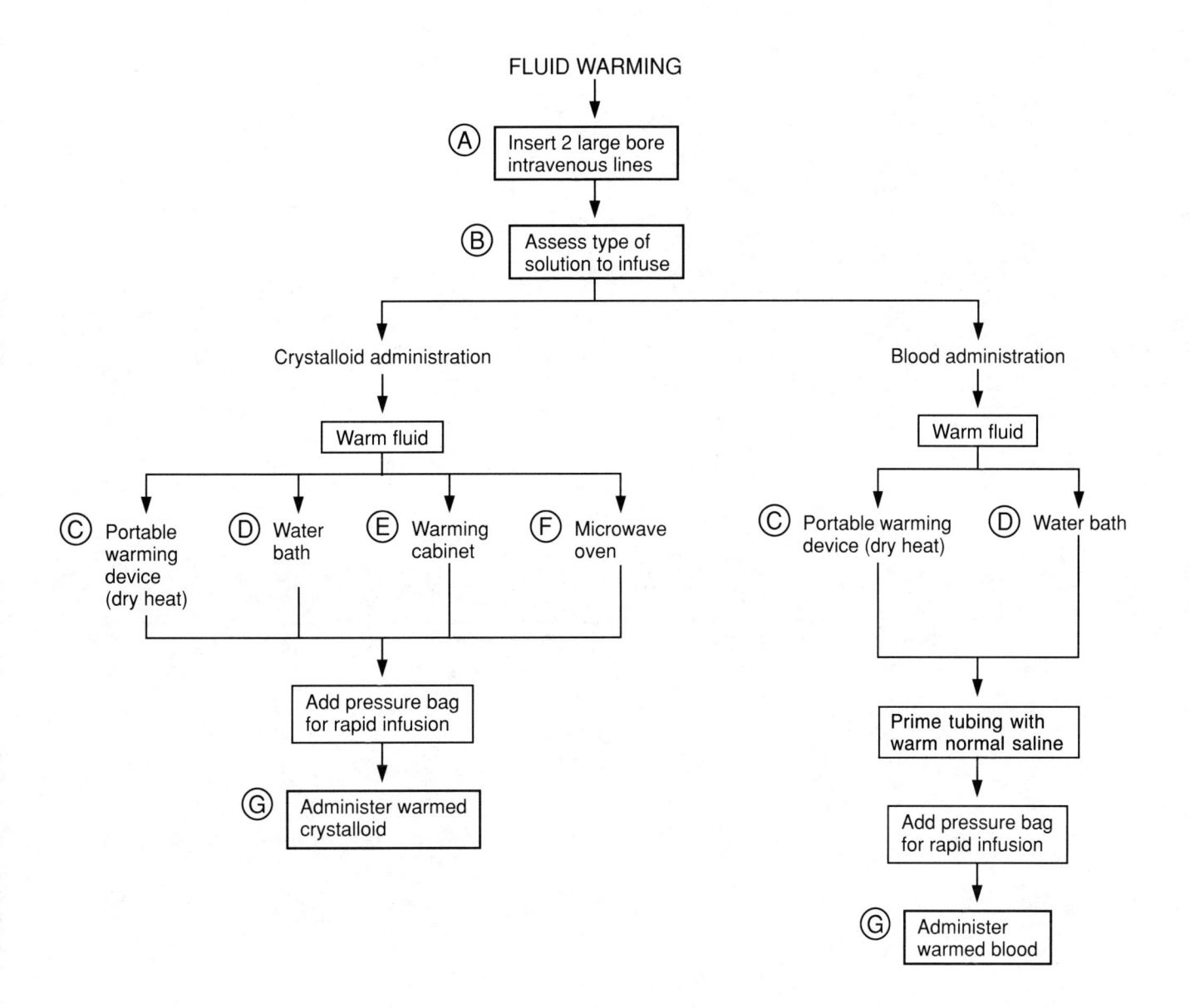

FLUID WARMING

- **A** Insert 2 large bore intravenous lines
- **B** Assess type of solution to infuse

Crystalloid administration

Warm fluid
- **C** Portable warming device (dry heat)
- **D** Water bath
- **E** Warming cabinet
- **F** Microwave oven

Add pressure bag for rapid infusion

G Administer warmed crystalloid

Blood administration

Warm fluid
- **C** Portable warming device (dry heat)
- **D** Water bath

Prime tubing with warm normal saline

Add pressure bag for rapid infusion

G Administer warmed blood

HEAD TRAUMA

Blunt Head Trauma
Penetrating Head Trauma
Skull Fracture

BLUNT HEAD TRAUMA

Gregory G. Stanford

Closed head trauma is the leading cause of early death after major trauma. Injury to the brain, like injury elsewhere in the body, causes swelling and edema. But unlike the rest of the body, there is no room for expansion to accommodate the increased cellular water. This increased swelling is a normal part of the inflammatory response but is counterproductive and dangerous within the closed cranial vault. As swelling of the brain progresses, decreased blood flow to the remaining viable neurons extends the injury and causes further swelling. A vicious circle is thus initiated, which progresses to CNS death by ischemia or herniation into the posterior fossa and foramen magnum. The goals of therapy in CNS trauma are to reduce edema to a minimum and to preserve oxygen and nutrient blood flow to the damaged brain.

A. A history of closed head trauma should alert medical personnel to the possibility of cervical spine injury. The cervical spine should be immobilized in all patients with closed head trauma until appropriate radiologic studies can be performed.

B. Closed head trauma includes a spectrum of CNS injuries, from a short loss of consciousness to major disruptions of cerebral function. Patients with a short loss of consciousness do not necessarily require a computed tomography (CT) scan but should be followed closely for 24 hours. Patients with reliable parents or loved ones who will be conscientious about examining the patient every 2 hours can be monitored at home. Patient education sheets can be very useful and help eliminate unnecessary visits and calls. More important, these sheets educate the patient and the patient's family about neurologic deterioration, so that the patient will return to the hospital before the patient is critical (Fig. 1). If there is any question about the ability or reliability of the family to monitor the neurologic status, the patient should be admitted to the hospital for observation.

C. CT scans should be done emergently for all patients with a focal neurologic deficit (i.e., localized to one area or region of the body on neurologic examination). If the CT scan cannot be performed expeditiously, exploratory burr holes may be indicated. The holes should be placed in the ipsilateral temporal region to a dilated pupil or on the contralateral temporal region to an abnormal motor response.

D. The indications for craniotomy are variable depending on the training and inclination of the neurosurgeon. Small mass lesions generally do not require intervention and can be followed closely. A lesion with a shift greater than 5 mm usually requires craniotomy.

E. Blunt carotid artery injury can produce focal neurologic deficits. It is probably a more common injury than is generally realized. All patients with a suspected closed head injury with a normal CT scan should undergo carotid angiography.

F. The management of blunt carotid artery injury is controversial. Many trauma surgeons explore these vessels surgically with repair or resection. However, many injuries extend to the intracranial portion of the carotid artery, thereby making surgical repair impossible. For this reason, many centers are treating these patients with anticoagulation therapy. Because these injuries are rare, no prospective studies have demonstrated an advantage of one technique over the other.

G. The Glasgow Coma Scale is a simple scale that attempts to quantitate the patient's level of consciousness. A patient with a Glasgow Coma Scale score of 8 or less has sustained a severe head injury. Scores between 9 and 12 are considered moderate, whereas minor injuries have values between 13 and 15. Patients with a moderate head injury should be admitted to an intensive care unit or neurosurgical care unit. Neurologic examinations should be performed at least every 2 hours, and any change should be evaluated with a CT scan. These patients have a good prognosis and should recover in time. Patients with a minor injury should be admitted and observed on the ward for at least 24 hours. Neurologic examination, every 2 hours for 24 hours, is indicated.

H. Patients with a severe head injury are at risk for increased intracranial pressure (ICP). Some centers place intracranial monitors in this patient population, whereas others believe that this invasive monitoring technique does not improve the morbidity or mortality rate. If not used, the neurologic status must be followed closely and any deterioration treated as an increase in ICP.

Patient with SUSPECTED CLOSED HEAD TRAUMA

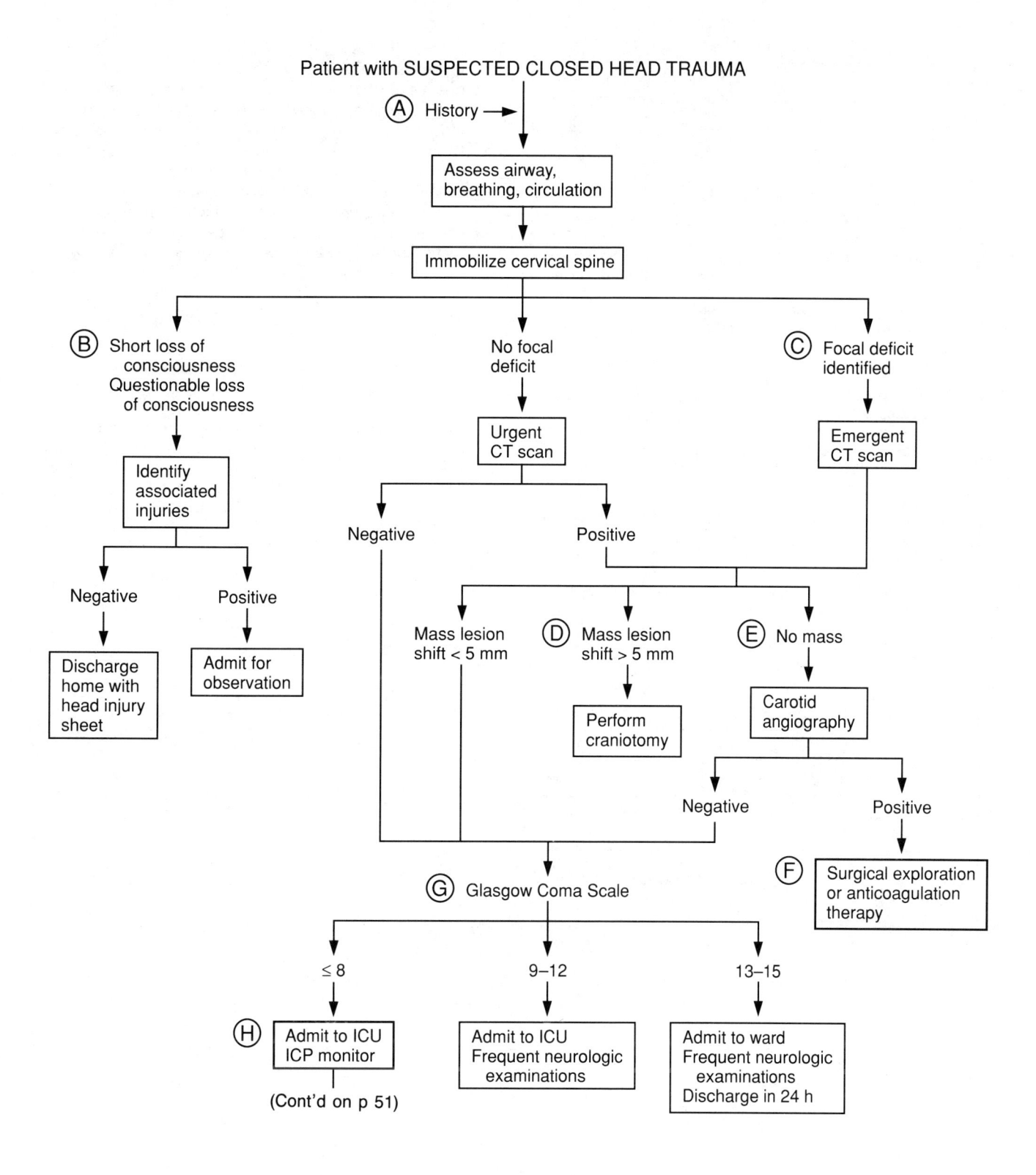

- (A) History →
- Assess airway, breathing, circulation
- Immobilize cervical spine

(B) Short loss of consciousness / Questionable loss of consciousness
- Identify associated injuries
  - Negative → Discharge home with head injury sheet
  - Positive → Admit for observation

No focal deficit
- Urgent CT scan
  - Negative → (G) Glasgow Coma Scale
  - Positive:
    - Mass lesion shift < 5 mm → (G) Glasgow Coma Scale
    - (D) Mass lesion shift > 5 mm → Perform craniotomy

(C) Focal deficit identified
- Emergent CT scan
  - Mass lesion shift < 5 mm
  - (D) Mass lesion shift > 5 mm → Perform craniotomy
  - (E) No mass → Carotid angiography
    - Negative → (G) Glasgow Coma Scale
    - Positive → (F) Surgical exploration or anticoagulation therapy

(G) Glasgow Coma Scale
- ≤ 8 → (H) Admit to ICU, ICP monitor (Cont'd on p 51)
- 9–12 → Admit to ICU, Frequent neurologic examinations
- 13–15 → Admit to ward, Frequent neurologic examinations, Discharge in 24 h

49

> You have had a head injury that is not severe enough to require hospitalization, and the following treatment and statements apply to you:
> 1. Limited activity for 24 hours.
>   a. No school for children.
>   b. No work for adults.
>   Your physician may ask for limited activity for more than 24 hours.
> 2. Clear, cold liquids for 8 hours (no milk), followed by reduced amounts of food for the next 24 hours.
> 3. Take only aspirin for headache or discomfort. Consult your physician before taking any other medicines you may have at home.
> 4. Be sure someone (family or friend) stays with you. They should be sure that you stay alert. They should check your breathing and pupils every 2 hours for 12 hours, then every 4 hours for the next 12 hours.
> 5. In a small number of cases, signs of serious injury may appear later, so keep your clinic appointment.
> 6. If any of the following things happen, you should consult your physician immediately or return to the emergency room:
>   a. Nausea and/or vomiting.
>   b. Unusual sleepiness or difficulty awakening. (Someone should be sure that the patient stays alert. Wake the patient up from sleep every 2 to 3 hours during the period of sleep or during the first night.)
>   c. One pupil much larger or different from the other; peculiar movements of the eyes; or difficulty focusing (blurred vision).
>   d. Weakness, paralysis, or numbness of arms or legs; peculiar gait; or stumbling.
>   e. Mental confusion or disorientation (excessive drowsiness, inattentiveness, incoherent thought, change in personality, inability to concentrate, stupor).
>   f. Irregular or labored breathing.
>   g. Persistent dizziness.
>
> Note: The interpretation of your x-ray film, as given to you by the physician in the emergency room, is only a preliminary report. The x-ray specialist reviews these films. If there is a change in the diagnosis, you and your physician will be notified within 24 hours. Sometimes fractures or abnormalities may not show up on x-ray films for several days; if symptoms persist or worsen, more x-ray films may have to be taken. If symptoms persist or worsen, call your physician or return immediately to the emergency room.

Figure 1 Dallas County Hospital District emergency suite follow-up patient care instruction sheet for head injuries.

I. Hyperventilation reduces the partial pressure of carbon dioxide in the blood ($PaCO_2$), which has profound effects on cerebral blood flow. A decreased $PaCO_2$ directly reduces intracranial blood volume, which subsequently reduces ICP. The $PaCO_2$ should be maintained between 25 and 30 mm Hg for patients at risk of, or with established, intracranial hypertension. Seizure activity should be aggressively controlled with benzodiazepines or phenytoin. Similarly, hyperthermia increases brain metabolic activity and should be treated with antipyretics and cooling blankets.

References

Clark WK. Trauma to the nervous system. In: Shires GT, ed. Principles of trauma care. New York: McGraw-Hill, 1985:232–266.

Dunham CM. Central nervous system assessment and stabilization. In: Siegel JH, ed. Trauma: emergency surgery and critical care. New York: Churchill Livingstone, 1987:813–818.

Pitts LH. Traumatic intracranial hemorrhage. In: Maull KI, ed. Advances in trauma. Vol. 1. Chicago: Yearbook, 1986:121–132.

(Cont'd from p 49)

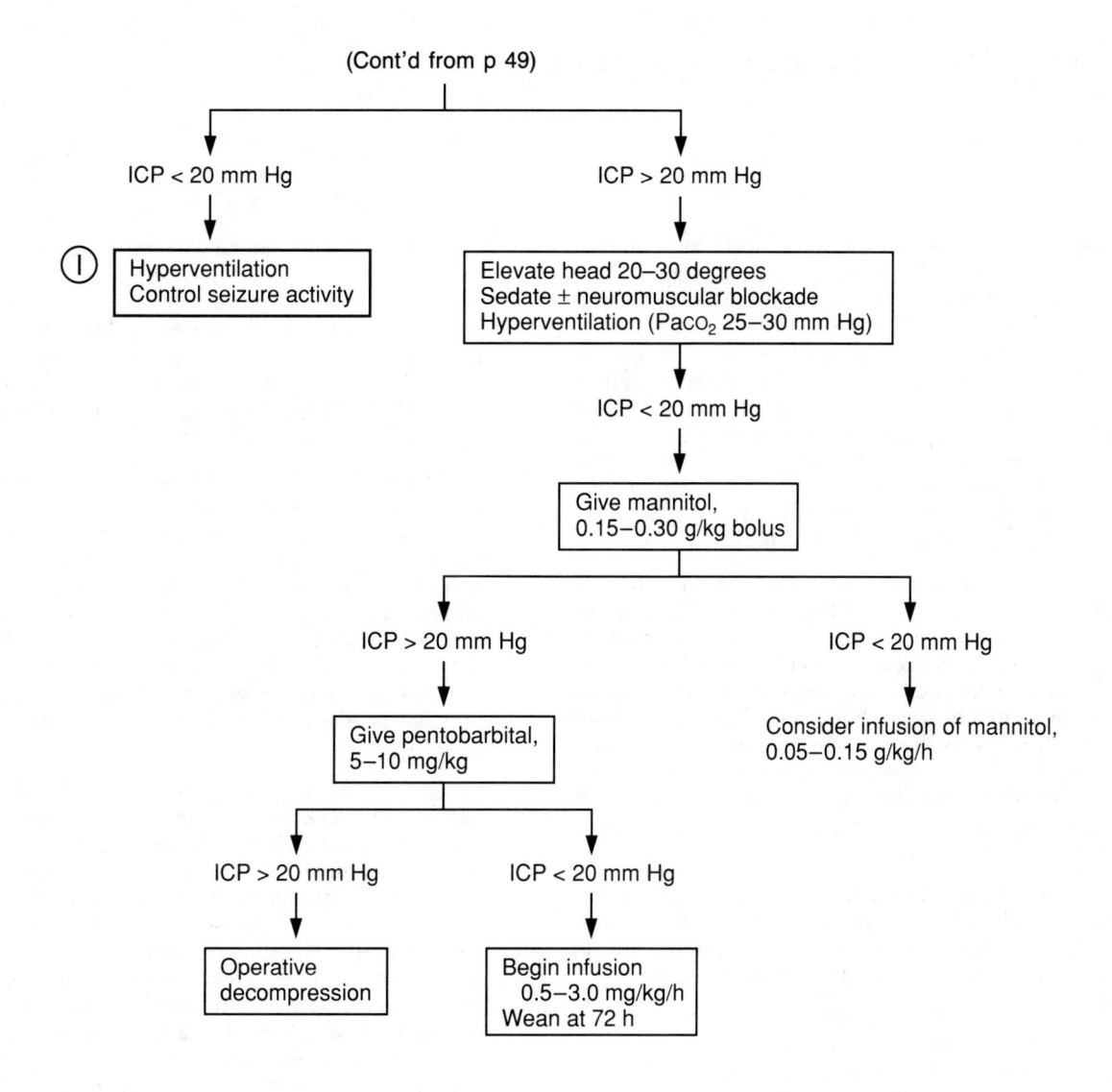

```
                          |
          ┌───────────────┴───────────────┐
     ICP < 20 mm Hg                  ICP > 20 mm Hg
          │                               │
    ┌─────────────────┐         ┌──────────────────────────────────┐
 ①  │ Hyperventilation │         │ Elevate head 20–30 degrees       │
    │ Control seizure  │         │ Sedate ± neuromuscular blockade  │
    │ activity         │         │ Hyperventilation (PaCO₂ 25–30 mm Hg)│
    └─────────────────┘         └──────────────────────────────────┘
                                              │
                                        ICP < 20 mm Hg
                                              │
                                   ┌──────────────────────┐
                                   │ Give mannitol,       │
                                   │ 0.15–0.30 g/kg bolus │
                                   └──────────────────────┘
                                       │              │
                                ICP > 20 mm Hg    ICP < 20 mm Hg
                                       │              │
                             ┌──────────────────┐   Consider infusion of mannitol,
                             │ Give pentobarbital,│  0.05–0.15 g/kg/h
                             │ 5–10 mg/kg        │
                             └──────────────────┘
                              │             │
                      ICP > 20 mm Hg    ICP < 20 mm Hg
                              │             │
                      ┌──────────────┐  ┌──────────────────┐
                      │ Operative    │  │ Begin infusion   │
                      │ decompression│  │ 0.5–3.0 mg/kg/h  │
                      └──────────────┘  │ Wean at 72 h     │
                                        └──────────────────┘
```

Algorithm for ICP management (continued). ICP < 20 mm Hg: ① Hyperventilation, Control seizure activity. ICP > 20 mm Hg: Elevate head 20–30 degrees; Sedate ± neuromuscular blockade; Hyperventilation (PaCO$_2$ 25–30 mm Hg). If ICP < 20 mm Hg, Give mannitol, 0.15–0.30 g/kg bolus. If ICP > 20 mm Hg, Give pentobarbital, 5–10 mg/kg. If ICP > 20 mm Hg, Operative decompression. If ICP < 20 mm Hg, Begin infusion 0.5–3.0 mg/kg/h, Wean at 72 h. If ICP < 20 mm Hg after mannitol bolus, Consider infusion of mannitol, 0.05–0.15 g/kg/h.

PENETRATING HEAD TRAUMA

Gregory G. Stanford

A. Penetrating injuries of the skull are usually fatal. Surprisingly, a small number of these patients survive long enough to arrive at the emergency room. Some of these patients may have relatively minor neurologic injuries in spite of having had a foreign body pass through the brain. The extent of the neurologic injury is dependent on those areas of the brain that are injured by the penetrating object itself, by the secondary effect of increased intracranial pressure (ICP), or by the mass effect from adjacent bleeding. Injuries to the brain stem usually result in death due to interruption of the major pathways controlling respiration and circulation.

B. Initial management of the patient with a penetrating injury to the skull involves following the ABCs (airway, breathing, and circulation) of trauma care by assuring a patent airway with adequate ventilation and correction of any circulatory abnormalities. These patients are frequently in hemorrhagic shock, and every effort should be made to restore the circulating blood volume as soon as possible to restore blood flow to the damaged brain. Brain injuries can cause the loss of a large amount of blood, and these patients frequently need rapid transfusion to restore circulation.

C. The cervical spine should be immobilized in all patients with a head injury until appropriate radiographs can be performed. The cervical spine can be injured by missile fragments or by the blast effect from the injury.

D. The wound should be covered with a sterile dressing as soon as possible to prevent further contamination of the cranial contents. Massive bleeding from a head wound should be examined to determine whether the bleeding is coming from the scalp or from within the skull. If the bleeding is coming from within the skull, pressure should not be applied because this will further increase intracranial pressure.

E. The primary survey should be completed by rapidly determining whether other life threatening injuries are present. Frequently patients with gunshot wounds to the brain have gunshot wounds to other parts of the body, and persons who have sustained a missile injury may have other injuries caused by blunt trauma. These other life threatening injuries should be treated when they are identified.

F. Monitor vital signs continuously in this patient population. Arterial hypertension and bradycardia are common in patients with CNS injury. Hypertension should be controlled to prevent increases in intracranial pressure that are damaging.

G. Computed tomography (CT) remains the evaluation of choice in patients with penetrating injuries to the head. Anteroposterior and lateral plain radiographs occasionally can be of benefit in localizing the site of injury. Anteroposterior and lateral cervical spine films should be reviewed to look for injuries to the cervical spine. Patients should be closely monitored during performance of the CT scan to prevent increases in the blood pressure or deterioration of vital signs secondary to the brain injury or associated injuries.

H. Open debridement in penetrating injury to the head remains controversial. Injuries in the area of the posterior fossa are usually not amenable to surgical treatment. Small injuries to the cerebrum do not require open debridement unless there is a mass lesion or significant foreign matter within the brain itself. Larger hemispheric lesions usually necessitate open debridement. Similarly, space occupying masses including subdural, epidural, and intracerebral hematomas usually cause shifts and need to be evacuated to prevent further damage to the brain.

I. Patients who do not require craniotomy should be admitted to the intensive care unit (ICU) for close neurologic observation. Other injuries should be treated as they are identified. Patients with a Glasgow Coma Scale score of less than 8 require intubation and mechanical ventilation for the purposes of hyperventilation. ICP monitoring should be considered in this patient population. These patients should be aggressively supported to maintain oxygenation to the damaged brain tissue. Hypotension should be avoided at all costs. Similarly, hypertension can also occur and should be aggressively treated. Increases in intracranial pressure should be treated as detailed on p 48.

J. Massive, nonsurvivable injuries are usually not treated with craniotomy. These patients should be considered potential candidates for organ donation.

References

Clark WK. Trauma to the nervous system. In: Shires GT, ed. Principles of trauma care. New York: McGraw-Hill, 1985:232–266.

Dunham CM. Central nervous system assessment and stabilization. In: Siegel JH, ed. Trauma: emergency surgery and critical care. New York: Churchill Livingstone, 1987:813–818.

Pitts LH. Traumatic intracranial hemorrhage. In: Maull KI, ed. Advances in trauma. Vol. 1. Chicago: Yearbook, 1986:121–132.

Swan KG, Swan RC. Gunshot wounds: pathophysiology and management. 2nd ed. Chicago: Yearbook, 1989:35–48.

Patient with PENETRATING HEAD TRAUMA

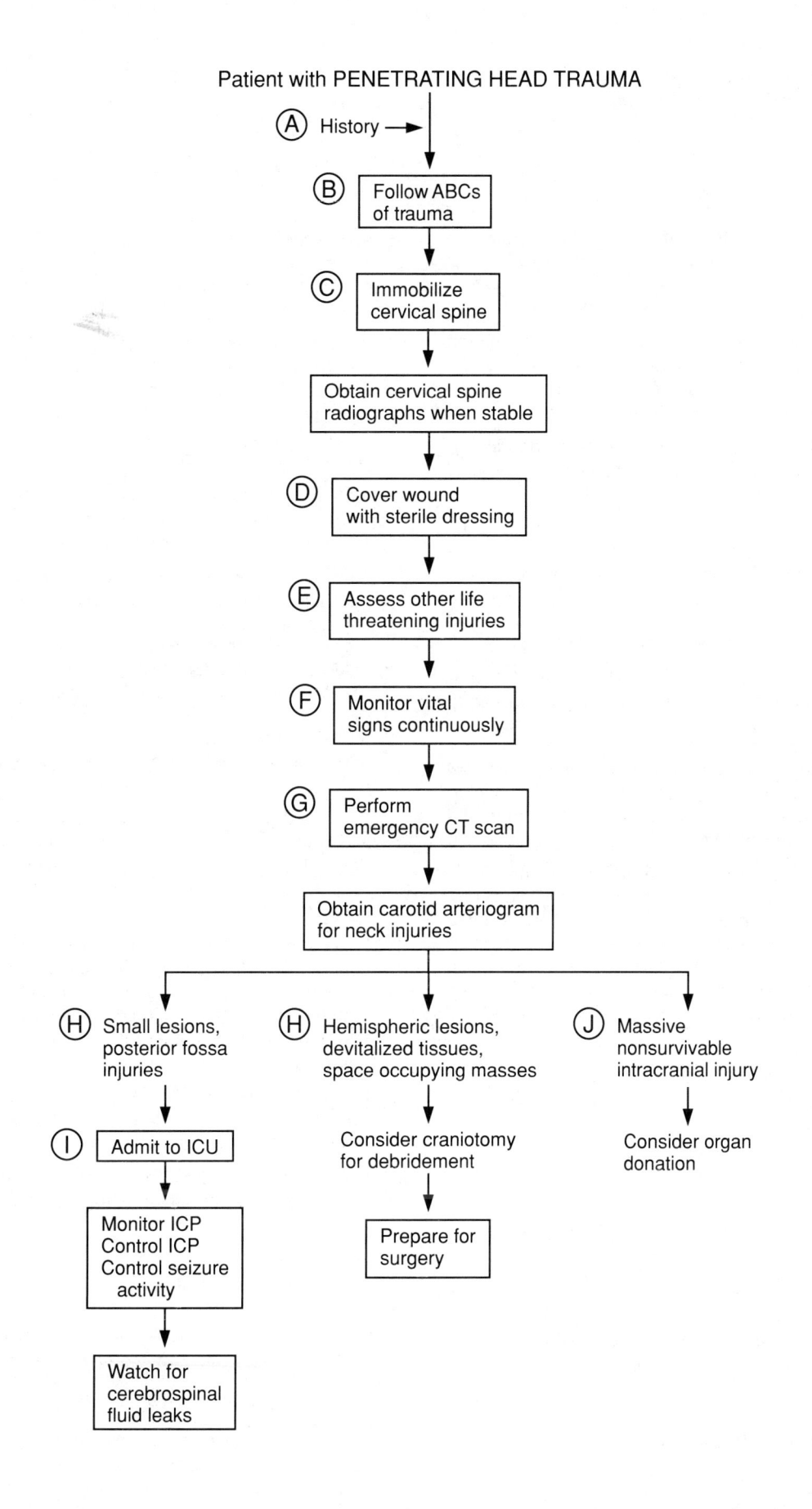

- (A) History
- (B) Follow ABCs of trauma
- (C) Immobilize cervical spine
- Obtain cervical spine radiographs when stable
- (D) Cover wound with sterile dressing
- (E) Assess other life threatening injuries
- (F) Monitor vital signs continuously
- (G) Perform emergency CT scan
- Obtain carotid arteriogram for neck injuries

- (H) Small lesions, posterior fossa injuries
  - (I) Admit to ICU
    - Monitor ICP, Control ICP, Control seizure activity
    - Watch for cerebrospinal fluid leaks
- (H) Hemispheric lesions, devitalized tissues, space occupying masses
  - Consider craniotomy for debridement
  - Prepare for surgery
- (J) Massive nonsurvivable intracranial injury
  - Consider organ donation

SKULL FRACTURE*

Jorie Klein

A. The type of skull fracture that follows a head injury depends on the velocity and mass of the object striking the head (Fig. 1).

B. Because hypercapnia increases intracranial pressure (ICP), anything that blocks the airway in the head injured patient is dangerous. Maintaining a patent airway and giving oxygen are among the most important early treatments of the head injured patient.

C. Assume that a cervical spine injury has occurred in anyone sustaining a major head injury. A lateral cervical spine film rules out injury to the neck.

D. The history should include the mechanism of injury, the site of impact on the head, the level of consciousness at the accident scene, and the vital signs as well as observation and assessment for other injuries. Note evidence of alcohol or drugs that alter mental status. Blood for toxicology screening should be drawn on admission.

E. A low velocity impact tends to produce linear fractures (simple breaks with no displacement). A fracture indicates that a substantial blow has occurred. Blood vessels may be damaged and an extradural hematoma may develop. Symptoms of increasing ICP include a decrease in the level of consciousness, usually accompanied by limb weakness on the side opposite the injury, and occasionally convulsions.

F. Depressed fractures are displacements of comminuted skull fragments, which if displaced sufficiently can compromise, bruise, or tear cerebral structures. With a depressed fracture less than the thickness of the skull and no signs of increased ICP, observation may be the only care indicated. If the fragment is displaced by more than 5 mm, surgery must be performed to elevate the depression, remove fragments, debride necrotic tissue, remove hematomas, repair lacerations, and decrease the possibility of infection.

G. A basilar fracture is not apparent on skull films. Clinical signs include raccoon eyes, Battle's sign, hemotympanum, rhinorrhea, and otorrhea. Disruption of the middle meningeal artery may cause a hematoma of the scalp, subarachnoid hemorrhage, an epidural hematoma, or intracerebral hemorrhage.

H. With dural penetration, a broad spectrum antibiotic that crosses the blood-brain barrier (e.g., ampicillin) should be used. Tetanus prophylaxis should be routine.

I. A dilated and fixed pupil in an unconscious head injured patient is presumed to be secondary to third cranial nerve compression caused by tentorial pressure. If pressure is not removed, irreversible damage will occur. Through the reduction of carbon dioxide by hyperventilation, cerebral vasoconstriction will occur, thus decreasing the blood volume in the brain. A $PaCO_2$ level reduced to 20 to 25 mm Hg is ideal. Mannitol (Osmitrol), 1 g/kg, or furosemide (Lasix), 1 mg/kg, may also be used to decrease the ICP.

J. Computed tomographic (CT) scanning identifies fractures and any subjacent injuries, such as intracranial hemorrhage, traumatic cerebral contusion and edema with midline shifts or herniations, or acute ventricular enlargements.

K. Penetrating wounds cause destruction of the cerebral contents. Cerebral damage from missiles, such as bullets, depends on the speed, size, and shape of the missile and on the brain structures injured. The larger the caliber of the missile and the higher the velocity, the more likely that death will occur.

L. Gunshot wounds of the head are a significant cause of open head injury. The prognosis depends on both the level of consciousness and the trajectory of the bullet.

M. Postcraniotomy monitoring and care are directed at detecting, avoiding, and treating increased ICP and recurrent hemorrhage.

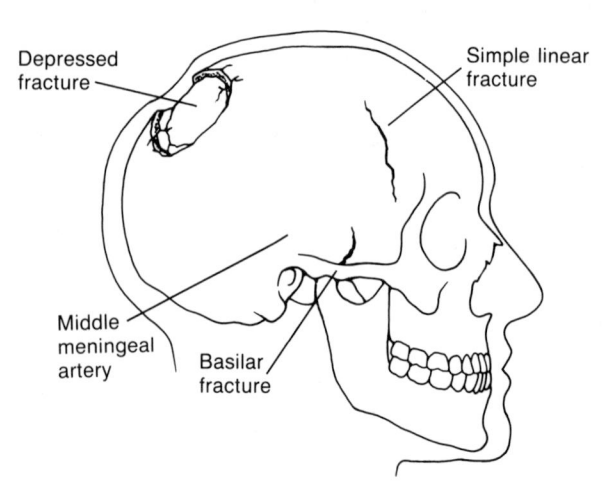

Figure 1 Types of skull fracture.

*Revised from Mancini ME. Decision making in emergency nursing. Toronto: BC Decker, 1987.

References

Budassi SA. Mosby's manual of emergency care practices and procedures. St. Louis: CV Mosby, 1984:349–371.

Cowley RA. Shock trauma critical care manual. Baltimore: University Park Press, 1983:215–227.

Lauros NE. Assessment and intervention in emergency nursing. Bowie, MD: Robert J Brady, 1983:215–227.

Scott J. Patient with a skull fracture. In: Mancini ME. Decision making in emergency nursing. Toronto: BC Decker, 1987:38.

Shires TG. Care of the trauma patient. New York: McGraw-Hill, 1979:207–257.

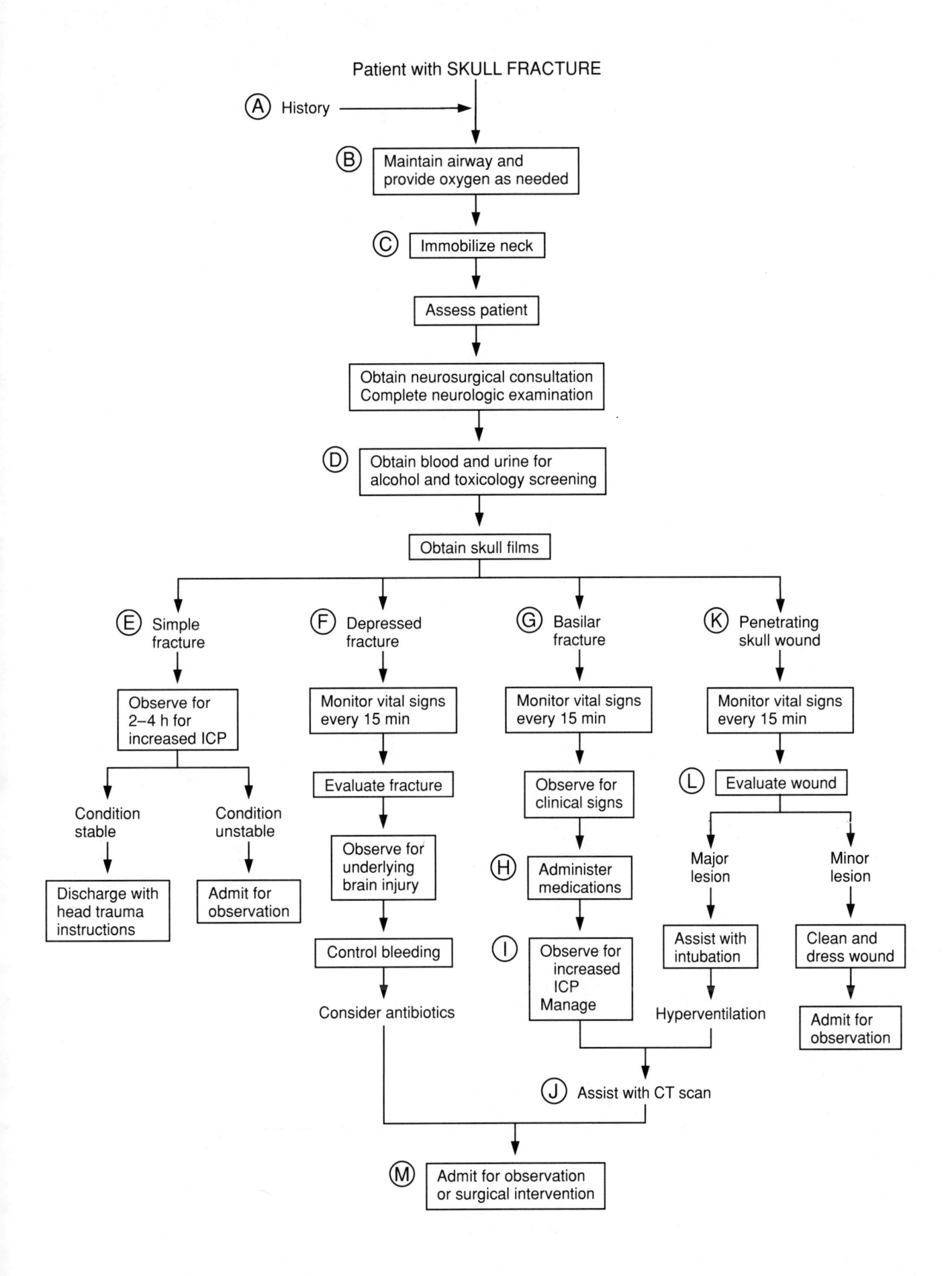

Patient with SKULL FRACTURE

```
                    Patient with SKULL FRACTURE
                              │
   (A) History ──────────────▶│
                              ▼
                   (B) ┌──────────────────────┐
                       │ Maintain airway and  │
                       │ provide oxygen as    │
                       │ needed               │
                       └──────────┬───────────┘
                                  ▼
                   (C) ┌──────────────────────┐
                       │ Immobilize neck      │
                       └──────────┬───────────┘
                                  ▼
                       ┌──────────────────────┐
                       │ Assess patient       │
                       └──────────┬───────────┘
                                  ▼
                       ┌──────────────────────────────┐
                       │ Obtain neurosurgical         │
                       │ consultation                 │
                       │ Complete neurologic          │
                       │ examination                  │
                       └──────────┬───────────────────┘
                                  ▼
                   (D) ┌──────────────────────────────┐
                       │ Obtain blood and urine for   │
                       │ alcohol and toxicology       │
                       │ screening                    │
                       └──────────┬───────────────────┘
                                  ▼
                       ┌──────────────────────┐
                       │ Obtain skull films   │
                       └──────────┬───────────┘
```

(E) Simple fracture	(F) Depressed fracture	(G) Basilar fracture	(K) Penetrating skull wound
Observe for 2–4 h for increased ICP	Monitor vital signs every 15 min	Monitor vital signs every 15 min	Monitor vital signs every 15 min
Condition stable → Discharge with head trauma instructions	Evaluate fracture	Observe for clinical signs	(L) Evaluate wound
Condition unstable → Admit for observation	Observe for underlying brain injury	(H) Administer medications	Major lesion → Assist with intubation → Hyperventilation
	Control bleeding	(I) Observe for increased ICP — Manage	Minor lesion → Clean and dress wound → Admit for observation
	Consider antibiotics		

(J) Assist with CT scan

(M) Admit for observation or surgical intervention

FACIAL TRAUMA

Maxillofacial Soft Tissue Trauma
Nasal Trauma
Dental Trauma
Ear Trauma

Eye Trauma
Maxillofacial Fractures: Airway Management
Maxillofacial Fractures: Treatment

MAXILLOFACIAL SOFT TISSUE TRAUMA

Kimberly L. Davies

The face is frequently subjected to trauma because of its exposed and unprotected anatomic position. The face is the most obvious physical characteristic of humans, playing a major role in personal identity, appearance, and emotional expressions. The face also functions as the vital center for smell, speech, eating, taste, vision, and hearing. Consequently, injuries that result in deformity often create complex problems for the patient. Although facial injuries are distracting, they are rarely life threatening unless associated with other serious injuries or complications. Goals of management are to restore function and to prevent and correct resultant deformity after all major injuries have been evaluated and stabilized.

A. History should include the circumstances, nature, and force of the injury; time injury occurred; observation for concurrent injuries; the patient's level of consciousness; and status of the airway at the accident site as well as prehospital interventions.

B. Airway obstruction is the leading cause of death in facial trauma. Obstruction can result from swelling, hemorrhage, bony disruption and/or deformity, and foreign objects. Massive intraoral bleeding, clots in the nasal passages, laryngeal edema, and soft tissue swelling all contribute to airway compromise. Interventions to establish and maintain a patent airway are described on p 362.

C. The face has a rich and generous blood supply, which can account for large losses of blood. Facial hemorrhage is usually readily controlled by direct pressure. If excessive bleeding occurs from the nasal or oral cavity, gauze packing may be required to stop the bleeding.

D. The likelihood of concurrent cervical spine injury with facial trauma must be considered. If any doubt exists, the best guideline is to immobilize the neck until radiologic examination has proved otherwise.

E. Primary focus of management must be directed toward airway, breathing, and circulation (ABCs). Nursing assessment for facial injuries should include inspection for any abrasions, contusions, lacerations, avulsions, loss of tissue, and amputation of structures from the face. It is equally important to note the location, size, and age of the wound. The patient's facial structures should be assessed for symmetry and sensory or motor deficits as well as for injuries to underlying bone or specialized structures.

F. Documentation should be accurate and descriptive in relation to soft tissue injuries. Because of the potential for permanent disfigurement, document type of injury, location, extent, structures involved, and wound care.

G. All facial wounds require vigorous, meticulous irrigation and cleaning to promote healing with minimal scarring. Heavily contaminated wounds or those imbedded with debris may require mechanical pulsating irrigation and debridement to prevent "tattooing," which can result in permanent scarring. Large tissue flaps should be irrigated and replaced to the tissue bed and covered with a sterile, moist dressing until repaired. Should the decision be made not to repair the wound in the emergency department because of patient condition or need for extensive repair, the wound should be cleaned and covered with a sterile saline-soaked gauze and an occlusive dressing applied.

H. Electrical burns of the mouth usually occur in small children. The oral mucosal burn may initially appear superficial; however, subsequent edema and tissue necrosis may increase the apparent size and depth of the injury. Wound care is conservative, consisting of the application of topical antibiotics and observation for complications.

I. Animal and human bites are considered "dirty wounds" with potential complications of cellulitis or abscess formation. Management of bite injuries includes copious irrigation and prophylactic antibiotic therapy. Depending on the extent of the injury and location, the wound may or may not be repaired immediately.

J. The circumstances of the bite and location of the animal responsible for the injury should be reported to the local authorities (i.e., animal control shelter, sheriff, or police department) for possible observation of the animal for the rabies virus. The decision to administer rabies postexposure prophylaxis is based on the circumstances of each individual exposure.

References

Behrman SJ, Behrman DA. Facial injuries. In: Shires TG, ed. Principles of trauma care. New York: McGraw-Hill, 1985:402–448.

Cantrill SV. Maxillofacial injuries. In: Kravis TC, Warner CG, eds. Emergency medicine. Rockville, MD: Aspen, 1983:1041–1052.

Edgerton MT, Kenny JG. Emergency care of maxillofacial and otological injuries. In: Zuidema GD, Rutherford RB, Ballinger W, eds. The management of trauma. Philadelphia: WB Saunders, 1985:275–344.

Kaban LB, Goldwyn RM. Facial injuries. In: May HL, ed. Emergency medicine. New York: John Wiley & Sons, 1984:323–352.

Lower J. Maxillofacial trauma. Emerg Nurs Clin North Am 1986; 21:611–628.

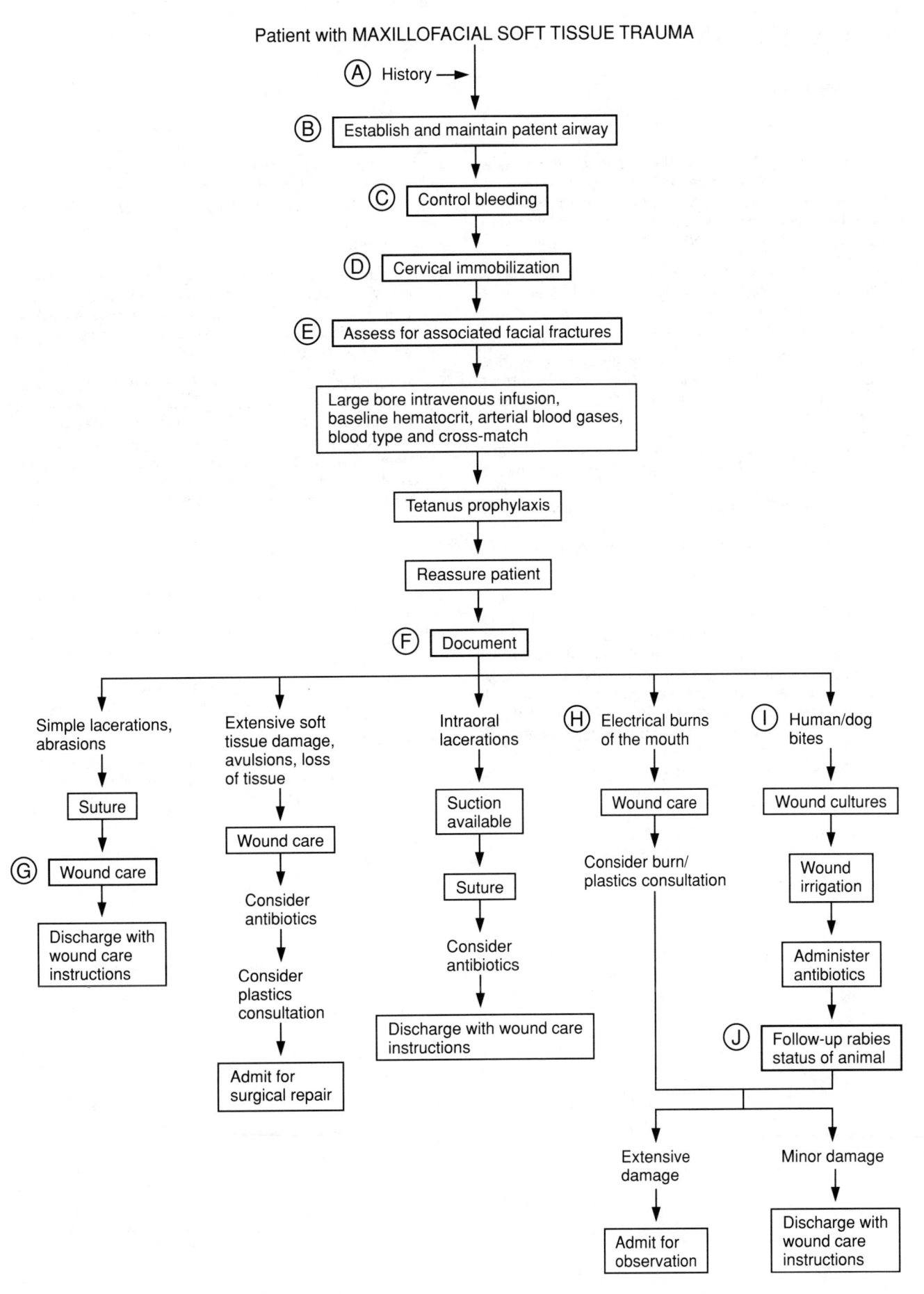

Patient with MAXILLOFACIAL SOFT TISSUE TRAUMA

- (A) History
- (B) Establish and maintain patent airway
- (C) Control bleeding
- (D) Cervical immobilization
- (E) Assess for associated facial fractures
- Large bore intravenous infusion, baseline hematocrit, arterial blood gases, blood type and cross-match
- Tetanus prophylaxis
- Reassure patient
- (F) Document

Simple lacerations, abrasions
- Suture
- (G) Wound care
- Discharge with wound care instructions

Extensive soft tissue damage, avulsions, loss of tissue
- Wound care
- Consider antibiotics
- Consider plastics consultation
- Admit for surgical repair

Intraoral lacerations
- Suction available
- Suture
- Consider antibiotics
- Discharge with wound care instructions

(H) Electrical burns of the mouth
- Wound care
- Consider burn/plastics consultation

(I) Human/dog bites
- Wound cultures
- Wound irrigation
- Administer antibiotics
- (J) Follow-up rabies status of animal

Extensive damage → Admit for observation

Minor damage → Discharge with wound care instructions

59

NASAL TRAUMA

Kimberly L. Davies

The projecting, fragile bony nasal framework is the weakest portion of the facial structure and thus a common site for facial fractures or injuries. Any time that nasal trauma is present it is imperative that the patient be evaluated thoroughly for possible associated CNS trauma or ocular injury.

A. History should document the direction and nature of the force that caused the nasal injury. It is helpful to determine any pre-existing nasal deformity or nasal obstruction the patient may have had.

B. The possibility of concurrent cervical spine injury must always be considered. Immobilization should be instituted if any suspicion of injury exists and continued until proved otherwise.

C. Assessment for nasal injuries should include inspection for any abrasions, lacerations, hematoma or edema formation, loss of tissue, or amputation of nasal structures. The nose should also be observed for any bleeding and/or CSF leakage. Assessment must also include evaluation for concurrent trauma such as head, ocular, or facial injuries.

D. Nasal fractures can be identified by depressions or deviation in the bony structure, ecchymosis, swelling, or bleeding. Intranasal examination may identify a constricted airway, septal deviation, or hematoma. Periorbital ecchymosis and edema or subconjunctival hemorrhage is common several hours postinjury. On manual palpation there is tenderness and/or crepitus at the injury site. Initial treatment is aimed to minimize post-traumatic swelling with the application of cold packs, elevation, antibiotics, and decongestants, with follow-up evaluation 5 to 7 days after swelling has subsided.

E. Full-thickness loss of the tip of the nose or nasal rim may be surgically replaced if the missing tissue is located and if wound margins are relatively smooth. The detached part should be kept in a cool, moist sterile gauze wrap until repair is attempted.

F. Epistaxis from nasal trauma generally abates spontaneously. Persistent nasal hemorrhage can usually be controlled with the application of firm anterior pressure. With severe epistaxis, intranasal packing may be required to arrest the bleeding.

G. A septal hematoma, if not recognized or treated, can result in infection or necrosis of the septum, becoming a cosmetic disaster months and years later. The septum should be visually inspected for a boggy appearance or swelling and tested for indentation with a cotton-tipped applicator. Aspiration relieves the hematoma with nasal packing inserted bilaterally to prevent reaccumulation.

References

Altreuter RW. Nasal trauma. Emerg Med Clin North Am 1987; 5:293–300.

Behrman SJ, Behrman DA. Facial injuries. In: Shires TG, ed. Principles of trauma care. New York: McGraw-Hill, 1985:402–448.

Cantrill SV. Maxillofacial injuries. In: Kravis TC, Warner CG, eds. Emergency medicine. Rockville, MD: Aspen, 1983:1041–1052.

Edgerton MT, Kenney JG. Emergency care of maxillofacial and otological injuries. In: Zuidema GD, Rutherford RB, Ballinger W, eds. The management of trauma. Philadelphia: WB Saunders, 1985:275–344.

Patient with NASAL TRAUMA

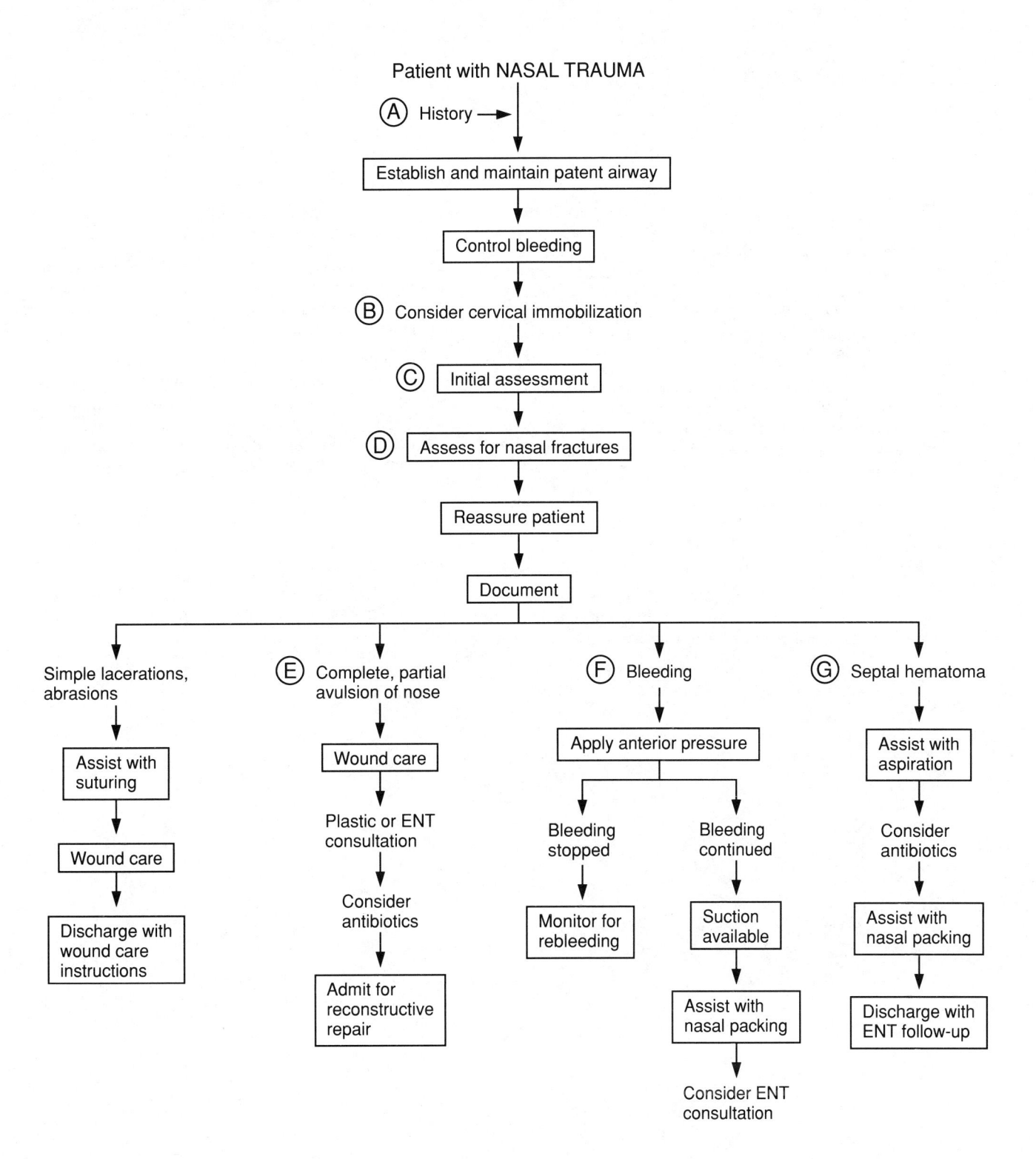

(A) History →

↓

Establish and maintain patent airway

↓

Control bleeding

↓

(B) Consider cervical immobilization

↓

(C) Initial assessment

↓

(D) Assess for nasal fractures

↓

Reassure patient

↓

Document

Simple lacerations, abrasions
↓
Assist with suturing
↓
Wound care
↓
Discharge with wound care instructions

(E) Complete, partial avulsion of nose
↓
Wound care
↓
Plastic or ENT consultation
↓
Consider antibiotics
↓
Admit for reconstructive repair

(F) Bleeding
↓
Apply anterior pressure
↓
- Bleeding stopped → Monitor for rebleeding
- Bleeding continued → Suction available → Assist with nasal packing → Consider ENT consultation

(G) Septal hematoma
↓
Assist with aspiration
↓
Consider antibiotics
↓
Assist with nasal packing
↓
Discharge with ENT follow-up

DENTAL TRAUMA

Kimberly L. Davies

A. Trauma to the teeth usually results from a blunt force to the mouth that fractures or avulses the teeth from the underlying bony segments. The most common area of injury is the anterior teeth and is often associated with intraoral and lip lacerations and/or mandibular fractures. History should include circumstances, nature, and force of the injury; time injury occurred; and observation for associated injuries.

B. Primary focus of management must be directed toward airway, breathing, and circulation. An aspirated tooth can cause partial or complete airway obstruction and requires immediate mechanical removal or surgical airway management.

C. The possibility of concurrent cervical spine injury with facial and/or dental trauma must be considered. If any doubt exists, cervical immobilization should be instituted.

D. The oral cavity must be carefully inspected to identify fractured or missing teeth, with avulsed segments removed to prevent aspiration or airway compromise.

E. Minor fractures of tooth enamel or dentin, although painful to the patient, require no emergency interventions. Routine dental measures are indicated to restore teeth to a comfortable and/or esthetic condition.

F. Partially avulsed teeth may initially be repositioned with light finger pressure. An oral surgeon or dentist should be consulted for evaluation and application of splinting mechanisms to salvage the tooth.

G. Replantation of completely avulsed teeth should be attempted if at all possible. To facilitate the procedure, the tooth should be kept clean and moist by wrapping it in moistened gauze and avoiding immersion or drying. An oral surgeon should be consulted to reposition and splint the tooth manually to prevent complete loss.

References

Kaban LB, Goldwyn RM. Facial injuries. In: May HL, ed. Emergency medicine. New York: John Wiley & Sons, 1984:323–352.

Kelly JP. Dental emergencies. In: Kravis TC, Warner CG, eds. Emergency medicine. Rockville, MD: Aspen, 1983:1053–1059.

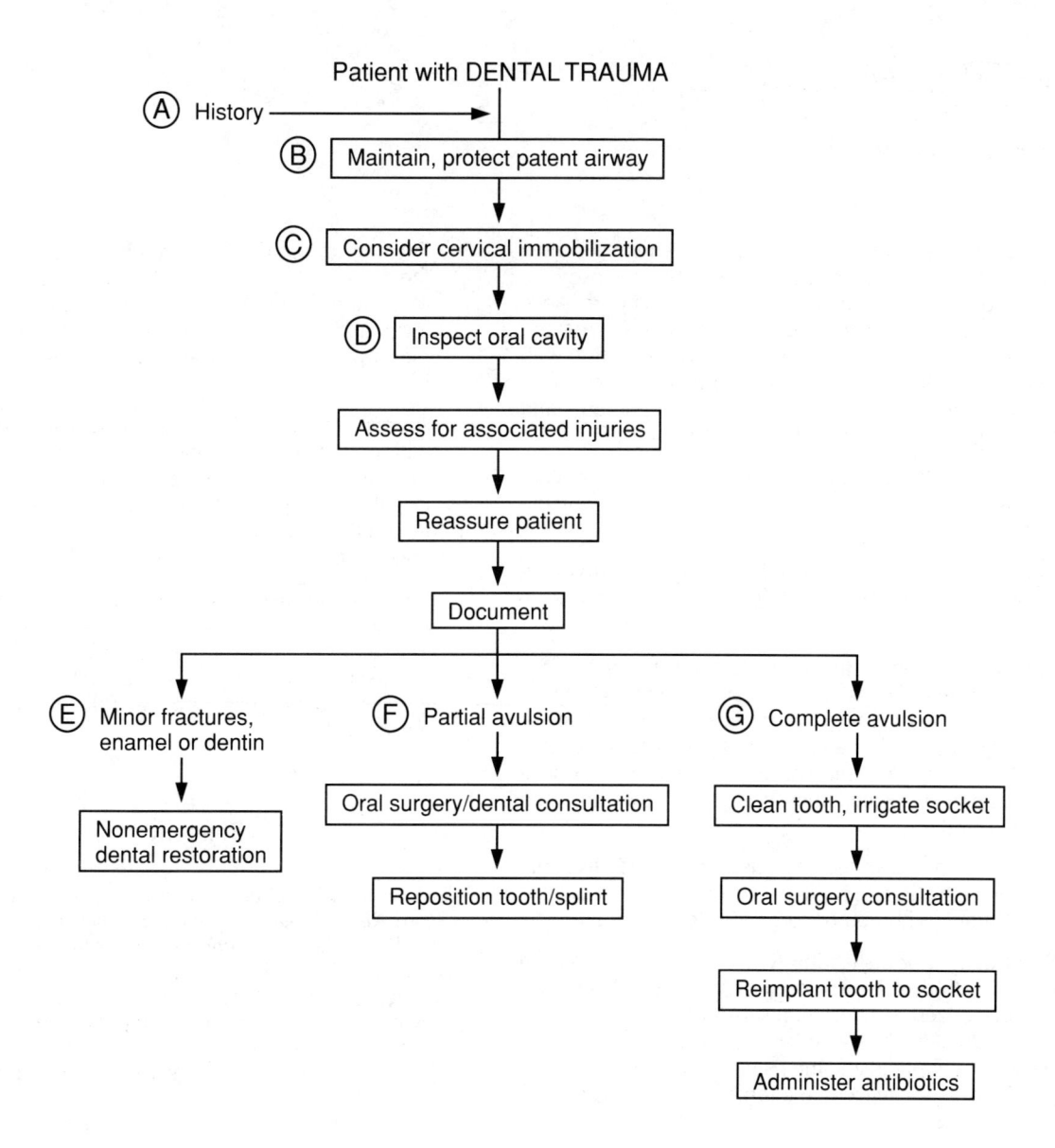

```
                    Patient with DENTAL TRAUMA
         Ⓐ History ─────────────►
                    Ⓑ  Maintain, protect patent airway
                                │
                                ▼
                    Ⓒ  Consider cervical immobilization
                                │
                                ▼
                    Ⓓ  Inspect oral cavity
                                │
                                ▼
                       Assess for associated injuries
                                │
                                ▼
                         Reassure patient
                                │
                                ▼
                            Document
            ┌───────────────────┼───────────────────┐
            ▼                   ▼                   ▼
    Ⓔ Minor fractures,   Ⓕ Partial avulsion   Ⓖ Complete avulsion
      enamel or dentin          │                   │
            │                   ▼                   ▼
            ▼          Oral surgery/dental    Clean tooth, irrigate socket
     Nonemergency         consultation                │
     dental restoration        │                      ▼
                               ▼             Oral surgery consultation
                      Reposition tooth/splint         │
                                                      ▼
                                             Reimplant tooth to socket
                                                      │
                                                      ▼
                                             Administer antibiotics
```

EAR TRAUMA

Kimberly L. Davies

The human ear is intricately designed and supported by a cartilaginous framework. The poorly protected, exposed ear is subject to a variety of injuries, as follows: as part of the skull base, as an appendage, and as an organ of hearing and balance. The ear is frequently traumatized in association with closed head injuries. Treatment goals for managing ear injuries are the preservation of the cartilaginous structures and identification of unobvious concomitant injuries.

A. History should include mechanism of injury, loss of consciousness, and changes in hearing ability following the insult.

B. The possibility of concurrent cervical spine injury must always be considered. Immobilization should be instituted if any possibility exists.

C. Initial assessment of the ear includes inspection of the auricle, external canal, and tympanic membrane. Signs and symptoms of otologic injury include bleeding and/or CSF drainage from the ear, pain, hearing loss, vertigo, and tinnitus. The external ear should be carefully inspected for abrasions, lacerations, ecchymosis, swelling, and foreign bodies.

D. Any time trauma to the ear exists, it is imperative that the patient be thoroughly assessed for possible associated CNS injury, with appropriate neurologic evaluation.

E. Blunt trauma or a shearing type of injury can result in the formation of a hematoma in the external pinna. If not recognized and treated, necrosis of the cartilage may result. Once the hematoma is aspirated, a firm pressure dressing is applied, and the patient is re-examined in 24 to 48 hours for reaccumulation of the hematoma.

F. Frostbite of the ear is treated with rapid rewarming of the tissue with moist heat (40°C). Depending on the extent of the injury, surgical debridement may be delayed for final demarcation of the injured tissue. Minor frostbite injuries of the ear are managed as minor burn injuries.

G. Animal and human bites are considered "dirty wounds" with potential complications of cellulitis or abscess formation. Management of bite injuries includes copious irrigation and prophylactic antibiotic therapy. Depending on the extent and location of the injury, the wound may or may not be repaired immediately.

H. Replantation may be considered in cases of complete auricle amputation if the detached part is located. Therefore, every attempt should be made to locate the missing tissue. To promote optimal replantation, the detached part should be preserved carefully to prevent tissue maceration.

References

Balkany TJ, Jafek BW. Otological trauma. In: Zuidema GD, Rutherford RB, Ballinger W, eds. The management of trauma. Philadelphia: WB Saunders, 1985:344–357.

Edgerton MT, Kenney JG. Emergency care of maxillofacial and otological injuries. In: Zuidema GD, Rutherford RB, Ballinger W, eds. The management of trauma. Philadelphia: WB Saunders, 1985:275–344.

Turbiak TW. Ear trauma. Emerg Med Clin North Am 1987; 5:243–251.

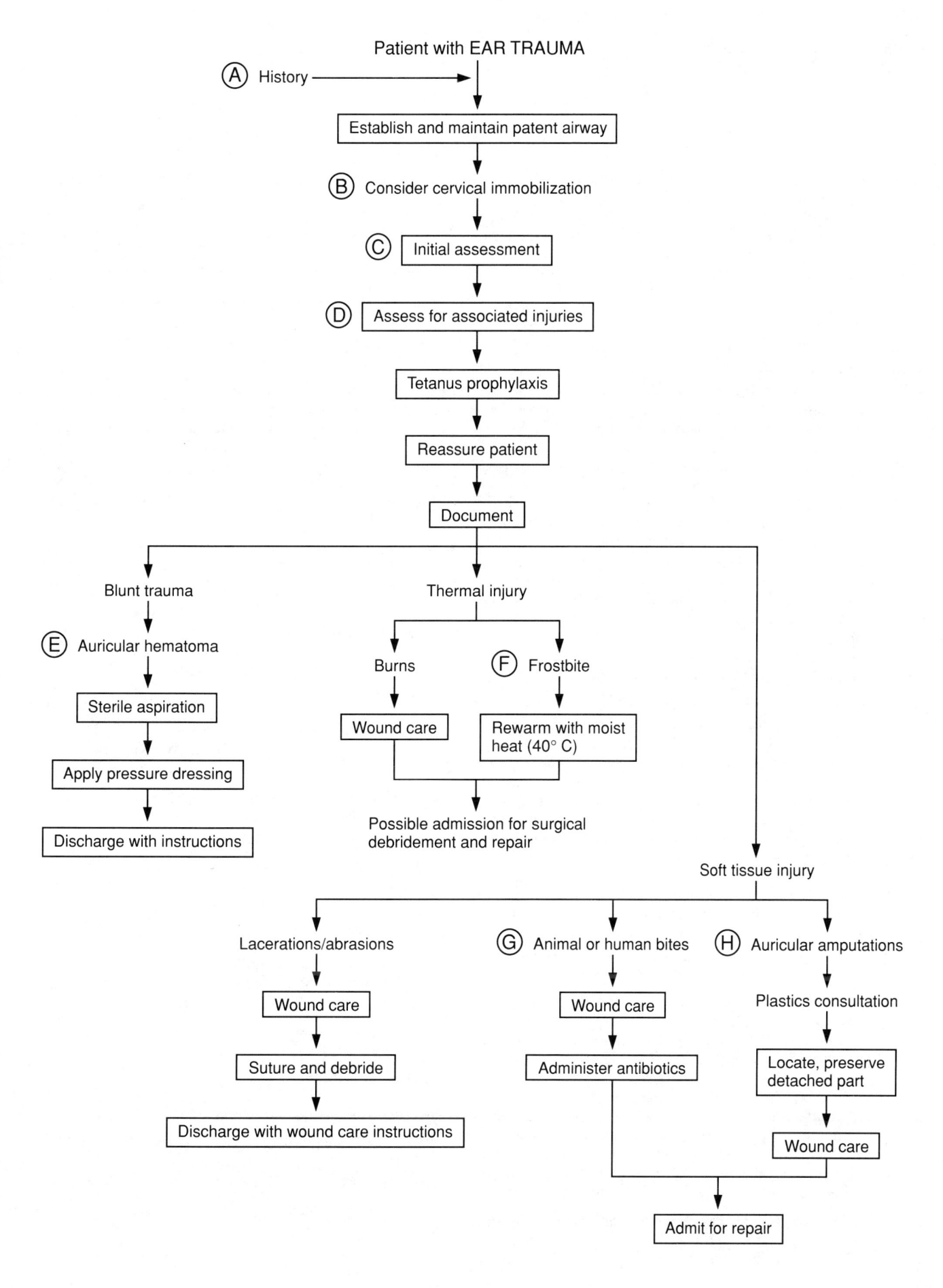

```
                          Patient with EAR TRAUMA
       Ⓐ History ──────────→│
                             ▼
                  ┌──────────────────────────────┐
                  │ Establish and maintain patent airway │
                  └──────────────────────────────┘
                             │
       Ⓑ Consider cervical immobilization
                             │
                             ▼
                  Ⓒ ┌──────────────────┐
                    │ Initial assessment │
                    └──────────────────┘
                             │
                             ▼
                  Ⓓ ┌──────────────────────────┐
                    │ Assess for associated injuries │
                    └──────────────────────────┘
                             │
                             ▼
                    ┌──────────────────┐
                    │ Tetanus prophylaxis │
                    └──────────────────┘
                             │
                             ▼
                    ┌──────────────────┐
                    │ Reassure patient │
                    └──────────────────┘
                             │
                             ▼
                    ┌──────────┐
                    │ Document │
                    └──────────┘
```

```
     Blunt trauma            Thermal injury

  Ⓔ Auricular hematoma       Burns    Ⓕ Frostbite

  ┌──────────────┐       ┌──────────┐  ┌──────────────────┐
  │ Sterile aspiration │  │ Wound care │  │ Rewarm with moist │
  └──────────────┘       └──────────┘  │ heat (40° C)      │
          │                              └──────────────────┘
          ▼
  ┌──────────────────┐         Possible admission for surgical
  │ Apply pressure dressing │       debridement and repair
  └──────────────────┘
          │
          ▼
  ┌────────────────────────┐
  │ Discharge with instructions │
  └────────────────────────┘

                                                    Soft tissue injury

      Lacerations/abrasions      Ⓖ Animal or human bites    Ⓗ Auricular amputations

         ┌──────────┐               ┌──────────┐            ┌──────────────────┐
         │ Wound care │               │ Wound care │            │ Plastics consultation │
         └──────────┘               └──────────┘            └──────────────────┘
              │                          │                          │
              ▼                          ▼                          ▼
       ┌──────────────────┐       ┌────────────────────┐      ┌──────────────────┐
       │ Suture and debride │       │ Administer antibiotics │      │ Locate, preserve │
       └──────────────────┘       └────────────────────┘      │ detached part    │
              │                                                └──────────────────┘
              ▼                                                         │
  ┌────────────────────────────────┐                                   ▼
  │ Discharge with wound care instructions │                          ┌──────────┐
  └────────────────────────────────┘                                  │ Wound care │
                                                                      └──────────┘
                                                                           │
                                              ┌────────────────┐           │
                                              │ Admit for repair │◄─────────┘
                                              └────────────────┘
```

EYE TRAUMA

Patricia C. Epifanio

A. All trauma patients require a primary and secondary assessment to identify any life threatening conditions. At this point, perform any life saving interventions. After control of airway, breathing, and circulation has been established, the eye trauma may be assessed and managed. Ocular trauma is generally not associated with a high mortality rate.

B. Continue with a focused assessment for the patient with ocular trauma.

C. History must include mechanisms of injury. The circumstances surrounding the incident may increase the index of suspicion for associated injuries and/or for the severity of the injury. Some types of injuries may require notification of the authorities. Signs and symptoms contribute to the diagnostic process. The history should also include past medical history, allergies, current tetanus immunization status, and treatment rendered before presenting to the hospital. If the patient has sustained a chemical burn to the eye(s), start immediate eye irrigation with copious amounts of normal saline, eye irrigating solution, or sterile water. Irrigation should be performed from the inner canthus to the outer canthus to prevent contamination of the other eye. This is a true eye emergency and requires immediate intervention. Maintain the irrigation until the pH of the eye has returned to normal (7.2 to 7.4).

D. Physical assessment must include assessment of visual acuity, visual fields, ocular mobility, and pupillary reactive and direct visualization. The eye should be observed for any gross abnormalities, including field deficit, diplopia and decreased vision, extraocular movement, hematomas, and facial asymmetry. A swollen eye may be opened gently to visualize the eyeball. When opening a swollen eye be certain that the examiner's hand rests on the patient's bony orbit so as not to place any undue pressure on the globe itself. Assessment for associated facial injuries, accomplished by performing a thorough examination of the head from the top to the chin, is essential. Palpate the orbital rim and the xygomatic arch for point tenderness and/or crepitus, irregularity, and movement, all of which may indicate a fracture site.

E. Complete loss of vision may result from these types of injury because of globe disruption and a retained intraocular foreign body. The most frequent offending objects may include sharp missiles (bullets, BBs, slivers of metal), knives, sticks, and glass. With high velocity missiles, suspect brain injury. Lid lacerations that transcend the lid margin require meticulous repair to prevent lid notches and corneal exposure. Lacerations that occur in the inner canthal area may involve the lacrimal system. Suspect lacrimal gland involvement when a laceration of the superior outer upper lid has been sustained.

F. The patient should sit or lie quietly with both eyes closed to reduce ocular movement, thus avoiding possible extension of the injury.

G. Any undue pressure on the globe may cause extrusion of the ocular contents.

H. Stabilize the impaled object. The unaffected eye is patched to decrease ocular movement. Patching is best accomplished by using one or more eye patches to fill the hollow without applying undue pressure on the globe. The patient should not be able to blink if the patches are placed correctly. Secure the patch in place with several strips of 2.5-cm wide tape placed diagonally from the forehead to the cheek.

I. If both eyes are patched because of extensive ocular trauma, provide reassurance to the patient. The possibility of visual loss produces a great deal of anxiety. Do not leave the patient alone. Consider allowing a calm individual to stay with the patient.

J. Patching the affected eye helps relieve pain associated with corneal abrasion.

K. Upon discharge, the patient needs instructions regarding the prescribed treatment plan, head injury precautions, plans for follow-up visits, and prevention.

L. The causes of blunt eye trauma are blows sustained from balls and fists. Physiologically the blow causes an increase in intraocular pressure, which displaces the intraocular structures (i.e., lens, retina).

M. Obtain radiographs or computed tomography (CT) scan as indicated. Prepare for funduscopic examination.

N. Hyphema is the presence of blood in the anterior chamber of the eye and is associated with secondary injury.

O. Hyphemic patients require admission because of the high incidence of a rebleed 3 to 7 days postinjury with more devastating consequences.

P. Blunt trauma is frequently associated with orbital or zygomatic injuries.

Q. Observe the patient for functional diplopia, unequal gaze and bleeding.

R. Intervention includes application of ice packs. Elevation of the head of the bed to 30 degrees is recommended to help decrease periorbital edema.

S. Refer to the appropriate consultant for disposition or admission.

References

Crowley R, Dunham C, eds. Shock trauma/critical care handbook. Rockville, MD: Aspen, 1986:103–119.

Kitt S, Kaiser J, eds. Emergency nursing: a physiologic and clinical perspective. Philadelphia: WB Saunders 1990:137–161.

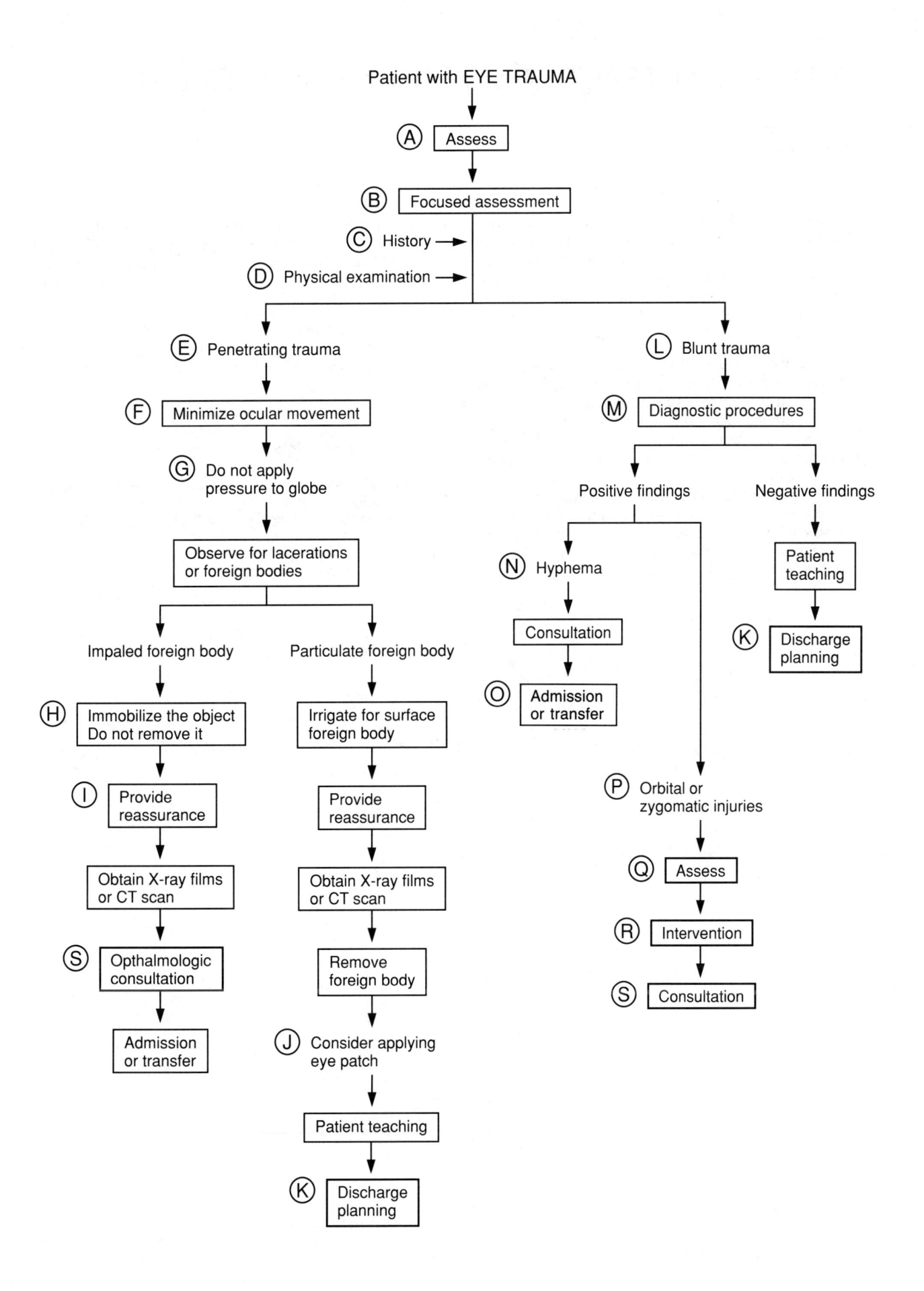

```
Patient with EYE TRAUMA
            │
      (A) Assess
            │
      (B) Focused assessment
            │
      (C) History ──▶
      (D) Physical examination ──▶
       ┌────────────┴────────────┐
       ▼                         ▼
(E) Penetrating trauma      (L) Blunt trauma
       │                         │
(F) Minimize ocular movement  (M) Diagnostic procedures
       │                    ┌────┴────────┐
(G) Do not apply       Positive findings   Negative findings
    pressure to globe        │                 │
       │               (N) Hyphema        Patient teaching
Observe for lacerations      │                 │
or foreign bodies       Consultation    (K) Discharge planning
   ┌────┴─────┐              │
Impaled    Particulate  (O) Admission or transfer
foreign     foreign
body        body
   │          │         (P) Orbital or zygomatic injuries
(H) Immobilize  Irrigate for            │
the object      surface foreign    (Q) Assess
Do not remove   body                    │
it              │                  (R) Intervention
   │         Provide                    │
(I) Provide  reassurance           (S) Consultation
reassurance     │
   │         Obtain X-ray films
Obtain X-ray or CT scan
films or CT     │
scan         Remove foreign body
   │            │
(S) Opthalmologic (J) Consider applying
consultation    eye patch
   │            │
Admission    Patient teaching
or transfer     │
             (K) Discharge planning
```

MAXILLOFACIAL FRACTURES: AIRWAY MANAGEMENT

Robert V. Walker
Ghali E. Ghali

A. Consistent with advanced trauma life support guidance, all patients who sustain significant supraclavicular trauma should be considered to have a cervical spine injury until proved otherwise. Inspect the oral cavity for debris, including loose teeth, bone, fillings, dentures, vomitus, and blood clots. Remove obstructing objects with a gloved hand or with high vacuum suction.

B. Depending on the patient's level of consciousness, one may choose the nasopharyngeal or the oropharyngeal airway as an adjunct to advanced airway control. Extension of the head, using only the chin lift or jaw thrust, facilitates placement of the airway. One should avoid hyperextension of the cervical spine. Assess the position of the maxilla and mandible relative to each other. If the mandible has relapsed posteriorly secondary to a fracture, placement of a bridle wire around the symphysis or stable teeth may be indicated. Often, this temporary stabilization may resolve an acute crisis by bringing the mandible and tongue forward.

C. The inability to intubate the trachea is the only true indication for creating a surgical airway. The surgical cricothyroidotomy is not recommended for children under 12 years of age; they are managed with needle cricothyroidotomy.

D. The presence of basilar skull fractures precludes the introduction of nasoendotracheal or nasogastric tubes except in cases of fiberoptic assisted intubation.

References

Assael LA. Oral Maxillofac Surg Clin North Am Trauma 1990; vol 2.

Dingman RO, Natuig P. Surgery of facial fractures. Philadelphia: WB Saunders, 1964.

Fonseca RJ, Walker RV. Oral and maxillofacial trauma. Philadelphia: WB Saunders, in press.

Rowe NL, Williams JL. Maxillofacial injuries. Vols. 1, 2. New York: Churchill Livingstone, 1985.

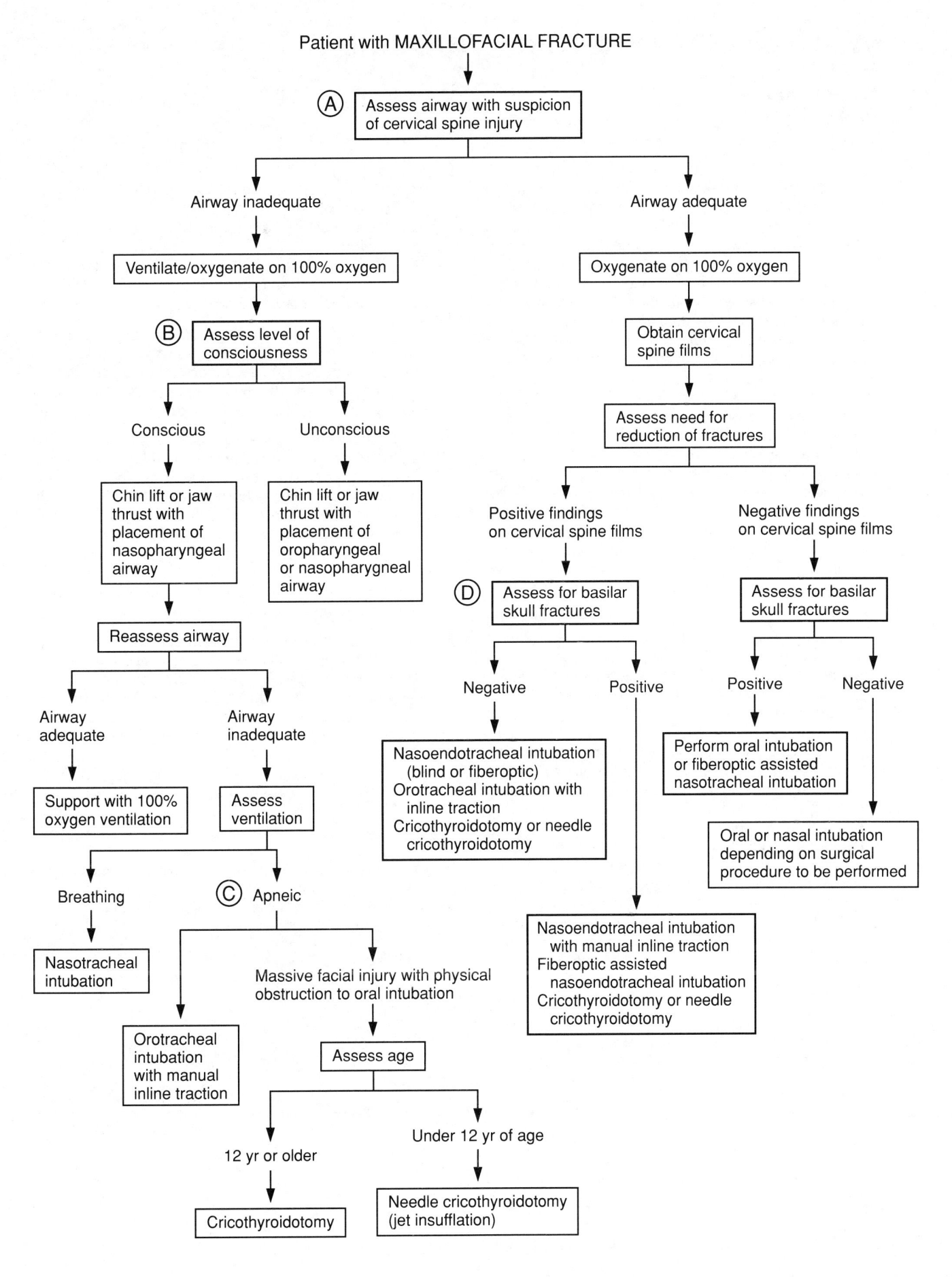

Patient with MAXILLOFACIAL FRACTURE

(A) Assess airway with suspicion of cervical spine injury

Airway inadequate

Ventilate/oxygenate on 100% oxygen

(B) Assess level of consciousness

- **Conscious**: Chin lift or jaw thrust with placement of nasopharyngeal airway → Reassess airway
- **Unconscious**: Chin lift or jaw thrust with placement of oropharyngeal or nasopharygneal airway

Reassess airway

- **Airway adequate**: Support with 100% oxygen ventilation
- **Airway inadequate**: Assess ventilation
  - **Breathing**: Nasotracheal intubation
  - **(C) Apneic**:
    - Orotracheal intubation with manual inline traction
    - Massive facial injury with physical obstruction to oral intubation → Assess age
      - **12 yr or older**: Cricothyroidotomy
      - **Under 12 yr of age**: Needle cricothyroidotomy (jet insufflation)

Airway adequate

Oxygenate on 100% oxygen

Obtain cervical spine films

Assess need for reduction of fractures

Positive findings on cervical spine films

(D) Assess for basilar skull fractures

- **Negative**: Nasoendotracheal intubation (blind or fiberoptic); Orotracheal intubation with inline traction; Cricothyroidotomy or needle cricothyroidotomy
- **Positive**: Nasoendotracheal intubation with manual inline traction; Fiberoptic assisted nasoendotracheal intubation; Cricothyroidotomy or needle cricothyroidotomy

Negative findings on cervical spine films

Assess for basilar skull fractures

- **Positive**: Perform oral intubation or fiberoptic assisted nasotracheal intubation
- **Negative**: Oral or nasal intubation depending on surgical procedure to be performed

MAXILLOFACIAL FRACTURES: TREATMENT

Robert V. Walker
Ghali E. Ghali

A. Patients who sustain facial trauma must be evaluated for more severe and potentially more life threatening injuries. These concomitant injuries include trauma to the chest, head, cervix, pelvis, abdomen, and extremities. Accordingly, general overall management of the trauma patient is of utmost importance. This management scheme is most favorably provided through a prioritized assessment and overall patient treatment plan. Using the American College of Surgeons Committee on Trauma protocol, treatment is divided into three main phases. Phase one involves a rapid survey of the patient's airway, breathing, circulation, and neurologic status (ABCDs). Phase two is a secondary survey that consists of a head-to-toe examination of the patient with great attention to detail. The third phase involves the definitive surgical care of the patient's injuries. Ideally, this last phase occurs after all specialty consultations are obtained, which will help shorten or minimize the number of anesthetics required for the patient. The definitive care of most facial fractures can be delayed until after the first two phases have been completed. An exception to this rule includes those fractures that directly contribute to airway obstruction.

B. A good clinical examination is the best method for detecting the presence of mandibular fractures. Additionally, a few key plain film radiographs are useful in the definitive diagnoses, as follows: a panoramic radiograph is the best general film; Towne's radiograph is the best to view condyles; an occlusal radiograph is the best to view symphysis; and lateral oblique and anteroposterior radiographs are useful for the body and angle region. Most condylar fractures are treated nonsurgically by closed reduction and intermaxillary fixation (IMF) for 10 to 14 days. This is followed by a 3-month period of physiotherapy to rehabilitate normal joint function. Open reduction of condylar fractures is always an option, and the method has appeal because of good plating fixation systems that currently exist. Mandibular fractures in children are generally treated nonsurgically with arch bars and IMF. The presence of developing tooth buds in the small mandible precludes the placement of most rigid fixation systems.

C. The clinical signs of orbital fractures are as follows:
  1. Enophthalmos
  2. Impairment of eye movement
  3. Diplopia
  4. Pseudoptosis and deepening of the supratarsal fold
  5. Orbital emphysema
  6. Infraorbital nerve paresthesia

D. The radiographic evaluation of zygomatic fractures should include the following radiographs: a submentovertex radiograph to view zygomatic arches and Waters' view for zygomatic buttresses and sinuses. A computer tomography (CT) scan should be done when indicated.

E. Fractures of the midface often defy classification owing to the severity of the force and the multidirectional source of the trauma. The LeFort classifications define the weakest areas of the midface complex when it is assaulted from a frontal direction at different levels. The LeFort type I fracture results from a force delivered above the level of the teeth. The LeFort type II fracture results from a force delivered at the level of the nasal bones. The LeFort type III fracture is caused by a force at the orbital level resulting in craniofacial dysfunction.

F. The radiographic evaluation of midface fractures should include a lateral skull view, a Waters view, and a reverse Waters view, together with a posteroanterior or anteroposterior view of the skull. For therapeutic reasons, a computed tomographic scan taken in the sagittal and, when indicated, in the coronal plane is obtained.

References

Assael LA, ed. Trauma. Oral Maxillofac Surg Clin North Am 1990; vol 2.

Dingman RO, Natvig P. Surgery of facial fractures. Philadelphia: WB Saunders, 1964.

Fonseca RJ, Walker RV. Oral and maxillofacial trauma. Philadelphia: WB Saunders, in press.

Rowe NL, Williams JL. Maxillofacial injuries. Vols. 1 & 2. New York: Churchill Livingstone, 1985.

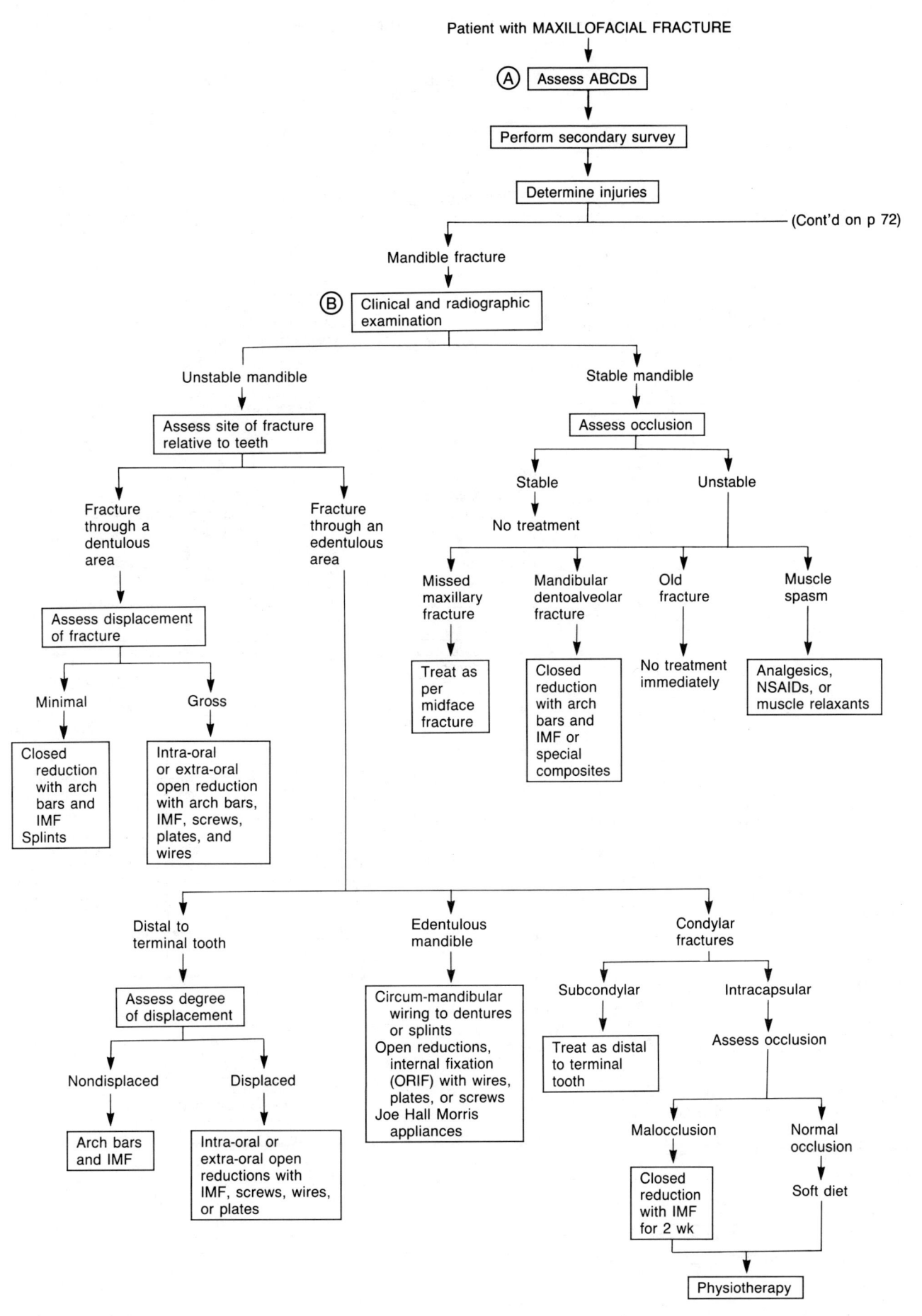

Patient with MAXILLOFACIAL FRACTURE

- (A) Assess ABCDs
- Perform secondary survey
- Determine injuries → (Cont'd on p 72)

Mandible fracture

(B) Clinical and radiographic examination

Unstable mandible

Assess site of fracture relative to teeth

Fracture through a dentulous area

Assess displacement of fracture

- **Minimal**: Closed reduction with arch bars and IMF Splints
- **Gross**: Intra-oral or extra-oral open reduction with arch bars, IMF, screws, plates, and wires

Fracture through an edentulous area

- **Distal to terminal tooth**: Assess degree of displacement
  - **Nondisplaced**: Arch bars and IMF
  - **Displaced**: Intra-oral or extra-oral open reductions with IMF, screws, wires, or plates
- **Edentulous mandible**: Circum-mandibular wiring to dentures or splints; Open reductions, internal fixation (ORIF) with wires, plates, or screws; Joe Hall Morris appliances
- **Condylar fractures**
  - **Subcondylar**: Treat as distal to terminal tooth
  - **Intracapsular**: Assess occlusion
    - **Malocclusion**: Closed reduction with IMF for 2 wk → Physiotherapy
    - **Normal occlusion**: Soft diet

Stable mandible

Assess occlusion

- **Stable**: No treatment
- **Unstable**:
  - Missed maxillary fracture → Treat as per midface fracture
  - Mandibular dentoalveolar fracture → Closed reduction with arch bars and IMF or special composites
  - Old fracture → No treatment immediately
  - Muscle spasm → Analgesics, NSAIDs, or muscle relaxants

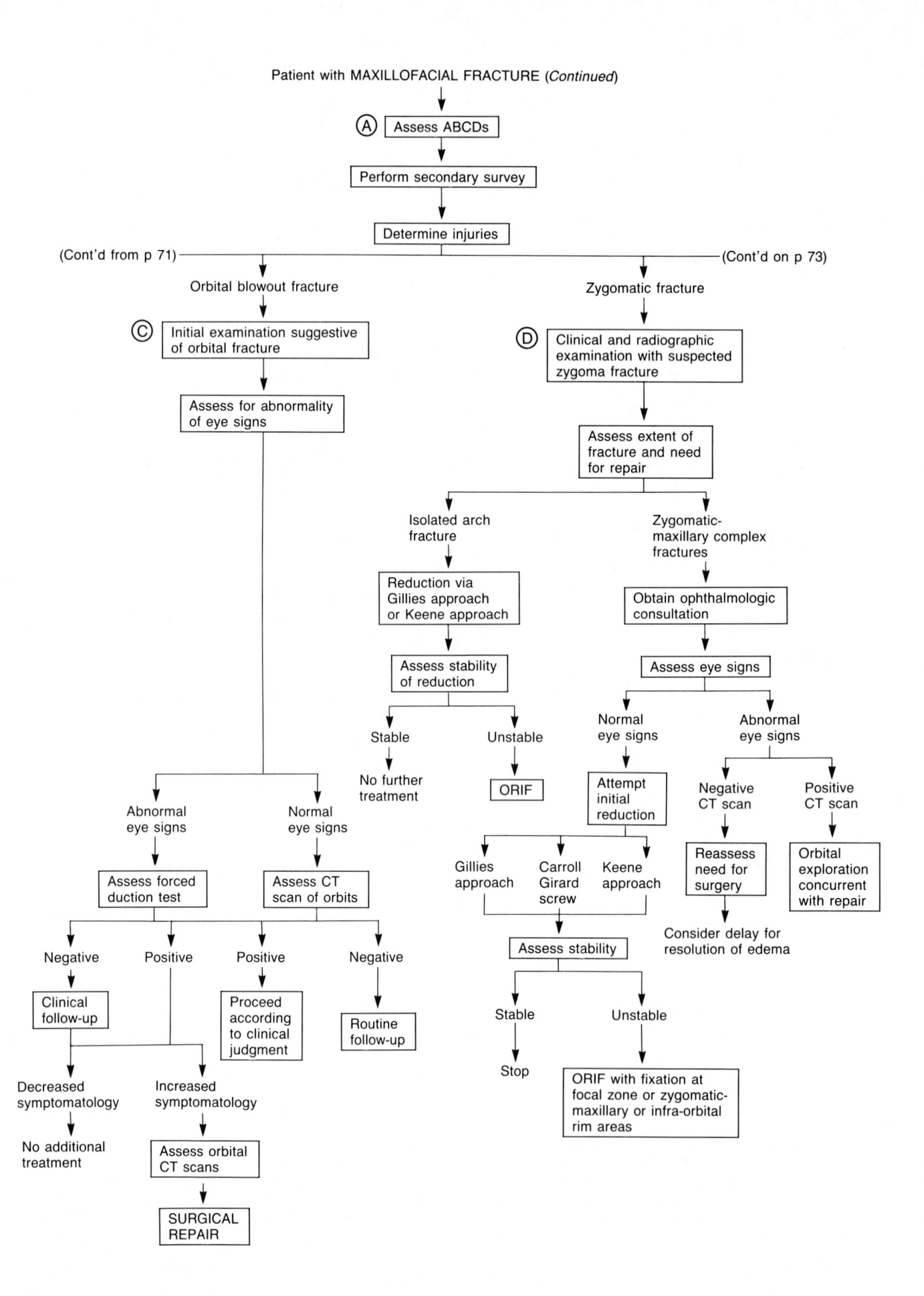

Patient with MAXILLOFACIAL FRACTURE (*Continued*)

- (A) Assess ABCDs
- Perform secondary survey
- Determine injuries

(Cont'd from p 71) ———— (Cont'd on p 73)

Orbital blowout fracture

- (C) Initial examination suggestive of orbital fracture
- Assess for abnormality of eye signs

Abnormal eye signs
- Assess forced duction test
  - Negative → Clinical follow-up
    - Decreased symptomatology → No additional treatment
    - Increased symptomatology → Assess orbital CT scans → SURGICAL REPAIR
  - Positive → Clinical follow-up (same branch as above)

Normal eye signs
- Assess CT scan of orbits
  - Positive → Proceed according to clinical judgment
  - Negative → Routine follow-up

Zygomatic fracture

- (D) Clinical and radiographic examination with suspected zygoma fracture
- Assess extent of fracture and need for repair

Isolated arch fracture
- Reduction via Gillies approach or Keene approach
- Assess stability of reduction
  - Stable → No further treatment
  - Unstable → ORIF

Zygomatic-maxillary complex fractures
- Obtain ophthalmologic consultation
- Assess eye signs

Normal eye signs
- Attempt initial reduction
  - Gillies approach
  - Carroll Girard screw
  - Keene approach
- Assess stability
  - Stable → Stop
  - Unstable → ORIF with fixation at focal zone or zygomatic-maxillary or infra-orbital rim areas

Abnormal eye signs
- Negative CT scan → Reassess need for surgery → Consider delay for resolution of edema
- Positive CT scan → Orbital exploration concurrent with repair

72

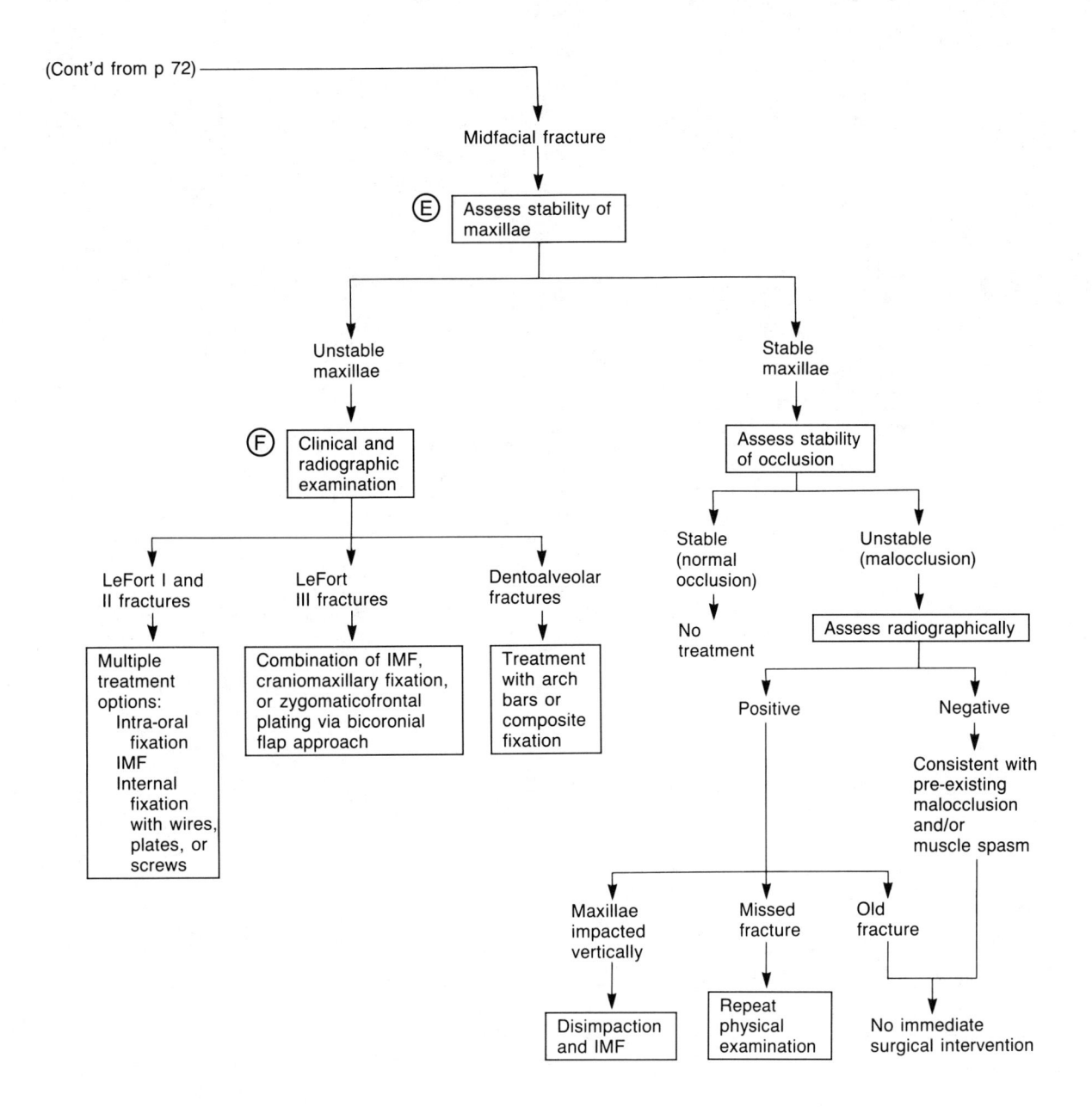

(Cont'd from p 72)
↓
Midfacial fracture
↓
(E) Assess stability of maxillae

- **Unstable maxillae**
  ↓
  (F) Clinical and radiographic examination
  - **LeFort I and II fractures**
    → Multiple treatment options:
       Intra-oral fixation
       IMF
       Internal fixation with wires, plates, or screws
  - **LeFort III fractures**
    → Combination of IMF, craniomaxillary fixation, or zygomaticofrontal plating via bicoronial flap approach
  - **Dentoalveolar fractures**
    → Treatment with arch bars or composite fixation

- **Stable maxillae**
  ↓
  Assess stability of occlusion
  - **Stable (normal occlusion)** → No treatment
  - **Unstable (malocclusion)**
    ↓
    Assess radiographically
    - **Positive**
      - Maxillae impacted vertically → Disimpaction and IMF
      - Missed fracture → Repeat physical examination
      - Old fracture → No immediate surgical intervention
    - **Negative** → Consistent with pre-existing malocclusion and/or muscle spasm → No immediate surgical intervention

73

NECK TRAUMA

Blunt Neck Trauma
Penetrating Neck Trauma

BLUNT NECK TRAUMA

Kimberly L. Davies

A. Blunt neck trauma is frequently associated with serious internal injuries to structures within the neck, which can present as immediate and life threatening or insidiously, with potentially devastating outcomes. The history should include mechanism of injury, type of blunt force or object striking the neck, status of the airway, level of consciousness, and vital signs as well as observation and assessment for other injuries.

B. The airway must be initially and continuously assessed for patency. The potential for hypoxia secondary to progressive partial or complete airway obstruction in nonpenetrating neck injuries is high; therefore, high-flow supplemental oxygen must be administered. For any airway intervention, hyperextension of the neck must be avoided.

C. Signs of laryngeal or tracheal injury with obstruction include stridor, inadequate air exchange, cyanosis, intercostal and supraclavicular retractions, and possible subcutaneous air. Intervention to establish an airway must be instituted immediately to prevent asphyxia and death.

D. Controversy exists over optimal airway management in partial or complete obstruction with known or suspected laryngeal trauma. Cricothyrotomy and blind intubation are definitely contraindicated. Controlled endotracheal intubation and emergency tracheostomy are options to relieve the obstruction. Needle tracheostomy with jet insufflation is probably the quickest, safest method to establish a tracheal airway.

E. Assume that a cervical spine injury exists in anyone who sustains blunt trauma to the neck. Cervical immobilization should be accomplished with sandbags and tape or lateral stabilizing devices rather than with a cervical collar; the latter can obstruct visual assessment of the anterior neck or interfere with surgical airway management. Anteroposterior and lateral cervical views, complete with C7, by radiologic examination are necessary to rule out cervical spine injury.

F. The initial assessment serves as the baseline for evaluation of changes in the patient's condition over time. Manifestations of blunt trauma to the neck are varied and related to the injured underlying structures. Assessment focuses on the airway; visual inspection should identify deformity, ecchymosis, abrasions, and swelling of the neck. The assessment should include palpation for subcutaneous air, tracheal or bony deformity, and masses.

G. As with any multisystem trauma patient, baseline laboratory studies should be obtained on admission. Initial arterial blood gas sampling assists in monitoring the effectiveness of the patient's oxygenation and ventilation, and if vascular injury is suspected, blood type and crossmatch are useful.

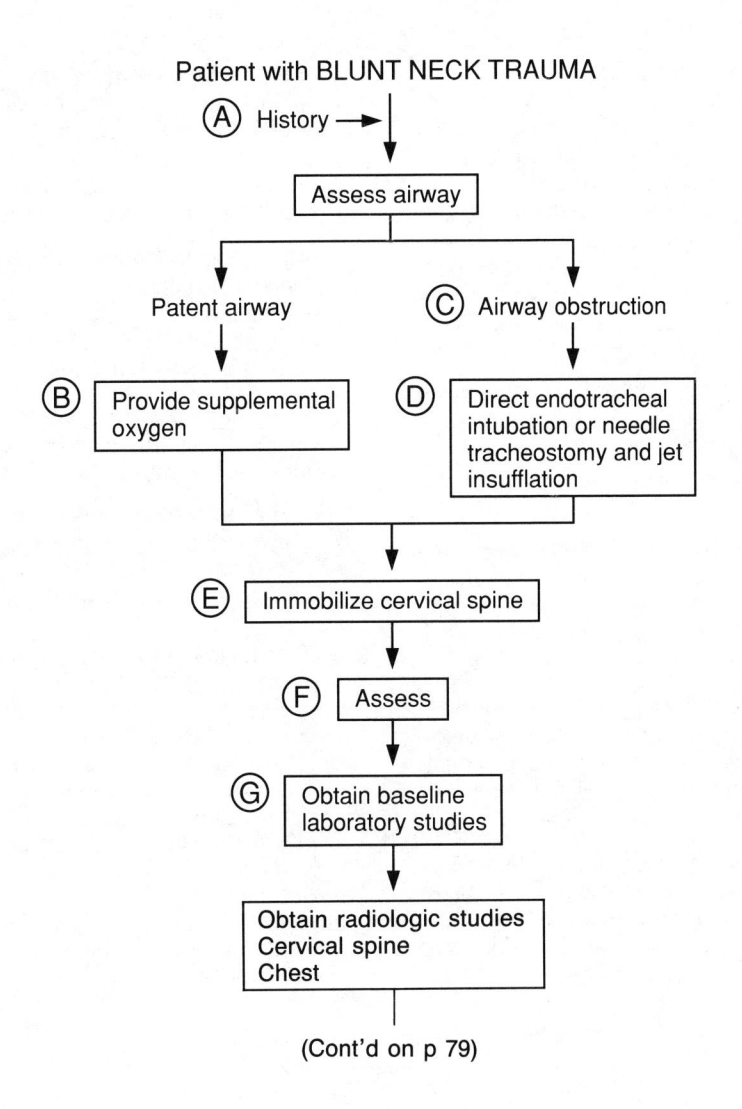

Patient with BLUNT NECK TRAUMA

(A) History ⟶

Assess airway

Patent airway   (C) Airway obstruction

(B) Provide supplemental oxygen

(D) Direct endotracheal intubation or needle tracheostomy and jet insufflation

(E) Immobilize cervical spine

(F) Assess

(G) Obtain baseline laboratory studies

Obtain radiologic studies
Cervical spine
Chest

(Cont'd on p 79)

H. The incidence of laryngeal or tracheal injuries is low; however, they can be overlooked or masked by other serious injuries. These injuries frequently occur when the anterior portion of the neck strikes an object (e.g., steering wheel, dashboard, or clothesline), thereby crushing these structures against the cervical vertebrae. Identifying laryngeal or tracheal injuries depends on maintaining a high index of suspicion. Common clinical findings of laryngeal tracheal injuries are symptoms of airway obstruction, subcutaneous air, aphonia or hoarseness, and loss of palpable landmarks of the neck.

I. Care of the patient with upper airway trauma is focused on continuous assessment for progressive worsening of any clinical finding identified in the initial assessment. Airway equipment must be readily available in anticipation of rapid intervention.

J. Injury to the esophagus secondary to blunt neck trauma is rare because the esophagus is relatively protected anatomically. Findings include tenderness of the neck, dysphagia, drooling, and crepitus. Mediastinitis and neck infections are later complications.

K. Contrast esophagograms and esophagoscopy are diagnostic tests employed to determine whether disruption of the cervical esophagus exists. Morbidity and mortality are directly related to the time interval between injury and surgical exploration and repair.

L. Suspected vascular injury that results from blunt trauma to the neck can be difficult to detect. Neurologic abnormalities frequently resemble signs of a cerebral vascular accident. These abnormalities can be difficult to differentiate from actual vascular injury, hypoxia, or direct injury to the nervous system. Prompt detection is essential because of the risk of prolonged cerebral ischemia and its devastating consequences. Assessment of the neck should include inspection for asymmetry, swelling, or discoloration in relation to the course of major vascular structures and evaluation of quality.

M. Neurologic deficits are characteristically delayed in onset. Therefore, initial assessment and continuously repeated examinations are necessary to detect any insidious or acute changes. If neurologic deterioration is identified, notify the physician immediately.

N. Acute cerebral deficits suggest carotid artery injury. Suspected carotid injury and expanding hematoma require immediate surgical intervention.

O. Actual injury to the cervical spine can result secondary to hyperextension or sharp rotation of the neck.

References

Balkany TJ, Rutherford RB, Narrod J, Jafek BW. The management of neck injuries. In: Zuidema GD, Rutherford RB, Ballinger W, eds. The management of trauma. Philadelphia: WB Saunders, 1985:359–378.

Healy GB, Koster JK. Neck injuries. In: May HL, ed. Emergency medicine. New York: John Wiley, 1984:363–364.

Shumrick KA, Shumrick DA. Laryngeal and tracheal foreign bodies and blunt trauma. In: Callaham ML, ed. Current therapy in emergency medicine. Toronto: BC Decker, 1987:235–238.

Sullivan PK, Jafek BW. Blunt cervical trauma. In: Moore EE, Eisman B, Van Way CW, eds. Critical decisions in trauma. St. Louis: CV Mosby, 1984:128–131.

(Cont'd from p 77)

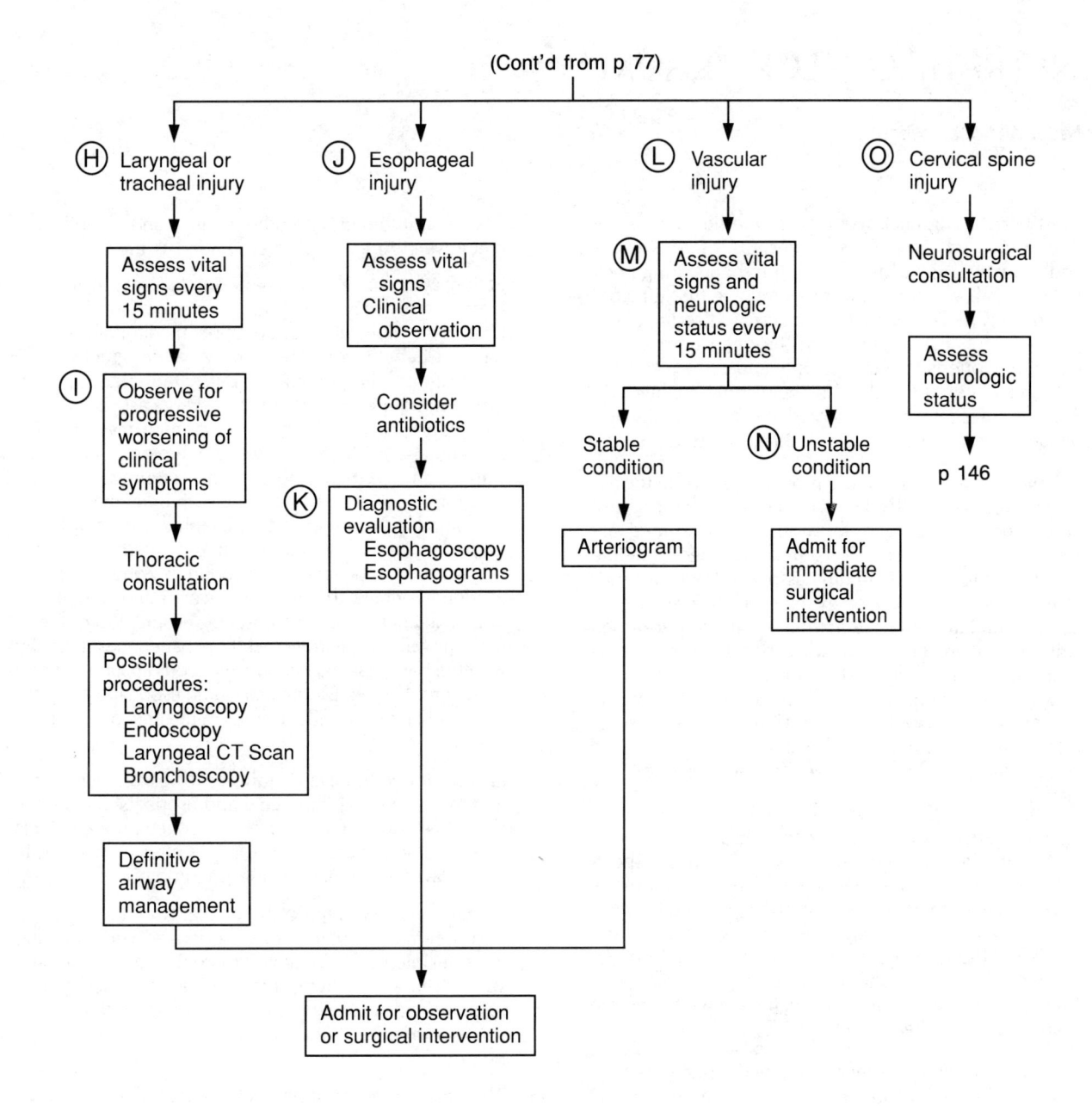

- **(H) Laryngeal or tracheal injury**
  - Assess vital signs every 15 minutes
  - **(I)** Observe for progressive worsening of clinical symptoms
  - Thoracic consultation
  - Possible procedures:
    - Laryngoscopy
    - Endoscopy
    - Laryngeal CT Scan
    - Bronchoscopy
  - Definitive airway management

- **(J) Esophageal injury**
  - Assess vital signs
  - Clinical observation
  - Consider antibiotics
  - **(K)** Diagnostic evaluation
    - Esophagoscopy
    - Esophagograms
  - Admit for observation or surgical intervention

- **(L) Vascular injury**
  - **(M)** Assess vital signs and neurologic status every 15 minutes
    - Stable condition → Arteriogram
    - **(N)** Unstable condition → Admit for immediate surgical intervention

- **(O) Cervical spine injury**
  - Neurosurgical consultation
  - Assess neurologic status
  - p 146

79

PENETRATING NECK TRAUMA

Miguel A. Lopez-Viego

A. Most penetrating neck wounds are the direct result of injuries caused by knives and gunshots. Motor vehicle and industrial accidents also result in penetrating neck trauma. Stab wounds more often involve the left side, are usually accompanied by external bleeding, and produce less severe damage to the deeper structures. Gunshot wounds penetrate deeply and more commonly produce serious bleeding and hematomas in the neck. Bullet injuries may indirectly produce injuries to the aerodigestive tract or to major vascular structures.

B. A rapid primary examination is performed while the airway is secured and bleeding is controlled with local pressure. The number and location of all wounds are recorded, and priorities of care are established. Penetrating neck trauma is commonly associated with wounds to the chest, abdomen, and extremities. The primary survey and initiation of resuscitation should be performed prior to focusing on the isolated cervical injury. Patients with neck wounds are particularly susceptible to acute airway embarrassment and vascular decompensation. All patients should have large caliber intravenous access established, equipment for immediate resuscitation and evaluation available, and experienced personnel on hand.

C. The stable trauma victim with neck injury should undergo a thorough evaluation if, on inspection, it is suspected that the wound has penetrated the platysma muscle. A complete secondary survey is done followed by chest films. A complete neurologic evaluation is performed and recorded. Placement of a nasogastric tube and direct or indirect laryngoscopy should not be done. The increased pressure generated by violent coughing or wretching can lead to uncontrolled bleeding.

D. The zone of injury in penetrating neck trauma is then determined. Zone I injuries occur at the area of the thoracic outlet extending superiorly to 1 cm above the clavicles. This location makes injuries to the great vessels at the thoracic outlet, trachea, and esophagus likely. The bony thorax (i.e., sternum, ribs, and clavicle) makes direct exposure and repair of injuries in this location impossible without a sternotomy or thoracotomy to allow for proximal control. Zone II injuries occur between the sternal notch and the angle of the mandible. Management of stable injuries in this area is controversial (operative management versus radiographic evaluation). Zone III injuries occur cephalad to the mandibular angle. Access to injured structures in Zone III may require anterior dislocation of the mandible, mandibular resections, craniotomies, and other lengthy and complicated maneuvers. Angiographic evaluation is the rule.

E. Patients who have injuries in Zone I are at greatest risk because they may have injuries to major arterial structures in the root of the neck or upper mediastinum. These patients benefit from preoperative arteriography.

Patients with penetrating injury in the Zone II area may not require arteriography in every case. Zone II arteriography may be helpful in planning the operative procedure. Zone II injuries with a neurologic deficit may warrant an arteriogram to evaluate cerebrovascular circulation. Cerebral arteriography with intracranial views combined with computed tomographic scans may be indicated in the patient who has an associated head injury.

Arteriography is recommended in Zone III injuries to identify where the injury is located and to plan the operative approach. Laryngoscopy, esophagoscopy, and barium swallow are indicated if the patient has difficulty breathing or speaking, has subcutaneous air, or has blood in the oropharynx. Esophagrams and esophagoscopy are especially likely to miss injuries in the area of the upper constrictions.

F. Patients found to have no injuries to vascular structures and to have normal laryngeal and esophageal anatomy should be admitted and observed. Zone I injury patients require a repeat chest film 6 hours after injury to rule out delayed presentation of a pneumothorax.

G. If any injury to a significant cervical structure is identified, operative repair with experienced surgeons and anesthesiologists is indicated to control the airway and vascular injuries. Attempting exploration of penetrating neck wounds outside the operating suite without adequate equipment, lighting, suction, or personnel is condemned.

H. The unstable penetrating neck trauma victim is at high risk for loss of airway and cardiovascular collapse. Once the determination of an unstable status is made, the airway should be secured. If it is evident that adequate gas exchange and oxygenation are not occurring in an apneic patient, or if obstruction or hemorrhage is present, immediate airway access is mandatory. Unless contraindicated or technically impossible, an endotracheal tube provides the fastest and safest airway control. When this route is not applicable, cricothyroidotomy (needle or surgical) becomes the most effective means of emergency airway control. Tracheostomy is reserved for the operating room and a more controlled setting, when the endotracheal and cricothyroid routes are not applicable.

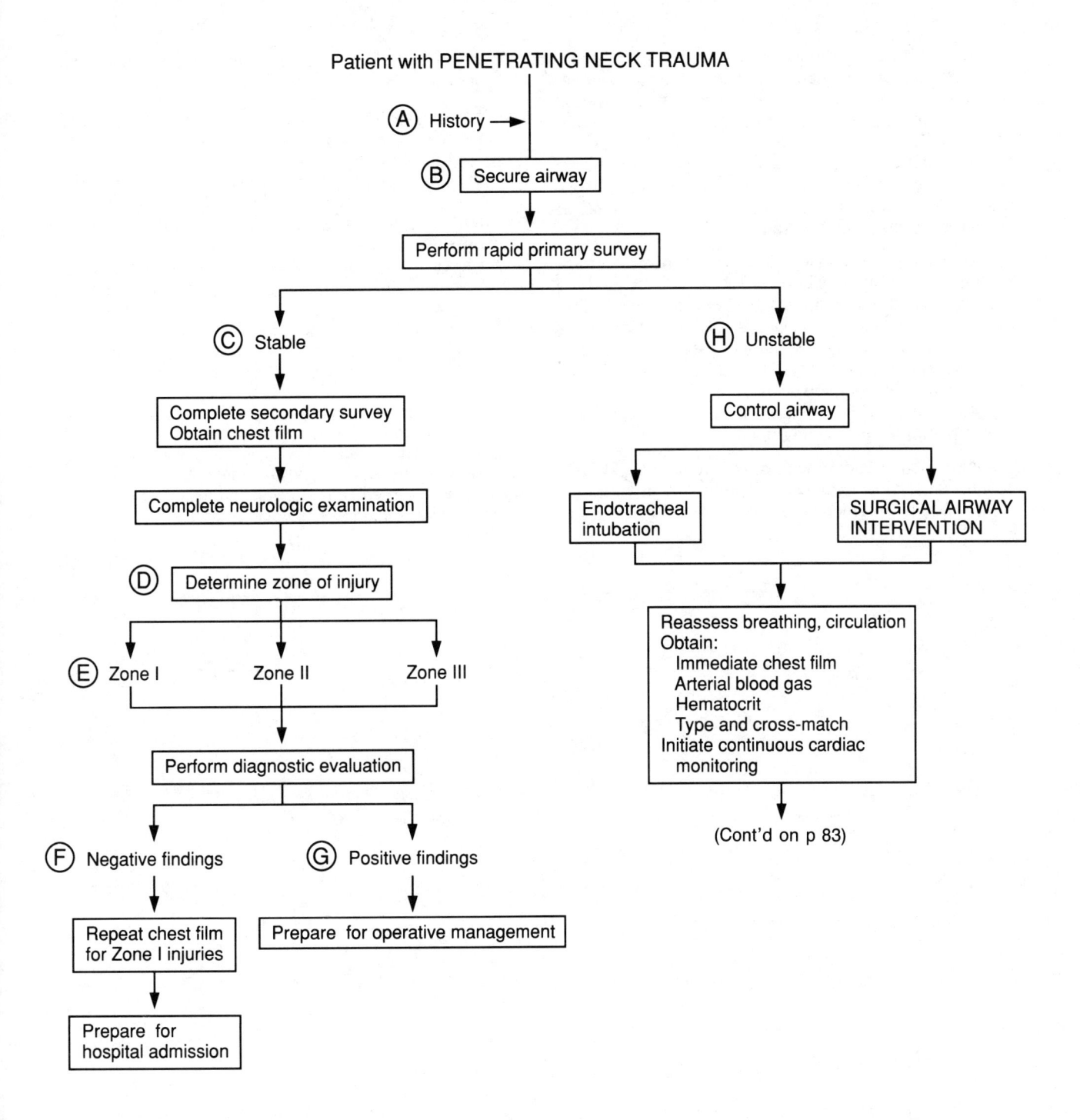

Patient with PENETRATING NECK TRAUMA

- (A) History →
- (B) Secure airway
- Perform rapid primary survey

(C) Stable
- Complete secondary survey
- Obtain chest film
- Complete neurologic examination
- (D) Determine zone of injury
  - (E) Zone I
  - Zone II
  - Zone III
- Perform diagnostic evaluation
  - (F) Negative findings
    - Repeat chest film for Zone I injuries
    - Prepare for hospital admission
  - (G) Positive findings
    - Prepare for operative management

(H) Unstable
- Control airway
  - Endotracheal intubation
  - SURGICAL AIRWAY INTERVENTION
- Reassess breathing, circulation
  Obtain:
  - Immediate chest film
  - Arterial blood gas
  - Hematocrit
  - Type and cross-match
  Initiate continuous cardiac monitoring

(Cont'd on p 83)

I. Two large bore intravenous lines should be established. Exsanguination from penetrating neck trauma is not uncommon. Patients with carotid, subclavian, or vertebral artery injuries may lose large volumes of blood through the visible external route or into occult space such as the pleural cavity or mediastinum. Rapid intravascular volume repletion with crystalloid and red cell components remains the mainstay of immediate stabilization enroute to the operating suite.

J. It is critical to recall that patients with penetrating neck trauma (particularly of Zone I) may have associated life threatening thoracic injuries (e.g., tension pneumothorax or massive hemothorax) as a result of their wound. These injuries may be the cause of their instability. The unstable patient is clearly not a candidate for angiographic, contrast, or endoscopic evaluation. These patients require aggressive intervention to control vascular and airway injuries in a timely manner.

K. Rapid vascular control with direct pressure for Zone II injuries can slow the rate of blood loss. Zone I injuries may require an emergency thoracotomy to access the intrathoracic organs and to gain control of the injured vessels.

L. Emergency operative management of Zone I injuries often requires median sternotomy for exposure and control of the thoracic outlet. Zone II injuries are approached typically via incisions along the anterior border of the ipsilateral sternocleidomastoid muscles. Management of unstable Zone III injuries can be extraordinarily difficult and often unrewarding. Control of inaccessible vessels may require balloon tamponade with inflatable vascular catheter or access via craniotomy or mandibular dislocation.

References

Larson DL, Cohn AM. Management of acute laryngeal injury: a critical review. J Trauma 1976; 16:858.

Liekweg WG, Greenfield LJ. Management of penetrating carotid artery injury. Ann Surg 1978; 188:587.

Roon AI, Christensen N. Evaluation and treatment of penetrating cervical injuries. J Trauma 1971; 19:391.

(Cont'd from p 81)

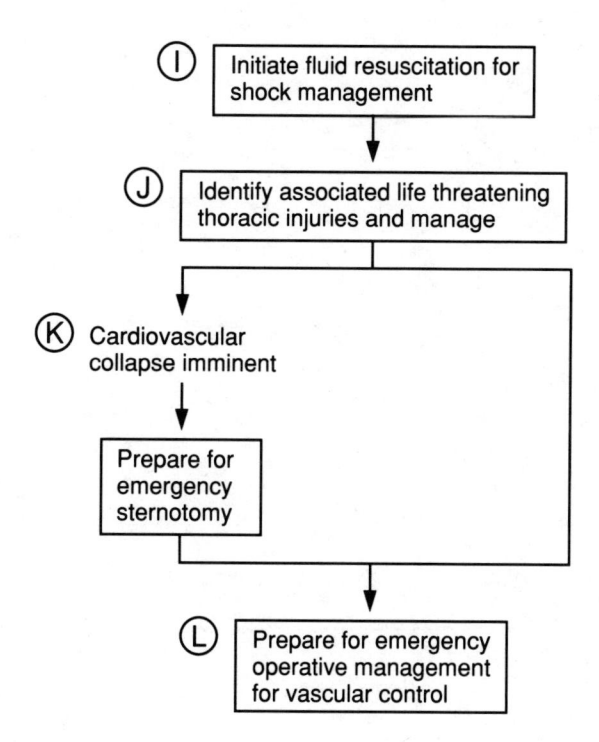

- (I) Initiate fluid resuscitation for shock management
- (J) Identify associated life threatening thoracic injuries and manage
- (K) Cardiovascular collapse imminent
  - Prepare for emergency sternotomy
- (L) Prepare for emergency operative management for vascular control

83

THORACIC TRAUMA: LIFE THREATENING INJURIES

Airway Obstruction
Tension Pneumothorax
Massive Hemothorax
Open Sucking Chest Wound

Flail Chest
Cardiac Tamponade
Emergency Thoracotomy

AIRWAY OBSTRUCTION

Kimberly L. Davies

A. Airway obstruction is a true life threatening emergency in which failure to identify or intervene has a disastrous or fatal outcome. Knowledge of the mechanism of injury is helpful when evaluating the potential for associated cervical spine injury. With blunt trauma it is imperative to manage the airway under the assumption that cervical injury exists (until proved otherwise).

B. General assessment of the airway involves level of consciousness, rate and pattern of respirations, and adequacy of respiratory effort. The conscious patient with partial obstruction may appear very apprehensive or restless, diaphoretic, pale, or cyanotic. Pooling of secretions, drooling, chest wall retractions, and audible stridor are likely clinical findings. Complete obstruction results in rapid loss of consciousness without detectable air exchange. In the early stages of obstruction the patient continues to have exaggerated respiratory movements, which quickly cease, and cyanosis becomes pronounced. Attempts to ventilate the patient are unsuccessful. With prolonged anoxia, cardiovascular and neurologic signs are present. Without immediate interventions to relieve the obstruction, the patient deteriorates to full cardiac arrest.

C. Airway management takes top priority. If the potential for cervical spine injury exists, cervical alignment should be manually maintained during all attempts to establish an airway, thereby preventing hyperextension of the neck. Definitive measures to immobilize the cervical spine should be deferred until an airway has been secured because immobilization devices may interfere with airway interventions.

D. The initial maneuver to open the airway of a trauma patient is the forward jaw thrust. The head tilt, chin lift method may be attempted if cervical spine injury has been excluded.

E. *All* victims of major trauma should receive supplemental oxygen. Delivery systems and flow rates are guided by overall patient condition.

F. Remove debris manually from the oral cavity and suction secretions. Suctioning of vomitus or blood can open the airway and prevent aspiration into the lungs. When obstruction is secondary to a lodged foreign body (i.e., tooth), direct laryngoscopy and McGill forceps should be used to remove the obstructive object. If this fails to relieve the obstruction, further options include cricothyrotomy or tracheostomy, depending on the location of the obstruction. Manual digital attempts to dislodge the object may be attempted if surgical airway interventions are not available.

G. Endotracheal intubation ensures a patent airway. Orotracheal intubation can be difficult or impossible without hyperextension of the neck, which is an impractical option with potential cervical spine injury. Alternative methods such as tactile intubation or blind oral intubation with a lighted stylet may be used. Nasotracheal intubation is an option with suspected associated cervical injury but is contraindicated with severe midfacial trauma and requires some spontaneous respiratory effort from the patient.

H. Once the patient has been intubated, placement must be verified with auscultation of bilateral lung fields to identify promptly right mainstem bronchus intubation or inadvertent esophageal intubation.

I. Cricothyrotomy is the fastest, safest surgical procedure for emergency airway management. It is indicated if all other attempts to establish an airway have failed or if status of the cervical spine is undetermined. Complications from emergency cricothyrotomy are rare, but it must be remembered that it does not protect against aspiration and is used only as a temporary airway until definitive measures are taken. The most common clinical indication for cricothyrotomy is the patient with massive facial trauma.

J. Emergency tracheostomy has limited indications for airway management because of potential complications, time, and skill required to complete the procedure. Tracheostomy is indicated with tracheal transection, severe anterior neck trauma, and pediatric patients who require a surgical airway (when the cricothyroid space is too small to insert an adequate size tube for effective ventilation).

References

Allo MD, Miller CF. Airway management. In: Zuidema GD, Rutherford RB, Ballinger W, eds. The management of trauma. Philadelphia: WB Saunders, 1985:379–390.

Callaham ML, ed. Current therapy in emergency medicine. Toronto: BC Decker, 1987:1–30.

Jorden RC, Rosen P. Airway management of the acutely injured. In: Moore EE, Eiseman B, Van Way CW, eds. Critical decisions in trauma. St. Louis: CV Mosby, 1984:128–131.

Menn SJ. Airway management. In: Kravis TC, Warner CG, eds. Emergency medicine. Rockville, MD: Aspen, 1983:821–830.

Moore EE. Resuscitation and evaluation of the injured patient. In: Zuidema GD, Rutherford RB, Ballinger W, eds. The management of trauma. Philadelphia: WB Saunders, 1985:1–26.

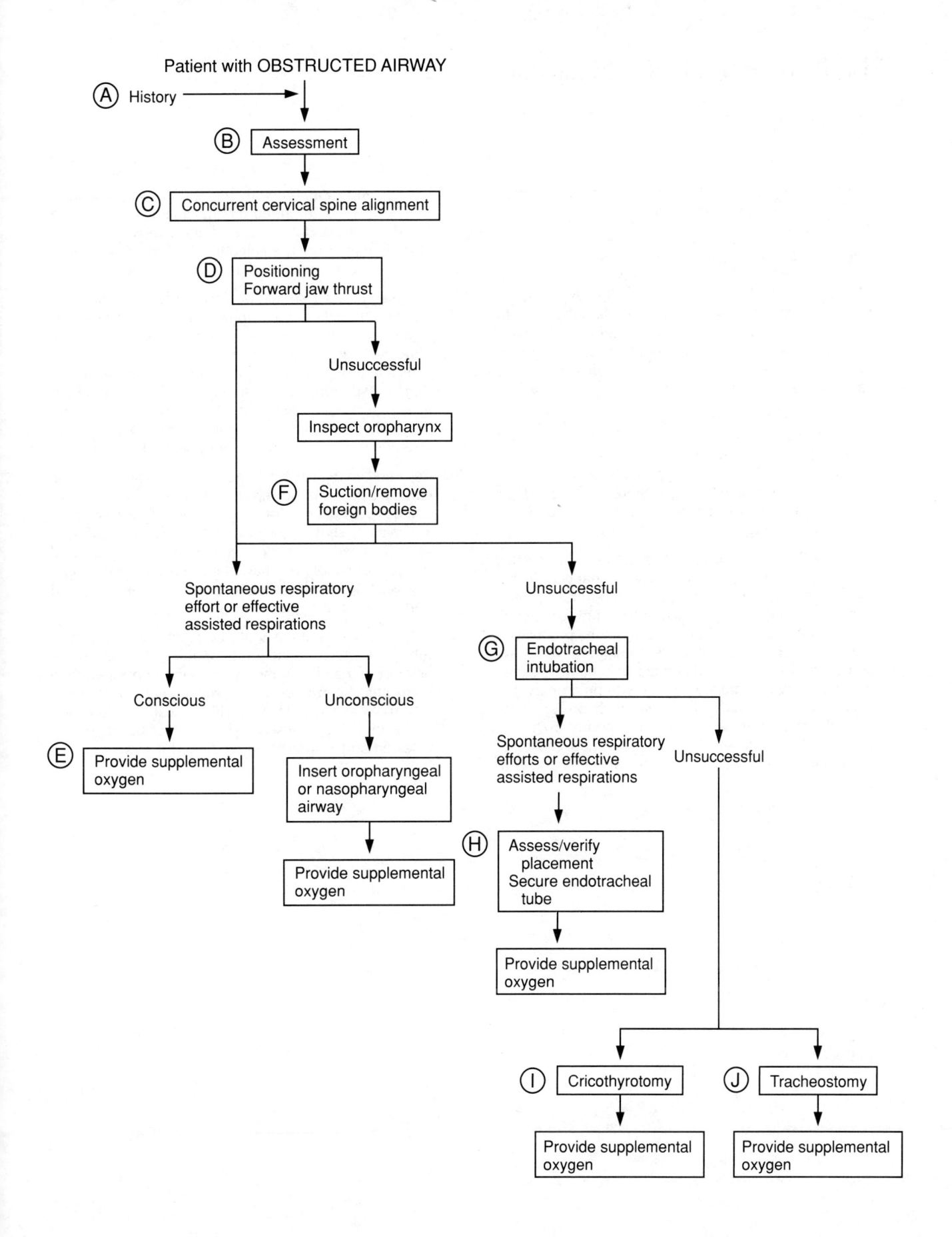

```
Patient with OBSTRUCTED AIRWAY
(A) History ─────────────▶
                    │
                    ▼
              (B) Assessment
                    │
                    ▼
   (C) Concurrent cervical spine alignment
                    │
                    ▼
         (D) Positioning
             Forward jaw thrust
                    │
          ┌─────────┴─────────┐
          │                   ▼
          │              Unsuccessful
          │                   │
          │                   ▼
          │           Inspect oropharynx
          │                   │
          │                   ▼
          │        (F) Suction/remove
          │            foreign bodies
          │                   │
          ▼                   ▼
  Spontaneous respiratory   Unsuccessful
  effort or effective           │
  assisted respirations         ▼
       │                  (G) Endotracheal
   ┌───┴────┐                  intubation
   ▼        ▼                     │
Conscious Unconscious      ┌──────┴──────┐
   │        │              ▼             ▼
   ▼        ▼         Spontaneous    Unsuccessful
(E) Provide  Insert oro-  respiratory
 supplemental pharyngeal  efforts or
 oxygen      or naso-     effective
             pharyngeal   assisted
             airway       respirations
               │              │
               ▼              ▼
           Provide       (H) Assess/verify
           supplemental      placement
           oxygen            Secure endotracheal
                             tube
                                │
                                ▼
                            Provide supplemental
                            oxygen
                                           │
                                    ┌──────┴──────┐
                                    ▼             ▼
                              (I) Cricothyrotomy (J) Tracheostomy
                                    │             │
                                    ▼             ▼
                              Provide         Provide
                              supplemental    supplemental
                              oxygen          oxygen
```

87

TENSION PNEUMOTHORAX

Lisa B. Jones

A. A patent upper airway is the first priority in a patient with suspected tension pneumothorax. It must be protected and maintained.

B. Adequate oxygenation and ventilation must include the delivery of adequate volume and inspired concentration of oxygen (e.g., FIO_2 greater than 0.85). A blood gas analysis should be obtained. The chest should be visually inspected both anteriorly and posteriorly. Signs of tracheal deviation, respiratory distress, unilateral absence of breath sounds, and distended neck veins are an indication of tension pneumothorax.

C. The patient with a normal respiratory status will have the primary and secondary initial assessment completed. If injuries that require hospitalization are identified, the patient and family should be prepared for admission. If no injuries that require hospitalization are identified, the patient should receive discharge instructions and be prepared for discharge.

D. A tension pneumothorax is a pneumothorax associated with progressive accumulation of air trapped in the pleural space. The pleural space is converted from a negative to an increasingly high positive pressure system that impairs venous return. The pressure produces a mediastinal shift that compresses the inferior vena cava as it passes through its diaphragmatic hiatus. A contralateral lung compression along with pulmonary collapse on the affected side results in hypoxia. These physiologic changes can result in hypoperfusion, hypoxia, and sudden death. The most common causes of tension pneumothorax are mechanical ventilation with positive end-expiratory pressure, spontaneous pneumothorax in which ruptured emphysematous bullae have failed to seal, and blunt chest trauma in which parenchymal lung injury has failed to seal. Tension pneumothorax is a clinical rather than a radiographic diagnosis.

E. The pleural space should be decompressed immediately with a needle thoracostomy. A needle is rapidly inserted into the second intercostal space in the midclavicular line of the affected hemithorax. This converts the tension pneumothorax into a simple pneumothorax. Aspirating with a syringe attached to a needle is helpful. The ability to aspirate air easily confirms the diagnosis. If air cannot be aspirated, withdraw the needle. The possibility of a subsequent pneumothorax exists.

F. Repeated reassessment is necessary. There should be clinical signs of improved respiratory exchange. Simultaneously the circulatory system should be evaluated. The patient should have cardiac monitoring and vital signs assessed. Two large bore intravenous lines should be established for potential volume replacement. A rapid assessment of the level of consciousness, skin color, and perfusion status should be done.

G. A tube thoracostomy should be performed. The chest tube is inserted into the fourth or fifth intercostal space, anterior midaxillary line. The chest tube should be connected to an underwater seal apparatus with 20 to 30 cm of water suction. This will re-expand the lung and drain any blood present. The patient should be reassessed and resuscitation continued if indicated.

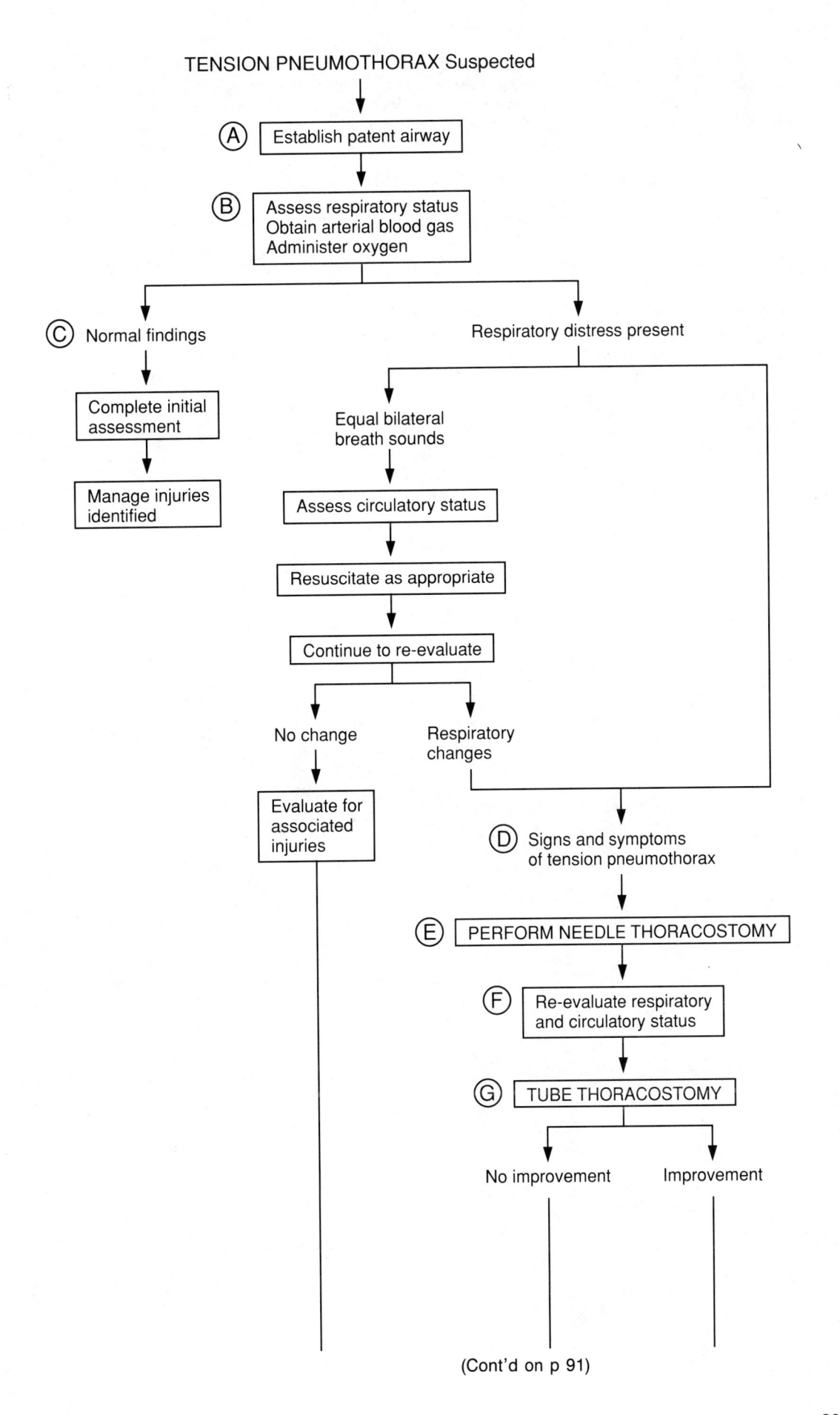

TENSION PNEUMOTHORAX Suspected

- (A) Establish patent airway
- (B) Assess respiratory status
  Obtain arterial blood gas
  Administer oxygen

(C) Normal findings
- Complete initial assessment
- Manage injuries identified

Respiratory distress present

Equal bilateral breath sounds
- Assess circulatory status
- Resuscitate as appropriate
- Continue to re-evaluate
  - No change → Evaluate for associated injuries
  - Respiratory changes

- (D) Signs and symptoms of tension pneumothorax
- (E) PERFORM NEEDLE THORACOSTOMY
- (F) Re-evaluate respiratory and circulatory status
- (G) TUBE THORACOSTOMY
  - No improvement
  - Improvement

(Cont'd on p 91)

H. Respiratory distress and tension pneumothorax may be confused with cardiac tamponade or massive hemothorax. If management of tension pneumothorax does not demonstrate an immediate clinical improvement, these injuries must be ruled out.

I. Obtain a chest film following chest tube insertion. The lung should rapidly re-expand. The air leak will be minimal unless associated injuries such as ruptured bronchus, lacerated lung, or esophageal perforation are present. If an air leak remains, these injuries must be ruled out.

J. The patient should have ongoing assessment and evaluation. Continuous cardiac monitoring, reassessment of vital signs, and continued resuscitation are imperative. A complete head-to-toe examination should be done to identify all suspected injuries.

K. The history should include the mechanism of injury, to assist in identifying any occult or associated injuries, and any pre-existing heart, lung, arterial, or renal disease that may complicate the hospital course. All routine medications and allergies must be addressed. The time of the last meal and any previous surgeries should be identified. The patient and family should be prepared for hospital admission. An explanation of the resuscitation and hospital course should be given to the patient and family.

References

Baxt W. Trauma: the first hour. Norwalk, CT: Appleton-Century-Crofts, 1985:111–114.

Knezevich B. Trauma nursing principles and practice. Norwalk, CT: Appleton-Century-Crofts, 1986:91–92.

Shires T. Principles of trauma care. New York: McGraw-Hill, 1985:267–274.

Strange J. Shock trauma care plans. Springhouse, PA: Springhouse, 1987:62–64.

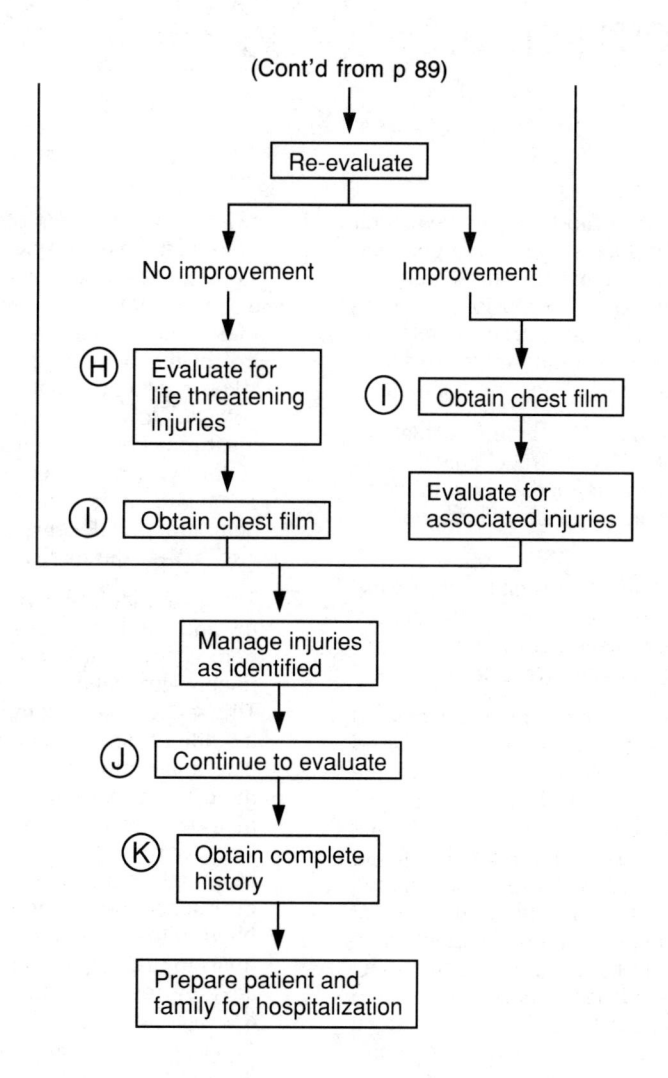

(Cont'd from p 89)
↓
Re-evaluate
├── No improvement
│   Ⓗ Evaluate for life threatening injuries
│   ↓
│   Ⓘ Obtain chest film
└── Improvement
    Ⓘ Obtain chest film
    ↓
    Evaluate for associated injuries

↓
Manage injuries as identified
↓
Ⓙ Continue to evaluate
↓
Ⓚ Obtain complete history
↓
Prepare patient and family for hospitalization

MASSIVE HEMOTHORAX

Gregory G. Stanford

A. A hemothorax is a collection of blood within the pleural space. The bleeding can be caused by blunt or penetrating chest trauma. In blunt trauma, the most frequent cause of bleeding is a pulmonary contusion; however, major and minor parenchymal injuries can lacerate pulmonary arteries and veins. Penetrating injuries usually result in direct damage to the pulmonary vasculature.

B. After an airway has been established, assess ventilation. If ventilation is inadequate, institute mechanical ventilation. Start fluid resuscitation immediately with blood given if there is no immediate response to fluid administration.

C. If the patient responds to fluid administration, the secondary survey should be completed. Baseline laboratory tests should be obtained. Constant reassessment is necessary to detect any change in cardiovascular status.

D. A hemothorax can be detected on a finding of decreased breath sounds and dullness to percussion in the involved hemithorax. Confirmatory evidence comes from the chest film; however, the radiograph is not necessary to make the diagnosis, and those patients who are unstable should have a chest tube placed immediately without waiting for the film. About 500 ml of blood are required to detect a hemothorax on the chest film. This amount of blood obliterates the lateral sulcus on the upright film. With supine patients, a hemothorax appears as a distinct haziness when the involved hemithorax is compared with the other hemithorax. If the patient has bilateral hemothoraces, the diagnosis can be very difficult. If possible, a lateral decubitus radiograph will demonstrate the blood in the chest, or a thoracentesis can be performed.

E. Those patients who have overt or impending cardiovascular collapse should have an emergency thoracotomy performed as a potentially life saving procedure. These patients have great vessel or cardiac injuries and rapidly exsanguinate into the chest unless the bleeding can be controlled immediately. Patients with suspected air embolism should also have an immediate thoracotomy for control of the hilar vessels. The thoracotomy should be performed immediately without attempting to transfer the patient to the operating room. Control of the hemorrhage should be obtained and the patient taken to the operating room for definitive treatment. This aggressive approach salvages the rare patient; most of these patients, however, have lethal injuries. Mechanisms are now available to retrieve in a sterile manner shed blood for reinfusion. These autotransfusion devices are safe and inexpensive and should be considered in those patients with continued blood loss from a hemothorax.

F. In the remaining patients, a large bore chest tube (larger than 36 F) should be placed. The optimal location is the fifth or sixth intercostal space at the anterior axillary line. This position allows adequate drainage and rapid placement. The tube should be directed posteriorly and superiorly. Placement in the posterior sulcus would provide the best drainage, but correct positioning is difficult in an acute situation, and the tube is frequently bent or twisted in futile attempts to reach the most dependent point in the pleural space. If the patient has greater than 1,000 ml of blood in the pleural space, there is usually a significant vascular injury to the great vessels or lung that cannot be expected to resolve without surgical control of the bleeding points. These patients should be taken expeditiously to the operating room for a thoracotomy. Occasionally, patients are transferred from other institutions or are otherwise several hours past the time of injury; a short period of observation is warranted. Some patients go into cardiovascular collapse when the hemothorax is decompressed, and these patients should also have an immediate thoracotomy.

G. The great majority of patients do not require thoracotomy and can be managed by chest tube drainage of the hemothorax. The chest tube should be connected to an underwater seal that prevents air from entering the chest. This seal can be accomplished by placing the tube into a bottle of sterile water with the water height placed at 20 cm. It is more easily performed, however, with commercial chest drainage systems that also provide a method of collecting the drainage without changing the negative pressure applied to the tube. Negative pressure is applied to the chest by maintaining a 20 cm column of water above the opening of the tube. Suction is applied to the air above the water level for a period of 24 hours to maintain a constant pressure to the chest, which aids in removing the blood and tamponading the damaged lung parenchyma. After 24 hours, external suction is removed, and the negative pressure is maintained by the water seal. If the patient has an air leak, external suction should be maintained until the air leak seals. When the daily drainage falls below 50 to 100 ml, the chest tube can be safely removed.

H. Continued bleeding from the chest tube may necessitate thoracotomy to control hemorrhage. The usual guidelines are to perform a thoracotomy on those patients with greater than 1,500 ml of output over the first 24 hours (not including the blood in the chest at the time the tube was placed), patients with greater than 500 ml of blood output for more than 1 hour, and patients with a continuous output of more than 200 ml of blood for 6 or more hours. These guidelines are not absolute and do not replace good surgical judgment.

I. If the unstable patient responds to resuscitation, a thorough search for associated injuries should be performed. All life threatening injuries should be treated when they are identified. Constant attention to chest tube output and vital signs is necessary to detect a deterioration in the patient's condition.

References

Blaisdell FW. Pneumothorax and hemothorax. In: Blaisdell FW, Trunkey DD, eds. Cervicothoracic trauma. New York: Thieme, 1986:157–165.

Gay WA, McCabe JR. Trauma to the chest. In: Shires GT, ed. Principles of trauma care. New York: McGraw-Hill, 1985:232–266.

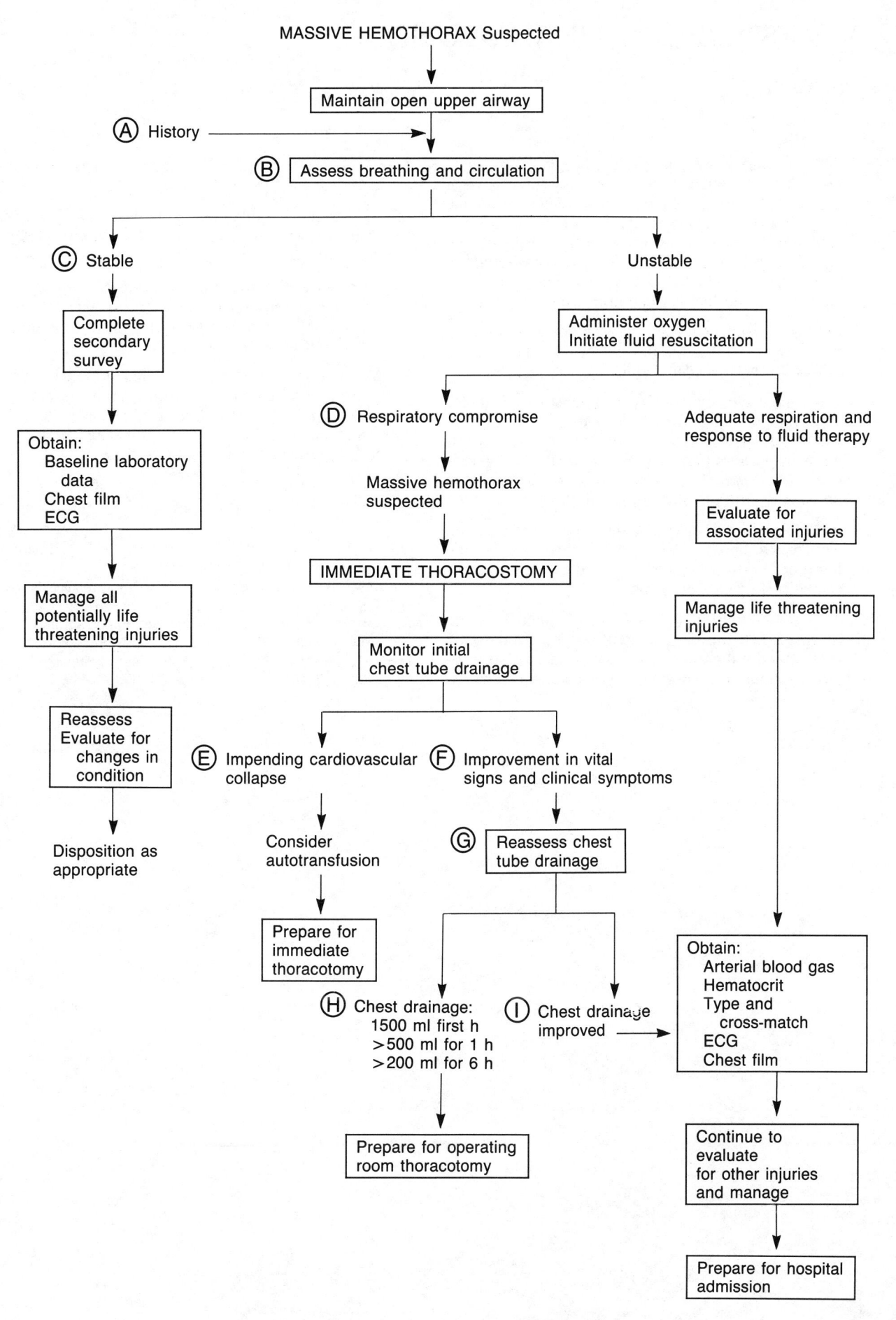

```
                    MASSIVE HEMOTHORAX Suspected
                                │
                                ▼
                    ┌─────────────────────────┐
   Ⓐ History ──────▶│ Maintain open upper airway │
                    └─────────────────────────┘
                                │
                                ▼
                    ┌─────────────────────────┐
                 Ⓑ │ Assess breathing and circulation │
                    └─────────────────────────┘
                       │                    │
            Ⓒ Stable  ▼                    ▼  Unstable
         ┌──────────────┐           ┌──────────────────────┐
         │ Complete     │           │ Administer oxygen    │
         │ secondary    │           │ Initiate fluid       │
         │ survey       │           │ resuscitation        │
         └──────────────┘           └──────────────────────┘
                │                       │                │
                ▼             Ⓓ Respiratory   Adequate respiration and
         ┌──────────────┐     compromise        response to fluid therapy
         │ Obtain:      │           │                │
         │ Baseline lab │           ▼                ▼
         │  data        │    Massive hemothorax  ┌──────────────┐
         │ Chest film   │    suspected           │ Evaluate for │
         │ ECG          │           │            │ associated   │
         └──────────────┘           ▼            │ injuries     │
                │          ┌─────────────────┐  └──────────────┘
                ▼          │ IMMEDIATE       │        │
         ┌──────────────┐  │ THORACOSTOMY    │        ▼
         │ Manage all   │  └─────────────────┘  ┌──────────────┐
         │ potentially  │           │           │ Manage life  │
         │ life         │           ▼           │ threatening  │
         │ threatening  │   ┌──────────────┐    │ injuries     │
         │ injuries     │   │ Monitor initial│  └──────────────┘
         └──────────────┘   │ chest tube    │          │
                │           │ drainage      │          │
                ▼           └──────────────┘           │
         ┌──────────────┐      │         │             │
         │ Reassess     │      ▼         ▼             │
         │ Evaluate for │ Ⓔ Impending  Ⓕ Improvement in│
         │ changes in   │ cardiovascular  vital         │
         │ condition    │ collapse    signs and clinical│
         └──────────────┘      │       symptoms         │
                │              ▼         │              │
                ▼         ┌──────────┐   ▼              │
          Disposition as  │ Consider │ Ⓖ┌────────────┐  │
          appropriate     │autotrans-│  │ Reassess   │  │
                          │ fusion   │  │ chest tube │  │
                          └──────────┘  │ drainage   │  │
                               │        └────────────┘  │
                               ▼           │      │     │
                          ┌──────────┐     │      │     │
                          │ Prepare  │     │      │     │
                          │ for      │     │      │     │
                          │ immediate│     │      │     │
                          │thoracotomy│    │      │     │
                          └──────────┘     │      │     │
                               │           │      │     │
                          Ⓗ Chest drainage:│     Ⓘ Chest drainage
                          1500 ml first h  │      improved ──────▶┌──────────────┐
                          >500 ml for 1 h  │                      │ Obtain:      │
                          >200 ml for 6 h  │                      │  Arterial    │
                               │           │                      │   blood gas  │
                               ▼           │                      │  Hematocrit  │
                          ┌──────────┐     │                      │  Type and    │
                          │ Prepare  │     │                      │   cross-match│
                          │ for      │     │                      │  ECG         │
                          │ operating│     │                      │  Chest film  │
                          │ room     │     │                      └──────────────┘
                          │thoracotomy│    │                             │
                          └──────────┘     │                             ▼
                                                                  ┌──────────────┐
                                                                  │ Continue to  │
                                                                  │ evaluate     │
                                                                  │ for other    │
                                                                  │ injuries     │
                                                                  │ and manage   │
                                                                  └──────────────┘
                                                                         │
                                                                         ▼
                                                                  ┌──────────────┐
                                                                  │ Prepare for  │
                                                                  │ hospital     │
                                                                  │ admission    │
                                                                  └──────────────┘
```

OPEN SUCKING CHEST WOUND

Jane Curran

A. Open sucking chest injuries occur secondary to penetrating trauma. An open chest wound allows free passage of air into and out of the pleural space. Effective ventilation is impaired, leading to hypoxia and hemodynamic compromise. A complete history must be taken, including the mechanism of injury (e.g., gunshot wound). Information to be illicited includes the type and size of the weapon and the distance from which it was fired.

B. As with all trauma patients, arterial blood gases must be rapidly assessed. The first priority is to maintain respiratory and cardiovascular stability.

C. The patient who presents with subcutaneous emphysema, dyspnea, tachycardia, decreased breath sounds, and the sound of air being sucked into the chest requires immediate intervention. Immediate treatment involves covering the wound with a sterile three corner occlusive dressing to stop the air from rushing in.

D. A complete blood cell count, electrolytes, and type and cross-match should be obtained simultaneously with the insertion of two large bore peripheral intravenous catheters (16 gauge or greater).

E. A chest tube must be inserted on the injured side, and a sterile airtight dressing should be applied. If the wound is large and if there is a continual air leak or an intrathoracic injury is suspected, a thoracotomy is required to repair the damage. The patient is transported emergently to the operating room.

F. The patient is admitted to the hospital, respiratory status is assessed frequently, and serial chest films are completed.

G. Management of a hemothorax involves inserting a chest tube and connecting the chest tube to 20 cm of suction. Autotransfusion immediately provides the patient with typed and cross-matched blood.

H. When a massive hemothorax (greater than 1500 ml) is present or when the chest tube output is greater than 200 ml per hour for 4 hours, major damage to the systemic and vascular system is suspected. The patient is taken immediately for a thoracotomy.

References

Cowley RA, Dunham MC. Shock trauma/critical care handbook. Rockville, MD: Aspen, 1988:145–187.

Knezevich B. Trauma nursing principles and practice. Norwalk, CT: Appleton-Century-Crofts, 1986:73–99.

Langfett D. Critical care certification, preparation, and review. Bowie, MD: Brady Communications, 1984:79–85.

Perdue P. Chest trauma. Cardona V, ed. Trauma nursing. Oradell, NJ: Medical Economics Books, 1985:123–139.

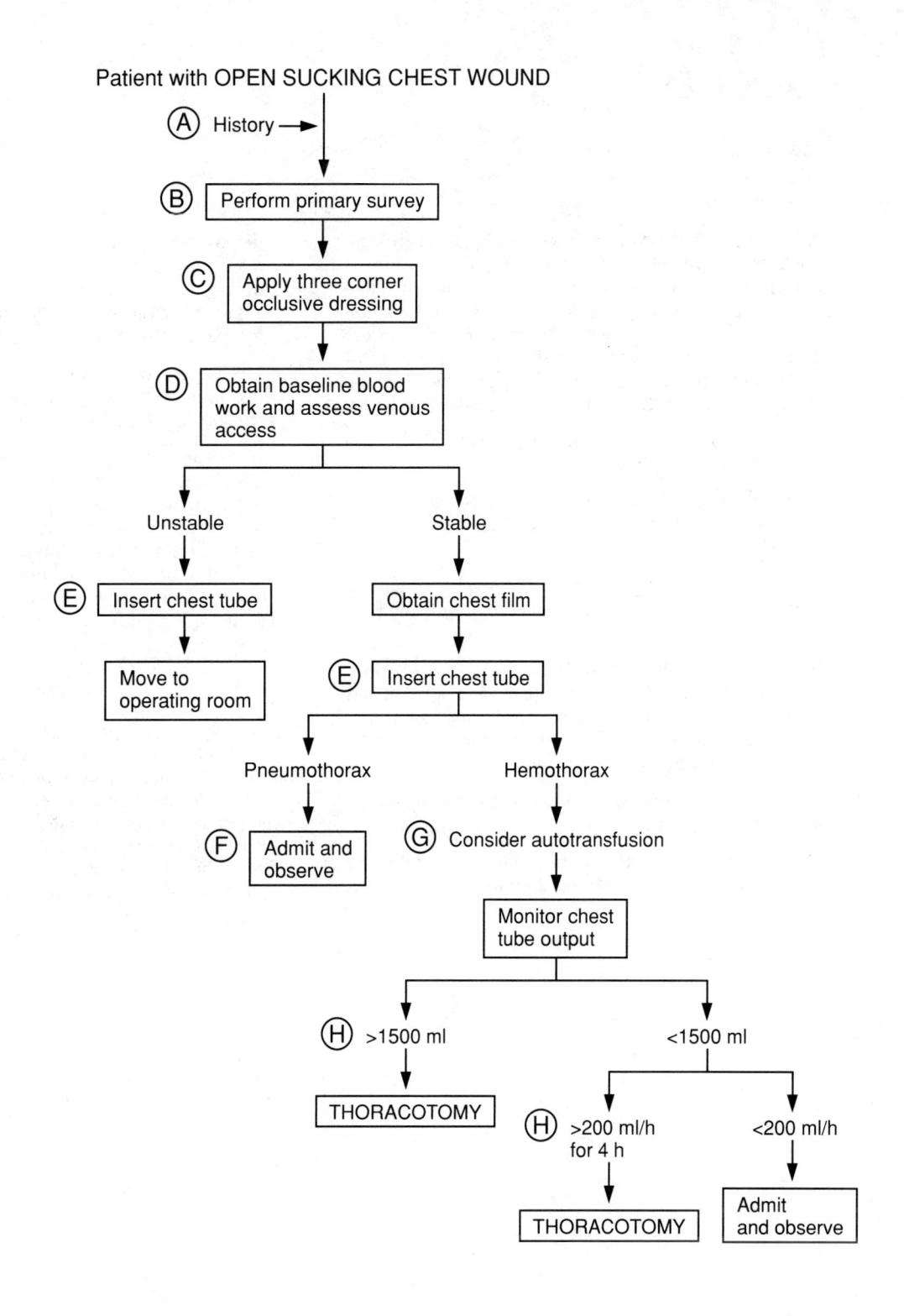

```
Patient with OPEN SUCKING CHEST WOUND
                 Ⓐ History ──→
                              ↓
                 Ⓑ  ┌─────────────────────┐
                    │ Perform primary survey│
                    └─────────────────────┘
                              ↓
                 Ⓒ  ┌─────────────────────┐
                    │ Apply three corner   │
                    │ occlusive dressing   │
                    └─────────────────────┘
                              ↓
                 Ⓓ  ┌─────────────────────┐
                    │ Obtain baseline blood│
                    │ work and assess venous│
                    │ access               │
                    └─────────────────────┘
                        ↓           ↓
                    Unstable       Stable
                        ↓           ↓
              Ⓔ ┌──────────────┐  ┌──────────────┐
                │Insert chest tube│ │Obtain chest film│
                └──────────────┘  └──────────────┘
                        ↓                ↓
                ┌──────────────┐  Ⓔ ┌──────────────┐
                │ Move to      │     │Insert chest tube│
                │ operating room│    └──────────────┘
                └──────────────┘      ↓           ↓
                                Pneumothorax  Hemothorax
                                      ↓           ↓
                              Ⓕ ┌─────────┐  Ⓖ Consider autotransfusion
                                │Admit and│           ↓
                                │observe  │     ┌──────────────┐
                                └─────────┘     │Monitor chest │
                                                │tube output   │
                                                └──────────────┘
                                                   ↓        ↓
                                            Ⓗ >1500 ml   <1500 ml
                                               ↓         ↓        ↓
                                          ┌──────────┐  Ⓗ>200 ml/h  <200 ml/h
                                          │THORACOTOMY│   for 4 h     ↓
                                          └──────────┘      ↓      ┌────────┐
                                                       ┌──────────┐│Admit   │
                                                       │THORACOTOMY││and observe│
                                                       └──────────┘└────────┘
```

FLAIL CHEST

Jane Curran

A. A flail chest develops if two or more adjacent ribs are fractured in two or more places or if the sternum is detached. The involved segment of the chest is unstable and has paradoxical movement, which results in impaired ventilation. As with all trauma patients, the mechanism must be ascertained if possible. The most common mechanisms of injury for a flail chest include motor vehicle accidents, falls, and aggravated assaults.

B. Two large bore peripheral intravenous (IV) catheters are inserted (16 gauge or larger).

C. A complete blood cell count with differential, electrolytes, type and cross-match, drug screen, and alcohol level should be obtained.

D. A baseline arterial blood gas (ABG) level is obtained, preferably on room air. These results determine the path of treatment.

E. All patients with flail chest do not require intubation. The patient is placed on 40 percent oxygen by mask and assessed frequently for hypoxia. This injury does not itself cause hypoxia; rather, it is damage to the underlying lung tissue that is the concern.

F. The IV fluid rate must be maintained at a keep open rate to avoid overhydration.

G. The patient's ABG levels must be evaluated carefully and frequently. The blunt force required for the injury predisposes the patient to pulmonary contusion, adult respiratory distress syndrome (ARDS), and/or cardiac contusion. Therefore, a chest film and ABG evaluation are a daily necessity. On the first sign of respiratory change, the patient must be re-evaluated.

H. The patient with hypoxia is defined as having a Pao_2 less than 60, $PaCO_2$ greater than 50, and/or respiratory rate greater than 25, on 40 percent oxygen concentration.

I. The patient is intubated and placed on a volume ventilator. Depending on the depths of hypoxia and the decrease in compliance, positive end-expiratory pressure may be employed. A Swan Ganz catheter is inserted to assess fluid status. The lungs are sensitive to either overhydration or underhydration, and a flail chest injury predisposes the patient to ARDS. The ultimate goal of treatment is prevention of hypoxia.

References

Cowley RA, Dunham MC. Shock trauma/critical care handbook. Rockville, MD: Aspen, 1988:145–187.

Knezevich B. Trauma nursing principles and practice. Norwalk, CT: Appleton-Century-Crofts, 1986:73–99.

Langfett D. Critical care certification, preparation, and review. Bowie, MD: Brady Communications, 1984:79–85.

Perdue P. Chest trauma. Cardona V, ed. Trauma nursing. Oradell, NJ: Medical Economics Books, 1985:123–139.

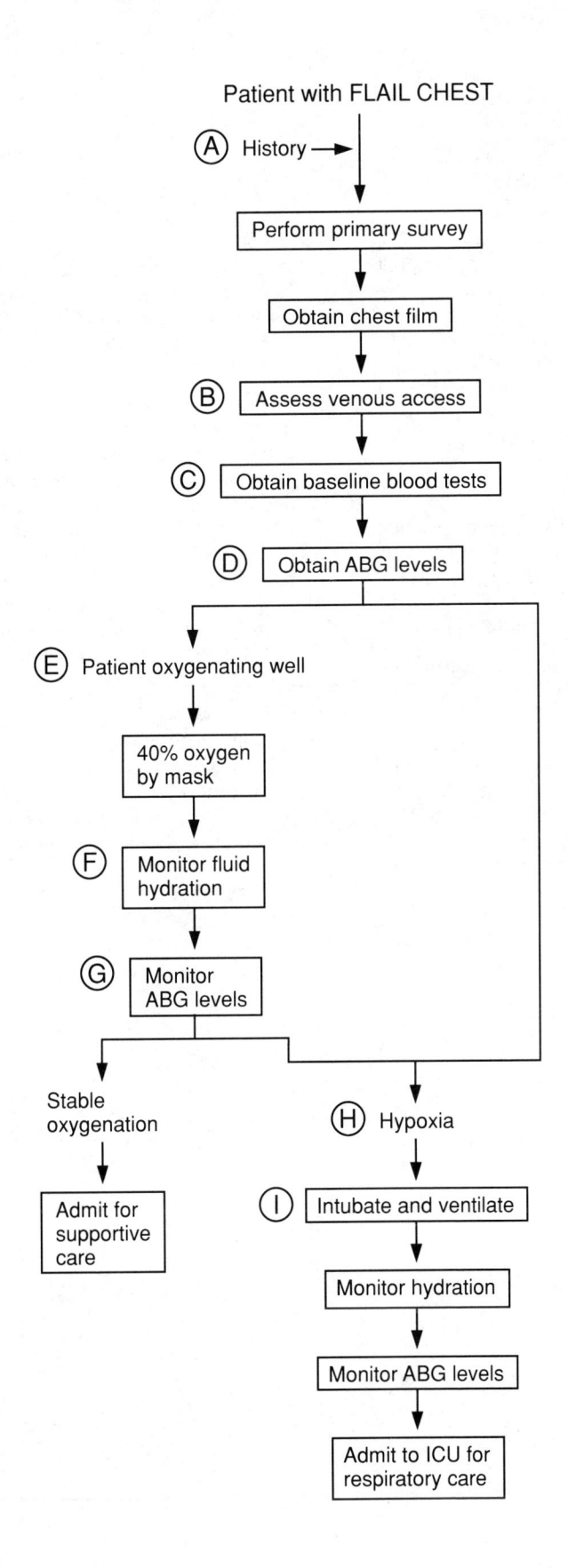

```
Patient with FLAIL CHEST
         │
    Ⓐ History →
         ↓
  ┌──────────────────┐
  │ Perform primary survey │
  └──────────────────┘
         ↓
  ┌──────────────────┐
  │ Obtain chest film │
  └──────────────────┘
         ↓
  Ⓑ ┌──────────────────┐
    │ Assess venous access │
    └──────────────────┘
         ↓
  Ⓒ ┌──────────────────┐
    │ Obtain baseline blood tests │
    └──────────────────┘
         ↓
  Ⓓ ┌──────────────────┐
    │ Obtain ABG levels │
    └──────────────────┘
         ↓
  Ⓔ Patient oxygenating well
         ↓
  ┌──────────────────┐
  │ 40% oxygen by mask │
  └──────────────────┘
         ↓
  Ⓕ ┌──────────────────┐
    │ Monitor fluid hydration │
    └──────────────────┘
         ↓
  Ⓖ ┌──────────────────┐
    │ Monitor ABG levels │
    └──────────────────┘
         ↓                        ↓
  Stable oxygenation        Ⓗ Hypoxia
         ↓                        ↓
  ┌──────────────────┐    Ⓘ ┌──────────────────┐
  │ Admit for        │      │ Intubate and ventilate │
  │ supportive care  │      └──────────────────┘
  └──────────────────┘              ↓
                            ┌──────────────────┐
                            │ Monitor hydration │
                            └──────────────────┘
                                    ↓
                            ┌──────────────────┐
                            │ Monitor ABG levels │
                            └──────────────────┘
                                    ↓
                            ┌──────────────────┐
                            │ Admit to ICU for  │
                            │ respiratory care  │
                            └──────────────────┘
```

CARDIAC TAMPONADE

Lisa B. Jones

A. Cardiac tamponade can be an injury or a symptom that is life threatening and requires immediate treatment. Cardiac tamponade most commonly results from penetrating injuries. Penetrating injuries to the "box" (sternal notch, nipple line to the subxyphoid process) should create a high index of suspicion for major vessel and heart injuries. Blunt injury may also cause the pericardium to fill with blood from the heart or great vessels. A complete history of the mechanism of injury should be obtained.

B. The upper airway should be assessed to ascertain patency and be secured. Specific attention should be given to the possibility of cervical spine fractures. Adequate oxygenation and ventilation must include the delivery of adequate volume and inspired concentrations of oxygen.

C. Rapid and accurate assessment of the trauma patient's hemodynamic status is essential. The state of consciousness, skin color, and heart rate should be immediately assessed. Rapid, thready pulses are early signs of hypovolemia. An irregular pulse is usually a warning of cardiac impairment. Absent central pulses at more than one site, without local injuries or other factors that preclude accurate palpation, signify the need for immediate resuscitative measures. The patient should have continuous cardiac monitoring.

D. Patients who arrive hemodynamically stable but who have a history of mechanism of injury that is significant to produce injury must have a complete initial assessment. Monitor closely for any changes in hemodynamic stability. All potential injuries must be ruled out.

E. If hemodynamic instability is identified, shock management must be initiated. Two large caliber intravenous catheters must be established for rapid crystalloid and blood administration. Blood should be drawn for type and cross-match and for baseline data (e.g., hematocrit [HCT]). Adequate resuscitation is assessed by improvement of physiologic parameters (i.e., respiratory rate, heart rate, blood pressure, pulse pressure, arterial blood gases [ABGs], and urinary output). Electromechanical dissociation may indicate a cardiac tamponade, tension pneumothorax, and profound hypovolemia.

F. Cardiac arrest on admission or shortly before demands that aggressive resuscitation measures be initiated. Cardiopulmonary resuscitation (CPR) is initiated with manual compression. Two large bore peripheral intravenous lines should be placed for rapid volume replacement with warmed fluid and blood. An ABG level should be obtained on arrival to identify base deficit.

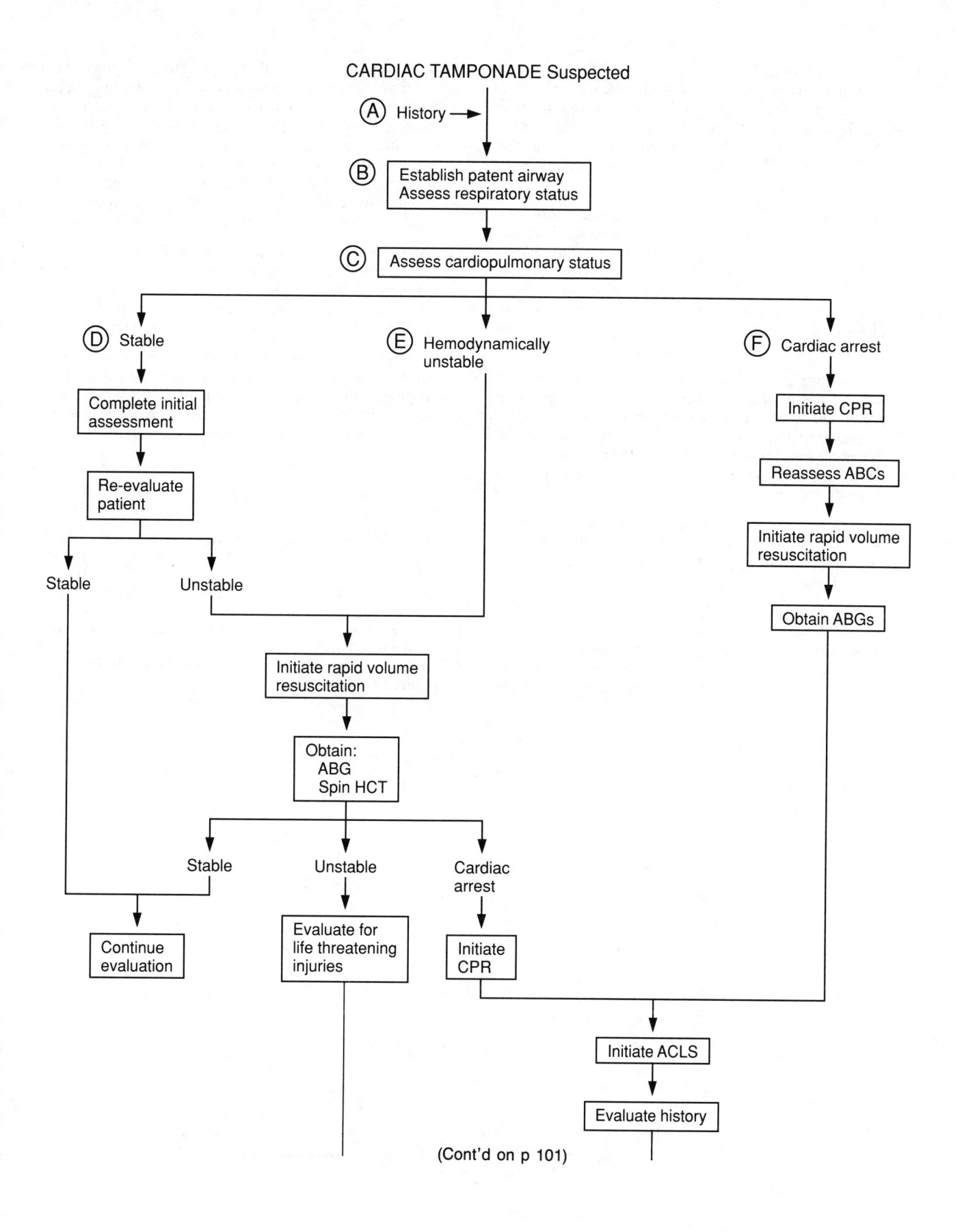

CARDIAC TAMPONADE Suspected

- **A** History →
- **B** Establish patent airway / Assess respiratory status
- **C** Assess cardiopulmonary status

D Stable
- Complete initial assessment
- Re-evaluate patient
  - **Stable** → Continue evaluation
  - **Unstable** → (see below)

E Hemodynamically unstable
- Initiate rapid volume resuscitation
- Obtain: ABG, Spin HCT
  - **Stable** → Continue evaluation
  - **Unstable** → Evaluate for life threatening injuries (Cont'd on p 101)
  - **Cardiac arrest** → Initiate CPR → Initiate ACLS → Evaluate history

F Cardiac arrest
- Initiate CPR
- Reassess ABCs
- Initiate rapid volume resuscitation
- Obtain ABGs
- Initiate ACLS
- Evaluate history

G. If cardiac tamponade is the suspected cause of hemodynamic instability, a pericardiocentesis is the immediate diagnostic tool. An 18-gauge over-the-needle 3-inch catheter attached to a stopcock is inserted below or along the left side of the xyphoid process into the pericardial sac. The pericardiocentesis is positive if nonclotting blood is aspirated.

H. Pericardiocentesis may be falsely negative. The needle may become obstructed on penetration. Pericardial aspiration may not be diagnostic or therapeutic if the blood in the pericardial sac is clotted, which might be the case after rapid bleeding. If findings are negative, the mechanism of injury and clinical symptoms are used to indicate the need for further diagnostic studies, or the negative pericardiocentesis results are accepted.

I. If the history for a cardiac tamponade is not present and the negative pericardiocentesis findings are accepted, a continued evaluation must be done. The airway, breathing, and circulation (ABCs) must be reassessed. All life threatening and potentially life threatening injuries must be identified and managed. A complete assessment and ongoing monitoring are imperative.

J. If any heart wound is suspected, a subxyphoid window is the treatment of choice. If definitive findings of tamponade are present, direct thoracotomy should be performed immediately.

K. Cardiac tamponade should be suspected in patients with inappropriately low cardiac performance in relationship to injuries. Beck's triad—systemic hypotension, muffled heart sounds, and elevated venous pressure reflected in neck vein distention—comprises the classic symptoms of cardiac tamponade. Pulsus paradoxus of greater than 15 mm Hg during inspiration is a significant finding but may be difficult to measure during a trauma resuscitation. An elevated central venous pressure, narrowed pulse pressure, and decreased cardiac output may be present. The electrocardiogram may demonstrate low voltage complexes. If the clinical symptoms of a cardiac tamponade are evident, the patient should be prepared for an immediate operating room (OR) thoracotomy.

L. An immediate OR thoracotomy is indicated in the case of a positive pericardiocentesis. The patient should be reassessed and closely monitored enroute to the OR. Aspiration of even a small amount of blood from the pericardial sac greatly improves cardiac output.

M. Emergency thoracotomy for trauma should be attempted in those patients with electrical activity either in the hospital or prehospital. Those patients presenting with agonal rhythm or rapidly deteriorating hemodynamic status have a more successful outcome.

References

American College of Surgeons. Advanced trauma life support course. Chicago: American College of Surgeons, 1989:97–98.

Baxt W. Trauma, the first hour. Norwalk, CT: Appleton-Century-Crofts, 1985.

Moylan J. Trauma surgery. Philadelphia: JB Lippincott, 1988:106–109.

Shires T. Principles of trauma care. New York: McGraw-Hill, 1985:274–286.

(Cont'd from p 99)

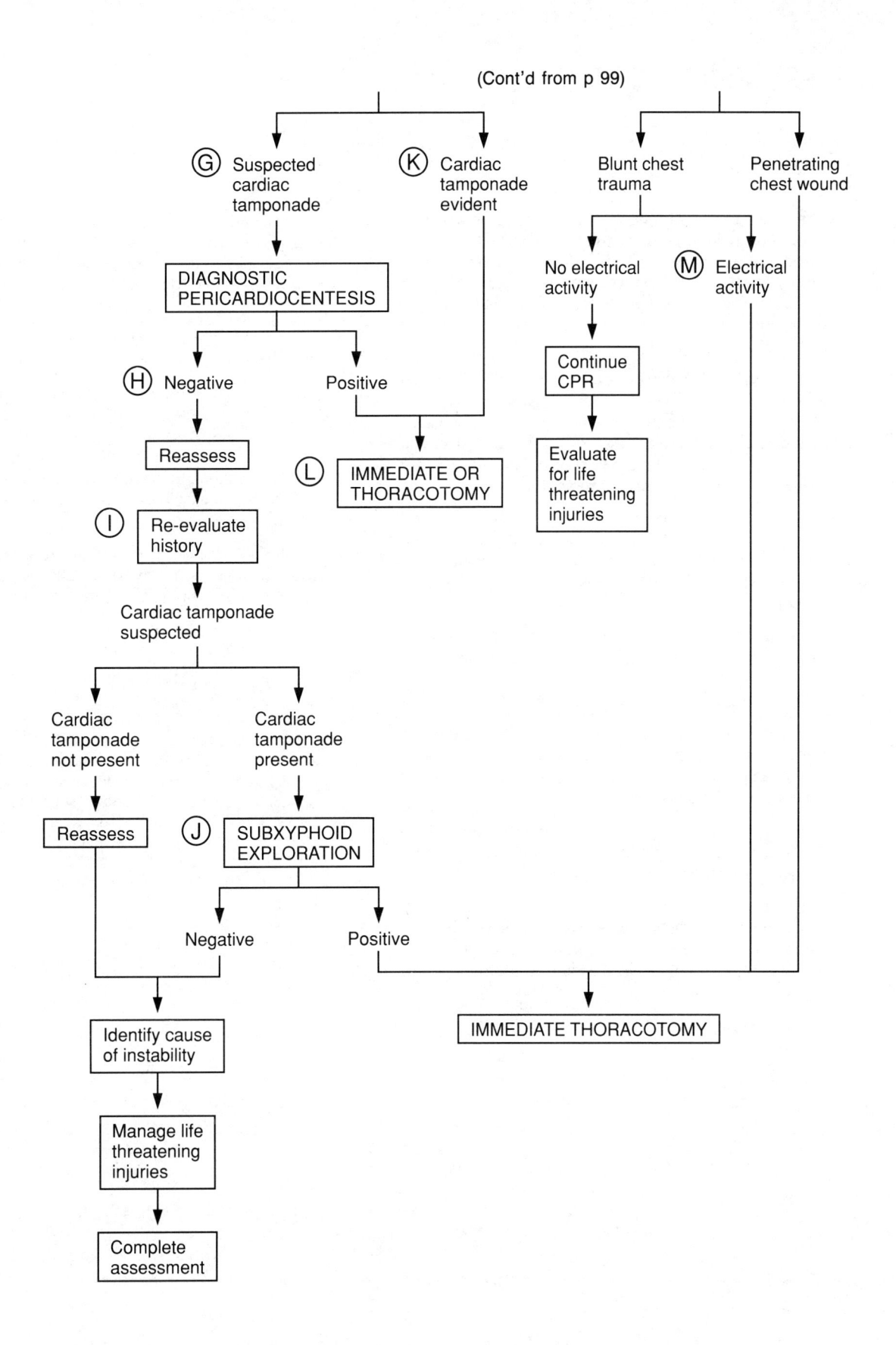

- **G** Suspected cardiac tamponade → **DIAGNOSTIC PERICARDIOCENTESIS**
  - **H** Negative → Reassess → **I** Re-evaluate history → Cardiac tamponade suspected
    - Cardiac tamponade not present → Reassess → Identify cause of instability → Manage life threatening injuries → Complete assessment
    - Cardiac tamponade present → **J** SUBXYPHOID EXPLORATION
      - Negative → Identify cause of instability (as above)
      - Positive → IMMEDIATE THORACOTOMY
  - Positive → **L** IMMEDIATE OR THORACOTOMY

- **K** Cardiac tamponade evident → **L** IMMEDIATE OR THORACOTOMY

- Blunt chest trauma
  - No electrical activity → Continue CPR → Evaluate for life threatening injuries
  - **M** Electrical activity → IMMEDIATE THORACOTOMY

- Penetrating chest wound → IMMEDIATE THORACOTOMY

EMERGENCY THORACOTOMY

John D. S. Reid

A. Emergency thoracotomy for trauma should be attempted only in those patients with signs of life either at the hospital or when in close proximity to the hospital with rapid transport. It is likely to be more successful in penetrating trauma than in blunt trauma and in those patients who are agonal or have rapidly deteriorating vital signs despite adequate resuscitation.

B. Subxyphoid pericardiocentesis may be helpful in those patients with cardiac tamponade. However, this is only a temporary measure that allows the patient to be transported to the operative room (OR) for thoracotomy. If there is no response to pericardiocentesis, the patient should undergo emergency thoracotomy.

C. A left fourth interspace thoracotomy is performed after rapid preparation of the skin. This is usually done at the level of the nipple and carried across and toward the axilla. A rib spreading retractor is required after the chest is opened.

D. The initial maneuver is cross-clamping of the descending thoracic aorta using a suitable vascular clamp.

E. If there is massive hemorrhage from the lung itself, it may be controlled by cross-clamping the entire hilum of the lung with a vascular clamp. If massive hemorrhage is coming from any of the great vessels inside the chest, manual compression and rapid transport to the OR for repair should be attempted.

F. If there is a penetrating cardiac injury, pericardial tamponade, or cardiac arrest, the pericardial sac should be opened with scissors anterior to the phrenic nerve.

G. If visualization is inadequate, or if there is a right chest injury, the thoracotomy may be extended across the sternum with a suitable bone cutting instrument (e.g., Lebsche knife or Gigli's wire saw) into the right chest.

H. If there is a penetrating injury to the heart, this should first be occluded manually or with an inflated Foley catheter balloon and then closed using pledgetted sutures. Cardiac massage, fluid resuscitation, and defibrillation should be continued as necessary. Inotropic drugs should be avoided to prevent rupture of the repaired area.

I. If there is no apparent injury or diffuse cardiac injury, fluid resuscitation, cardiac massage, cardiac drugs, and defibrillation should be continued as necessary.

J. If there is no abnormality of the heart itself and if cardiac activity is present, continue fluid resuscitation, cardiac massage, cardiac drugs, and defibrillation as necessary. Treatment should be directed toward conditions precipitating the cardiovascular collapse (e.g., massive hemorrhage from extremity trauma or cardiac arrest prior to traumatic event).

K. If there is a response to cardiac massage, the patient should be moved rapidly to the OR for definitive repair of injuries, declamping of the thoracic aorta, and closure of the chest.

References

Feliciano DV, Bitondo CG, Cruse PA. Liberal use of emergency center thoracotomy. Am J Surg 1986; 151:654–659.

Moreno C, Moore EE, Majure JA, Hopeman AR. Pericardial tamponade: a critical determinant for survival following penetrating cardiac wounds. J Trauma 1986; 26:821–825.

Schwab CW, Adcock OT, Max MH. Emergency department thoracotomy (EDT). A 26-month experience using an "agonal" protocol. Am J Surg 1986; 52:20–29.

Shorr RM, Crittenden M, Indeck M, Hartunian SL, Rodriguez A. Blunt thoracic trauma, analysis of 515 patients. Ann Surg 1987; 205:200–205.

Wilson SM, Au FC. In extremis use of a Foley catheter in a cardiac stab wound. J Trauma 1986; 26:400–402.

Patient Requiring EMERGENCY THORACOTOMY

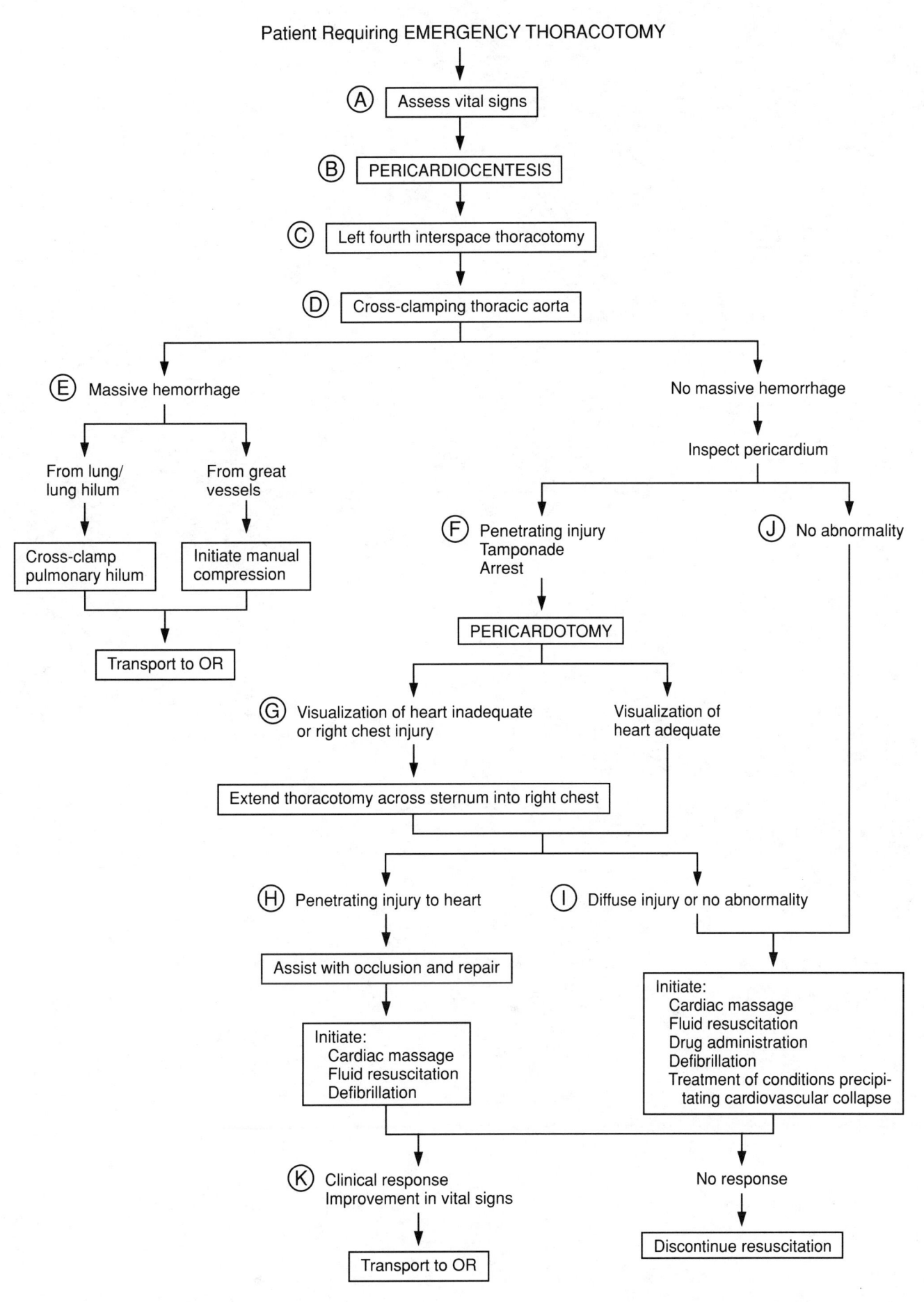

- **A** Assess vital signs
- **B** PERICARDIOCENTESIS
- **C** Left fourth interspace thoracotomy
- **D** Cross-clamping thoracic aorta

E — Massive hemorrhage

- From lung/lung hilum → Cross-clamp pulmonary hilum → Transport to OR
- From great vessels → Initiate manual compression → Transport to OR

No massive hemorrhage

Inspect pericardium

- **F** Penetrating injury, Tamponade, Arrest → PERICARDOTOMY
  - **G** Visualization of heart inadequate or right chest injury → Extend thoracotomy across sternum into right chest
  - Visualization of heart adequate
    - **H** Penetrating injury to heart → Assist with occlusion and repair → Initiate: Cardiac massage, Fluid resuscitation, Defibrillation
    - **I** Diffuse injury or no abnormality → Initiate: Cardiac massage, Fluid resuscitation, Drug administration, Defibrillation, Treatment of conditions precipitating cardiovascular collapse
- **J** No abnormality → Initiate: Cardiac massage, Fluid resuscitation, Drug administration, Defibrillation, Treatment of conditions precipitating cardiovascular collapse

- **K** Clinical response / Improvement in vital signs → Transport to OR
- No response → Discontinue resuscitation

THORACIC TRAUMA: POTENTIALLY LIFE THREATENING INJURIES

Myocardial Contusion
Pulmonary Contusion
Aortic Trauma
Laryngotracheal Trauma
Traumatic Diaphragmatic Hernia
Esophageal Trauma

MYOCARDIAL CONTUSION

Johnese Spisso
Edward W. Pottmeyer

A. Myocardial contusion is a lesion that occurs primarily from blunt trauma to the torso. The spectrum of injury may vary from localized areas of ecchymosis to significant myocardial fiber disruption. Contusion is the most common finding in patients with severe chest trauma, with a reported incidence of 20 percent. Subendocardial hemorrhages and rupture of the ventricular wall are less prevalent but can be fatal in relation to other associated injuries.

B. The initial assessment must focus on the airway, breathing, and circulation priorities (ABCs) of resuscitation. During the primary survey, life threatening conditions are treated prior to assessment for this lesion.

C. Assessment of the patient for a myocardial contusion begins during the secondary survey with an index of suspicion, based on the history and/or mechanism of injury. Patients who present with blunt chest trauma, chest wall contusions, or sternal and upper rib fractures are evaluated for this lesion. Presenting signs and symptoms may include precordial chest pain, dyspnea, and hypotension.

D. The hemodynamically unstable patient with multiple system injuries can be significantly compromised by an underlying cardiac contusion and loss of myocardial reserve. Associated injuries must be identified and treated to stabilize the patient.

E. Twelve-lead ECG and continuous cardiac rhythm monitoring are a diagnostic priority for the patient with suspected myocardial contusion. ECG abnormalities that are characteristic of this injury range from nonspecific ST-T wave changes and/or inversion associated with myocardial ischemia to rhythm disturbances of paroxysmal atrial tachycardia, right bundle branch block, ventricular tachycardia, and premature ventricular contractions.

F. The initial ECG may appear normal, and the patient may be asymptomatic. It is important to continue to observe and assess the patient who, based on mechanism of injury, has a high index of suspicion for this injury because injured areas with decreased microcirculation can progress to myocardial necrosis. If symptoms occur, a repeat ECG, echocardiogram, serial cardiac isoenzymes, and continuous cardiac monitoring for 48 hours are usually indicated.

G. Patients who have apparent ECG abnormalities consistent with myocardial ischemia and/or contusion warrant an echocardiogram. This noninvasive diagnostic study identifies areas of pericardial fluid collections and evaluates myocardial wall function. A multiple gated acquisition study (MUGA) scan may be used for further evaluation of ventricular wall motion and right ventricular ejection fraction. Continual assessment of cardiac rhythm is essential, and these patients usually require telemetry or intensive care monitoring and nursing assessment. Serial cardiac isoenzymes and serial 12-lead ECGs are also needed to monitor progression of this injury.

H. The patient with the confirmed diagnosis of myocardial contusion requires ongoing assessment for signs and symptoms of extension of myocardial damage or coronary artery injury. Complications of ventricular rupture, aneurysm, or thrombus can be life threatening sequelae of myocardial contusion.

References

Hurley ET, Mayfield W. Aortic injuries. In: Blaisdell FW, Trunkey DD, eds. Trauma management, cervicothoracic trauma. Vol. III. New York: Theime, 1986:205–206.

Hurn PL. Thoracic injuries. In: Cardona V, et al, eds. Trauma nursing from resuscitation through rehabilitation. Philadelphia: WB Saunders, 1988:477.

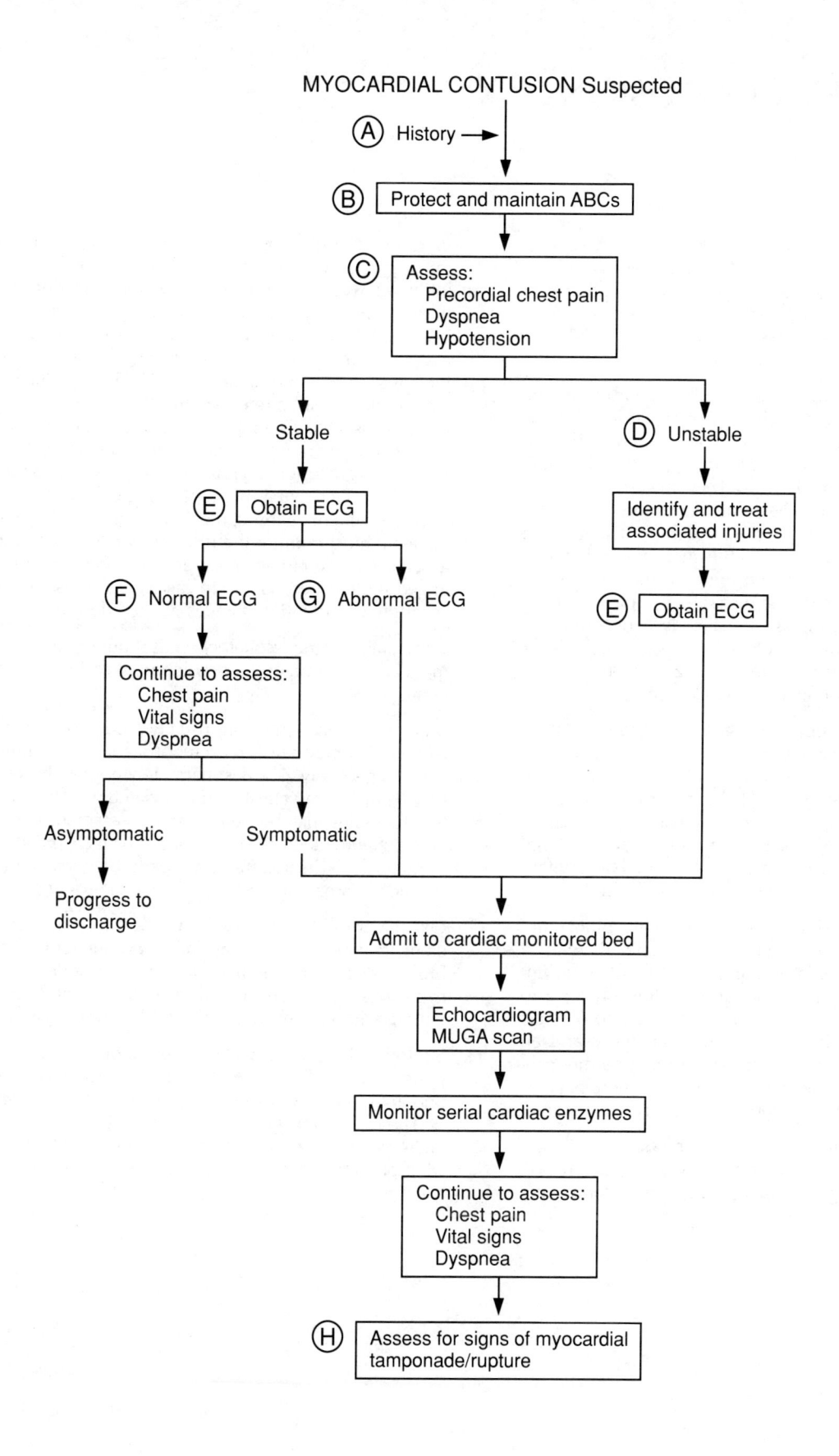

MYOCARDIAL CONTUSION Suspected

- (A) History →
- (B) Protect and maintain ABCs
- (C) Assess:
    - Precordial chest pain
    - Dyspnea
    - Hypotension

Stable:
- (E) Obtain ECG
    - (F) Normal ECG → Continue to assess: Chest pain, Vital signs, Dyspnea
        - Asymptomatic → Progress to discharge
        - Symptomatic → Admit to cardiac monitored bed
    - (G) Abnormal ECG → Admit to cardiac monitored bed

(D) Unstable:
- Identify and treat associated injuries
- (E) Obtain ECG → Admit to cardiac monitored bed

Admit to cardiac monitored bed
↓
Echocardiogram
MUGA scan
↓
Monitor serial cardiac enzymes
↓
Continue to assess:
- Chest pain
- Vital signs
- Dyspnea
↓
(H) Assess for signs of myocardial tamponade/rupture

PULMONARY CONTUSION

Lisa B. Jones

Pulmonary contusions are the most common injury seen in North America. They are potentially lethal because of the resulting respiratory failure that develops over time rather than occurs instantly. Severe pulmonary contusions are almost indistinguishable from adult respiratory distress syndrome (ARDS).

A. Pulmonary contusions are usually characterized by damage to the lung parenchyma that results in localized edema and hemorrhage. They are associated with more acute chest trauma, such as pneumothorax, hemothorax, rib fractures, and flail chest. They may, however, be present without other chest trauma. Pulmonary contusions develop after the lungs, which contain a large volume of blood, strike against the rigid chest wall, thereby producing a compression injury to the lung tissue. Patients with pre-existing disease or injury such as chronic pulmonary disease, impaired level of consciousness, abdominal injury, skeletal injuries that require immobilization, or renal failure are more susceptible to the development of a pulmonary contusion.

B. A patent airway, adequate oxygenation, and ventilation (ABCs) must be maintained to allow the delivery of an adequate volume and an inspired concentration of oxygen. Accurate assessment of hemodynamic status is essential. Adequate resuscitation is evaluated by ventilatory rate, heart rate, blood pressure, pulse pressure, arterial blood gases, and urinary output. All actual and potential life threatening injuries must be addressed.

C. Pulmonary contusions can occur with blunt and penetrating trauma. Contusions associated with a hemothorax, fractured ribs, and flail chest often go unnoticed. Contusions may not appear clinically for 2 to 24 hours after chest injury, with a lag of 4 to 6 hours frequently found between the time of injury and an abnormal chest film. A complete history and mechanism of injury history are needed to identify those patients with a potential to develop a pulmonary contusion.

D. In the early development of a pulmonary contusion, dyspnea and tachycardia are noted with a relatively normal Pao_2. No lung abnormalities may be evident. Within 12 to 24 hours, chest films may shown evidence of initial parenchymal changes (patchy areas of ill defined infiltrate), which can progress to well defined opacities. In the severest contusion, the classic "white lung" may be seen. Minor auscultatory findings may be present. The progressive obstruction of the alveoli and bronchioles, increased mucus production, and ineffective coughing lead to atelectasis, altered ventilation and/or perfusion ratios, resistance to air flow, and respiratory acidosis, thereby producing the clinical signs and symptoms of pulmonary contusion. Hypoxia may appear up to 6 hours postinjury. Tachypnea, hemoptysis, rales, and dyspnea become evident as the contusion progresses. The trauma team must monitor the respiratory rate and rhythm, auscultate for developing rales, and observe for any blood tinged sputum. Arterial blood gas evaluations should be scheduled to identify changes as they develop.

E. Any changes in the respiratory status should alert the trauma team to the potential development of a pulmonary contusion.

F. Mild pulmonary contusions usually produce tachypnea, tachycardia, blood tinged secretions, and an inability to cough effectively. The last-named symptom, however, may be due to the chest pain associated with the initial trauma. Rales may be heard. ABC assessment may reveal a slightly decreased Po_2 caused by tachypnea. The primary goals in treatment are early diagnosis, maintenance of a patent airway, and adequate oxygenation.

G. Oxygen by mask with good humidification may be sufficient treatment. Chest physiotherapy, suctioning, and bronchoscopy may facilitate the removal of debris and secretions. Pain management may be indicated to encourage the patient to cough and breath deeply.

H. Sputum culture and sensitivity tests should be obtained periodically to detect any developing infectious process, and antibiotic coverage should be adjusted accordingly. The patient must be closely observed for signs of increasing hypoxemia as the contusion processes develop.

I. Mild pulmonary contusions rapidly resolve within 3 to 4 days.

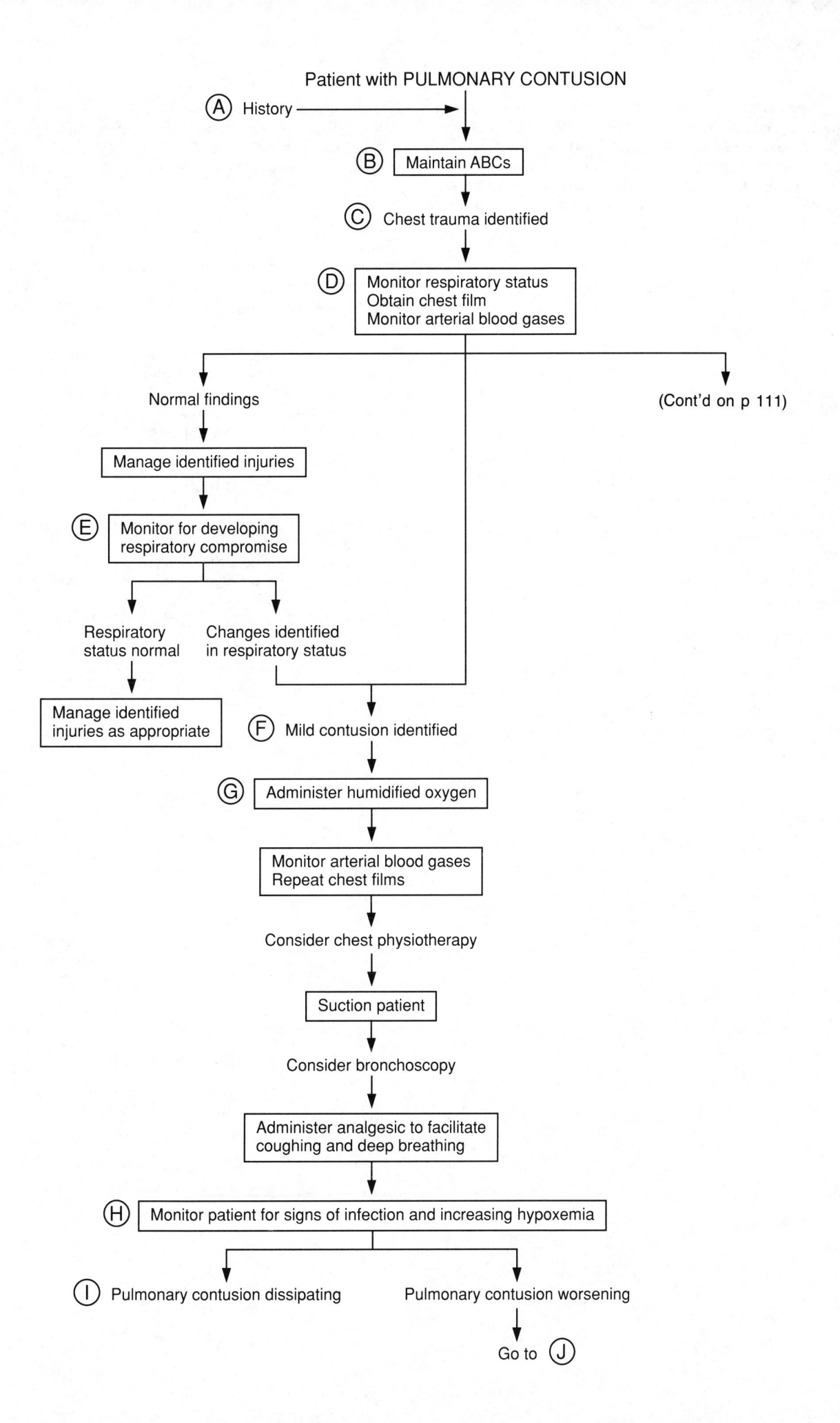

Patient with PULMONARY CONTUSION

- **(A)** History
- **(B)** Maintain ABCs
- **(C)** Chest trauma identified
- **(D)** Monitor respiratory status
  Obtain chest film
  Monitor arterial blood gases

Branches:
- Normal findings
- (Cont'd on p 111)

Normal findings → Manage identified injuries → **(E)** Monitor for developing respiratory compromise
- Respiratory status normal → Manage identified injuries as appropriate
- Changes identified in respiratory status → **(F)** Mild contusion identified

(F) Mild contusion identified → **(G)** Administer humidified oxygen → Monitor arterial blood gases / Repeat chest films → Consider chest physiotherapy → Suction patient → Consider bronchoscopy → Administer analgesic to facilitate coughing and deep breathing → **(H)** Monitor patient for signs of infection and increasing hypoxemia

- **(I)** Pulmonary contusion dissipating
- Pulmonary contusion worsening → Go to **(J)**

109

J. The patient with severe pulmonary contusion demonstrates tachypnea, tachycardia, and persistent rales. Secretions are more copious, and frank blood may become evident. Severe hypoxemia and CO_2 retention with a widening alveolar-arterial gradient indicate severe respiratory failure. Chest films usually exhibit some abnormal findings but often do not correlate with the extensive damage. "White lung" may appear on repeat chest films.

K. Severe contusions show progressive evidence of still, wet lungs and increased work of breathing. Measured pulmonary compliance falls; peak airway pressure increases. The degree of deterioration in PaO_2 and pH level is usually a function of failure to recognize the extent of the contusion and to institute early ventilation support and pulmonary hygiene.

L. Severe contusions can be managed with intermittent mandatory ventilation (IMV) and positive end-expiratory pressure (PEEP) and/or continuous positive airway pressure (CPAP). Pharmacologic paralysis may be indicated with controlled mechanical ventilation or high frequency ventilation to aerate the poorly compliant damaged lungs.

M. Barotrauma development can be reduced by maintaining adequate sedation.

N. Early institution of chest physiotherapy, postural drainage, and percussion is important. Treatment should be specific to the area of lung involved. Bloody mucus should become thinner and darker in 48 to 72 hours and eventually clear. Routine sputum cultures and daily chest films are helpful in monitoring developing infection.

O. A pulmonary artery catheter is advantageous in monitoring the patient. An oxygen saturation exceeding 90 percent should be maintained. Fluid overload should be avoided while adequate tissue perfusion is maintained.

P. Anticipate a hypermetabolic catabolic state. Adequate nutritional support should be provided with calories and protein. Carbohydrates in excess should be avoided.

Q. Care should focus on pulmonary hygiene and on regaining respiratory reserve. The patient will be at risk for developing a traumatic cyst and will need continued observation and follow-up.

R. The severe contusion that shows little or no improvement may develop post-traumatic respiratory distress syndrome. The presence of associated injuries (shock with massive transfusion, prolonged hypoventilation, and sepsis) may potentiate the development of ARDS.

References

American College of Surgeons. Early care of the injured patient. Philadelphia: WB Saunders, 1976:125–126.

Hurn P. Thoracic injuries. In: Cardona V et al, eds. Trauma nursing from resuscitation through rehabilitation. Philadelphia: WB Saunders, 1988:472–476.

Shires T. Principles of trauma care. New York: McGraw-Hill, 1985:267–274.

Strange J. Shock trauma care plans. Springhouse, PA: Springhouse, 1987:73–75.

(Cont'd from p 109)

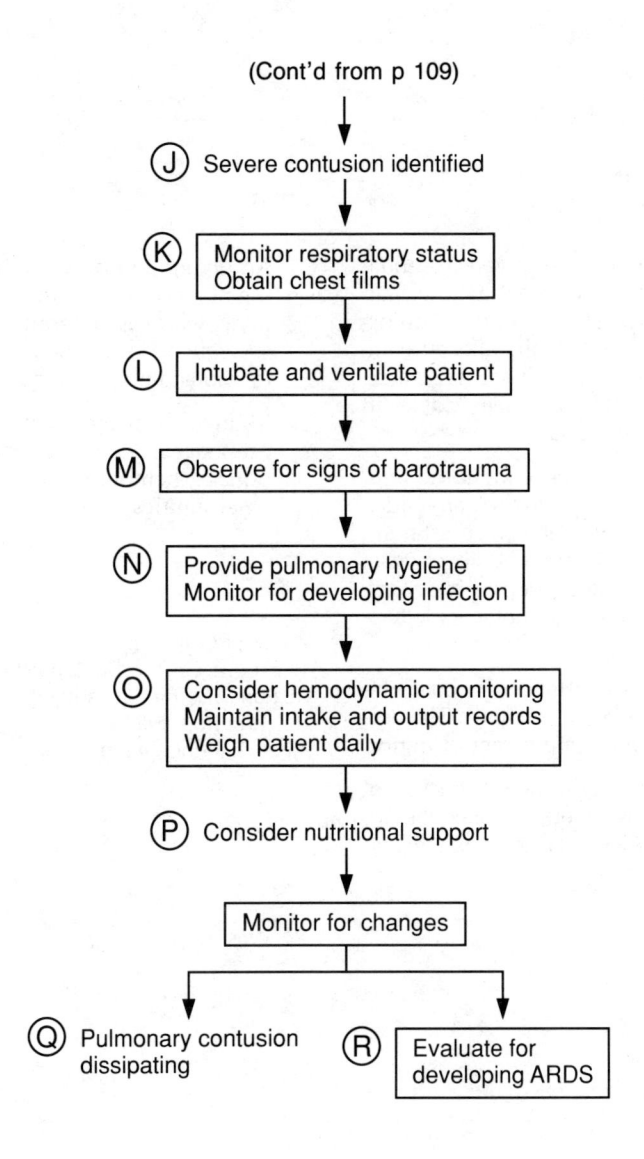

↓

Ⓙ Severe contusion identified

↓

Ⓚ Monitor respiratory status
Obtain chest films

↓

Ⓛ Intubate and ventilate patient

↓

Ⓜ Observe for signs of barotrauma

↓

Ⓝ Provide pulmonary hygiene
Monitor for developing infection

↓

Ⓞ Consider hemodynamic monitoring
Maintain intake and output records
Weigh patient daily

↓

Ⓟ Consider nutritional support

↓

Monitor for changes

↓   ↓

Ⓠ Pulmonary contusion dissipating

Ⓡ Evaluate for developing ARDS

AORTIC TRAUMA

Lisa B. Jones

A. A high index of suspicion for aortic rupture is essential in rapid deceleration injuries. Most patients who sustain aortic injuries die before arrival at the hospital. Approximately 20 percent survive the initial injury because the hemorrhage is contained by mediational structures. Therefore, time is of the utmost importance. A delay in diagnosis and treatment could be fatal.

B. Although a chest film is not diagnostic for aortic injuries, certain findings can be suggestive of an injury. Theses findings include a widened mediastinum; tracheal deviation; fracture of first or second rib, clavicle, or scapula; abnormal aortic contour; depression of left mainstem bronchus; massive left hemothorax; or left apical hematoma.

C. Because a delay in diagnosis and treatment could be fatal, an aortogram should be done promptly. The aortogram can identify the location and extent of injury.

D. Injuries associated with blunt trauma include fracture of the sternum, clavicle, or ribs; pneumothorax, hemothorax, or cardiac injury and/or cardiac tamponade; and tracheobronchial injuries.

E. An urgent thoracotomy should be performed to repair the blunt or penetrating aortic injury. Because most patients who sustain aortic injuries arrive at the hospital severely hypovolemic or in cardiac arrest, an emergency thoracotomy may be necessary.

F. Injuries associated with penetrating trauma include esophageal injury, cardiac injury and/or cardiac tamponade, hemothorax, pneumothorax, and tracheobronchial injuries.

References

Moore E, Eisman B, VanWay C. Critical decision in trauma. St. Louis: CV Mosby, 1984:164–167.

Mozlan J. Trauma surgery. Philadelphia: JB Lippincott, 1988:183–195.

Shires T. Principles of trauma care. New York: McGraw-Hill, 1985:277–289.

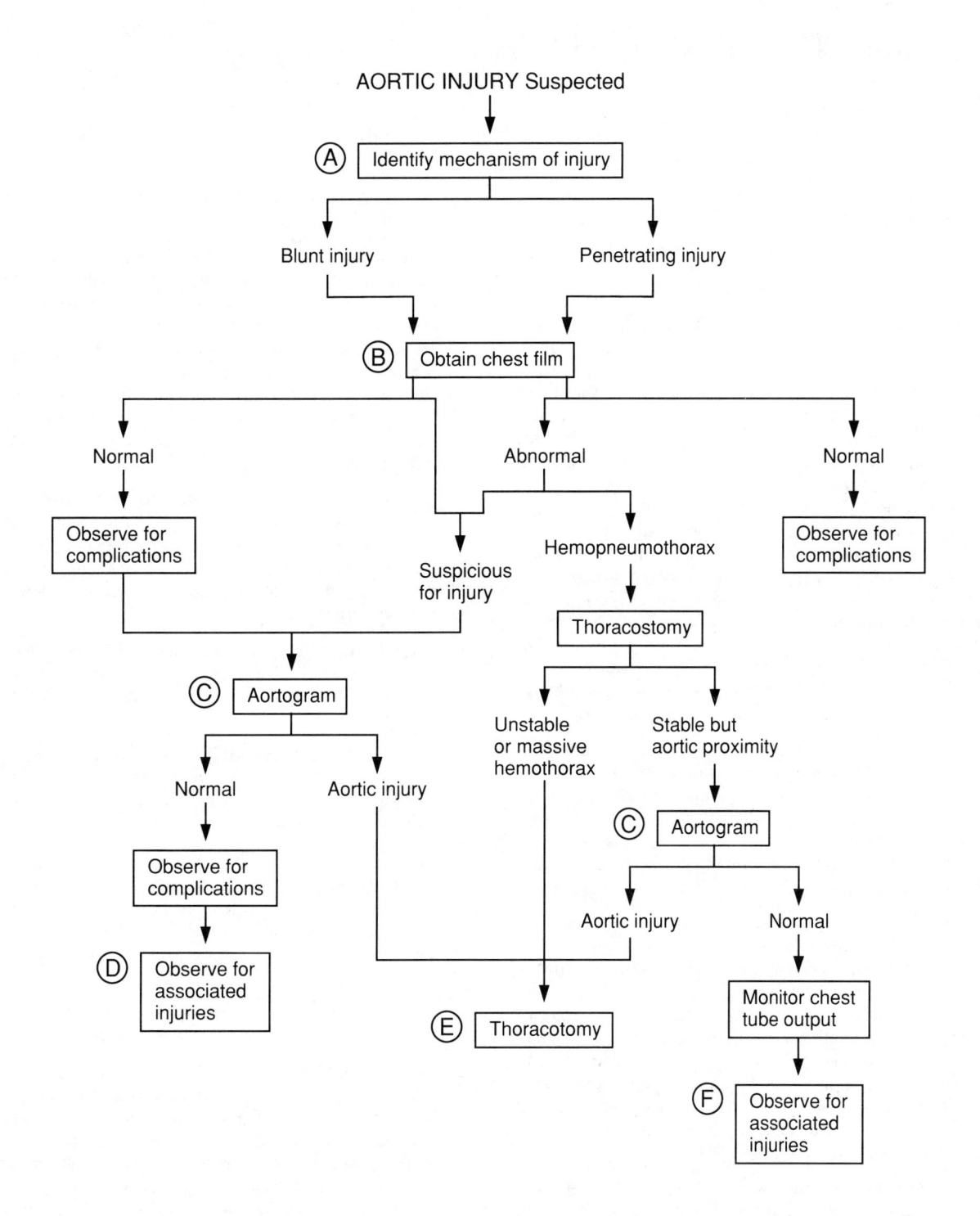

```
                    AORTIC INJURY Suspected
                              ↓
                   ⒶIdentify mechanism of injury
                      ↙              ↘
                Blunt injury      Penetrating injury
                      ↓              ↓
                   ⒷObtain chest film
         ↙         ↓         ↓              ↘
      Normal              Abnormal           Normal
         ↓         ↓         ↓                 ↓
    Observe for        Hemopneumothorax    Observe for
    complications           ↓              complications
         │      Suspicious   ↓
         │      for injury   ↓
         │         │      Thoracostomy
         │         │      ↙        ↘
         ↓         ↓   Unstable    Stable but
      ⒸAortogram     or massive   aortic proximity
         ↙    ↘     hemothorax         ↓
      Normal  Aortic injury            ⒸAortogram
         ↓         │                  ↙        ↘
     Observe for   │             Aortic injury  Normal
     complications │                  ↓            ↓
         ↓         │                  │        Monitor chest
     ⒹObserve for  │                  │        tube output
     associated    │                  │            ↓
     injuries      └──────→ ⒺThoracotomy      ⒻObserve for
                                               associated
                                               injuries
```

113

LARYNGOTRACHEAL TRAUMA

Gregory G. Stanford

Laryngotracheal trauma is relatively uncommon compared with other injuries of the head and neck. The reason for this disparity is unknown, but these injuries are commonly fatal because of the disruption of the airway.

A. Injuries to the larynx and trachea can be from blunt or penetrating trauma. The most common injury results from a blunt force applied to the anterior neck from a fist or steering wheel that traps the laryngotracheal structures against the rigid cervical spine. The amount of damage relates to the amount of energy applied to the neck and the area over which this force is distributed. Penetrating trauma is usually from a missile or a knife but can result from any sharp object, including flying glass fragments in an automobile accident. As a result of the intricate network of interacting cartilaginous structures, injury frequently disrupts the integrity of the airway, which can result in partial or total airway obstruction. Treatment of laryngotracheal injuries is also complicated by the importance of restoring normal anatomic relationships to ensure normal phonation, which is important to both the quality and the preservation of life. Early treatment is thus directed at establishing and maintaining airway patency without sacrificing future function.

B. Signs and symptoms of laryngotracheal trauma are related to airway dysfunction, including hemoptysis, airway obstruction, and leakage of air from the disrupted airway into surrounding tissues. Patients are generally anxious and confused. Disruption of the mucosa causes bleeding that can manifest by coughing, frank hemoptysis, or vomiting of swallowed blood. Injury to the larynx causes dysphonia or aphonia.

C. Airway obstruction may be complete or incomplete. Incomplete obstruction may appear as wheezing or stridor. The clinical signs related to laryngotracheal injuries include deformity of the normal contours of the anterior neck and, especially, of the thyroid cartilage. Leakage of air from the damaged airway results in subcutaneous emphysema and crepitus. If the patient is conscious, tenderness on palpation is almost always present. The possibility of cervical spine injury should always be considered in patients with laryngotracheal trauma.

D. The first priority of treatment is the establishment and maintenance of an adequate airway. Any evidence of actual or impending airway obstruction should be treated by an emergency tracheostomy. A cricothyroidotomy is contraindicated in laryngeal injuries because of (1) potential damage to the laryngeal cartilages and (2) possible airway placement in the retropharyngeal space. Similarly, endotracheal intubation may result in further damage to the larynx and can convert partial obstruction to complete obstruction. Swelling is the rule and not the exception in laryngeal trauma, and the spontaneously breathing patient can have sudden airway compromise from edema or hematoma. It is much safer to perform a tracheostomy in a patient who may not have required it than not to perform a tracheostomy in a patient who did require it.

E. The severity of a laryngeal or tracheal injury can distract the examiner from other life threatening injuries. These injuries need to be evaluated and treated concurrently with the laryngeal or tracheal injuries.

F. Anteroposterior and lateral radiographs should be obtained on all patients. These films not only evaluate the cervical spine but also give valuable information as to the nature and extent of injury to the larynx and trachea. The optimal examination should consist of initial overpenetration to delineate the bony structures, followed by soft tissue views. Signs of laryngotracheal trauma are displacement of the epiglottis, disruption of the air column, subcutaneous emphysema, endolaryngeal swelling, and retropharyngeal edema or hematoma.

G. Indirect mirror laryngoscopy can be helpful in the stable and cooperative patient but is usually inadequate or impossible in most laryngeal injuries. Direct laryngoscopy can increase the damage or induce complete airway obstruction and should not be done until a tracheostomy has been performed.

H. A contrast laryngogram is performed by slowly instilling a radiopaque dye into the upper airway. This study is helpful in assessing minor and less-than-obvious injuries.

I. Computed tomography (CT) is now the study of choice in evaluating laryngeal injuries because of its excellent resolution and its ability to detect injuries to the surrounding soft tissues.

J. The main therapeutic decision in laryngotracheal injuries is whether to manage a patient nonoperatively or operatively. Many injuries can be managed nonoperatively with spontaneous resolution. If the injury cannot be expected to resolve, operative intervention is warranted.

K. If an esophageal or carotid injury is possible, appropriate contrast studies or exploration is indicated.

L. Nonoperative therapy is possible in those patients with a stable larynx, no obstruction, and nondisplaced fractures. Bed rest and voice rest are mandatory to allow the injured tissues to heal. Humidified air keeps the mucosa moist and helps mobilize secretions. With mucosal disruption, prophylactic antibiotics with a first-generation cephalosporin are indicated for the first 24 hours postinjury. Voice therapists can be valuable consultants in helping the patient regain normal phonation.

References

Caro J Jr, Leonard G, Tzadik A. Laryngeal trauma. In: Maull KI, ed. Advances in trauma. Vol. 1. Chicago: Yearbook, 1986:157–165.

Gallia LJ. Laryngotracheal trauma. In: Blaisdell FW, Trunkey DD, eds. Cervicothoracic trauma. New York: Thieme, 1986:117–128.

Perry MO. Penetrating wounds of the neck. In: Shires GT, ed. Principles of trauma care. New York: McGraw-Hill, 1985:365–369.

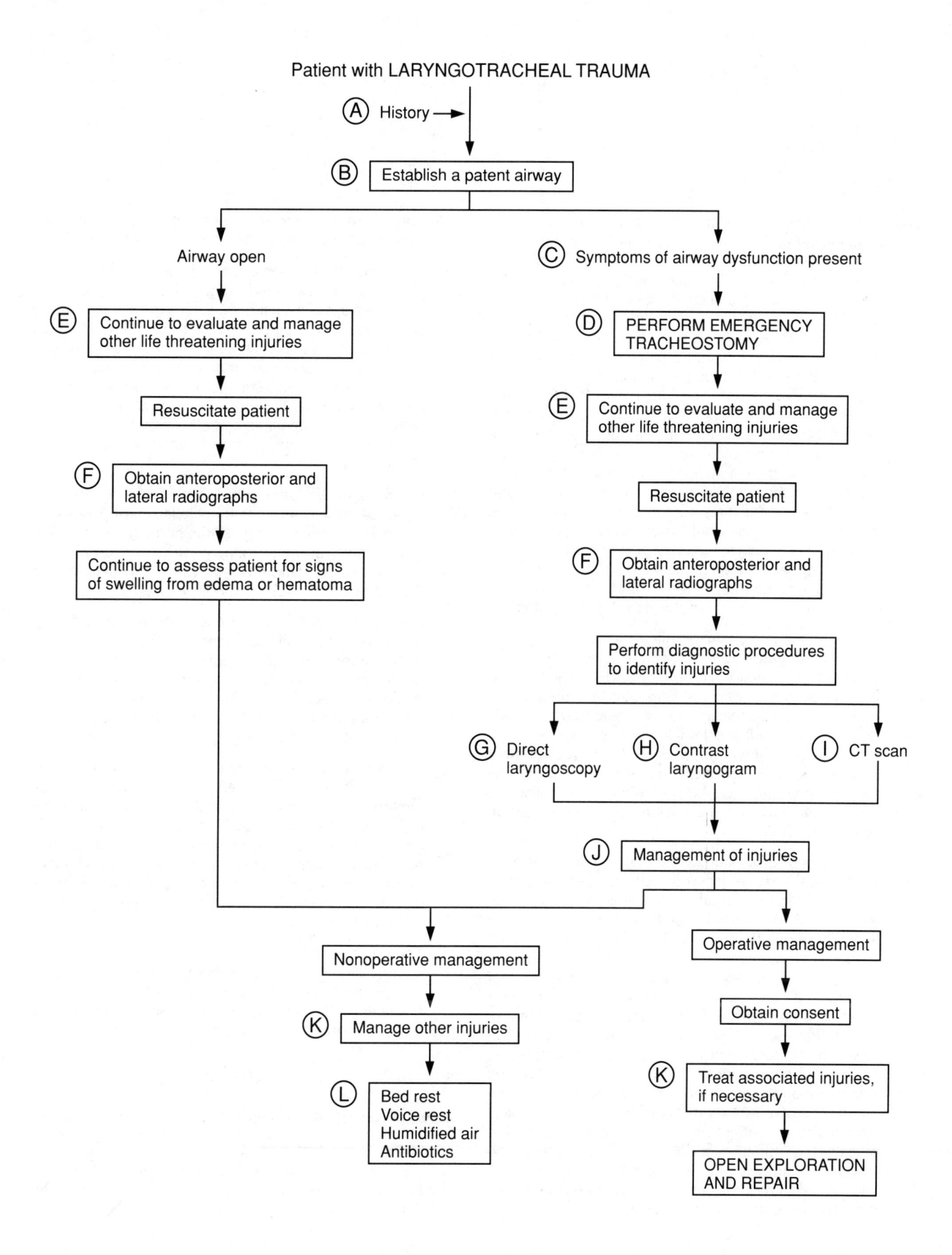

```
Patient with LARYNGOTRACHEAL TRAUMA
         Ⓐ History →
              ↓
         Ⓑ Establish a patent airway
         ↙                    ↘
   Airway open          Ⓒ Symptoms of airway dysfunction present
        ↓                          ↓
Ⓔ Continue to evaluate and    Ⓓ PERFORM EMERGENCY
  manage other life              TRACHEOSTOMY
  threatening injuries             ↓
        ↓                    Ⓔ Continue to evaluate and manage
   Resuscitate patient          other life threatening injuries
        ↓                          ↓
Ⓕ Obtain anteroposterior      Resuscitate patient
  and lateral radiographs         ↓
        ↓                    Ⓕ Obtain anteroposterior and
 Continue to assess patient      lateral radiographs
 for signs of swelling from       ↓
 edema or hematoma           Perform diagnostic procedures
                             to identify injuries
                          ↙        ↓        ↘
                      Ⓖ Direct  Ⓗ Contrast  Ⓘ CT scan
                      laryngoscopy laryngogram
                             ↓
                      Ⓙ Management of injuries
                       ↙              ↘
          Nonoperative management   Operative management
                ↓                        ↓
          Ⓚ Manage other injuries    Obtain consent
                ↓                        ↓
          Ⓛ Bed rest               Ⓚ Treat associated injuries,
             Voice rest              if necessary
             Humidified air            ↓
             Antibiotics           OPEN EXPLORATION
                                   AND REPAIR
```

115

TRAUMATIC DIAPHRAGMATIC HERNIA

Jorie Klein
Thomas Drury

A. Traumatic herniation of the diaphragm is most commonly associated with blunt trauma. Automobile accidents are responsible for over 80 percent of traumatic diaphragmatic disruptions. Falls, direct blows (e.g., animal kicks, aggravated assaults), and crushing injuries (e.g., run-over accidents, cave-ins) are other causes of diaphragmatic injuries. Ninety-five percent of diaphragmatic hernias occur on the left side, and 5 percent involve the right hemidiaphragm. It is thought that dense liver and right kidney protect the right hemidiaphragm far better than the stomach, left lobe of the liver, spleen, and left kidney protect the left hemidiaphragm. Because a force of great magnitude is needed to injure the diaphragm, there is a high incidence of associated injuries with traumatic disruption of the diaphragm. Associated injuries include rib and skeletal fractures, ruptured spleen, major head injuries, liver injuries, small bowel perforations, pancreatic injuries, and stomach injuries. An injury to the spleen and kidney should alert the team to a potential left sided diaphragmatic injury. Hepatic and renal injuries require careful evaluation of the right hemidiaphragm.

B. Traumatic diaphragmatic hernia is considered a potentially life threatening thoracic injury because of the potential for respiratory compromise. The patient should have a complete initial evaluation, and life threatening injuries should be managed appropriately. The resuscitation phase should be initiated with oxygen administration, establishment of two large bore precautionary intravenous lines, adequate fluid resuscitation, and placement of a nasogastric tube and Foley catheter. The patient should have ongoing assessment and re-evaluation of all intervention.

C. Symptoms of disruption of the diaphragm are directly related to the space occupying effects of the herniated viscera within the pleural cavity. Initial signs and symptoms vary. Approximately one-third of the patients have a small perforation without herniation and do not demonstrate associated symptoms. Ten percent of the patients have massive herniation of intra-abdominal contents into the chest, which produces a severe compression of the lung and contralateral displacement of the mediastinum. This group of patients may exhibit severe respiratory distress, cyanosis, and hypotension. Frequently, other patients complain of pain in the left upper abdomen quadrant, left lower thorax, and left shoulder as well as shortness of breath. The physical examination of patients with large tears and herniation reveals a combination of dullness and tympany to percussion, decreased or absent breath sounds, or bowel sounds in the chest. Patients with massive herniation have a deviated trachea, and apical heart sounds are shifted. Caution should be taken when performing a thoracostomy when diaphragmatic injury is suspected.

D. The typical findings on a chest film associated with diaphragmatic hernia include an arch-like shadow that suggests elevation of the left hemidiaphragm, the appearance of an opacity or irregularity of the left hemidiaphragm, gas densities or bubbles above the level of the diaphragm, and atelectasis. Other common radiographic findings associated with diaphragmatic injury include varying amounts of pleural fluid, the presence of air-fluid levels within the left hemidiaphragm, displacement of the heart and mediastinal structures, and coiled nasogastric tube in the chest.

E. Gastrografin by mouth or nasogastric tube confirms the presence of the stomach within the left chest. Swallowed Gastrografin may either enter the herniated stomach or stop abruptly at the esophagogastric junction because of the acute angulation. Contrast studies with barium in the colon or stomach may be indicated.

F. Penetrating wounds of the chest and upper abdomen should alert the evaluating team to a potential diaphragmatic injury. Unless the diaphragmatic defect is large, herniation may not occur immediately, and the injury may be missed. To identify any missed injuries, it is recommended that the diaphragm be evaluated when an exploration of the chest or abdomen is undertaken.

G. Blunt chest trauma has a higher incidence of diaphragmatic hernia (refer to paragraph A) than does penetrating chest trauma and is associated with a combination of injuries. The absence of these associated injuries in no way excludes the possibility of diaphragmatic disruption. The evaluating team must evaluate the mechanism of injury and create an "index of suspicion." If the index of suspicion is high, all attempts to rule out the injury should be made.

H. The treatment of every diaphragmatic injury is surgical repair. Patients with massive herniation require immediate operative intervention. If no injury to the diaphragm is identified, the patient must be reassessed and continuously monitored to identify occult or delayed injuries.

References

American College of Surgeons. Advanced trauma life support course. Chicago: American College of Surgeons, 1989:99.

Gay WA Jr, McCabe JC. Trauma to the chest: principles of trauma care. 3rd ed. New York: McGraw-Hill, 1985:S81–82.

Hill LD. Injuries of the diaphragm following blunt trauma. Surg Clin North Am 1972; 52:611.

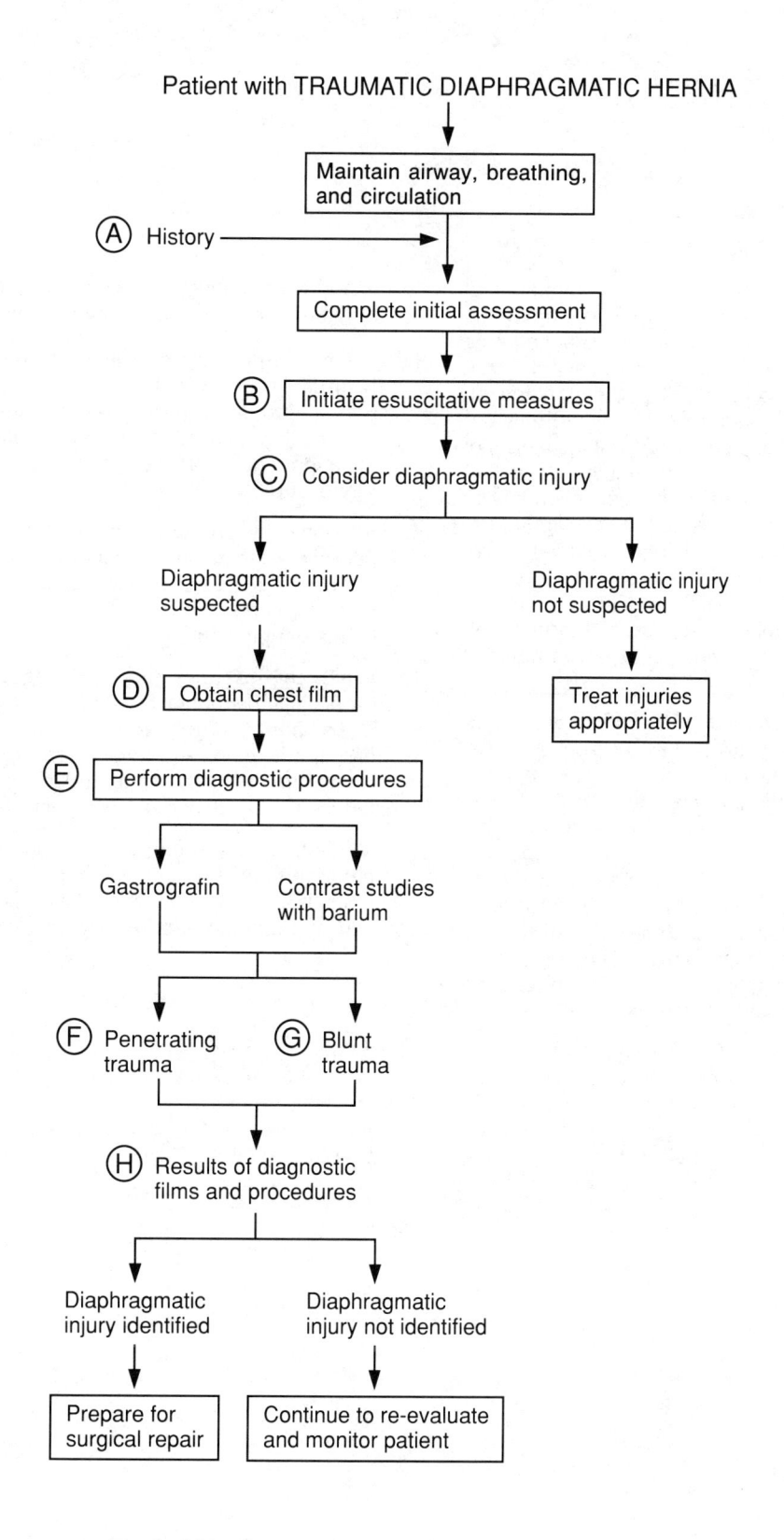

```
                  Patient with TRAUMATIC DIAPHRAGMATIC HERNIA
                                      │
                                      ▼
                          ┌───────────────────────┐
                          │ Maintain airway,       │
                          │ breathing,             │
                          │ and circulation        │
          (A) History ───▶└───────────────────────┘
                                      │
                                      ▼
                          ┌───────────────────────┐
                          │ Complete initial       │
                          │ assessment             │
                          └───────────────────────┘
                                      │
                                      ▼
                       ┌──────────────────────────────┐
                   (B) │ Initiate resuscitative        │
                       │ measures                      │
                       └──────────────────────────────┘
                                      │
                                      ▼
                   (C) Consider diaphragmatic injury
                          ┌───────────┴───────────┐
                          ▼                       ▼
                Diaphragmatic injury     Diaphragmatic injury
                suspected                not suspected
                          │                       │
                          ▼                       ▼
                 ┌──────────────────┐   ┌──────────────────┐
             (D) │ Obtain chest film │   │ Treat injuries    │
                 └──────────────────┘   │ appropriately     │
                          │              └──────────────────┘
                          ▼
                 ┌────────────────────────┐
             (E) │ Perform diagnostic      │
                 │ procedures              │
                 └────────────────────────┘
                          │
                   ┌──────┴──────┐
                   ▼             ▼
              Gastrografin    Contrast studies
                              with barium
                   │             │
                   ▼             ▼
             (F) Penetrating  (G) Blunt
                 trauma           trauma
                   └──────┬──────┘
                          ▼
                 ┌────────────────────┐
             (H) │ Results of diagnostic│
                 │ films and procedures │
                 └────────────────────┘
                          │
                 ┌────────┴────────┐
                 ▼                 ▼
          Diaphragmatic       Diaphragmatic
          injury identified   injury not identified
                 │                 │
                 ▼                 ▼
         ┌──────────────┐  ┌──────────────────────┐
         │ Prepare for   │  │ Continue to re-evaluate│
         │ surgical repair│  │ and monitor patient   │
         └──────────────┘  └──────────────────────┘
```

117

ESOPHAGEAL TRAUMA

Johnese Spisso
Edward W. Pottmeyer

A. Esophageal disruption is the most life threatening of all digestive perforations. The majority of traumatic esophageal perforations are attributable to penetrating injuries; blunt trauma accounts for less than 10 percent of incidents. The diagnosis of esophageal perforation following blunt trauma is often difficult. Determining the diagnosis requires a careful correlation of mechanism of injury, physical findings, and patient symptoms. Penetrating injuries to the esophagus may occur secondary to gunshot wounds or stab wounds to the neck and upper chest. The injury most commonly occurs at the pharyngoesophageal junction. Blunt rupture of the esophagus is exceedingly rare and usually occurs at the cervicothoracic region (proximal esophagus to carina). Cervical spine injuries are a common associated finding of esophageal trauma.

B. Esophageal injuries are difficult to identify during the initial assessment. The hallmark findings of esophageal disruption include subcutaneous emphysema, crepitation of the neck and mediastinum, chest pain, dysphagia, cervical tenderness, and hemoptysis. Patient symptoms vary accordingly with location of the rupture (e.g., cervicothoracic, midthoracic, lower thoracic), degree of bacterial contamination, and gastric enzyme erosion at the site of the disruption. A high index of suspicion for esophageal injury should be recognized in any patient with blunt or penetrating neck or torso trauma, and the symptom complex should be described.

C. Patient outcome is dependent on early detection of esophageal ruptures. Delay in diagnosis leads to further corrosion and contamination of tissues by the digestive juices and bacteria. Diagnostic evaluation includes chest and abdominal films to detect air in the mediastinum or abdomen. Endoscopy and esophagography are used to define the anatomic location of the tear.

D. In the multiple trauma patient who is hemodynamically unstable and warrants emergency operative exploration, endoscopy and esophagography may be delayed because they could contribute to mortality. In these cases, the abdominal esophagus is inspected during exploratory laparotomy.

E. If esophagography and endoscopy are initially negative, periodic assessments are performed to monitor patient symptoms. Repeat esophagography and endoscopy or operative exploration may be indicated if the patient remains symptomatic.

F. When endoscopy and esophagography confirm esophageal disruption, rapid intervention is indicated. Decompression of gastric contents via insertion of nasogastric tubing and surgical repair of the tear are performed immediately. Antibiotic therapy is instituted to reduce the incidence of postoperative infection.

G. Mediastinitis, fistula formation, esophageal strictures, and peritonitis are all potential complications. Patient morbidity is dependent on rapid diagnosis of the disruption and on minimalization of bacterial contamination.

References

Beal S, Pottmeyer E, Spisso J. Esophageal perforation following external blunt trauma. Trauma 1988; 28:1425–1432.

Hurn P. Thoracic Injuries. In: Cardona V, et al, eds. Trauma nursing: resuscitation through rehabilitation. Philadelphia: WB Saunders, 1988:505–506.

Patient with SUSPECTED ESOPHAGEAL INJURY

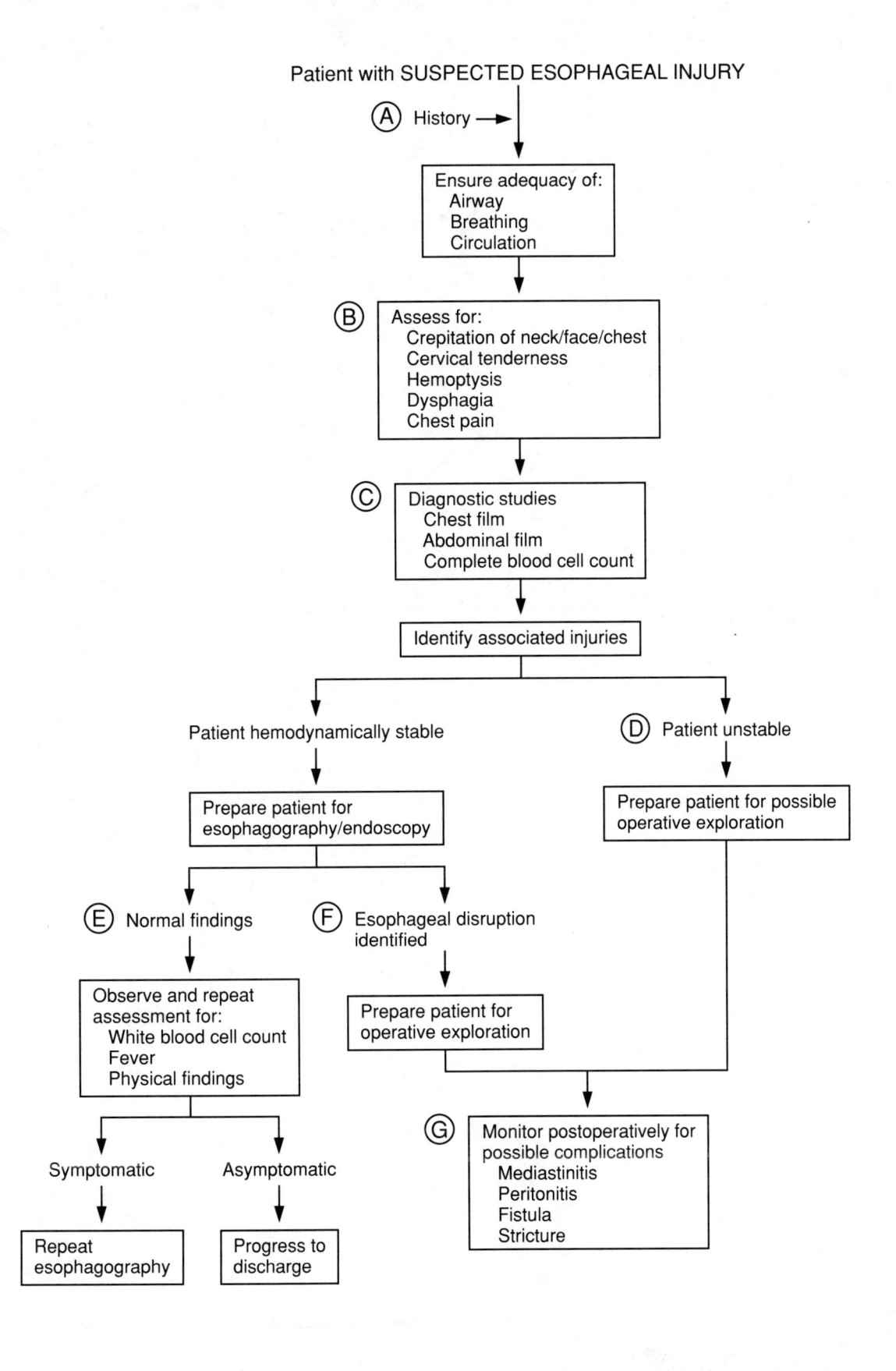

(A) History →

↓

Ensure adequacy of:
- Airway
- Breathing
- Circulation

↓

(B) Assess for:
- Crepitation of neck/face/chest
- Cervical tenderness
- Hemoptysis
- Dysphagia
- Chest pain

↓

(C) Diagnostic studies
- Chest film
- Abdominal film
- Complete blood cell count

↓

Identify associated injuries

├── Patient hemodynamically stable
│   ↓
│   Prepare patient for esophagography/endoscopy
│   ├── **(E)** Normal findings
│   │   ↓
│   │   Observe and repeat assessment for:
│   │   - White blood cell count
│   │   - Fever
│   │   - Physical findings
│   │   ├── Symptomatic → Repeat esophagography
│   │   └── Asymptomatic → Progress to discharge
│   └── **(F)** Esophageal disruption identified
│   ↓
│   Prepare patient for operative exploration
│
└── **(D)** Patient unstable
    ↓
    Prepare patient for possible operative exploration

↓

(G) Monitor postoperatively for possible complications
- Mediastinitis
- Peritonitis
- Fistula
- Stricture

THORACIC TRAUMA: OTHER MANIFESTATIONS

Simple Hemothorax or Pneumothorax
Subcutaneous Emphysema
Rib Fractures

SIMPLE HEMOTHORAX OR PNEUMOTHORAX

Lisa B. Jones

A. Patients are assessed and treatment priorities are established based on injuries and vital signs. Logical sequential treatment priorities must be established based on a rapid, primary evaluation of the patient. Adequate oxygenation and ventilation of the trauma patient must include the delivery of adequate volume and inspired concentrations of oxygen (i.e., FIO_2 greater than 0.85). Rapid and accurate assessment of the patient's hemodynamic status must be done by evaluating the state of consciousness, skin color, and heart rate. A minimum of two large bore intravenous lines and continuous cardiac monitoring (ECG) should be established.

B. Visual inspection of the chest, both anterior and posterior, must be done to identify all potential injuries. Palpation of the entire chest cage will identify rib fractures and clavicular and sternal injuries. Any fracture, contusion, or hematoma to the chest wall should indicate potential occult injuries. Breath sounds should be auscultated high on the anterior chest to assess for a pneumothorax and at the posterior bases to assess for a hemothorax. Hypertympanic percussion of the chest may indicate a hemothorax.

C. The history should include the mechanism of injury. Information such as the speed of the vehicle, wearing of a seatbelt, whether patient was driver or passenger, point of impact, and extent of compartment intrusion should be obtained in motor vehicle accidents. The height of the fall, breaks in fall, how victim landed, and the surface on which victim landed should be obtained in all fall accidents. Penetrating injury mechanisms should also be obtained. Identify any pre-existing heart, lung, arterial, or renal disease and whether the patient is taking any routine medications. All allergies and the time of last meal should be identified.

D. Chest films demonstrate any apparent peripheral lucent rim that results from visceral and parietal pleural separation. If there is equivocation, inspiratory-expiratory views should be obtained. A relatively small pneumothorax may be missed on a supine chest film. The films should be obtained in the upright position when possible. Increased lucency superimposed over the diaphragm in the supine film suggests the presence of a pneumothorax. A small hemothorax will result in blunting of the castophrenic angle, and a moderately sized hemothorax will produce partial opacification of the hemothorax and a lateral meniscus. A large hemothorax will produce opacification of the hemothorax. It is difficult to identify a hemothorax on a supine film, but increased density is usually noted in the affected hemothorax. If there is any question regarding the presence of a hemothorax, a lateral decubitus chest film is obtained.

E. A pneumothorax results from air entering the potential space between the visceral and parietal pleurae. Lacerations with air leakage are the most common cause of pneumothorax developing from blunt trauma. A laceration to the intercostal vessel or internal mammary artery may also produce a hemothorax. Treatment for a simple hemothorax or pneumothorax is a thoracostomy.

F. The unstable patient should be reassessed for missed life threatening injuries. The patient should be assessed for intercostal and supraclavicular muscle retractions. The patient should be monitored for signs of impending hypoxia, an increased respiratory rate, a change in breathing pattern, and cyanosis (i.e., patient must have a hemoglobin level of at least 5 g/100 ml of blood to produce cyanosis).

G. Continue evaluation to identify any missed injuries. Intrathoracic and extrathoracic injuries must be ruled out. The patient should be assessed for any developing signs of respiratory distress. Injuries associated with hemothorax and pneumothorax include rib fractures, aortic and great vessel injuries, and lung lacerations.

H. The chest film should be repeated in 6 hours to identify a delayed pneumothorax development. If the repeat films are normal and no other injuries are identified, the patient may be discharged home. The patient should be instructed to return to the hospital if shortness of breath, increased pain, increased heart rate, or weakness develops.

I. A chest tube should be placed in the fourth or fifth intercostal space, anterior to the midaxillary line. The chest tube should be connected to an underwater seal apparatus within 20 to 30 cm of water suction and a sterile occlusive dressing applied to the insertion site. The patient should have an immediate reassessment following the procedure.

J. It is imperative to monitor and document the initial chest tube output. A liter of blood is an indication to initiate a thoracic surgery consultation. A persistent drainage of more than 200 ml of blood per hour for 4 hours may indicate the need for a thoracotomy. The drainage system should be kept below the level of the tube. The chest tube drainage should be monitored and documented.

K. A chest film should be repeated after the thoracostomy to ensure correct placement and to observe for lung re-expansion and fluid evacuation.

L. The patient should have a continued assessment to rule out any missed injuries or developing complications. The vital signs and cardiac status should be monitored and documented. The patient and family should be prepared for hospital admission. An explanation of the resuscitation and hospital course should be given to the patient and family.

References

American College of Surgeons. Early care of the injured patient. Philadelphia: WB Saunders, 1976:120–125.

Bart W. Trauma: the first hour. Norwalk, CT: Appleton-Century-Crofts, 1985:115–116.

Seaman M. Pneumothorax and hemothorax. In: Mancini M, ed. Decision making in emergency nursing. Toronto: BC Decker, 1987:50–51.

Shires T. Principles of trauma care. New York: McGraw-Hill, 1985:267–274.

Strange J. Shock trauma care plans. Springhouse, PA: Springhouse, 1987:67–68.

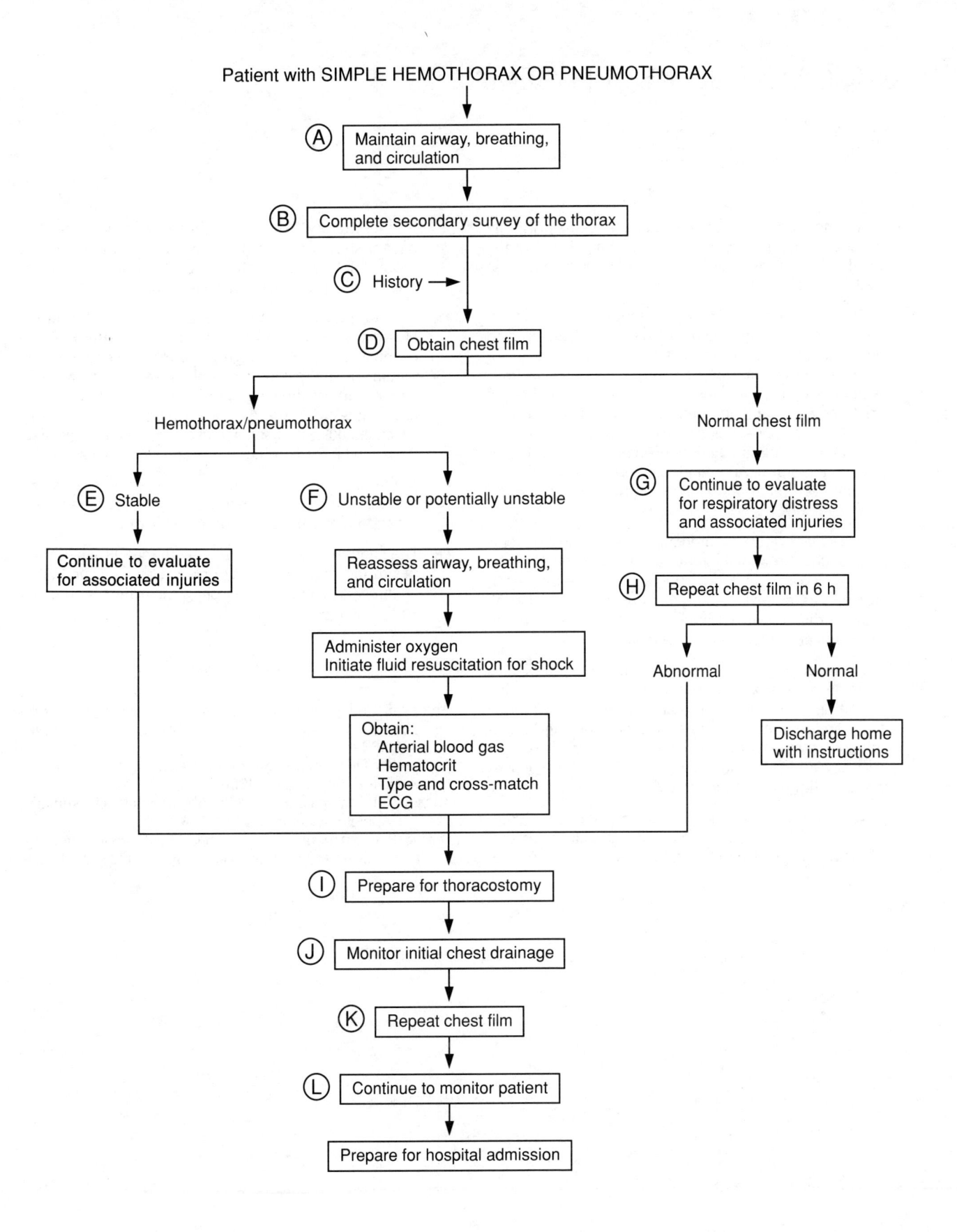

Patient with SIMPLE HEMOTHORAX OR PNEUMOTHORAX

- **A** Maintain airway, breathing, and circulation
- **B** Complete secondary survey of the thorax
- **C** History
- **D** Obtain chest film

Hemothorax/pneumothorax

- **E** Stable
  - Continue to evaluate for associated injuries
- **F** Unstable or potentially unstable
  - Reassess airway, breathing, and circulation
  - Administer oxygen
  - Initiate fluid resuscitation for shock
  - Obtain:
    - Arterial blood gas
    - Hematocrit
    - Type and cross-match
    - ECG

Normal chest film

- **G** Continue to evaluate for respiratory distress and associated injuries
- **H** Repeat chest film in 6 h
  - Abnormal
  - Normal → Discharge home with instructions

- **I** Prepare for thoracostomy
- **J** Monitor initial chest drainage
- **K** Repeat chest film
- **L** Continue to monitor patient
- Prepare for hospital admission

123

SUBCUTANEOUS EMPHYSEMA

Jane Curran
Thomas Drury

A. Nonpenetrating or blunt chest trauma occurs primarily in motor vehicle accidents and falls. Knowledge of the mechanism of injury and a high index of suspicion in evaluating chest trauma are essential.

B. Assessing the chest or thoracic injuries involves the following four steps: inspection, palpation, percussion, and auscultation. During inspection, an assessment for bilateral chest expansion, contusions, and open wounds is done. Palpation includes evaluating for sternal or rib fractures, subcutaneous emphysema, and tracheal deviations. The process of percussion can assess abnormalities in underlying structures (i.e., nonresonance indicates evidence of fluid). Auscultation determines presence or absence of breath and heart sounds, including sound characteristics.

C. Injuries that involve the bronchus are rare. Most patients with tracheobronchial injuries die at the scene. Presenting symptoms include subcutaneous emphysema, hemoptysis, or tension pneumothorax (p 88). Intubation may be difficult, if not impossible; therefore, immediate surgical intervention is necessary.

D. Subcutaneous emphysema is a symptom that indicates an injury to an aspect of the respiratory system or esophagus; it needs to be assessed and reassessed frequently for changes. The airway must be established and maintained to complete definitive treatment, such as barium swallow and bronchoscopy. Related injuries such as pneumothorax must be treated.

E. Injuries to the trachea and larynx are infrequent. Symptoms include hoarseness, palpable subcutaneous emphysema, dyspnea, and respiratory distress. If the patient is in respiratory distress, a tracheotomy is indicated. The patient should be taken immediately to the operating room (OR). When an airway is established, an evaluation by diagnostic tests can be completed.

F. The esophagus is rarely injured by blunt trauma. However, blunt injury to the lower one-third of the esophagus causes spillage of gastric contents into the pleura. The patient often complains of difficulty and discomfort in swallowing. Furthermore, rupture of the esophagus can cause dyspnea, cyanosis, hematemesis, subcutaneous emphysema, and pneumothorax. The diagnosis can be made by barium swallow or esophagoscopy.

G. A fiberoptic bronchoscopy is done to assess the respiratory tract for injuries. It can be done under intravenous sedation if the patient's condition permits.

H. The patient is taken immediately to the OR when injuries to the respiratory tract or esophagus occur. When no injury is determined by testing, the patient is observed and discharged accordingly.

References

American College of Surgeons. Advanced trauma life support course. Chicago: American College of Surgeons. 1988:89–111.

Cowley RA, Dunham MC. Shock trauma/critical care handbook. Rockville, MD: Aspen, 1986:145–187.

Knezevick B. Trauma nursing: principles and practice. Norwalk, CT: Appleton-Century-Crofts, 1986:73–99.

Perdue P. Chest trauma. In: Cardona V, ed. Trauma nursing. Oradell, NJ: Medical Economics Books, 1985:123–139.

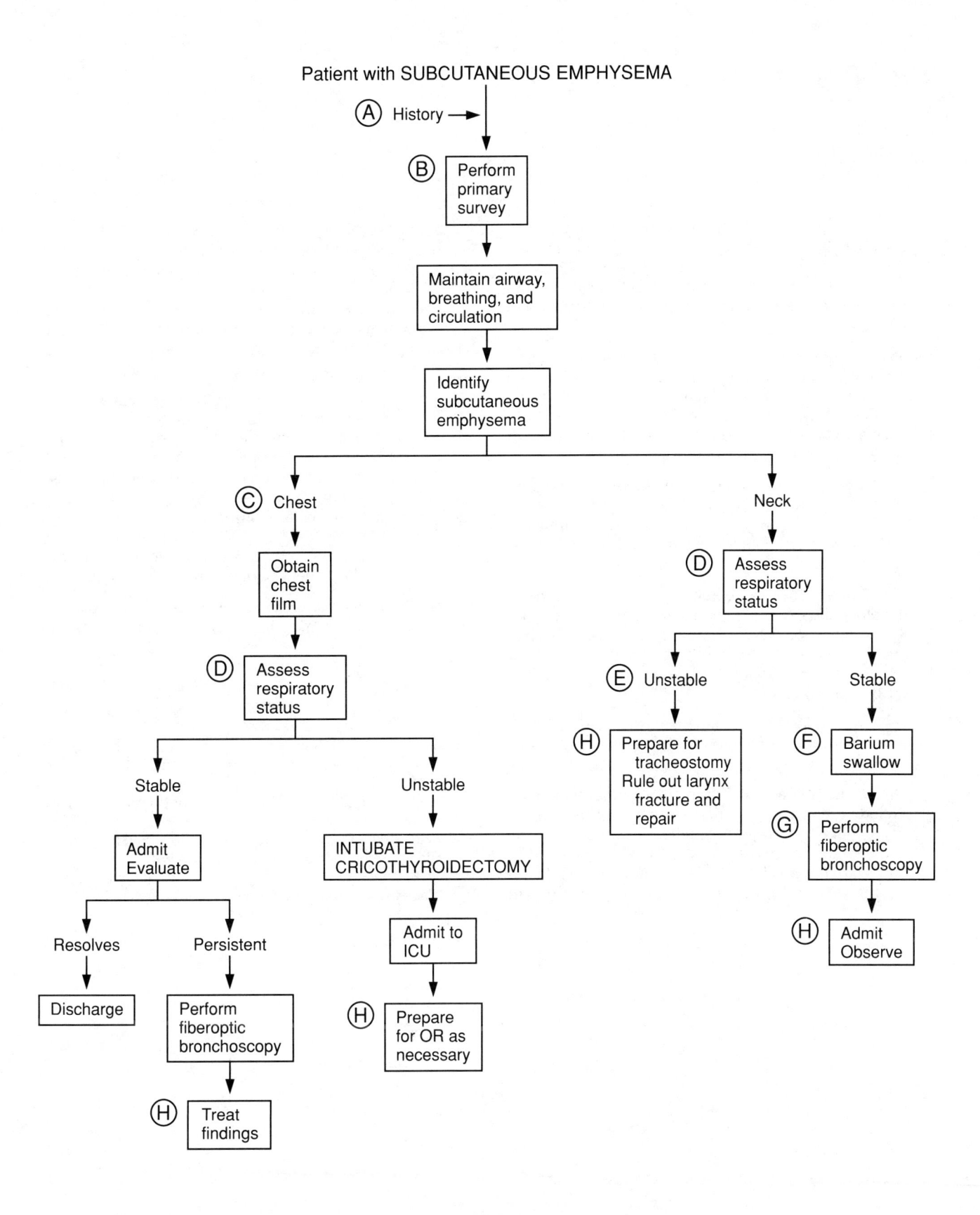

Patient with SUBCUTANEOUS EMPHYSEMA

(A) History →

(B) Perform primary survey

↓

Maintain airway, breathing, and circulation

↓

Identify subcutaneous emphysema

(C) Chest

↓

Obtain chest film

↓

(D) Assess respiratory status

- **Stable** → Admit Evaluate
  - Resolves → Discharge
  - Persistent → Perform fiberoptic bronchoscopy → (H) Treat findings
- **Unstable** → INTUBATE CRICOTHYROIDECTOMY → Admit to ICU → (H) Prepare for OR as necessary

Neck

↓

(D) Assess respiratory status

- (E) **Unstable** → (H) Prepare for tracheostomy. Rule out larynx fracture and repair
- **Stable** → (F) Barium swallow → (G) Perform fiberoptic bronchoscopy → (H) Admit Observe

125

RIB FRACTURES

Jane Curran
Thomas Drury

A. Upon completion of the primary survey, a description of the mechanism of injury will assist in determining the extent of injury. This will guide the assessment and intervention. The three most common mechanisms of injuries are motor vehicle accidents, aggravated assaults, and falls.

B. Sternal fractures are often associated with severe thoracic injuries. Because a major force is required to fracture the sternum, injuries to the heart and great vessels must be considered. Obtain an ECG, cardiac enzymes, and isoenzymes to evaluate for cardiac contusion. An aortogram is obtained to rule out great vessel injuries.

C. Fractures of ribs 1 to 4 require the same consideration as sternal fractures. The force required to fracture ribs 1 to 4 may result from deceleration or crush injuries. A high index of suspicion for underlying thoracic injuries must be maintained.

D. Ribs 5 to 9 sustain most blunt thoracic trauma and are therefore the most commonly fractured ribs. Hemothorax, pneumothorax, or rupture of the tracheobronchial tree can occur. Therefore, bilateral breath sounds and bilateral chest expansion must be assessed and continuously re-evaluated.

E. Fractures in ribs 10 to 12 are often associated with kidney, spleen, and liver injuries because of their close proximity to these organs.

F. Once major thoracic and abdominal injuries have been excluded, the major priority becomes pain relief. The titrating of analgesics should relieve pain but not interfere with the cough mechanism. The elderly patient or one with pre-existing pulmonary disease should be hospitalized and observed. Stringent pulmonary care should consist of incentive spirometry, routine coughing, and deep breathing and analgesics as required. There are several methods of pain relief available to the patient with multiple rib fractures, the obvious being parenteral or oral medication. However, intercostal nerve blocks, transcutaneous electrical nerve stimulator (TENS), and intermittent thoracic epidural instillation with morphine have recently been used.

G. The elderly and those with pre-existing respiratory disease require stringent pulmonary care. Routine care consists of chest films to evaluate for atelectasis and arterial blood gases to assess for hypoxia. The pain from inspiration can lead to hypoventilation and eventually atelectasis. Congruent with a pre-existing disease, atelectasis can lead to respiratory insufficiency. An assessment should be made for character of breath sounds, bilateral chest expansion, and capillary refill to determine any change in the patient's condition.

H. Simple rib fractures require analgesics. These patients are discharged home with instructions and follow-up appointments.

References

American College of Surgeons. Advanced trauma life support course. Chicago: American College of Surgeons, 1988:89–111.

Crowley RA, Dunham MC. Shock trauma/critical care handbook. Rockville, MD: Aspen, 1988:145–187.

Knezevich B. Trauma nursing: principles and practice. Norwalk, CT: Appleton-Century-Crofts, 1986:73–99.

Perdue P. Chest trauma. In: Cardona V, ed. Trauma nursing. Oradell, NJ: Medical Economics Books, 1985:123–139.

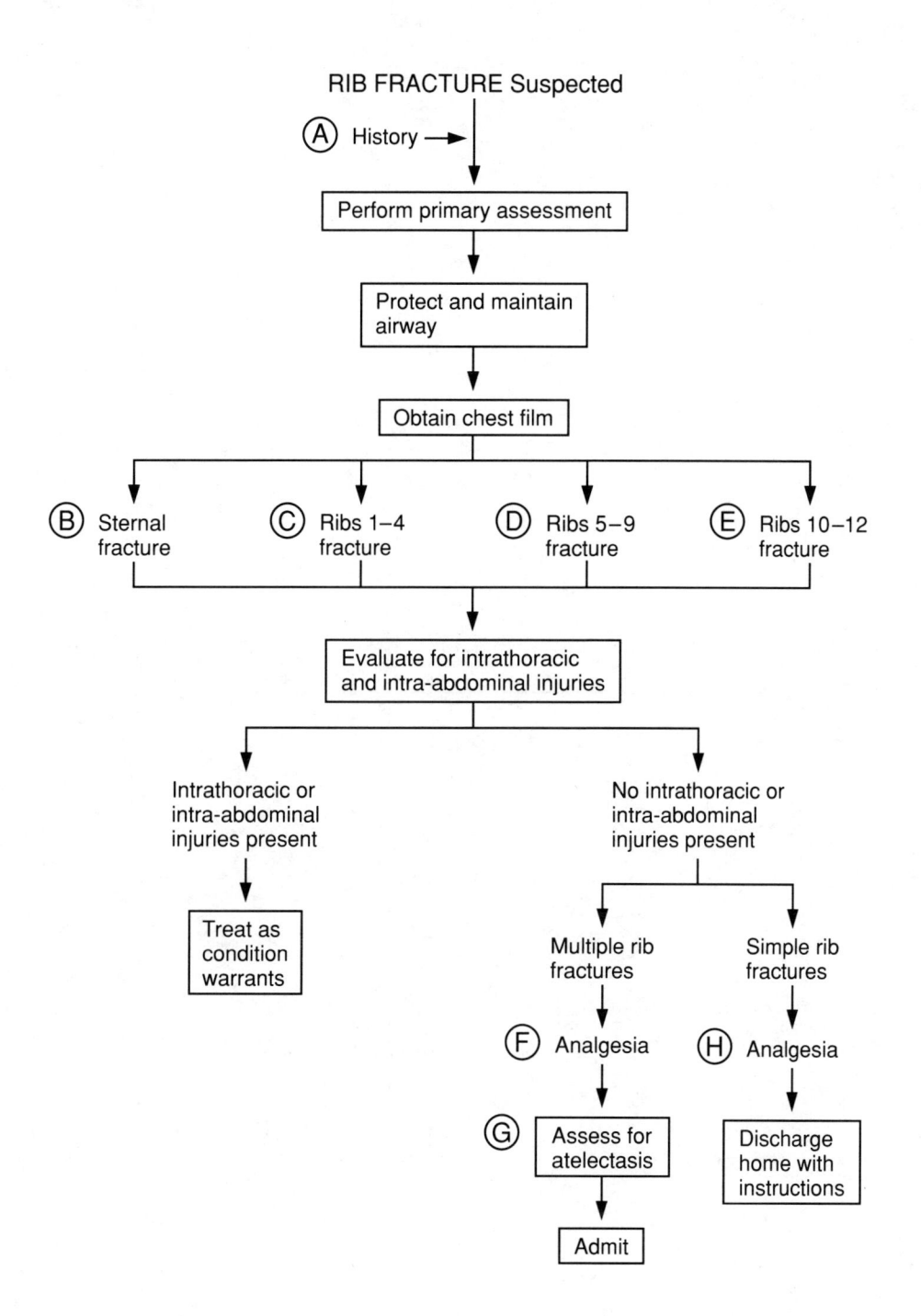

```
                    RIB FRACTURE Suspected
              (A) History ──►
                              │
                              ▼
                   ┌──────────────────────┐
                   │ Perform primary      │
                   │ assessment           │
                   └──────────┬───────────┘
                              ▼
                   ┌──────────────────────┐
                   │ Protect and maintain │
                   │ airway               │
                   └──────────┬───────────┘
                              ▼
                   ┌──────────────────────┐
                   │ Obtain chest film    │
                   └──────────┬───────────┘
         ┌──────────┬─────────┼─────────┬──────────┐
         ▼          ▼         ▼         ▼          ▼
      (B) Sternal (C) Ribs 1–4 (D) Ribs 5–9 (E) Ribs 10–12
          fracture    fracture    fracture     fracture
                              │
                              ▼
                   ┌──────────────────────┐
                   │ Evaluate for         │
                   │ intrathoracic and    │
                   │ intra-abdominal      │
                   │ injuries             │
                   └──────────┬───────────┘
              ┌───────────────┴───────────────┐
              ▼                               ▼
      Intrathoracic or              No intrathoracic or
      intra-abdominal               intra-abdominal
      injuries present              injuries present
              │                   ┌───────────┴───────────┐
              ▼                   ▼                       ▼
      ┌──────────────┐      Multiple rib             Simple rib
      │ Treat as     │      fractures                fractures
      │ condition    │          │                       │
      │ warrants     │     (F) Analgesia          (H) Analgesia
      └──────────────┘          │                       │
                                ▼                       ▼
                       (G) ┌──────────────┐      ┌──────────────┐
                           │ Assess for   │      │ Discharge    │
                           │ atelectasis  │      │ home with    │
                           └──────┬───────┘      │ instructions │
                                  ▼              └──────────────┘
                           ┌──────────────┐
                           │ Admit        │
                           └──────────────┘
```

ABDOMINAL TRAUMA

Blunt Abdominal Trauma
Penetrating Abdominal Trauma
Trauma to the Pelvis

BLUNT ABDOMINAL TRAUMA

Thomas Drury

A. Obtaining information on the mechanism of injury is extremely important in blunt abdominal trauma. The most common mechanisms of injury are motor vehicle accidents, falls, and aggravated assaults. The time and mechanism of injury, estimated speed of impact, damage to involved vehicles, use and types of restraining devices, position and location of the victims after the accident, and the condition of other occupants must be elicited from prehospital personnel. When the patient has pelvic fractures, a major chest injury, hypotension on arrival, or hypotension in the field, an abdominal injury must be suspected. The most commonly injured organs are the spleen and liver.

B. Baseline blood studies are important in determining trends in specific levels (e.g., hematocrit, amylase). A complete blood cell count (CBC) with differential, electrolytes, amylase, type and cross-match, and drug and alcohol levels (if appropriate) should be attained.

C. Insert at least two large bore (16 gauge or greater) intravenous catheters peripherally or via cutdown. The subclavian route is contraindicated in trauma patients.

D. A complete abdominal examination must be undertaken in the following order: inspection, auscultation, percussion, and palpation. Evaluate for guarding, rigidity, distention, and pain. Remember that hollow organs can burst and cause early signs of peritonitis and late signs of hypovolemia, whereas ruptured solid organs cause early signs of hypovolemia and late signs of peritonitis.

E. A Foley catheter is inserted to assess hourly output and to evaluate for shock. Insertion of a Foley catheter is contraindicated when blood is present at the urinary meatus, when there is a scrotal or perineal hematoma (butterfly), or when a high riding prostate is present. A suprapubic cystostomy may be necessary.

F. Urine should be tested with a hematest. If positive, an intravenous pyelogram, urethrogram, or cystogram may be necessary, depending on the suspected area of injury.

G. A nasogastric tube is inserted to prevent aspiration and to decompress the upper gastrointestinal tract. The aspirate should be evaluated for blood, which is a sign of disruption to the tract.

Patient with BLUNT ABDOMINAL TRAUMA

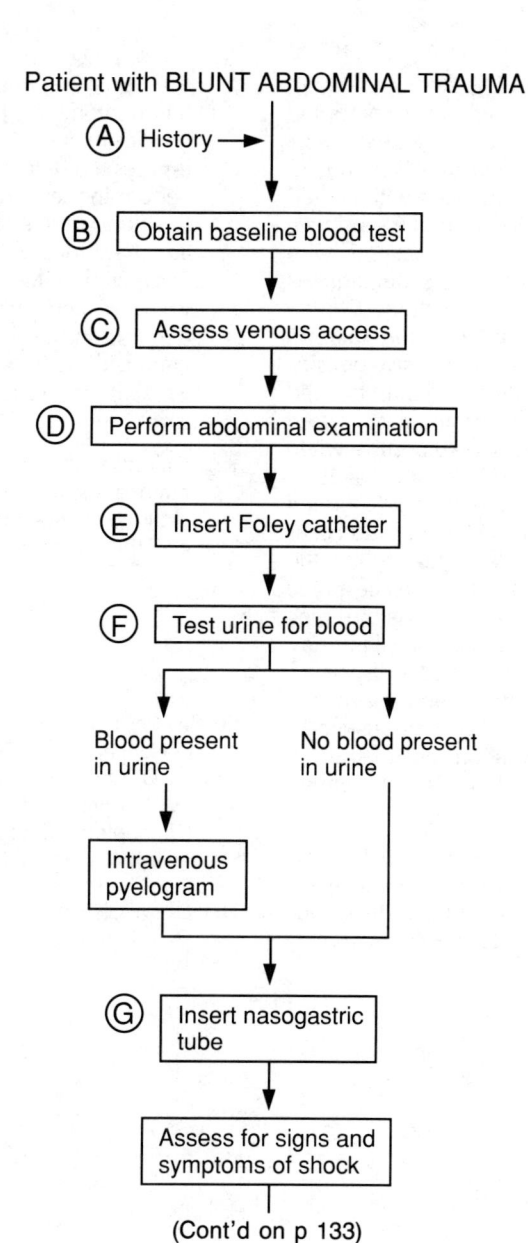

- (A) History →
- (B) Obtain baseline blood test
- (C) Assess venous access
- (D) Perform abdominal examination
- (E) Insert Foley catheter
- (F) Test urine for blood
  - Blood present in urine → Intravenous pyelogram
  - No blood present in urine
- (G) Insert nasogastric tube
- Assess for signs and symptoms of shock

(Cont'd on p 133)

H. Controversy exists regarding diagnostic studies for evaluation of abdominal injuries. The use of a computed tomography (CT) scan or a diagnostic peritoneal lavage (DPL) is a physician's preference. Indications for DPL include (1) spinal cord or head injuries along with altered mental status, (2) any altered mental status, (3) substance or alcohol abuse, and (4) polytrauma patients who require anesthesia but for whom examination is impossible and anesthesia will mask symptoms. Contraindications for DPL include existing need for laparotomy, multiple abdominal surgeries, and massive obesity. An alternative approach (i.e., open method) must be used for the gravida uterus, and a suprapubic approach is used with pelvic fractures. A DPL is considered positive when any of the following are present: (1) aspiration of 10 to 20 ml of nonclotted blood, (2) greater than 100,000 red blood cells (RBCs), (3) greater than 500 white blood cells (WBCs), (4) bacteria, bile, or amylase greater than 100 units per liter, and (5) lavage fluid exiting the chest tube or Foley catheter. A CT scan is noninvasive, defines type and extent of injury, and detects retroperitoneal injuries. A diaphragm injury is not determined reliably by physical examination or DPL and is often found during surgery. However, diaphragm injuries should be suspected when an abnormal air shadow is present in the left hemithorax or when irregular or indistinct hemidiaphragm is present on chest film.

I. A hypotensive patient with positive physical findings indicates the need for immediate exploratory laparotomy. The patient should not undergo further testing, such as DPL or CT scan, but should instead go immediately to the operating room.

J. A CT scan can define structures at risk for injury in the retroperitoneum. The CT scan better defines solid organ injuries than it does hollow viscous injuries. Pancreatic injuries are determined by monitoring amylase and by performing serial examinations. Renal injuries including the kidney, ureter, bladder, and urethra are evaluated by an intravenous pyelogram, cystogram, and urethrogram. Deceleration injuries often cause injuries to the inferior vena cava and aorta. These injuries have a high mortality rate, and many patients die at the scene. An arteriogram is done to evaluate for retroperitoneal injury, and a high index of suspicion and knowledge of the mechanism of injury are key.

K. Patients with unimpaired levels of consciousness and no major associated injury may be safely observed with serial blood studies and repeat CT scans. Patients who undergo DPL are admitted and observed for 24 hours.

References

Cowley RA, Dunham MC. Shock trauma/critical care handbook. Rockville, MD: Aspen, 1986:201–253.

Gibson D. Abdominal trauma. Trauma Q 1987; 4:11–25.

Knezevick B. Trauma nursing: principles and practice. Norwalk, CT: Appleton-Century-Crofts, 1986:99–112.

Strange JM. Abdominal trauma. In: Cordona V, ed. Trauma nursing. Oradell, NJ: Medical Economics Books, 1985:87.

Thal ER, McClelland RN, Shires TA. Abdominal trauma. In: Shires TA, ed. Principles of trauma care. New York: McGraw-Hill, 1985:291.

(Cont'd from p 131)

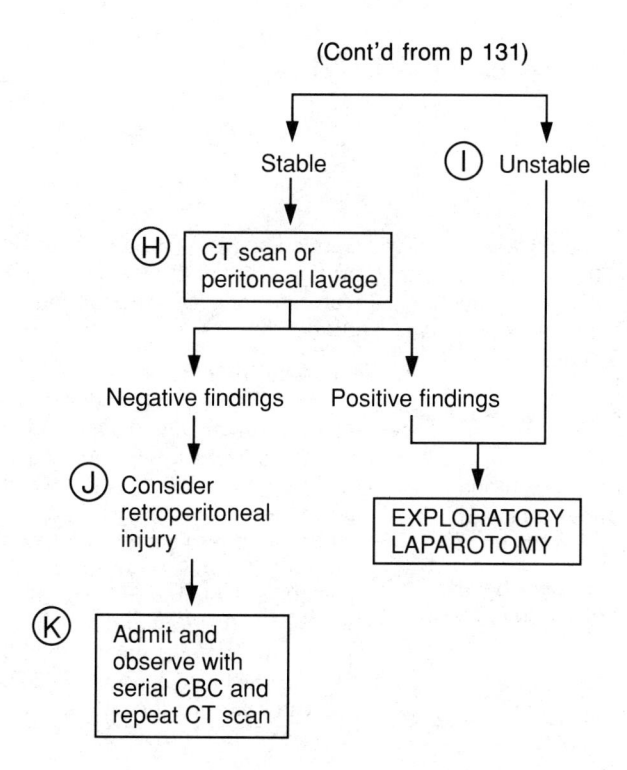

```
                Stable              Ⓘ Unstable
                  │                      │
                  ▼                      │
           ┌──────────────┐              │
        Ⓗ │  CT scan or  │              │
           │  peritoneal  │              │
           │   lavage     │              │
           └──────────────┘              │
              │       │                  │
              ▼       ▼                  │
        Negative    Positive             │
        findings    findings             │
              │       │                  │
              │       └──────────┬───────┘
              ▼                  ▼
        Ⓙ Consider         ┌──────────────┐
          retroperitoneal  │ EXPLORATORY  │
          injury           │ LAPAROTOMY   │
              │            └──────────────┘
              ▼
           ┌──────────────┐
        Ⓚ │ Admit and    │
           │ observe with │
           │ serial CBC and│
           │ repeat CT scan│
           └──────────────┘
```

PENETRATING ABDOMINAL TRAUMA

Thomas Drury

A. Information regarding the history of injury should be obtained, including the time of injury, type of weapon, handgun caliber, knife length, distance of victim from assailant, number of gunshot or stab wounds noted, and amount of blood at scene. The organs most often injured with stab wounds include the liver, diaphragm, and spleen. With gunshot wounds, the small bowel, liver, and large bowel are most often injured.

B. The initial blood work should include a complete blood cell count (CBC) with differential, electrolytes, amylase, type and cross-match, and alcohol and drug screen.

C. As with all trauma patients, two large bore peripheral (16 gauge or greater) intravenous catheters should be inserted.

D. A Foley catheter is inserted to monitor urinary output. The urine is hematested for the possibility of renal injury. Before catheter insertion, the patient must be evaluated for urethral or bladder damage if any of the following is present: blood at the meatus, scrotal or perineal hematoma, or a high riding prostate. Either an intravenous pyelogram, urethrogram, or cystogram is ordered, depending on the suspected area of injury.

E. A nasogastric tube is inserted to decompress the gastrointestinal tract and to prevent aspiration. The aspirate is assessed for blood, the presence of which is a possible sign of gastrointestinal injury.

F. Treatment depends on the location of the stab wounds.

G. The anteroposterior area is that area below the costal cartilages to the inguinal ligament and below the inferior tip of the scapula to the superior tip of the iliac crest. Treatment includes a local wound exploration to determine whether peritoneal penetration did occur. The area is anesthetized locally and extended if necessary. When the wound does not enter the peritoneum (i.e., the injury does not extend past the posterior rectus fascia or the internal oblique muscle), irrigation, debridement, and closure are performed.

H. If the wound enters the peritoneum or if the depth of the tract cannot be determined, further diagnostic evaluation is necessary.

I. In thoracoabdominal injuries, that region from the nipple line to the costal cartilages, both the chest and the abdomen can be injured because of the raising of the diaphragm during expiration. Local wound explorations are contraindicated because of the possibility of creating a pneumothorax. However, an abdominal injury must be ruled out, and thus a computed tomography (CT) scan or diagnostic peritoneal lavage (DPL) is in order. A CT scan can often define the wound tract in a retroperitoneal injury.

J. A nasogastric tube and Foley catheter are prerequisites for DPLs. There is much debate regarding what constitutes a positive DPL in stab wound patients. Some physicians consider a DPL positive with a red blood cell (RBC) count of 1,000 cells, which ensures that small lacerations to hollow organs are detected. However, standard positive result criteria include the following: (1) aspiration of 10 to 20 ml of nonclotting blood; (2) greater than 100,000 red blood cells; (3) greater than 500 white blood cells (WBCs); and (4) presence of bile, bacteria, or an amylase level greater than 100 units per liter. In the case of thoracoabdominal stab wounds, some sources advocate lowering the criteria level for RBCs to 5,000 to incorporate the possibility of a diaphragm injury.

K. In the case of evisceration, the patient requires an exploratory laparotomy to determine the extent of injury. DPL, CT scan, and local wound exploration are not done.

L. All unstable patients are taken immediately to the operating room. Evaluation with local wound exploration, DPL, or CT scan is unnecessary because the abdomen must be explored to determine the exact cause of hypotension. As is the case with all penetrating injuries, a tetanus toxoid is given as well as a broad-spectrum antibiotic prior to departing for the operating room.

M. The treatment of gunshot wounds to the abdomen is the same regardless of whether the patient is stable. All patients undergo an exploratory laparotomy. The degree of injury is dependent on the distance, speed, and size of the missile and on the organs involved. A bullet can hit bony prominences and change direction. Therefore, the bullet cannot be assumed to have traveled a straight path.

References

Cowley RA, Dunham MC. Shock trauma/critical care handbook. Rockville, MD: Aspen, 1986:201–253.

Gibson D. Abdominal trauma. Trauma Q 1987; 4:11–25.

Knezevick B. Trauma nursing: principles and practice. Norwalk, CT: Appleton-Century-Crofts, 1986:99–112.

Strange JM. Abdominal trauma. In: Cardona V, ed. Trauma nursing. Oradell, NJ: Medical Economics Books, 1985:87.

Thal ER, McClelland RN, Shires TA. Abdominal trauma. In: Shires TA, ed. Principles of trauma care. New York: McGraw-Hill, 1985:291.

Patient with PENETRATING ABDOMINAL TRAUMA

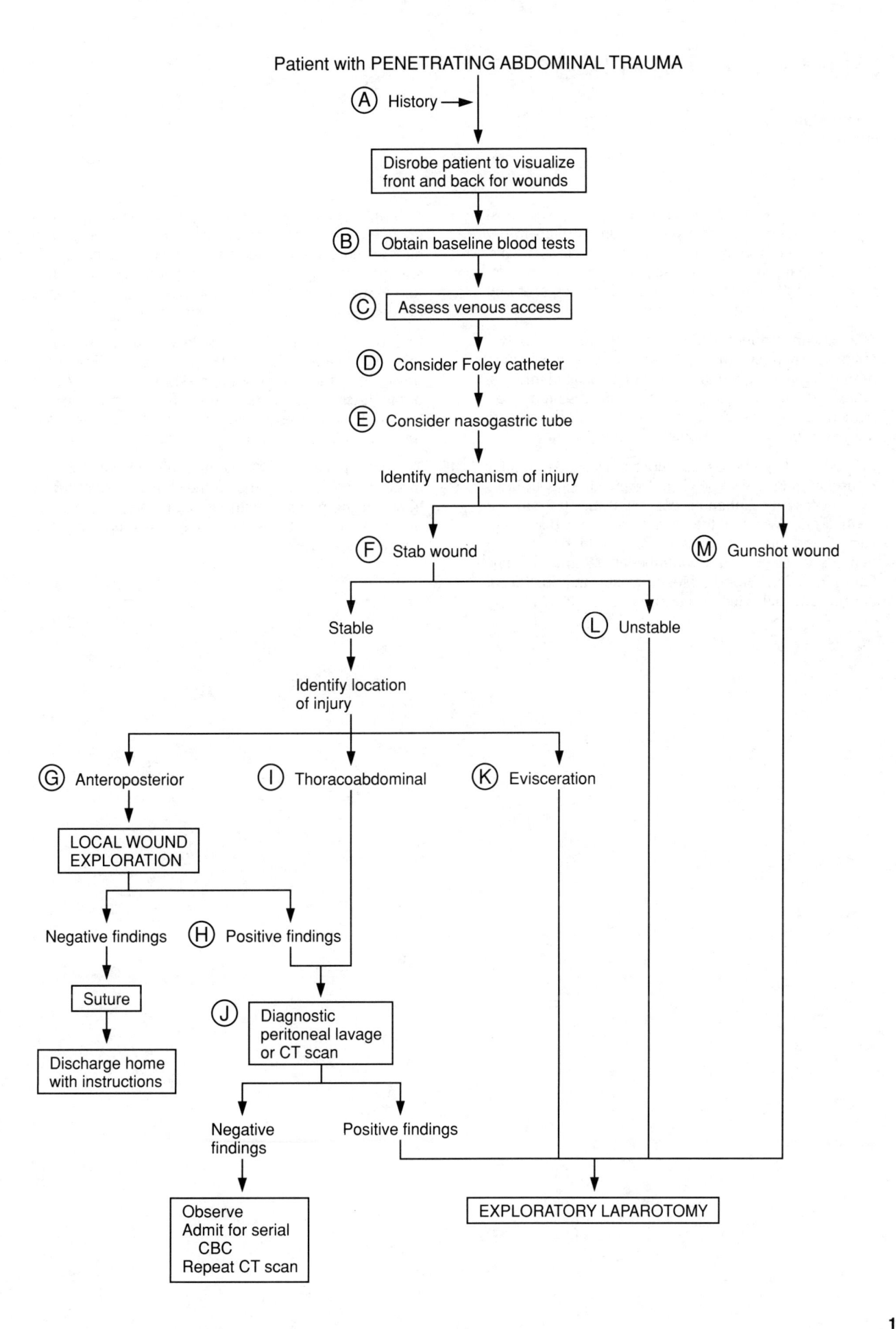

(A) History →

↓

Disrobe patient to visualize front and back for wounds

↓

(B) Obtain baseline blood tests

↓

(C) Assess venous access

↓

(D) Consider Foley catheter

↓

(E) Consider nasogastric tube

↓

Identify mechanism of injury

- (F) Stab wound
  - Stable
    - Identify location of injury
      - (G) Anteroposterior → LOCAL WOUND EXPLORATION
        - Negative findings → Suture → Discharge home with instructions
        - (H) Positive findings
      - (I) Thoracoabdominal → (J) Diagnostic peritoneal lavage or CT scan
        - Negative findings → Observe, Admit for serial CBC, Repeat CT scan
        - Positive findings → EXPLORATORY LAPAROTOMY
      - (K) Evisceration → EXPLORATORY LAPAROTOMY
  - (L) Unstable → EXPLORATORY LAPAROTOMY
- (M) Gunshot wound → EXPLORATORY LAPAROTOMY

135

TRAUMA TO THE PELVIS

Connie Mattice
Nathan Coates

A. Pelvic fractures can be devastating injuries. The most common mechanism of pelvic fracture is blunt injury such as caused by motor vehicle or motorcycle accidents. Penetrating injuries rarely cause pelvic fractures. History should include the etiology, speed of impact, seat belt use, and extrication time.

B. A significant amount of force is needed to cause pelvic fractures. Therefore, these patients have a relatively high mortality rate from hemorrhage and associated injuries. Open fractures can have a mortality rate as high as 50 percent. Signs of shock or associated injuries indicate the need for immediate operative intervention.

C. At least two large bore intravenous lines are needed for resuscitation. If severe pelvic or lower extremity injuries exist, access via saphenous cut-downs may not provide central circulation if the iliac vessels are disrupted. Packed red blood cells (PRBCs) should be given if hemodynamic instability continues after 2 to 3 L of crystalloid infusion. Blood losses of greater than 6,000 ml are not unusual with severe injuries.

D. A simple anteroposterior view of the pelvis provides enough information to detect most fractures. Specialized films are not usually needed. Computed tomography (CT) scanning may be of value, especially if an acetabular fracture is suspected. Careful hemodynamic monitoring is needed while the patient is in the radiology suite.

E. Physical examination is vital to the assessment of pelvic injuries. If pain is elicited by pushing the iliac crests down, by compression of the crests toward each other, or by pressing against the pubis, a fracture must be suspected. Unfortunately, physical examination alone may miss up to 25 percent of pelvic fractures.

F. The determination of a potential injury is vital. Ecchymosis or hematoma around the penis or scrotum or blood at the penile meatus is highly suggestive of an injury. A Foley catheter cannot be placed until urethral integrity is assured.

Patient with TRAUMA TO THE PELVIS

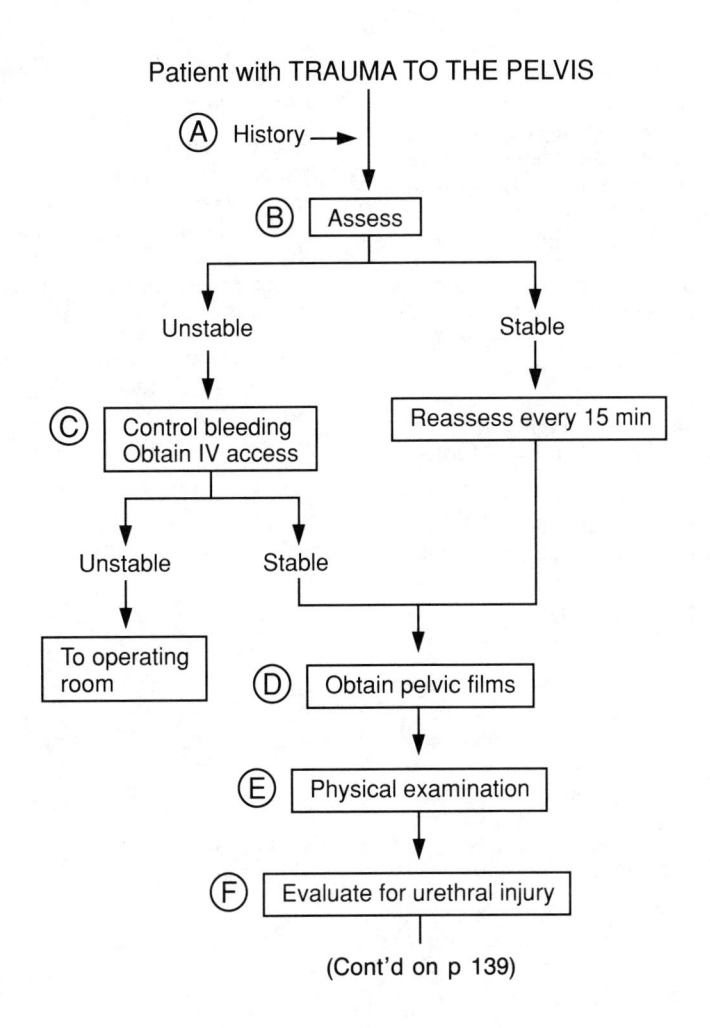

(A) History →

(B) Assess
- Unstable
  - (C) Control bleeding / Obtain IV access
    - Unstable → To operating room
    - Stable →
- Stable → Reassess every 15 min →

(D) Obtain pelvic films

(E) Physical examination

(F) Evaluate for urethral injury

(Cont'd on p 139)

G. Rectal and vaginal examinations determine the existence of an open fracture. Assessment of rectal tone is also important. Inability to palpate the prostate suggests a membranous urethral disruption and the need for a retrograde urethrogram. As the hematoma accumulates, the prostate gland is displaced superiorly. Blood may indicate rectal trauma, possibly caused by a bony fragment.

H. Fifteen to 20 ml of water soluble contrast is injected into the meatus in a sterile manner. Voiding is prevented by urethral compression until a plain film is obtained. Any evidence of extravasation indicates the need for further studies (i.e., intravenous pyelogram [IVP], cystogram) to exclude other urologic injuries. If urethral integrity is disrupted, a Foley catheter is precluded to prevent further urethral injury.

I. Hematuria is the best indicator of renal trauma. A count of greater than 40 red blood cells per high power field suggests the need for an IVP and a cystogram to exclude other injuries.

J. Because contrast is used for IVP, knowledge of the patient's renal function is vital. Increasing the intravenous infusion rate may promote a renal dye "washout." Films obtained 8 to 10 minutes after dye infusion demonstrate the parenchyma and collecting systems. CT scanning is an alternative diagnostic procedure for complex injuries but is not a good initial screening test.

K. Urologic input is valuable in planning the patient's potential operative sequence. Suprapubic catheter placement is mandatory for urethral injuries. Controversy continues, however, regarding placement of a Foley catheter at the same time.

(Cont'd from p 137)

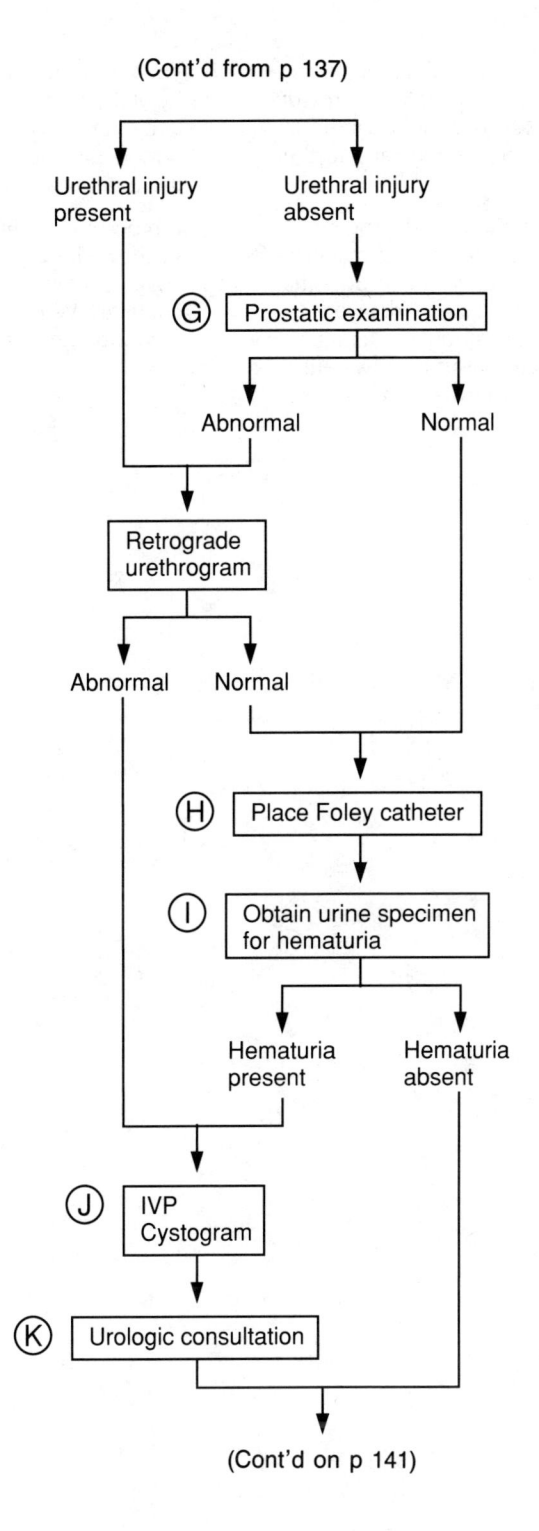

```
         ┌──────────────┬──────────────┐
         ▼                             ▼
   Urethral injury              Urethral injury
      present                       absent
         │                             │
         │                             ▼
         │                    ⓖ  Prostatic examination
         │                      ┌──────────┬──────────┐
         │                      ▼                     ▼
         │                   Abnormal              Normal
         │                      │                     │
         ▼                      ▼                     │
                                                      │
   ┌──────────────┐                                   │
   │ Retrograde   │                                   │
   │ urethrogram  │                                   │
   └──────────────┘                                   │
      ┌────┬────┐                                     │
      ▼         ▼                                     │
  Abnormal   Normal                                   │
      │         │                                     │
      │         └─────────────────┬───────────────────┘
      │                           ▼
      │                  ⓗ  Place Foley catheter
      │                           │
      │                           ▼
      │                  ⓘ  Obtain urine specimen
      │                      for hematuria
      │                      ┌────────┬────────┐
      │                      ▼                 ▼
      │                 Hematuria          Hematuria
      │                  present             absent
      │                      │                 │
      └──────────┬───────────┘                 │
                 ▼                             │
         ⓙ  IVP                                │
            Cystogram                          │
                 │                             │
                 ▼                             │
         ⓚ  Urologic consultation              │
                 └──────────────┬──────────────┘
                                ▼
```

(Cont'd on p 141)

139

L. If an open fracture is noted by rectal, vaginal, or skin assessment, operative intervention is needed to provide fecal, and possibly urinary, diversion. Orthopaedic input is essential in determining fracture type and further therapy.

M. Fixation by internal or external methods can be considered. Internal fixation risks disruption of the tamponading fascial planes of the retroperitoneum and potential exsanguination, and therefore it is usually delayed. External fixation methods allow rapid ambulation; patients can go home with them in place. Unfortunately, neither form of fixation halts massive hemorrhage nor reduces markedly displaced fractures.

N. The key to nonoperative therapy is assessing the stability of the fracture. A stable, or minimally displaced, fracture such as a pubic or single ischial ring can be managed nonoperatively. Early ambulation is vital in preventing the complications of bed rest.

O. If blood loss continues, further PRBC administration is needed. Transfusions of greater than 10 units risk a coagulopathy; therefore, clotting times are monitored accordingly. Warming the hypothermic patient may prevent a continuing coagulopathy.

(Cont'd from p 139)

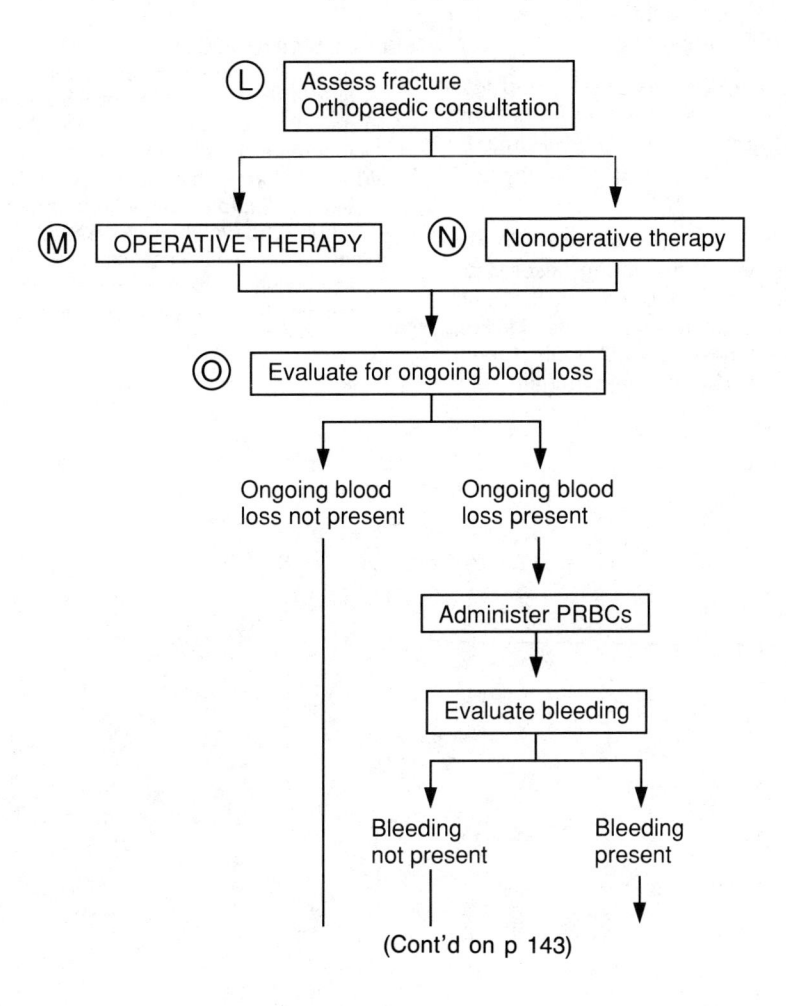

```
                    Ⓛ ┌─────────────────────────┐
                      │ Assess fracture          │
                      │ Orthopaedic consultation │
                      └─────────────────────────┘
                           │              │
                           ▼              ▼
              Ⓜ ┌──────────────────┐  Ⓝ ┌──────────────────┐
                │ OPERATIVE THERAPY│    │ Nonoperative therapy│
                └──────────────────┘    └──────────────────┘
                           │
                           ▼
                  Ⓞ ┌─────────────────────────────┐
                    │ Evaluate for ongoing blood loss│
                    └─────────────────────────────┘
                         │              │
                         ▼              ▼
                 Ongoing blood    Ongoing blood
                 loss not present  loss present
                         │              │
                         │              ▼
                         │      ┌──────────────────┐
                         │      │ Administer PRBCs │
                         │      └──────────────────┘
                         │              │
                         │              ▼
                         │      ┌──────────────────┐
                         │      │ Evaluate bleeding│
                         │      └──────────────────┘
                         │          │        │
                         │          ▼        ▼
                         │      Bleeding   Bleeding
                         │      not present present
                         │          │        │
                         └──────────┘        ▼
                         (Cont'd on p 143)
```

141

P. Pneumatic antishock garments (PASGs) or military antishock trouser (MAST) suits may stabilize fractures, but they do not prevent further blood loss.

Q. Angiography may be useful for continued blood loss. Delineation of a single vessel allows embolization; however, single vessel injury as the source of ongoing blood loss occurs in only 1 percent of these patients, approximately.

R. If the above modalities fail, operative intervention may be needed. Large single vessel disruption necessitates repair. If there is no single vessel injury, packing the pelvis and closing may tamponade further losses. Packing removal must occur in the next 48 to 72 hours. Operative intervention is associated with a high mortality rate.

References

Burke J, Boyd R, McCabe C. Trauma management: early management of visceral nervous system and musculoskeletal system injuries. Chicago: Year Book, 1988.

Campbell J. Basic trauma life support: advanced pre-hospital care. Baltimore: Brady Communication, 1985.

Cardona V, Hurn P, Bastangel-Mason P, Scanlon-Schilpp A, Veise-Berry S. Trauma nursing from resuscitation through rehabilitation. Philadelphia: WB Saunders, 1988:527–539.

Moreno C, Moore EE, Rosenberger A, Cleveland H. Hemorrhage associated with major pelvic fractures: a multispecialty challenge. J Trauma 1986; 26:987–994.

(Cont'd from p 141)

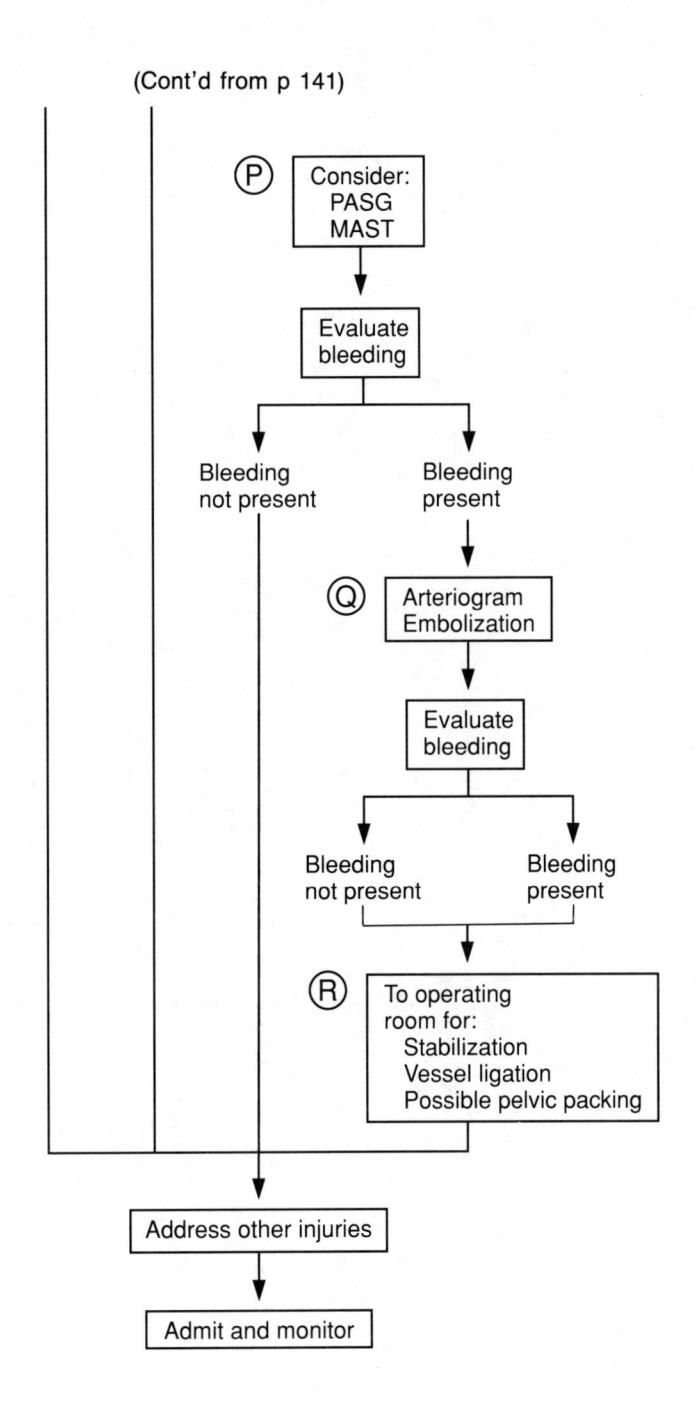

Ⓟ Consider:
PASG
MAST

↓

Evaluate bleeding

↓ ↓
Bleeding not present / Bleeding present

↓
Ⓠ Arteriogram Embolization

↓

Evaluate bleeding

↓ ↓
Bleeding not present / Bleeding present

↓
Ⓡ To operating room for:
  Stabilization
  Vessel ligation
  Possible pelvic packing

↓

Address other injuries

↓

Admit and monitor

SPINAL TRAUMA

Cervical Spinal Trauma
Thoracolumbar Spinal Trauma

CERVICAL SPINAL TRAUMA

Suzy Baulch
Jeffrey M. Lobosky

A. All patients with multisystem trauma, head injury, or altered mental status from any cause (e.g., alcohol or drug intoxication) should be assumed to have suffered a cervical spine injury until such is ruled out. Complaints of neck pain, numbness or tingling in the extremities, weakness, or paralysis are indications of a spinal cord injury until proved otherwise. Certain injuries such as diving accidents, head trauma, and other acceleration-deceleration injuries predispose to vertebral column and/or spinal cord injury. Both should be considered with a high index of suspicion. Flexion may result in a wedge fracture of the vertebrae, whereas hyperextension can cause disruption of the intervertebral disk. A high distance fall can result in a compression fracture.

B. Airway, breathing, and circulation must be secured and maintained. The spine must be immobilized with spine boards, rigid collars, towel rolls and/or sand bags, and tape to avoid damage or further injury to the spinal cord. It is estimated that 10 to 15 percent of all spinal cord injuries actually occur *after* the patient has received assistance from bystanders or medical personnel.

C. Careful clinical evaluation of the patient is mandatory for both the patient's well-being and medicolegal documentation. Any neurologic deficit should be noted and pertinent negatives included. Neurologic deficits depend on location and severity of the injury. Injury that completely disrupts the spinal cord results in total paralysis and loss of sensation below the level of the lesion. With the incomplete injury there is some preservation of sensory and/or motor function below the level of the lesion. Categorization of the incomplete transection is made according to the area of damage, i.e., central, anterior, lateral, or peripheral. A thorough review of other organ systems and close monitoring of vital signs should be carried out.

D. Initial radiographic studies should include lateral cervical spine films that provide adequate visualization from the skull base to the C7, T1 interspace. An arteroposterior "open mouth" odontoid view should be obtained, and a "swimmer's view" may be required to evaluate the lower cervical spine.

E. Review of the radiographic studies should determine the presence of a spinal fracture. However, factors such as poor patient cooperation, thick soft tissues, or other injuries may prevent verification. For this reason treatment for spinal cord injury should be initiated without delay.

F. There are instances when the patient can suffer damage to the spinal cord or nerve roots without a fracture. This situation most often arises in the very young and very old. These patients should be treated as promptly as patients with a spinal fracture. Those patients with negative films and no neurologic injury can be managed conservatively.

G. All patients with a confirmed fracture or with a neurologic deficit, and all patients whose radiographs are equivocal, need vigilant maintenance of spinal immobilization. Intravenous access with a large bore catheter should be established because patients with spinal cord injury may be hypotensive and bradycardic as a result of sympathetic nervous system disruption. A Foley catheter is inserted to help monitor fluid balance. A nasogastric tube is inserted to prevent abdominal distention from interfering with respiratory efforts. Careful evaluation of vital signs and neurologic function is mandatory every 45 minutes.

CERVICAL SPINAL TRAUMA Suspected

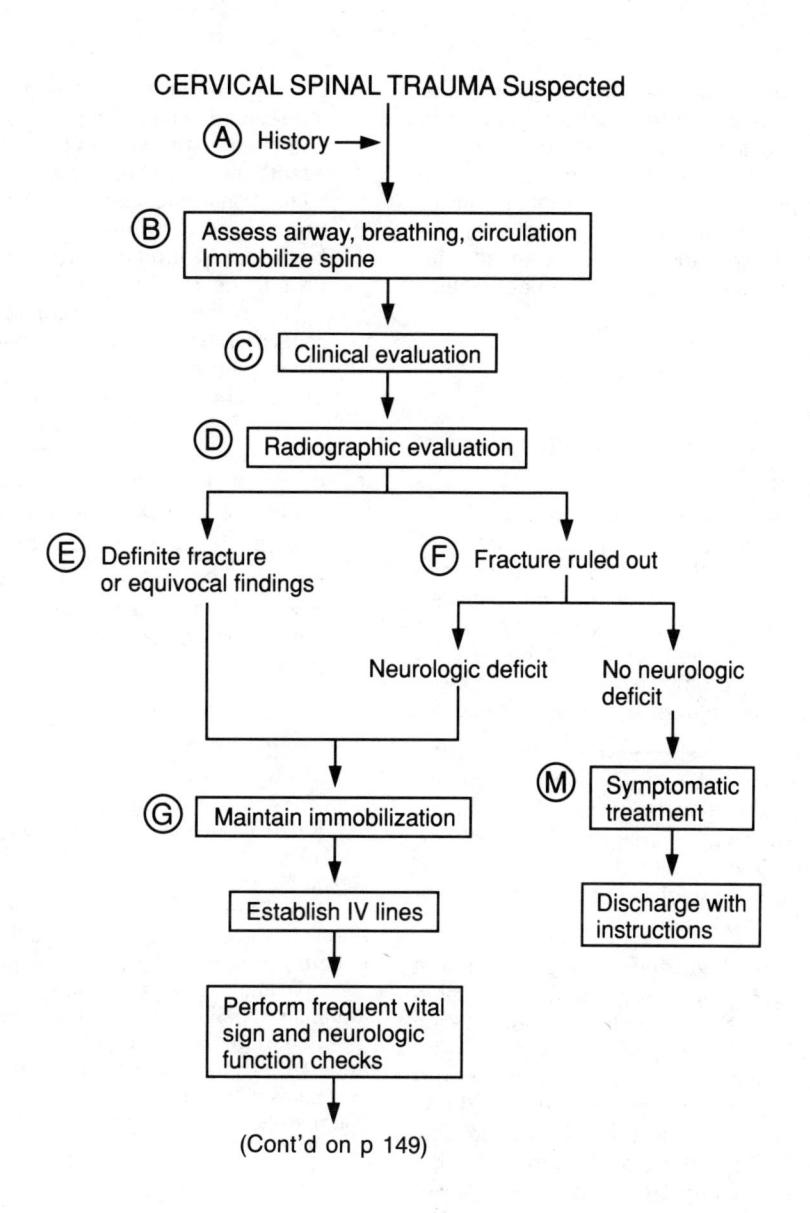

- **A** History
- **B** Assess airway, breathing, circulation; Immobilize spine
- **C** Clinical evaluation
- **D** Radiographic evaluation
  - **E** Definite fracture or equivocal findings
  - **F** Fracture ruled out
    - Neurologic deficit
    - No neurologic deficit
      - **M** Symptomatic treatment
        - Discharge with instructions
- **G** Maintain immobilization
  - Establish IV lines
  - Perform frequent vital sign and neurologic function checks

(Cont'd on p 149)

H. Additional radiographic studies are usually required to define the extent of osseous interruption, the stability of the damaged segment, and the degree of spinal cord or nerve root compromise. Flexion-extension views of the lateral spine, computed tomography scanning with or without intrathecal contrast material, magnetic resonance imaging, polytomography, and myelography are all valuable adjuncts in this evaluation. Strict immobilization must be maintained.

I. Once the above studies are completed, the clinical team should be able to define accurately the extent of the fracture and to determine the stability of the fracture. These studies should also rule out a fracture in the patient whose initial studies were equivocal.

J. Stable fractures are those in which the osseous disruption was insufficient to compromise spinal alignment or to allow abnormal mobility. Patients who have stable fractures but are neurologically intact may be managed symptomatically (see paragraph M). Any patient with a neurologic deficit, even if the fracture is stable or if no fracture exists, warrants prompt entry into a treatment protocol for spinal cord injuries.

K. Unstable fractures pose the greatest risk to both the patient and the clinical team. These patients may be neurologically normal or have minimal initial deficits, but imprudent management or improper immobilization may be catastrophic. Therefore strict, defined immobilization protocols must be established and frequent neurologic re-evaluation monitored.

L. All patients with a neurologic deficit and those without a deficit but with a radiographically confirmed unstable fracture need immediate attention in an intensive care unit (ICU) staffed by qualified personnel who care for the spinal injured patient. An arterial line, central venous monitor, and cardiac monitor are required in addition to intravenous lines, Foley catheter, and nasogastric tube. Those patients suffering a spinal cord injury invariably experience respiratory compromise from loss of intercostal muscle groups. Thus, careful monitoring of pulse oximetry, blood gases, tidal volume, and vital capacity is essential. Hypotension and bradycardia from sympathetic nervous system disruption may require pressor agents and atropine. These patients often require skeletal traction for maintenance of immobilization and reduction of bony deformity. Most frequently this is achieved by the application of Gardner-Wells skull tongs or Halo orthotic device. Many patients may require direct surgical intervention to decompress the spinal cord or nerve roots or to provide rapid, permanent bony stabilization. Finally, these injuries affect not only the patient but his or her family, friends, and the clinical treatment team as well. Strong psychological support and early intervention by trained counselors and rehabilitation physiatrists minimize the difficulties suffered by these patients and maximize their potential for a reasonable recovery.

M. Patients who are neurologically intact and have normal radiographic studies are to be treated symptomatically. A soft collar for musculoskeletal support and the administration of analgesics and muscle relaxants are appropriate.

References

Cooper PR. Management of posttraumatic spinal instability. Park Ridge, IL: American Association of Neurological Surgeons, 1990.

Gazna ER, Harrington IJ. Biomechanics of musculoskeletal injury. Boston: Williams & Wilkins, 1982:163–222.

Hanak M, Scott A. Spinal cord injury. New York: Springer, 1983.

Roberts JM. Trauma of the cervical spine: TEM/priorities in multiple trauma. Germantown, MD: Aspen Systems, 1979:63–77.

Rothman RH, Simeone FA. The spine. Philadelphia: WB Saunders, 1982:647–756.

Ruby EB. Advanced neurologic and neurosurgical nursing. St. Louis: CV Mosby, 1984:394–424.

Youmans JR. Neurological surgery. Philadelphia: WB Saunders, 1990:2378–2402.

(Cont'd from p 147)

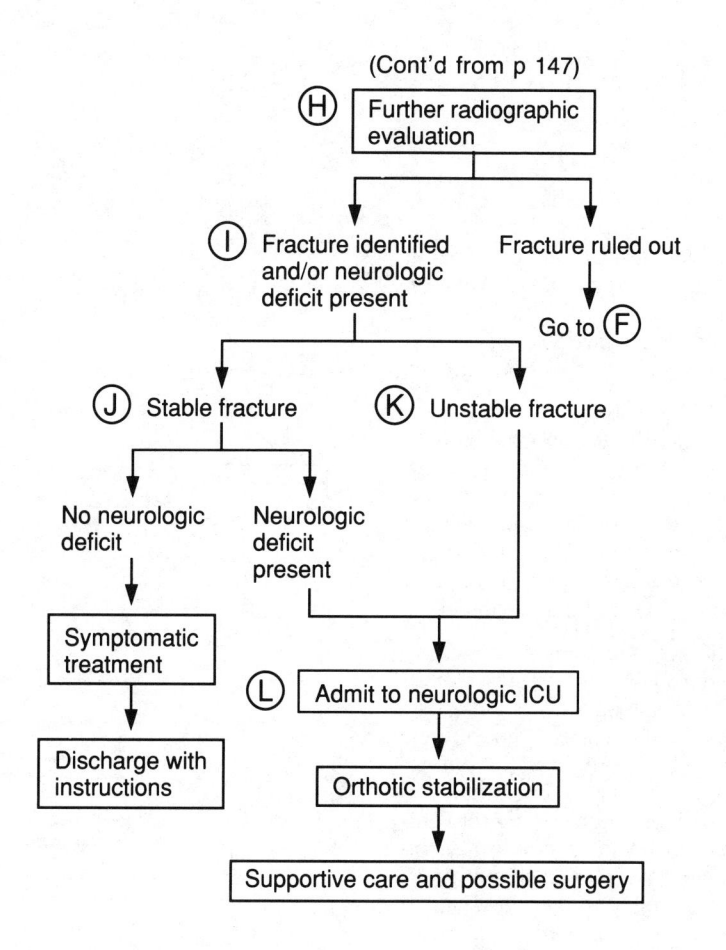

- **H** Further radiographic evaluation
  - **I** Fracture identified and/or neurologic deficit present
    - **J** Stable fracture
      - No neurologic deficit → Symptomatic treatment → Discharge with instructions
      - Neurologic deficit present → **L** Admit to neurologic ICU
    - **K** Unstable fracture → **L** Admit to neurologic ICU → Orthotic stabilization → Supportive care and possible surgery
  - Fracture ruled out → Go to **F**

THORACOLUMBAR SPINAL TRAUMA

Jorie Klein

A. Thoracolumbar spine injuries result from hyperflexion or compression trauma. Most are of the flexion-rotation or fracture-dislocation type. A complete history should be obtained, including the mechanism of injury and whether the patient was able to sit or stand after the accident.

B. A patient suspected of having a thoracolumbar spine injury should be immobilized in the recumbent position on a backboard. All procedures performed prior to and during radiographic examination must be done with the patient immobilized. No attempt should be made to sit the patient up. Turning should be done in log roll fashion, with traction maintained on the legs and shoulders.

C. Securing the airway, breathing, and circulation (ABCs), complete monitoring of vital signs, and physical examination are necessary as with any patient who has sustained trauma. Frequently there are associated injuries. A calcaneal fracture should be ruled out in the patient who has sustained a fall; blunt chest and abdominal trauma must be ruled out in patients injured in motor vehicle accidents. Pelvic and hip fractures should also be ruled out. Examination of the spine should be done with the patient carefully log rolled on his or her side. A large gap between the spinous process may indicate a tear of the interspinous ligaments. Hematomas, tenderness, and ability or inability to void after the injury should be noted. A thorough neurologic examination should be carried out, including documentation of voluntary movements and strength in the extremities. The sensory evaluation should include the response to pinprick, proprioception, deep tendon reflexes, the bulbocavernous reflex, sphincter tone, and perianal sensation.

D. Adequate radiographic examination, including well exposed anteroposterior and lateral views of the thoracolumbar spine, is mandatory before a treatment plan can be initiated. Computed tomographic (CT) scanning is the best adjunctive test for identifying disease.

E. Most classification systems are based on the mechanism of injury. Stable injuries generally include an isolated compression and wedge fracture of the vertebral body, rare hyperextension injuries such as traumatic spondylolisthesis, and transverse or spinous process fractures secondary to direct trauma or muscular contractions; there is usually acceptable alignment and stability (Fig. 1).

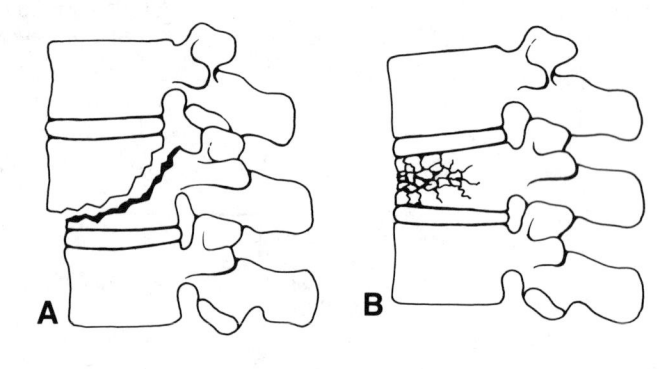

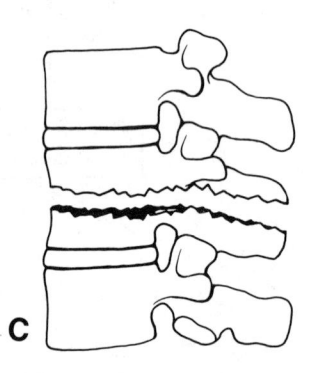

Figure 1 Fractures of the thoracolumbar spine. *A*, Fracture-dislocation; *B*, wedge fracture; *C*, chance fracture. (Reprinted with permission from Scott J. Thoracolumbar spinal fracture. In: Mancini ME, ed. Decision making in emergency nursing. Toronto: BC Decker, 1988:42.)

F. Nearly all major injuries of the thoracolumbar spine result in a vertebral body fracture. If posterior osseous or ligamentous disruption is sufficient to permit significant spinal displacement with real or potential neurologic compromise, the injury is defined as unstable. Spinal cord injury with an unstable fracture-dislocation of the thoracolumbar spine can result from cord compression (burst fracture), cord crushing (flexion-rotation and shear fractures), or cord traction (flexion-distraction dislocation).

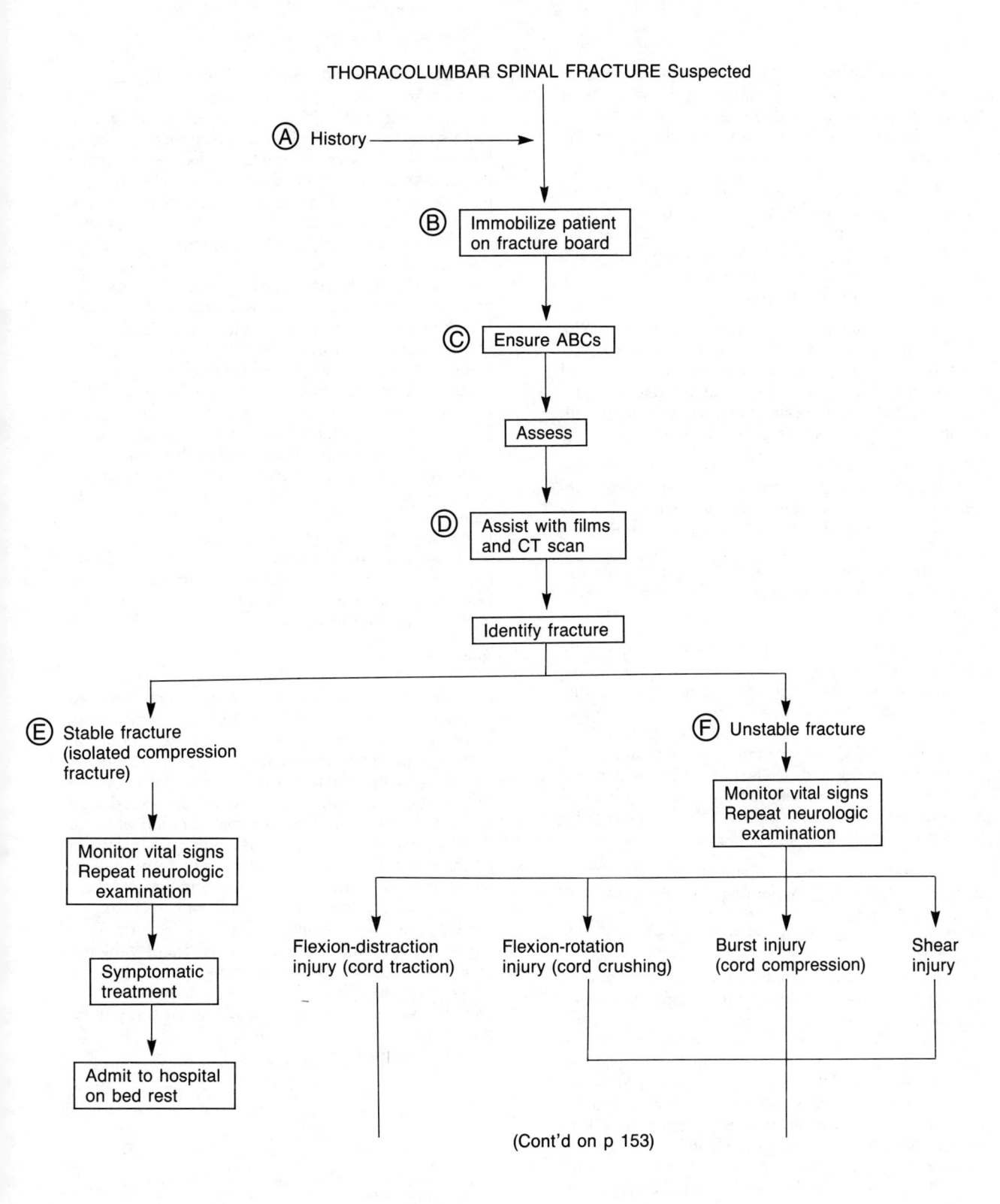

THORACOLUMBAR SPINAL FRACTURE Suspected

(A) History →

↓

(B) Immobilize patient on fracture board

↓

(C) Ensure ABCs

↓

Assess

↓

(D) Assist with films and CT scan

↓

Identify fracture

├──────────────────────────────┬────────────────────────────────────┤

(E) Stable fracture (isolated compression fracture)

↓

Monitor vital signs
Repeat neurologic examination

↓

Symptomatic treatment

↓

Admit to hospital on bed rest

(F) Unstable fracture

↓

Monitor vital signs
Repeat neurologic examination

↓

- Flexion-distraction injury (cord traction)
- Flexion-rotation injury (cord crushing)
- Burst injury (cord compression)
- Shear injury

(Cont'd on p 153)

G. Flexion-distraction forces, often experienced by persons wearing lap seat belts, can cause transverse fractures through both anterior and posterior spinal elements (chance fracture; see Fig. 1). These fractures heal readily and are not prone to instability.

H. Patients with unacceptable alignment or in whom the fracture is grossly unstable require immediate intervention. Decompression of the neural elements is best accomplished by realignment and stabilization. This could involve postural reduction by hyperextending the spine or open reduction and internal fixation.

I. Open reduction and internal fixation with Harrington instrumentation are preferred over closed techniques. Fractures with unstable patterns that result in a partial neurologic deficit should be reduced and stabilized immediately. Stabilization can be delayed in patients with no neural deficit or with a complete lesion.

J. Spinal cord injuries are described as complete, incomplete (partial), or root. A complete cord injury demonstrates loss of conscious sensorimotor function below the level of the injury. An incomplete injury spares some motor or sensory function. A root injury impairs function of the sensorimotor ability in the distribution of one root. Incomplete injuries occur more often than complete injuries.

K. Patients with complete cord injuries associated with thoracic vertebrae one through four demonstrate good to normal upper extremity muscle function. Patients with cord injuries at thoracic vertebrae five to lumbar vertebrae two have partial to good trunk stability. Patients with lumbar vertebrae three to four injuries demonstrate good control of the trunk and pelvis, hip flexors, adductors, and quadriceps. Patients with cord injuries at lumbar vertebrae five or below have control of the hip extensors, abductors, knee flexors, and ankles.

L. Management of the patient with thoracolumbar cord injuries necessitates close monitoring. Most paraplegic patients demonstrate some degree of respiratory insufficiency. This insufficiency may be associated with other traumatic injuries, thereby producing airway obstruction, intercostal or diaphragmatic respiratory muscle paralysis, associated thoracic or tracheal trauma, or aspiration. The evaluating team must closely monitor the airway, breathing, and circulation of the patient with spinal cord injuries. Prevention of potential complications begins when the life-threatening injuries are addressed. Further deterioration of vertebra stability is prevented by immobilization. Immobilization techniques should be re-evaluated after every procedure that requires log roll movements (e.g., therapeutic procedures, radiologic films). The patient must be carefully monitored for spinal shock and managed appropriately. The patient should have a nasogastric tube inserted to prevent the development of a paralytic ileus, which allows fluid and gas to accumulate in the bowel. The pH level of the gastric content should also be monitored because these individuals are especially prone to stress ulcers caused by the increased acidity of gastric content. Antacids should be administered if the pH level is less than 4. The evaluating team should initiate steps to prevent the complication of thrombosis. If the initial evaluation and diagnostic work-up are prolonged, the team may want to consider early placement of an antiembolization stocking or alternate compression device. Venous punctures should be avoided in the lower extremities to decrease the potential for development of thrombosis. The evaluating team must be sensitive to the potential breakdown of skin integrity. The lack of sensory warning mechanisms, the inability to move freely, and the circulatory changes potentiate breakdown of skin integrity with cord injuries at any level. The prolonged pressure of being in one position for the lengthy diagnostic evaluation must also be addressed by the team. The team should be aware of the shearing forces, produced by pulling the patient across a sheet, that can disrupt skin integrity. The team should also be aware of the psychosocial impacts the injury may have on the patient. The patient's fear of paralysis may be accompanied by anxiety generated by the unfamiliar hospital surroundings and by diagnostic procedures (e.g., CT scan, magnetic resonance imaging). The caregivers should use good eye contact and reassure the patient. The patient should be informed about the injury, the diagnostic evaluation and its outcome, and potential prognosis. The patient's significant other or family members should be included in all discussions. This will provide the patient and family with some reality to begin to deal with their emotions.

M. Autonomic dysreflexia is a life threatening complication for the paraplegic patient. This phenomenon can occur any time after spinal shock dissipates. The causes of autonomic dysreflexia are a full rectum, an overdistended bladder, or a decubitus ulcer. These causes produce an overexaggerated response of the sympathetic nervous system attributable to the lack of control from higher centers. Autonomic dysreflexia is characterized by a sudden severe headache secondary to elevated blood pressure, which can produce a cerebral hemorrhage or myocardial infarction if untreated. Other symptoms include bradycardia or tachycardia, sweating and flushing above the level of the lesion and pallor and coolness below the level of injury, nasal stuffiness, and apprehension. Treatment includes removal of the causative agent, ganglionic blocking agents to disrupt the hyperreflexic state, and hydralazine hydrachloride for the hypertension. This complication occurs most frequently in the first year following injury but may occur at any time throughout the paraplegic's life span.

References

American College of Surgeons. Early care of the injured patient. Philadelphia: WB Saunders, 1976:120–131.
Cowley RA. Shock trauma/critical care manual. Baltimore: University Park Press, 1983:73–143.
Rudy E. Advanced neurological and neurosurgical nursing. St. Louis: CV Mosby, 1984:398–409.
Scott J. Thoracolumbar spinal fracture. In: Mancini ME, ed. Decision making in emergency nursing. Toronto: BC Decker, 1988:423.
Shires CT. Care of the trauma patient. New York: McGraw-Hill, 1979:349–395.

(Cont'd from p 151)

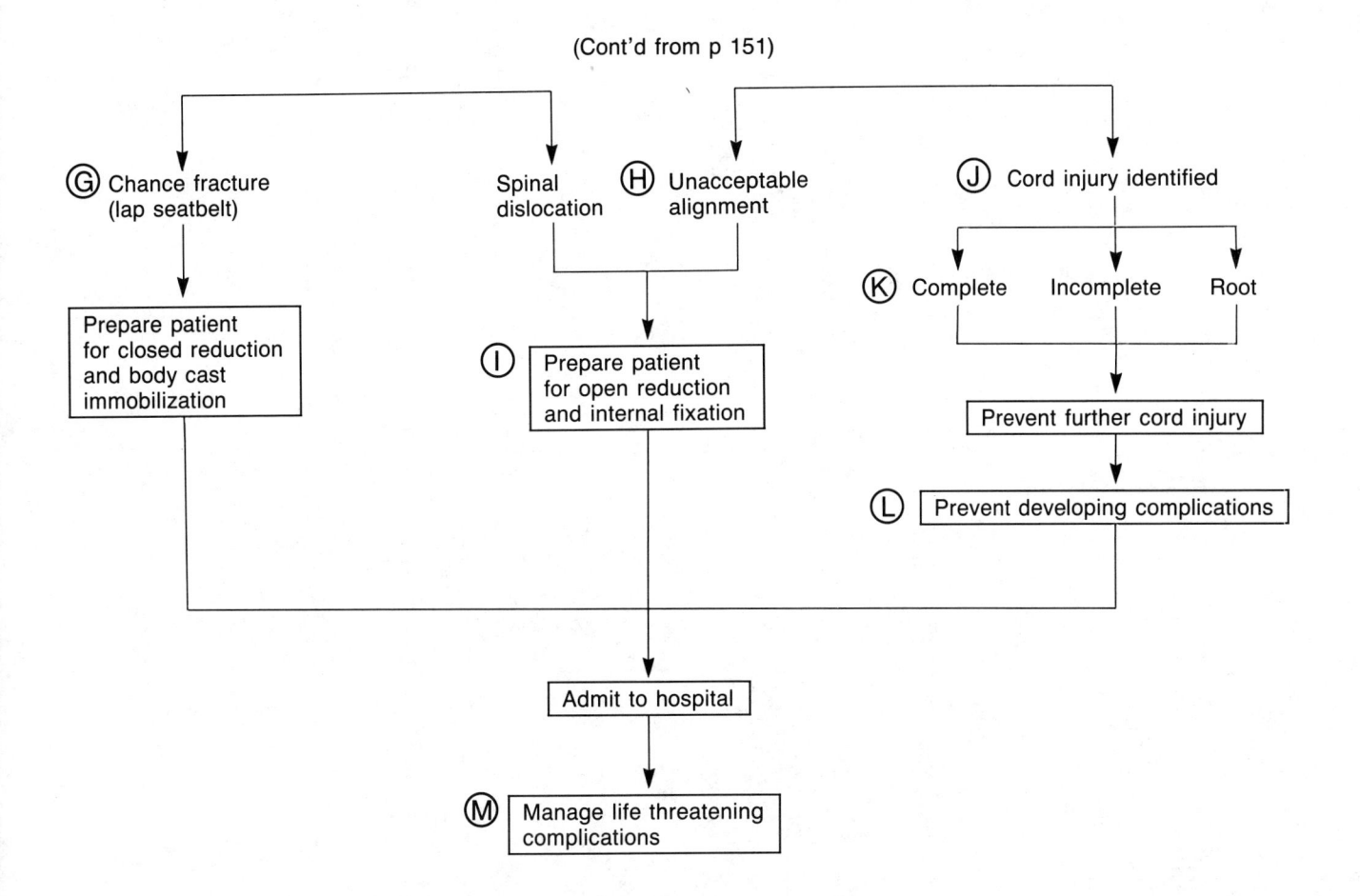

- **G** Chance fracture (lap seatbelt) → Prepare patient for closed reduction and body cast immobilization
- Spinal dislocation
- **H** Unacceptable alignment → **I** Prepare patient for open reduction and internal fixation
- **J** Cord injury identified
  - **K** Complete / Incomplete / Root → Prevent further cord injury → **L** Prevent developing complications

→ Admit to hospital → **M** Manage life threatening complications

UPPER EXTREMITY TRAUMA

Shoulder and Clavicle Trauma
Humeral Head, Elbow, Upper Arm, Forearm,
 and Wrist Trauma
Hand Trauma

SHOULDER AND CLAVICLE TRAUMA

Johnese Spisso

A. Clavicular fractures may result from blunt trauma to the anterior chest and/or direct force of impact to the shoulders. Scapular fractures and shoulder dislocations are known to result from forces that cause a displacement (i.e., abduction force or external rotation) of the shoulder joint or from a direct blow force to the scapula.

B. Initial assessment of the patient reveals tenderness over the affected region and limited mobility of the fractured shoulder.

C. Neurovascular function is assessed to determine axillary nerve and/or arterial injury. Particular attention should be paid to a finding of diminished sensation in the lateral shoulder area, which is associated with axillary nerve lesions.

D. Diagnosis is usually confirmed on radiographic examination, with the most definitive views being anteroposterior chest films and tangential lateral scapular films.

E. When scapular fractures are confirmed, reassessment of the shoulder joint should be performed to check for the presence of a glenoid process fracture. Treatment of scapular fractures involves application of a sling and swathe for immobilization of the upper arm and shoulder. Patients should be discharged and scheduled for follow-up examination in 3 to 5 days. Instructions should be given to return for examination if the joint becomes subluxated, if sensation decreases, or if skin abrasions occur from sling application.

F. Should dislocations can be further classified as anterior or posterior. Anterior dislocation is more common and is often associated with humeral tuberosity fractures. Posterior dislocation is often characterized by the inability to rotate the shoulder beyond the neutral position and can be confirmed by tangential lateral scapular radiographic views.

Treatment of shoulder dislocations requires immediate closed reduction. Analgesia is required prior to the application of sustained traction along the humerus of the dislocated side. Pain that is caused by muscle spasms can be reduced by intravenous narcotics in combination with continuous countertraction of the humerus. After closed reduction is completed, a repeat film is indicated to confirm successful reduction. A sling and swathe are then applied, and the patient can be discharged with follow-up orthopaedic examination in 3 to 5 days.

G. Initial assessment of the patient may reveal point tenderness and swelling over the clavicular region. The mechanism of injury can cause associated upper extremity trauma; thus, it is important to assess nerve function to rule out brachial plexus damage. Quality of pulses and venous congestion must also be assessed to rule out vascular injury to the upper extremity.

H. The diagnosis of clavicular fracture is confirmed by x-ray films. Optimal views for visualization and identification of fracture are anteroposterior chest and apical lordotic views.

I. Contusions and bruising of the clavicle require only symptomatic treatment of discomfort.

J. When a clavicular fracture or dislocation is identified, the application of a figure-of-eight sling is appropriate treatment. Caution should be taken to avoid applying the sling too tightly because this can lead to swelling and neuropathy.

K. Upon discharge, the patient should be instructed to monitor the upper extremity and shoulder for swelling and to notify the physician upon its occurrence. Follow-up examination should be performed 1 to 2 weeks post injury.

References

Gustillo RB. Management of open fractures and complications. In: American Association of Orthopedic Surgeons, ed. Instructional course lectures. Vol 31. St. Louis: CV Mosby, 1982:64–74.

Trafton PG, Chapman MW. Orthopedic emergencies. In: Mills J, Ho M, Trunkey D, eds. Current emergency diagnosis and treatment. Los Angeles: Lange, 1983:293–314.

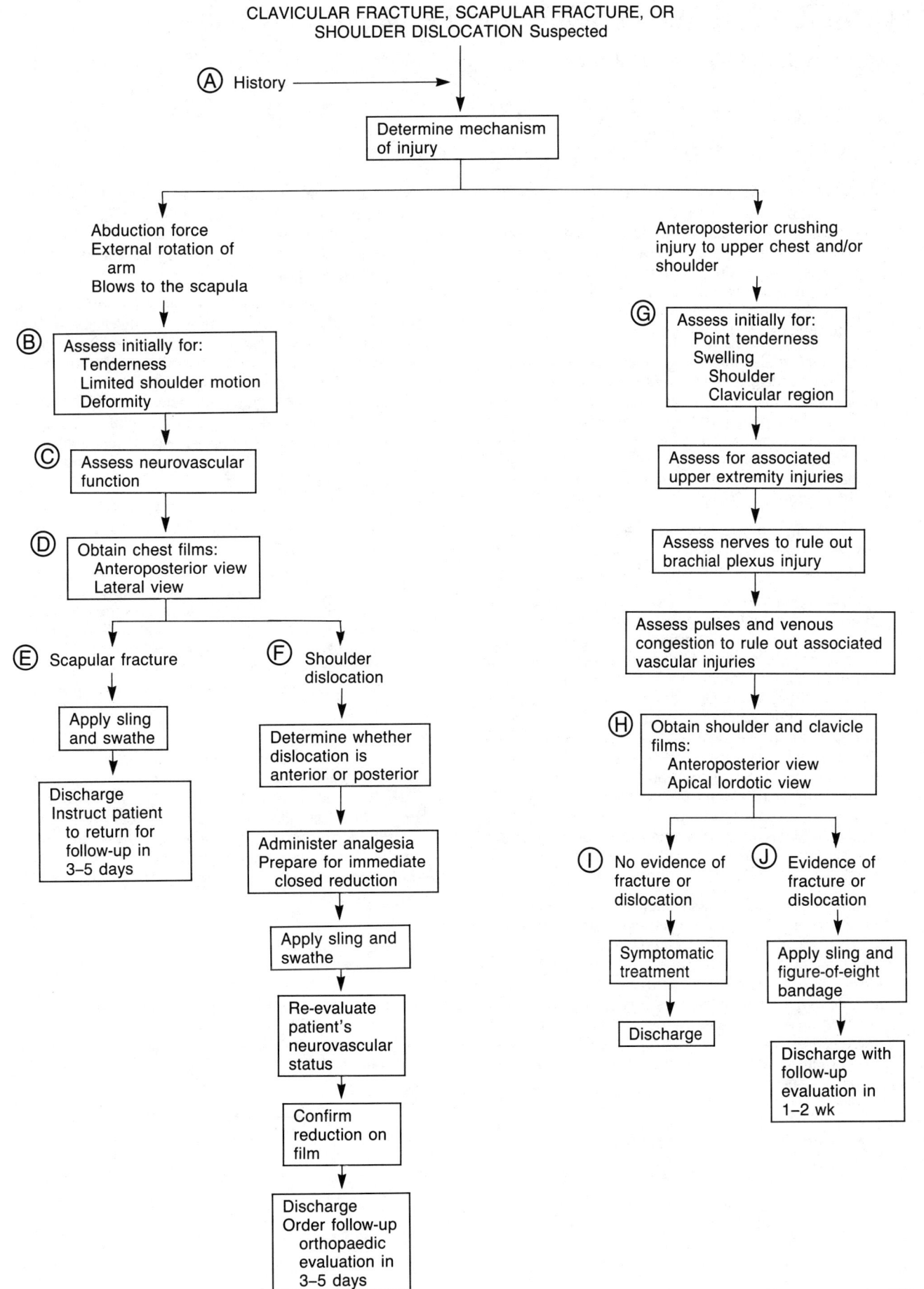

CLAVICULAR FRACTURE, SCAPULAR FRACTURE, OR SHOULDER DISLOCATION Suspected

(A) History

↓

Determine mechanism of injury

Abduction force / External rotation of arm / Blows to the scapula

(B) Assess initially for:
- Tenderness
- Limited shoulder motion
- Deformity

(C) Assess neurovascular function

(D) Obtain chest films:
- Anteroposterior view
- Lateral view

(E) Scapular fracture
- Apply sling and swathe
- Discharge. Instruct patient to return for follow-up in 3–5 days

(F) Shoulder dislocation
- Determine whether dislocation is anterior or posterior
- Administer analgesia. Prepare for immediate closed reduction
- Apply sling and swathe
- Re-evaluate patient's neurovascular status
- Confirm reduction on film
- Discharge. Order follow-up orthopaedic evaluation in 3–5 days

Anteroposterior crushing injury to upper chest and/or shoulder

(G) Assess initially for:
- Point tenderness
- Swelling
- Shoulder
- Clavicular region

Assess for associated upper extremity injuries

Assess nerves to rule out brachial plexus injury

Assess pulses and venous congestion to rule out associated vascular injuries

(H) Obtain shoulder and clavicle films:
- Anteroposterior view
- Apical lordotic view

(I) No evidence of fracture or dislocation
- Symptomatic treatment
- Discharge

(J) Evidence of fracture or dislocation
- Apply sling and figure-of-eight bandage
- Discharge with follow-up evaluation in 1–2 wk

HUMERAL HEAD, ELBOW, UPPER ARM, FOREARM, AND WRIST TRAUMA

Johnese Spisso

A. Upper extremity fractures are a common injury associated with blunt trauma. They can produce morbidity and long-term disability if not recognized and treated promptly. Soft tissue damage progresses rapidly after bone fractures and the resulting tearing of the periosteum, surrounding blood vessels, and lymphatics. Early reduction and fixation of the fracture stabilize the injury, prevent further tissue disruption, and reduce morbidity.

B. Following initial primary assessment of the trauma patient, a secondary assessment of the upper extremity is performed. The limb is examined for evidence of deformity, swelling, pain, passive and active range of motion difficulties; neurovascular status and peripheral nerve status. Positive findings indicate the need for radiographs of the affected area to determine the extent and location of the fracture.

C. Fractures caused by a blunt force are further identified as open or closed. Open fractures require operative irrigation and debridement within 8 hours post injury.

D. Penetrating injuries are often associated with vascular injuries, and they require prompt angiography if the wound is in proximity to a major vessel or if neurovascular examination reveals a deficit. If angiography is positive for vessel injury, the patient should be prepared for operative revascularization. Upper extremity vascular injuries can result in devastating functional loss if all efforts are not made to salvage the limb. As ischemia persists, functional muscle mass loss increases; thus, revascularization is imperative 6 to 8 hours post injury. Postoperatively the patient is at risk for the development of compartment syndrome secondary to reperfusion of the limb. Neurovascular status and compartment pressures are assessed and fasciotomies are performed if compartment pressures reach critical levels that compromise the limb.

E. Humeral fractures are associated with pain and deformity and are confirmed on radiographic examination. Neurovascular status is examined to determine whether vascular or peripheral nerve damage exists. Nondisplaced fractures of the humerus are managed by splinting. Proximal humeral fractures are best immobilized by application of a sling and swathe, whereas humeral shaft fractures require a plaster U splint. Following application of the splint device, neurovascular reassessment is indicated. Displaced humeral fractures frequently require operative open reduction and internal fixation (ORIF). Assessment for glenohumeral fractures (i.e., dislocation of the shoulder) should be performed; this is often an associated injury.

F. Elbow and olecranon injuries can be associated with neurovascular injuries and require early diagnosis and treatment to prevent disabling complications. Volkmann's contracture can occur secondary to forearm ischemia and is attributable to arterial occlusion or compartment syndrome. Elbow dislocations are treated with closed reduction, application of a splint, and elevation of the limb. Olecranon fractures associated with dislocation of the elbow are more extensive injuries and may require surgical open reduction and fixation.

G. Fractures of the radius and ulna require assessment of the radial, median, and ulnar nerves and for possible flexion or extension deficits secondary to compartment syndrome. Radiographic views must include the wrist and elbow regions to confirm the extent and level of forearm fracture. Most displaced fractures of the forearm require open reduction and internal fixation. Postoperative neurovascular status is reassessed and monitored to rule out compartment syndrome. Nondisplaced fractures respond to provisional reduction and application of a splint.

H. Wrist joint fractures can be associated with median and ulnar nerve injury and command thorough sensory motor assessment. The severity of wrist fractures ranges widely. Application of spica splints to the volar thumb is indicated for mild dislocations, whereas ORIF may be needed for more severe fractures. Frequent assessment of the area of continued swelling and possible neurovascular compromise is indicated. Prompt intervention minimizes potential disability.

References

Blaisdell F, Trunkey DD. Trauma to extremities: general principles. Sci Am 1988; 1:1–11.

Trafton PG. Fractures. In: Trunkey DD, Lewis FR, eds. Current therapy of trauma–2. Toronto: BC Decker, 1986:335–362.

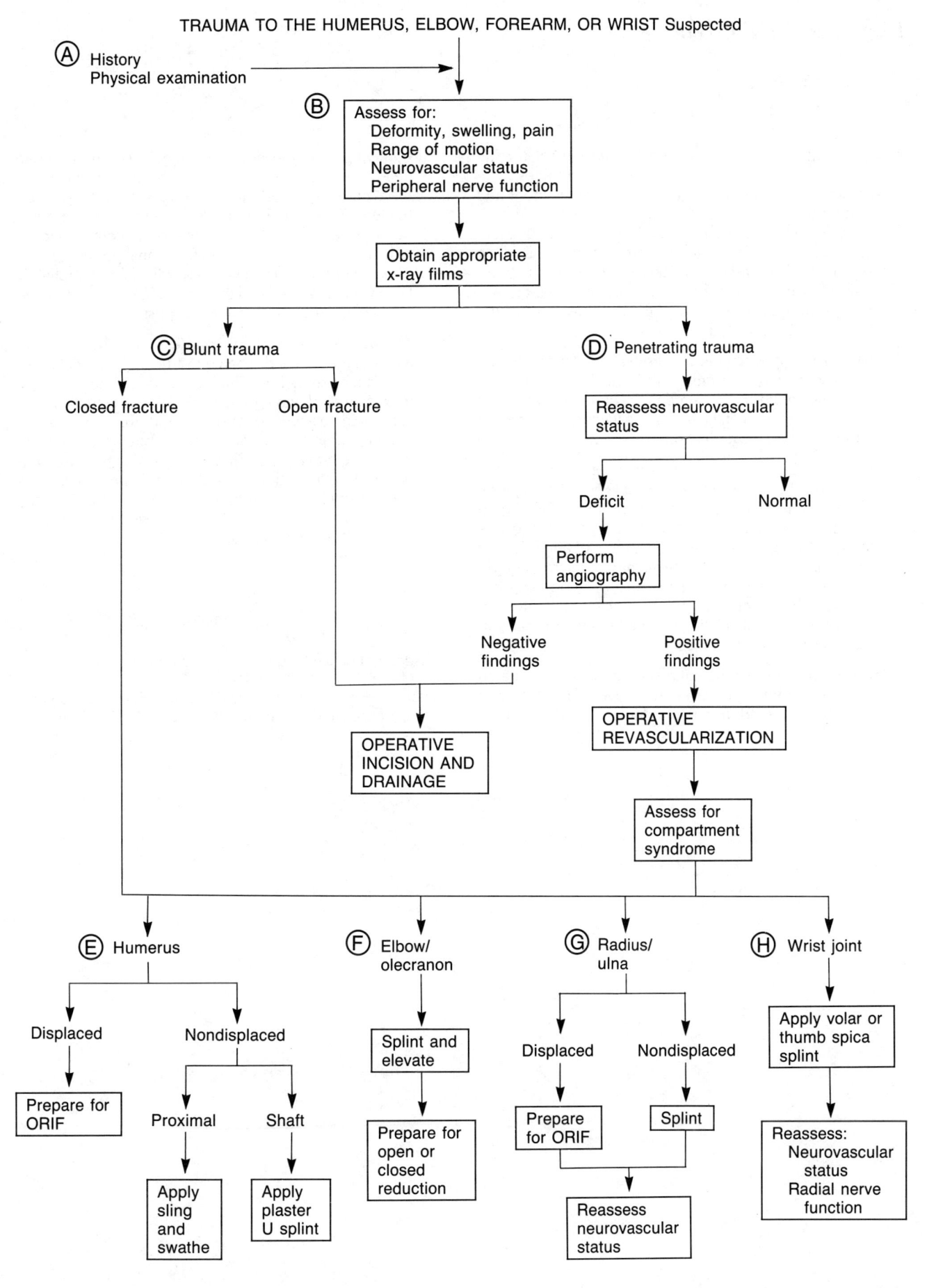

TRAUMA TO THE HUMERUS, ELBOW, FOREARM, OR WRIST Suspected

(A) History, Physical examination

(B) Assess for:
- Deformity, swelling, pain
- Range of motion
- Neurovascular status
- Peripheral nerve function

Obtain appropriate x-ray films

(C) Blunt trauma
- Closed fracture
- Open fracture

(D) Penetrating trauma
- Reassess neurovascular status
  - Deficit → Perform angiography
    - Negative findings → OPERATIVE INCISION AND DRAINAGE
    - Positive findings → OPERATIVE REVASCULARIZATION → Assess for compartment syndrome
  - Normal

(E) Humerus
- Displaced → Prepare for ORIF
- Nondisplaced
  - Proximal → Apply sling and swathe
  - Shaft → Apply plaster U splint

(F) Elbow/olecranon
- Splint and elevate
- Prepare for open or closed reduction

(G) Radius/ulna
- Displaced → Prepare for ORIF → Reassess neurovascular status
- Nondisplaced → Splint

(H) Wrist joint
- Apply volar or thumb spica splint
- Reassess: Neurovascular status, Radial nerve function

HAND TRAUMA

Johnese Spisso

A. After initial assessment of the trauma patient for life threatening injuries, evaluation of the extremities is indicated. Hand injuries require prompt assessment and appropriate intervention to minimize the extent of disability. Simultaneous evaluation of structural and functional components of the hand is necessary because of the proximity of the vasculature, nerves, tendons, and bones. Careful assessment of the integrity of the skin that overlies the injured region and of the mobility level of the hand is also indicated.

B. Closed and open fractures or dislocation of the hand can occur secondary to trauma. This is usually evidenced by swelling, deformity, impaired range of motion, and pain elicited on motion of the hand. The fracture is confirmed by radiographic examination.

C. Open fractures are those in which a break in the integrity of the overlying skin has occurred. These fractures require open reduction and internal fixation (ORIF). Open fractures of the hand also require prompt evaluation for tendon damage. If tendon injuries are identified, further orthopaedic assessment is necessary to determine indications for suture or primary repair. Tendon injuries threaten the functional ability of the hand; thus orthopaedic hand specialists should be involved early in the decision making process.

D. Closed fractures of the hand should also be evaluated for tendon injuries by assessing active range-of-motion limitations. If tendon injury is demonstrated, consultation with an orthopaedic hand specialist is indicated to determine the level of extension or flexion injury and the type of repair required. The closed fracture is best treated with initial immobilization of the hand in functional position. While preparing the patient for closed reduction, correct splinting in functional position places the wrist in a dorsiflexed position, with the thumb slightly flexed and abducted and the fingers flexed slightly. Neurovascular status is re-examined post splinting.

E. The patient who sustains injuries to the hand should receive appropriate discharge instructions after definitive care is rendered. These include teaching the patient to recognize signs and symptoms of possible complications, such as increased pain or discomfort, loss of sensation, swelling, or loss of motor function. Patients are to be instructed to return for evaluation if any of these symptoms occurs. Routine follow-up evaluation as an outpatient is needed to monitor the hand's return to functional status and the patient's need for occupational therapy or rehabilitation consultations.

References

Blaisdell F, Trunkey DD. Trauma to extremities: general principles. Sci Am 1988; 1:1–11.

Trafton PG. Fractures. In: Trunkey DD, Lewis FR, eds. Current therapy of trauma–2. Toronto: BC Decker, 1986:335–362.

TRAUMA TO THE HAND Suspected

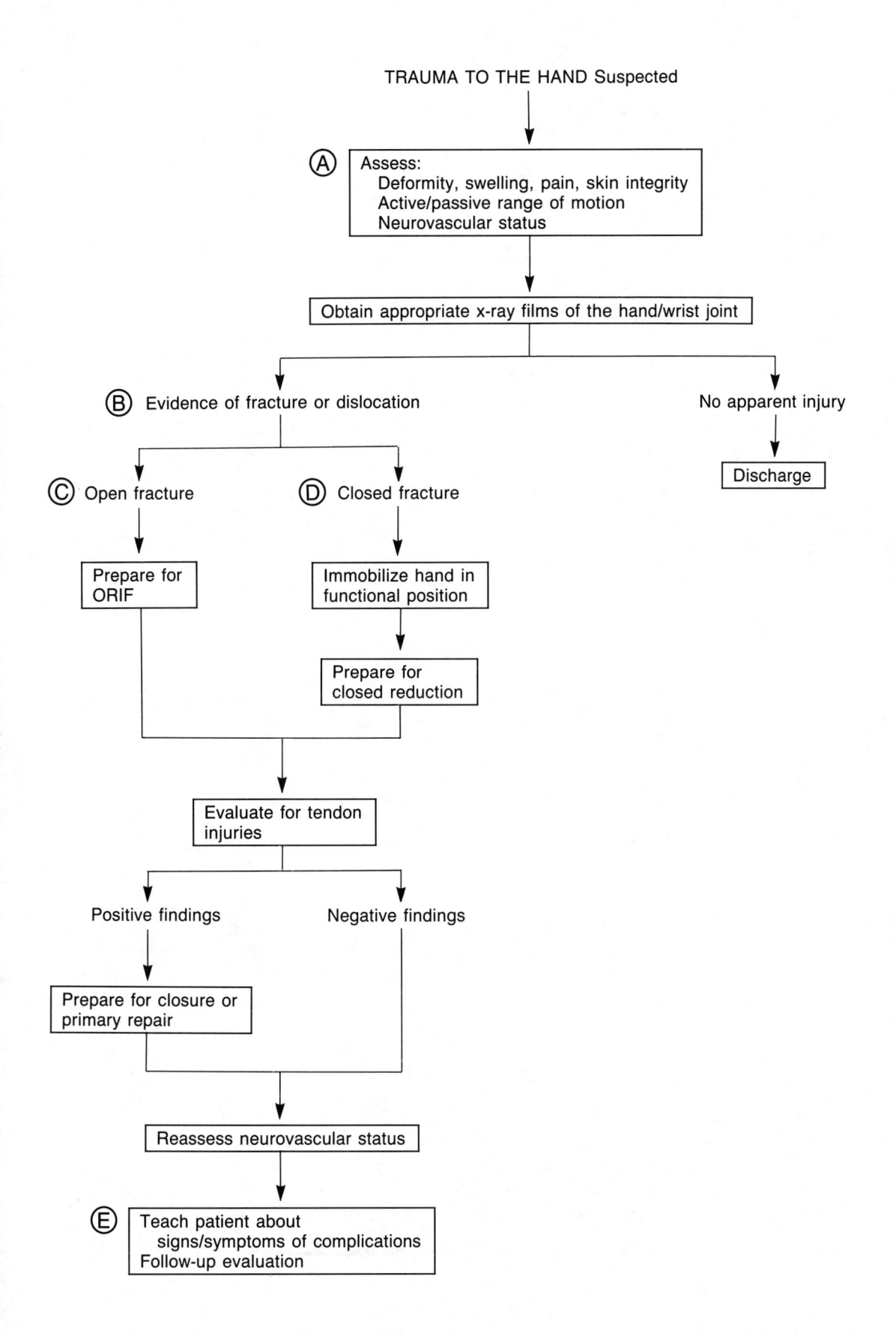

- **(A) Assess:**
  - Deformity, swelling, pain, skin integrity
  - Active/passive range of motion
  - Neurovascular status

Obtain appropriate x-ray films of the hand/wrist joint

- **(B) Evidence of fracture or dislocation**
  - **(C) Open fracture** → Prepare for ORIF
  - **(D) Closed fracture** → Immobilize hand in functional position → Prepare for closed reduction
- **No apparent injury** → Discharge

Evaluate for tendon injuries
- Positive findings → Prepare for closure or primary repair
- Negative findings

Reassess neurovascular status

- **(E)** Teach patient about signs/symptoms of complications
  Follow-up evaluation

161

LOWER EXTREMITY TRAUMA

Acetabular, Hips, and Femur Trauma
Knee Trauma
Lower Leg, Ankle, and Foot Trauma
Mangled or Amputated Extremity

ACETABULAR, HIP, AND FEMUR TRAUMA

William I. Sterett
J. Kenneth Burkus

A. An appropriate history including time of injury should be obtained. Fractures and injuries about the pelvis, hip, and femur are generally high velocity injuries, and a careful examination for associated injuries should be performed. A neurovascular examination and appropriate x-ray films are required. All patients involved in high energy trauma should routinely have an anteroposterior (AP) pelvis x-ray film done as part of their evaluation.

B. For a penetrating or crush injury, angiography should routinely be performed when the injury is in proximity to major vascular structures. If an expanding arterial hematoma is recognized, immediate operation is indicated. Intimal damage may be created by the shock of a close pass by a bullet. In the emergency room, direct pressure should be used to tamponade arterial active bleeding.

C. A high velocity bullet is one that travels at a speed greater than approximately 700 m per second (or 2100 ft per second). A high velocity bullet may cause extensive tissue damage or necrosis in addition to missile tract damage. Fractures caused by low velocity bullets may be treated with local wound care, ellipsing of the skin edges, and definitive fracture management. Patients with type I and II injuries (see p 168) should receive a cephalosporin, whereas an aminoglycoside should be added for type III injuries.

D. Arterial injury trails only fractures and blunt soft tissue trauma as the leading cause of acute compartment syndrome, owing to postischemic swelling. Following a revascularization procedure about the hip where warm ischemic time has been prolonged, distal compartment pressures should be measured and followed closely. If pressures exceed 30 mm Hg, immediate fasciotomies of involved compartments should be performed. If the leg compartments are tense but pressures are below critical values, consideration should be given to continuous monitoring with a Wick catheter.

E. In the case of an acetabular fracture, Judet or oblique views should be obtained to assess stability. From these, a computed tomography (CT) scan for preoperative planning and traction to decrease pressure on the articular cartilage may be considered. Operative reduction and internal fixation (ORIF), if necessary, should be done after careful preoperative planning.

F. Ten percent of posterior dislocations incur sciatic nerve palsy, which is tested more effectively by firing the gastroc-soleus complex. Slow but spontaneous recovery can be expected in the majority of cases. A thorough physical examination reveals fractures elsewhere on the body associated with sciatic nerve palsy. Timely reduction of the dislocation is required because the incidence of avascular necrosis of the femoral head is directly related to the duration of dislocation. This is an orthopaedic emergency and should be relocated in the operating room to assess postreduction stability.

References

Blaisdell FW, Trunkey DD. Trauma to extremities: general principles. Sci Am 1988; 5:1–14.

Hennessy MJ, Banks HH, Leach RB, Quigley TB. Extremity gunshot wound and gunshot fracture in civilian practice. Clin Orth Rel Res 1976; 114:296–303.

Rockwood CA, Green DP, eds. Fractures in adults. Vol. 2. Philadelphia: JB Lippincott, 1984:1287–1335.

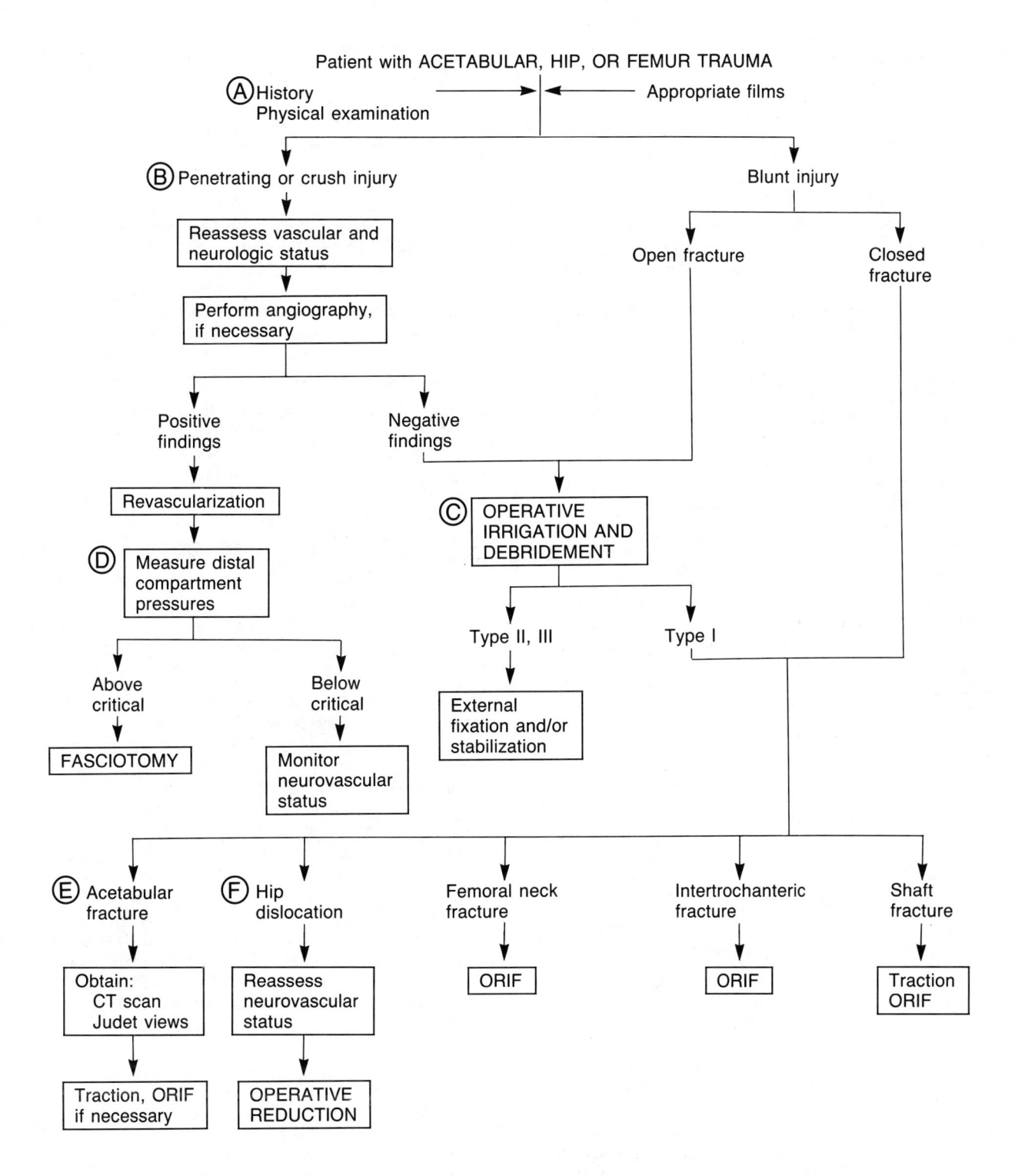

```
                    Patient with ACETABULAR, HIP, OR FEMUR TRAUMA
        (A) History                    →      ←    Appropriate films
            Physical examination
                    │                                    │
        ┌───────────┴──────────┐                         │
        ▼                                                ▼
    (B) Penetrating or crush injury                  Blunt injury
        │                                                │
        ▼                                       ┌────────┴────────┐
    Reassess vascular and                       ▼                 ▼
    neurologic status                       Open fracture      Closed
        │                                                      fracture
        ▼
    Perform angiography,
    if necessary
        │
    ┌───┴────┐
    ▼        ▼
Positive   Negative
findings   findings
    │          │
    ▼          └──────────────┐
Revascularization             ▼
    │                    (C) OPERATIVE
    ▼                        IRRIGATION AND
(D) Measure distal            DEBRIDEMENT
    compartment                   │
    pressures                ┌────┴────┐
    │                        ▼         ▼
┌───┴───┐                Type II, III  Type I
▼       ▼                    │
Above   Below                ▼
critical critical        External
│       │                fixation and/or
▼       ▼                stabilization
FASCIOTOMY  Monitor
            neurovascular
            status

(E) Acetabular  (F) Hip         Femoral neck    Intertrochanteric   Shaft
    fracture        dislocation  fracture        fracture            fracture
    │               │               │               │                   │
    ▼               ▼               ▼               ▼                   ▼
Obtain:         Reassess          ORIF            ORIF               Traction
CT scan         neurovascular                                         ORIF
Judet views     status
    │               │
    ▼               ▼
Traction, ORIF  OPERATIVE
if necessary    REDUCTION
```

165

KNEE TRAUMA

William I. Sterett
J. Kenneth Burkus

A. This chapter primarily discusses knee injuries with positive radiographic findings, lacerations with questionable arthrotomy, and penetrating or crush injuries with altered vascular or neurologic status. If a history of a gunshot wound is obtained by the emergency room personnel, information regarding the caliber and speed of the missile should be obtained to help in the decision making process. Inspection and palpation of the involved area should be performed first, and if normal, range of motion of the knee should be tested. Crepitance or pain is an indication for radiologic examination. Films should include the joints above and below the knee or, if the joint is involved, the long bones above and below. Specifically, it should be established whether the quadriceps mechanism is intact and whether the knee flexors are functioning. The popliteal artery can typically be palpated directly in the posterior popliteal fossa.

B. All open fractures created by the bone piercing the skin need to be irrigated and debrided in the operating room. Any open fracture created by a high velocity gunshot (i.e., traveling at a speed greater than 700 m or 2100 ft per second) or any gunshot wound that is intra-articular needs to be debrided in the operating room. Only the low velocity gunshot wounds that are not intra-articular may be irrigated and debrided in the emergency room. This debridement includes elliptical excision of the involved skin edges. Distal arterial insufficiency or excessively tight compartments caused by hematoma formation are indications for surgical exploration of low velocity gunshot wounds. Neurologic deficit is not an indication for operative exploration because it is typically caused by contusion injuries to the nerve that resolve on their own. When severed by a bullet, however, these nerves can rarely be reanastomosed.

C. Although there are approximately five collateral vessels that stem from the popliteal artery, this area is particularly sensitive to disruption of flow. Any differences from the contralateral side should be investigated with angiography. Dorsalis pedis and tibialis posterior pulses should be assessed, as should capillary refill. Injuries in proximity to the major vessel should also be explored. Small intimal flaps, which thrombose int he first 48 to 72 hours, may initially appear normal on vascular examination. However, if these do clot and are not repaired within 8 hours, they invariably require amputation. The peroneal nerve crosses inferior to the knee over the lateral aspect of the proximal fibula. Injury to this nerve can be assessed by active dorsiflexion of the great toe (EHL) and sensation in the first web space.

D. Type I wounds (less than 1 cm in size), and some type II wounds (1 to 10 cm in size) that are clean, may be treated similarly to closed injuries, whereas type III injuries (greater than 10 cm or with extensive soft tissue damage) are generally treated with external fixation. Despite the size, a type I wound may be classified as a type III wound if there is either extensive soft tissue damage, such as from high energy impact, or gross contamination of the wound, such as from a farm or from oil and automobile parts. The grading of the open fracture in this way provides a direct correlation with the risk of infection.

E. Lacerations about the knee often look benign when in fact they have violated the joint or ruptured the extensor mechanism. These are usually on the anteriosuperior portion of the knee. The first maneuver that should be performed is evaluation of the extensor mechanism. This can be done by having the patient lift his or her leg off the bed with the knee straight. Approximately 100 ml of normal saline is injected into the knee joint well away from the laceration. If the wound is not completely dry prior to injection, methylene blue should be added to the saline. If there is no fluid extravasation from the wound, the saline may be reaspirated and the wound irrigated and primarily closed.

F. Of knee dislocations, 30 to 40 percent are associated with disruption of the popliteal artery. With an anterior dislocation the artery is stretched and particularly prone to disruption. When peroneal nerve disruptions are included, more than 50 percent of patients with this injury have neurovascular compromise. Even after a normal neurovascular examination, a small intimal flap may have been raised that may not thrombose for 48 to 72 hours. Most physicians recommend angiography for all patients who have a dislocated knee, particularly with an anterior dislocation, which is a hyperextension injury. If a vascular injury in this area is not treated within the first 8 hours, the amputation rate is 86 percent. Although it is not unreasonable to monitor a hospitalized patient closely, conservative treatment comprises giving an angiogram to all those with traumatic knee dislocation despite a normal neurovascular examination.

References

Chapman MW. Open fractures. In: Chapman's operative orthopaedics. Philadelphia: JB Lippincott, 1988:173–178.

Green NE, Allen BL. Vascular injuries associated with dislocation of the knee. J Bone Joint Surg 1977; 59-A:236–239.

Hennessy MJ, Banks HH, et al. Extremity gunshot wound and gunshot fracture in civilian practice. Clin Orth Rel Res 1976; 114:296–303.

Hohl M, Larson RL, Jones DC. Fractures and dislocation of the knee. In: Rockwood CA, Green DP, eds. Fractures in Adults. Vol. 2. Philadelphia: JB Lippincott, 1984:1429–1508.

TRAUMA ABOUT THE KNEE Suspected

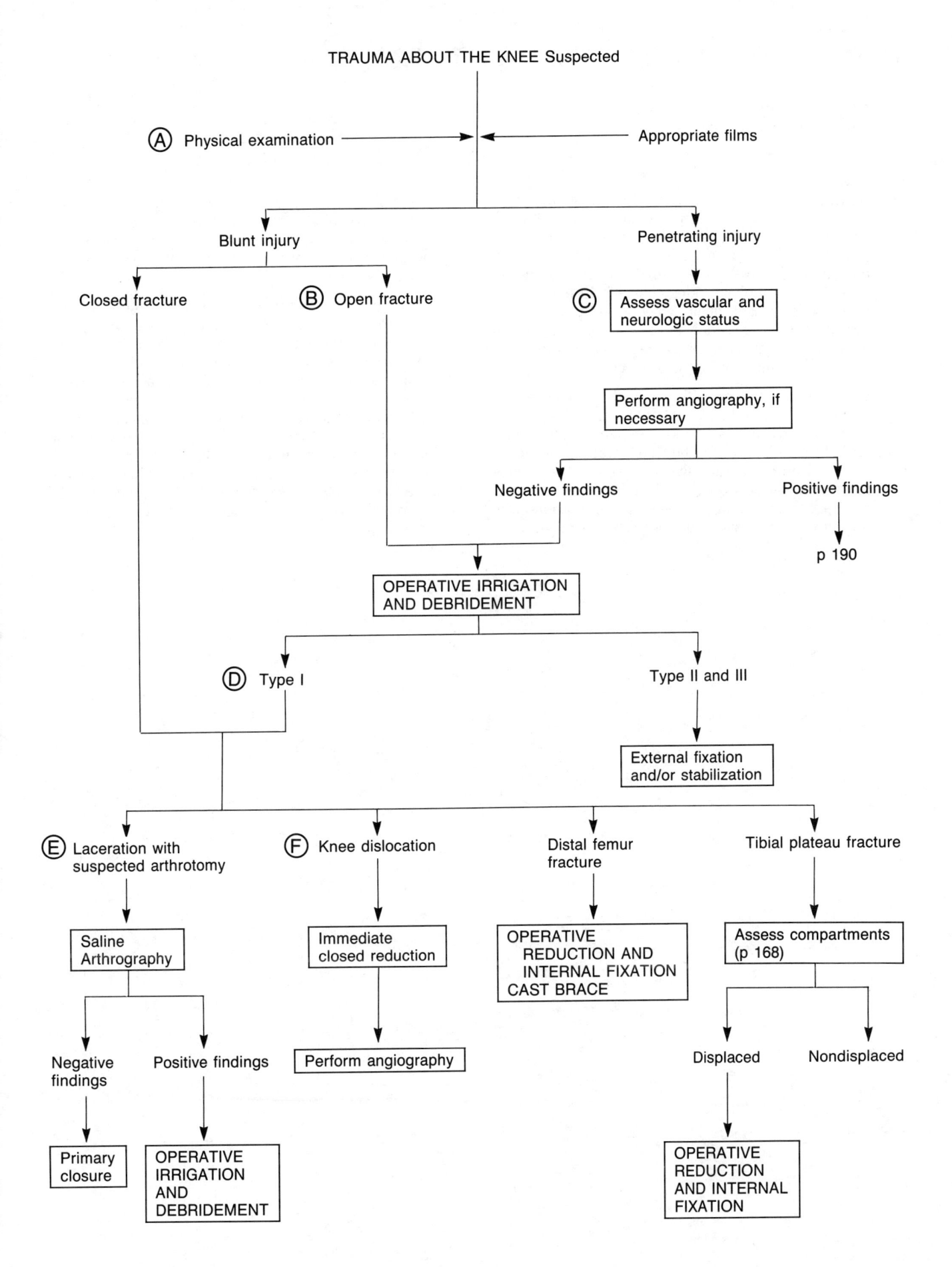

- (A) Physical examination
- Appropriate films

Blunt injury
- Closed fracture
- (B) Open fracture

Penetrating injury
- (C) Assess vascular and neurologic status
  - Perform angiography, if necessary
    - Negative findings → OPERATIVE IRRIGATION AND DEBRIDEMENT
    - Positive findings → p 190

After OPERATIVE IRRIGATION AND DEBRIDEMENT:
- (D) Type I
- Type II and III → External fixation and/or stabilization

Categories:
- (E) Laceration with suspected arthrotomy
  - Saline Arthrography
    - Negative findings → Primary closure
    - Positive findings → OPERATIVE IRRIGATION AND DEBRIDEMENT
- (F) Knee dislocation
  - Immediate closed reduction
  - Perform angiography
- Distal femur fracture
  - OPERATIVE REDUCTION AND INTERNAL FIXATION CAST BRACE
- Tibial plateau fracture
  - Assess compartments (p 168)
    - Displaced → OPERATIVE REDUCTION AND INTERNAL FIXATION
    - Nondisplaced

LOWER LEG, ANKLE, AND FOOT TRAUMA

William I. Sterett
J. Kenneth Burkus

A. A history of mechanism of injury including time of accident is obtained. Vascular examination includes palpation of dorsalis pedis, posterior tibial arteries, and assessment of capillary refill. Sensory examination should include the first web space (i.e., deep peroneal nerve). Motor examination includes clinically involved structures, especially EHL, tibialis anterior, and gastroc-soleus complex. Anteroposterior and lateral radiographs and three-dimensional views of involved areas should be obtained if the ankle or foot is involved.

B. Open fractures are generally classified based on the size of the wound and the extent of soft tissue destruction. Type I wounds are less than 1 cm in size, type II wounds are between 1 and 10 cm, and type III wounds are greater than 10 cm or have extensive soft tissue damage. Type III wounds may be further classified based on periosteal stripping or vascular injuries. Any type I or II wound with excessive contamination, such as a farm wound, immediately becomes a type III wound. In one study, 44 percent of type III wounds eventually became infected. In our institution we use a first-generation cephalosporin for type I and II wounds and add an aminoglycoside for type III wounds.

C. Angiography is required if the vascular examination is abnormal, including pulse rate or capillary refill, or if the area of penetration is in proximity to major vascular structures. Auscultation that reveals a systolic bruit may isolate the area of vessel injury. Despite a normal vascular examination, an angiogram should be performed in suspicious areas to locate reparable intimal flaps. Major vessels of the lower extremity include those proximal to the trifurcation in the leg. A quick motor examination may be performed by firing the EHL or tibialis anterior (deep peroneal nerve), peroneus longus (superficial peroneal nerve), and gastroc-soleus (tibial nerve).

Patient with LOWER LEG, ANKLE, OR FOOT TRAUMA

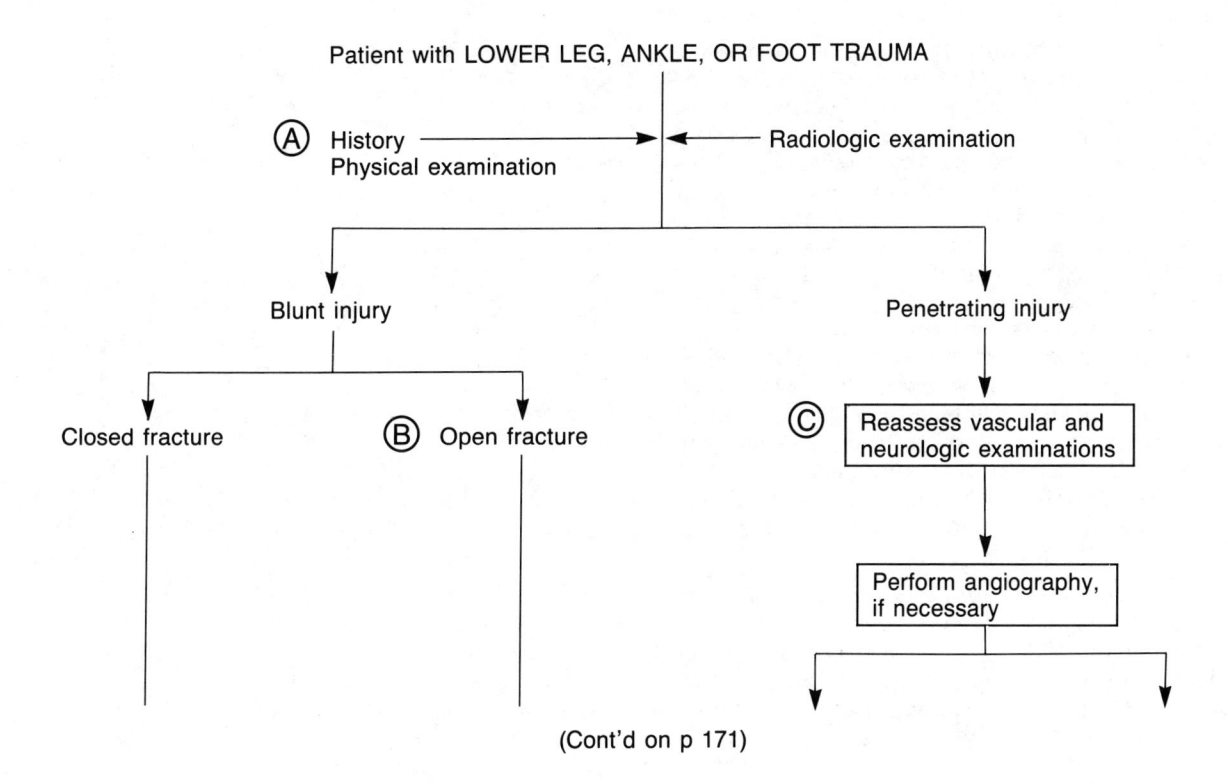

(A) History — Physical examination ←— Radiologic examination

- Blunt injury
  - Closed fracture
  - (B) Open fracture
- Penetrating injury
  - (C) Reassess vascular and neurologic examinations
  - Perform angiography, if necessary

(Cont'd on p 171)

169

D. Inordinate pain or dysesthesia is the hallmark of symptoms in a compartment syndrome. Signs include hypesthesia, pain with passive stretching of the involved muscles, and muscle weakness. Vascular examination is entirely normal in all but the most advanced cases because pressures are elevated only to a point well below arterial perfusion pressure and generally below venous return pressures. Irreversible nerve or muscle damage occurs with elevated pressures within 6 to 8 hours. Any indeterminate examination or tight compartment in a patient with an altered mental status warrants a measurement of intracompartmental pressures. Common causes of a compartment syndrome include major vascular injury, fractures with intracompartmental hemorrhage, postischemic swelling, constrictive dressings, and burns (Fig. 1). When assessing acute compartment syndromes, it is easiest to think in terms of "P"s, as follows: pressure, pain with stretch, paresis, paresthesia, pulses, and intact pink colour (Fig. 2).

E. There are many ways to measure the compartmental pressures of an extremity, the most common of which involves either the Wick or Slit catheter techniques. In our institution we have recently begun using a disposable, portable Stryker measuring device that may be utilized in the emergency room or operating room. Normal resting intracompartmental pressure is ±4 mm Hg. Although a variety of threshold levels for fasciotomy have been described, we generally recommend a pressure of 30 mm Hg as a relative indication for fasciotomy, depending on peripheral perfusion and compartment trends.

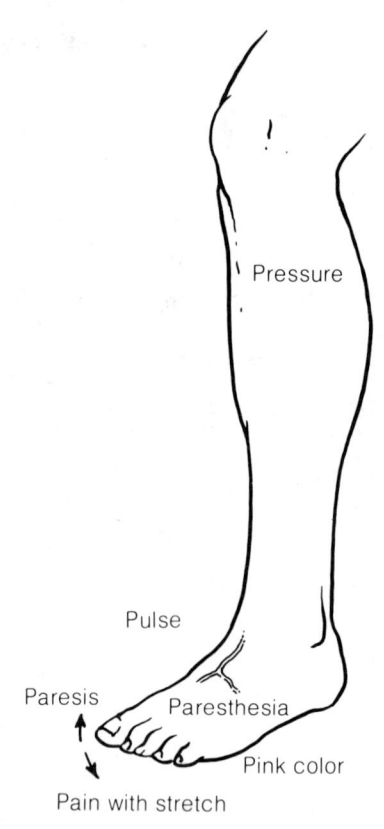

Figure 2 The "P"s in assessing compartment syndrome.

F. Clinical examination of the distal compartments must be performed following revascularization of a limb. Postischemic swelling is a major cause of compartment syndrome secondary to capillary leak. Following 6 hours of warm ischemia time, irreversible muscle necrosis occurs. Compartment pressures should *always* be measured following revascularization procedures of major vessels. If pressures are below critical value, neurovascular status may be closely monitored.

References

Gustillo RB. Management of open fractures and complications. In: American Association of Orthopedic Surgeons. Instructional course lectures. Vol. 31. St. Louis: CV Mosby, 1982:64–74.

Hargens AR, Schmidt AA, Evans KL, et al. Quantitation of skeletal muscle necrosis in a model compartment syndrome. J Bone Joint Surg 1981; 63-A:631–636.

Mubarak SJ. Compartment syndromes. In: Chapman's operative orthopaedics. Vol. 1. Philadelphia: JB Lippincott, 1988:179–195.

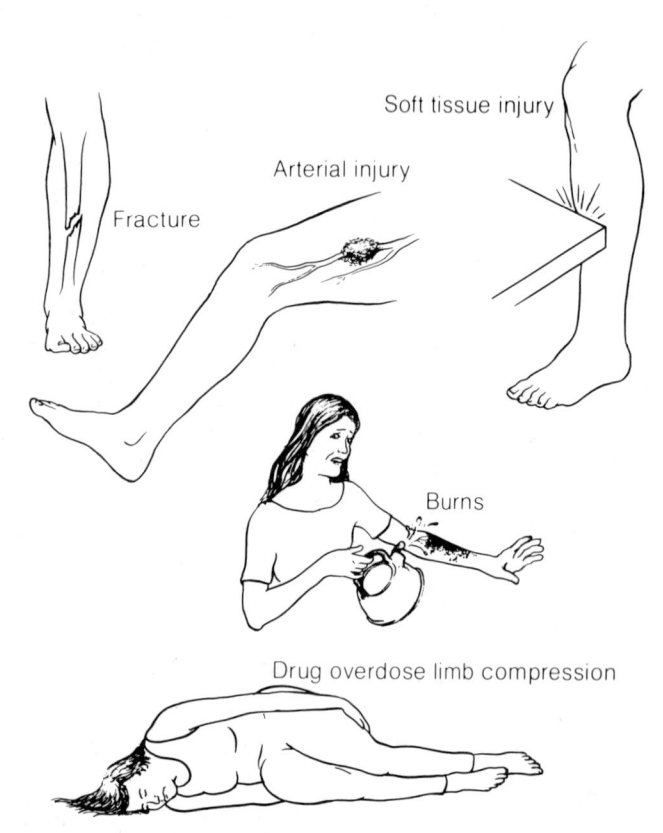

Figure 1 Leading causes of compartment syndrome.

(Cont'd from p 169)

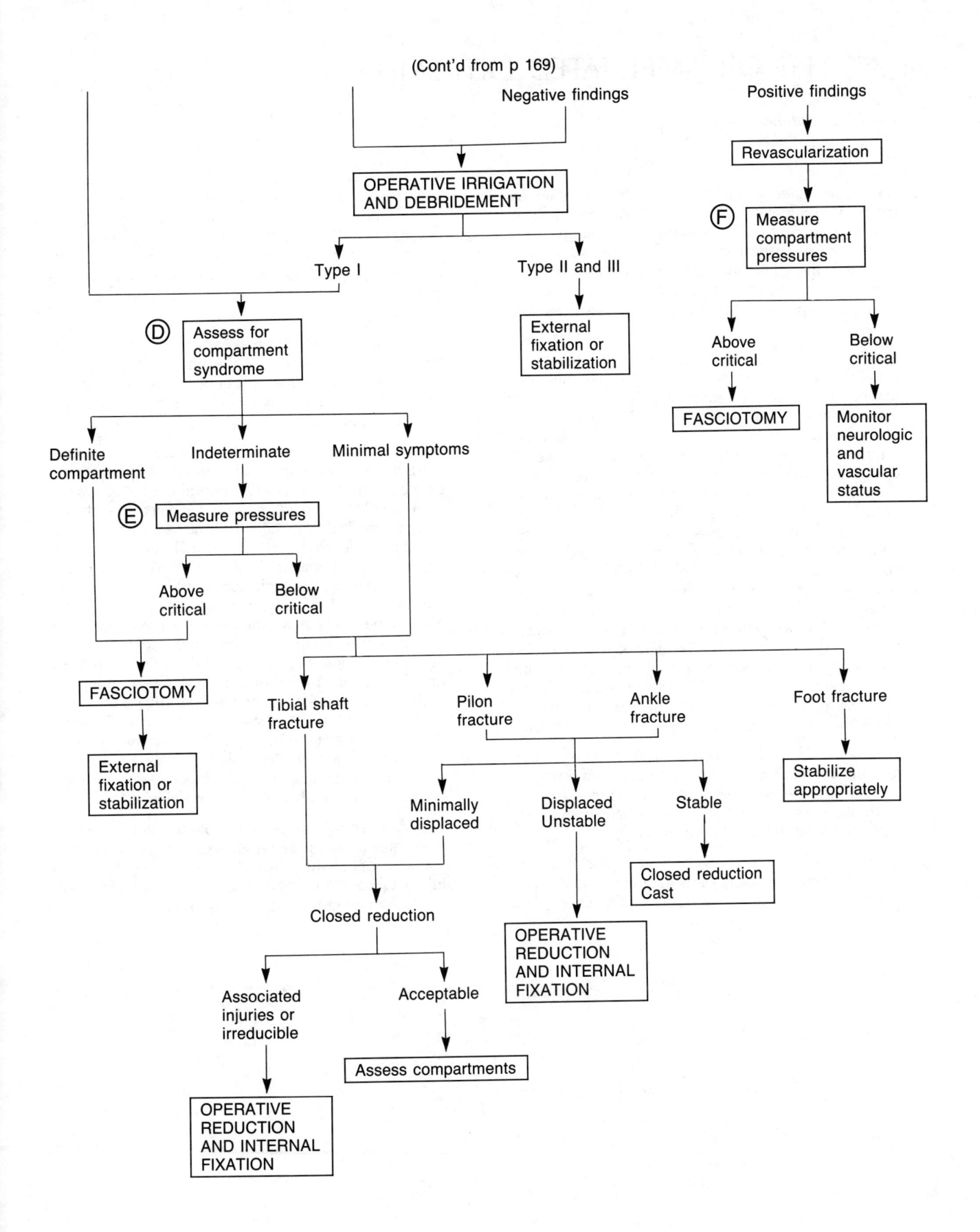

```
                                    Negative findings          Positive findings
                                           │                          │
                                           ▼                          ▼
                                  ┌──────────────────┐        ┌──────────────────┐
                                  │ OPERATIVE        │        │ Revascularization│
                                  │ IRRIGATION       │        └──────────────────┘
                                  │ AND DEBRIDEMENT  │                 │
                                  └──────────────────┘                 ▼
                                    │            │            Ⓕ ┌──────────────┐
                                 Type I      Type II and III     │ Measure      │
                                    │            │               │ compartment  │
                                    ▼            ▼               │ pressures    │
                              Ⓓ ┌──────────┐  ┌──────────┐       └──────────────┘
                                │ Assess for│ │ External │          │         │
                                │ compart-  │ │ fixation │       Above      Below
                                │ ment      │ │ or       │       critical   critical
                                │ syndrome  │ │ stabili- │          │         │
                                └───────────┘ │ zation   │          ▼         ▼
                                              └──────────┘    ┌──────────┐ ┌──────────┐
                                                              │FASCIOTOMY│ │ Monitor  │
                                                              └──────────┘ │ neurologic│
                                                                           │ and      │
                                                                           │ vascular │
                                                                           │ status   │
                                                                           └──────────┘
```

- Definite compartment → FASCIOTOMY → External fixation or stabilization
- Indeterminate → Ⓔ Measure pressures
  - Above critical → FASCIOTOMY
  - Below critical
- Minimal symptoms

- Tibial shaft fracture → Closed reduction
  - Associated injuries or irreducible → OPERATIVE REDUCTION AND INTERNAL FIXATION
  - Acceptable → Assess compartments
- Pilon fracture
  - Minimally displaced
  - Displaced Unstable → OPERATIVE REDUCTION AND INTERNAL FIXATION
- Ankle fracture
  - Displaced Unstable → OPERATIVE REDUCTION AND INTERNAL FIXATION
  - Stable → Closed reduction Cast
- Foot fracture → Stabilize appropriately

171

MANGLED OR AMPUTATED EXTREMITY

Patricia C. Epifanio

A. All trauma patients require primary and secondary assessments to identify any life threatening conditions. At this point, perform any life saving interventions. After control of airway, breathing and circulation has been established, the extremity injury may be assessed and managed. Extremity trauma is generally not associated with a high mortality. Manage any other associated injuries.

B. Continue with a focused assessment of the patient with extremity trauma. Patients with mangled extremity trauma require careful assessment of their injuries because some of these injuries that appear minor may actually be disastrous, and the opposite may also be true: those injuries that appear terrible may be minor in nature. Of critical importance in assessment are the elapsed time since the injury and the amount of ischemia. Assessment of the neurovascular status of the extremity should include circulation and innervation. Circulation in the extremity may be assessed by pulse presence and quality, color, temperature, and capillary refill. Early detection of vascular compromise is important to the patient's ultimate treatment outcome. Innervation assessment includes both movement and sensation. Have the patient flex and extend each joint of the affected extremity. Test for sensation in the web space of the thumb, tip of the index finger, tip of the little finger, web space between the great toe and the second toe, heel, and plantar surface of the foot. Careful documentation is essential.

C. History should include time of injury, mechanisms of injury, environment where the injury occurred, immunization history, pertinent previous medical history, present medications, patient's age, occupation, hand dominance, and emergency transport information.

D. Control bleeding with a pressure dressing and elevation. Dress the wound with dry sterile dressings and position the extremity in an anatomic position of function when splinting. To avoid any possible damage to severed vessels, do not probe the wound to clamp any bleeding blood vessels. Do not use a tourniquet. It will increase tissue destruction and may interfere with possible replantation and may require a more extensive amputation. The goal of treatment is to preserve and restore maximum function.

E. All trauma patients should have two large bore intravenous lines initially. At the time of line insertion, blood should be drawn for routine admission laboratory studies, including a type and cross-match for possible blood transfusion.

F. The extremity should be elevated to help to decrease edema formation, to reduce pain, and to decrease tissue damage. Cooling extends the period of time allowable for revascularization and repair of the defect. Assist with wound care, including copious irrigation. The amputated part should be rinsed with normal saline to remove large particulate matter, wrapped in a dry sterile dressing, and placed in a sterile cup or plastic zip-lock bag. Place the container with the part on top of ice in a larger container. Be sure that the melting ice water does not seep into the container with the amputated part. Do not freeze the amputated part. Label and store in a safe place until it is needed for surgery. In caring for the stump, remove any visible foreign bodies and irrigate with normal saline or Ringer's lactate. Cover the area with a dry sterile dressing. Do not cover the open wound with povidone-iodine (Betadine) solution; it may be harsh on exposed nerve endings and small blood vessels. Support the extremity on a board. Cool and elevate.

G. X-ray films should be taken of both the stump and the amputated part(s). In all orthopaedic injuries it is important to visualize the joints above and below the site of injury. Good anteroposterior and lateral films are helpful in evaluating the extent of the injury.

Patient with **MANGLED OR AMPUTATED EXTREMITY**

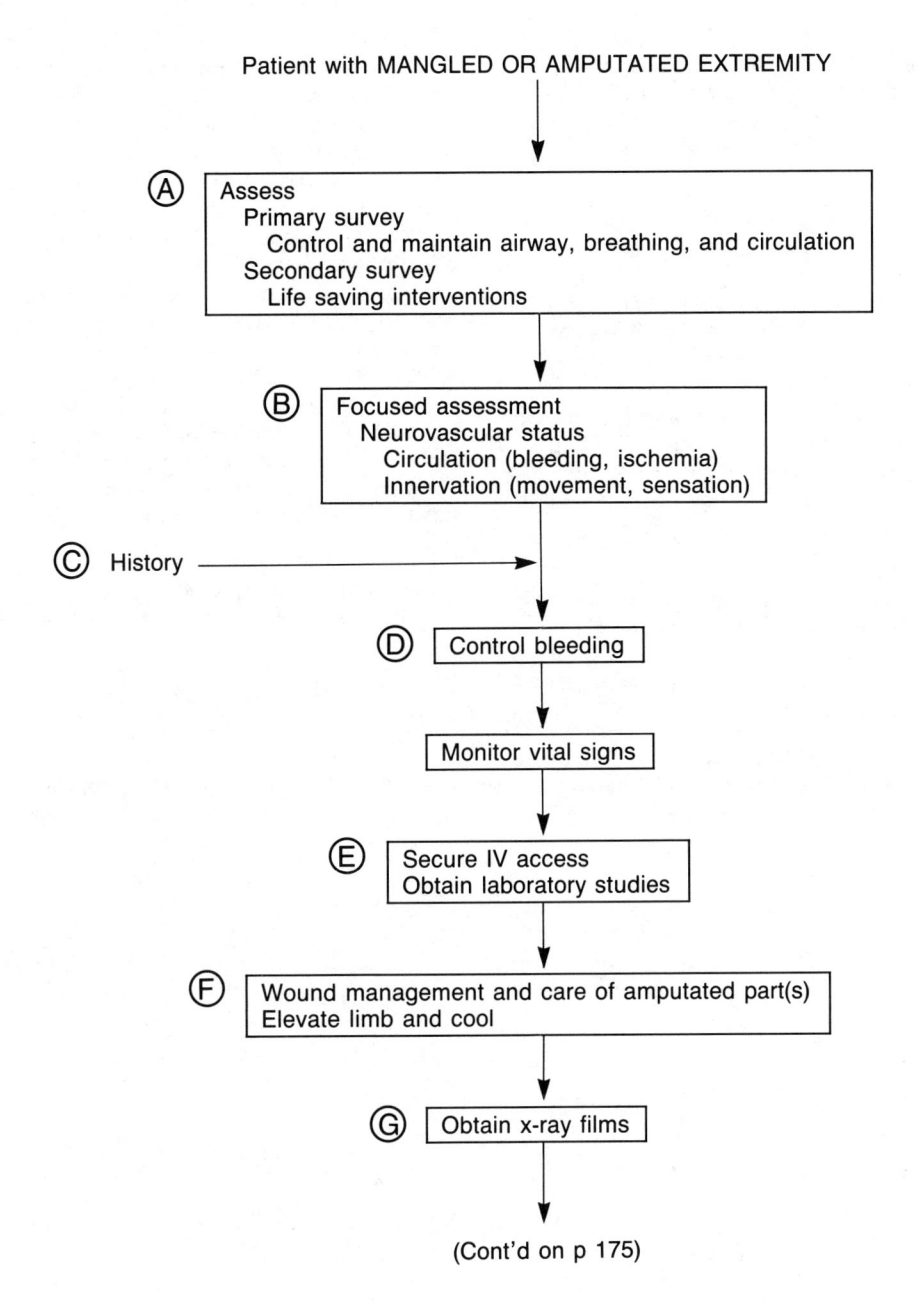

- (A) Assess
  - Primary survey
    - Control and maintain airway, breathing, and circulation
  - Secondary survey
    - Life saving interventions

- (B) Focused assessment
  - Neurovascular status
    - Circulation (bleeding, ischemia)
    - Innervation (movement, sensation)

- (C) History →

- (D) Control bleeding

- Monitor vital signs

- (E) Secure IV access
  Obtain laboratory studies

- (F) Wound management and care of amputated part(s)
  Elevate limb and cool

- (G) Obtain x-ray films

(Cont'd on p 175)

173

H. Administration of broad-spectrum antibiotics is indicated for all patients with extremity trauma because of the open nature of the wound and the mechanism of injury. A large portion of these injuries are caused by industrial and motor vehicle accidents.

I. Monitor vital signs for changes in the patient's hemodynamic status. Vital signs include compartment pressures. Observe for compartment syndrome, which may results from a crush injury, often associated with mangle type injuries of the forearm or leg. Possible signs and symptoms include pain that is out of proportion to the nature of the injury, palpable tension of the compartment, decreased pulse, motor weakness, and extreme tenderness on passive stretching of the muscles within the affected compartment. Assist with direct measurement of compartment pressure. It may be necessary to prepare the patient for fasciotomy to facilitate decompression.

J. Immediate revascularization is required in an ischemic extremity to ensure neurovascular function and limb salvage. If the ischemic time is greater than 6 hours, saving the limb becomes questionable, particularly if associated muscle crush injury also is present.

K. With current microvascular techniques, it is possible to anastomose 1-mm vessels together, which makes replantation of digits possible. Replantations have been successful with thumb, multiple finger, transmetacarpal, wrist, forearm, upper arm, and some lower limb amputations, particularly those proximal to the transmetatarsal level. Decisions to attempt replantation are made on an individual basis. A detailed discussion should be held with the patient regarding the risks and expected results. The chances of a successful outcome are improved with a guillotine type of injury and are decreased in those injuries with avulsed or severely crushed amputation. Immediate revascularization is required in an ischemic extremity to ensure neurovascular function and limb salvage. If the ischemic time is greater than 6 hours, saving the limb becomes questionable, particularly with associated muscle crush injury. Two microvascular surgical teams must usually perform the replantation. The first team works on the patient, and the other team identifies the structures on the amputated part.

L. If the patient is not in a facility that has microvascular surgical and specialized rehabilitation capabilities, prepare the patient for transfer to a definitive care center.

References

Crowley R, Dunham C, eds. Shock trauma/critical care handbook. Rockville, MD: Aspen, 1986:354–358; 363–364; 367–411.

(Cont'd from p 173)

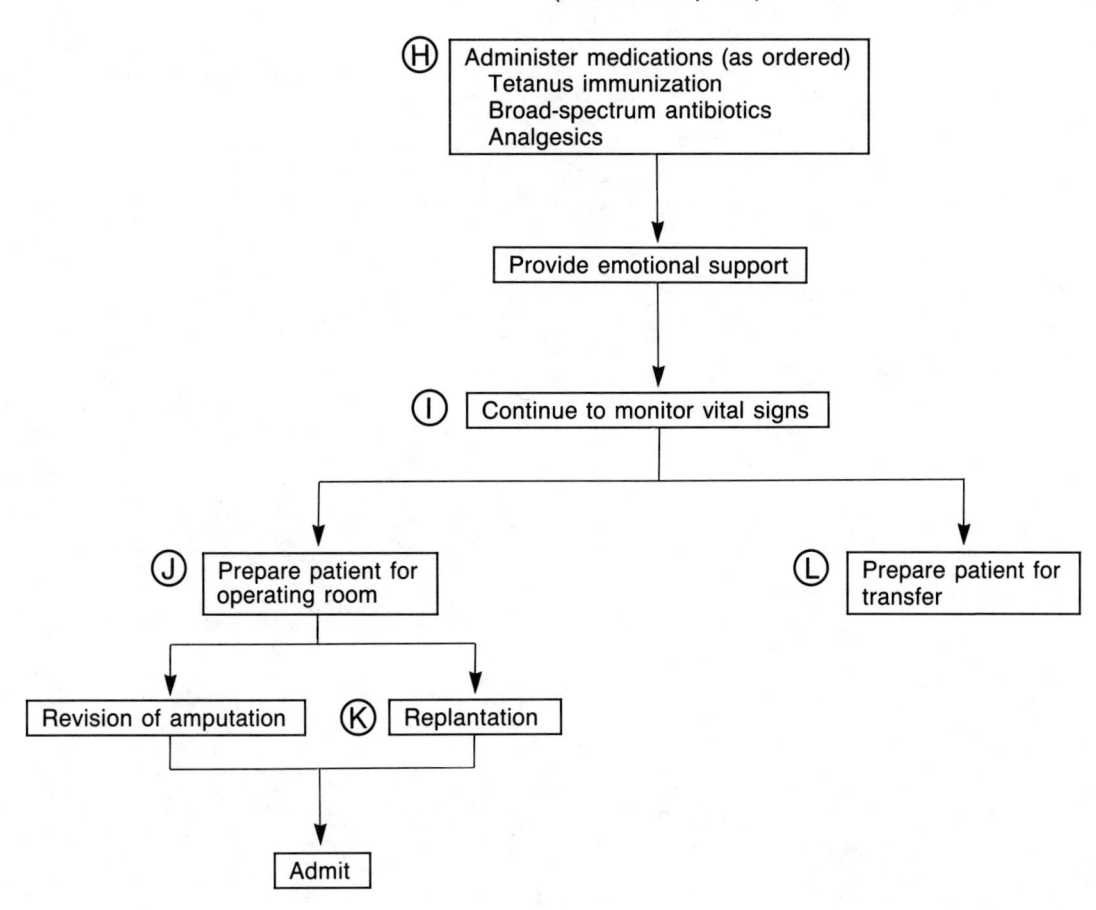

- **H** Administer medications (as ordered)
  - Tetanus immunization
  - Broad-spectrum antibiotics
  - Analgesics

↓

Provide emotional support

↓

- **I** Continue to monitor vital signs

↓ ↓

- **J** Prepare patient for operating room
- **L** Prepare patient for transfer

↓ ↓

Revision of amputation | **K** Replantation

↓

Admit

PERIPHERAL NERVE TRAUMA

PERIPHERAL NERVE TRAUMA

Jan Bear

A. A complete history including how the injury took place, trauma involved, forces involved, and time of injury is necessary. The level of injury is determined by a complete motor and sensory examination; the nerve or nerves involved are identified (Figs. 1 through 6). If a wound is present, its condition and age are documented. Complete documentation of the motor and sensory levels of the nerve injury is important to follow the recovery process. Do not use local anesthetics to infiltrate wounds for exploration or repair until nerve injury has been ruled out.

B. Rule out other causes of paresthesia, anesthesia, paresis, or paralysis because these injuries, if left untreated, can cause irreversible damage. Compartment syndrome and arterial injury are the most common injuries that can mimic nerve injury (Table 1).

C. Peripheral nerves can be damaged as a result of traction, compression, contusion, or laceration.

D. The types of closed injuries encountered are traction, compression, and contusion. Traction injuries can occur in association with fractures at the time of injury, during reduction or fixation, and in dislocations. Stretching of a nerve trunk up to 15 percent of its length can occur without injury. The tensile strength of the perineurium is exceeded when the nerve is stretched about 20 percent, which results in tearing at the elastic limit of stretch. Spontaneous recovery is typical in these lesions. Contusion and compression injuries typically show spontaneous recovery.

E. Neuropraxia is a minor injury that results from traction or compression where ischemia and/or local demyelination interferes with nerve function. Motor function damage is usually more severe than that of sensory function; recovery occurs within hours to days. Axonotmesis is an injury in which continuity of the nerve axons is disrupted. The endoneural tube remains intact so that the regenerating axons can re-establish functional connections. Prognosis is good, and recovery usually occurs within a year. Neurotmesis is a disruption of the axons and of the nerve connective tissue. Healing results in fibrosis, loss of coaptation, and loss of continuity, which mitigate against spontaneous recovery. Surgical repair is indicated.

F. The extremity should be immobilized in a neutral position, midway between the pull of the flexors and extensors of the involved extremity.

G. Consult a peripheral nerve surgeon as to preferences regarding management while the patient is in the emergency department. The initial physical examination should be well documented. This is the most important part of the emergency department management of peripheral nerve injuries.

H. The rest of this decision tree gives a brief outline of how the peripheral nerve surgeon will handle the injury. This is meant to give an overview of the treatment options for better understanding of nerve injuries. There are a number of adjunctive tests that can be used to monitor patients with peripheral nerve injuries in addition to a detailed physical examination, which includes evaluation of motor and sensory injury levels.

I. Open injuries primarily include gunshot wounds (GSWs) and lacerations. GSWs can be separated into high velocity (greater than 2000 ft per second), low velocity (less than 2000 ft per second), and shotgun injuries. The prognosis of conservative treatment in high velocity wounds is up to 68 percent spontaneous recovery and is about the same in low velocity civilian handgun wounds. Spontaneous recovery from shotgun wounds is reported to be only about 45 percent. Lacerations should be diagnosed clinically as severed nerve lesions (i.e., neurotmesis) until proved otherwise by operative intervention.

J. Treat the wound as any other open wound in terms of tetanus status and tendon, arterial, or bony injury and consult the appropriate physicians. A peripheral nerve surgeon should be consulted immediately and given a complete rundown of the history and physical examination. The limb should be splinted in a neutral position.

TABLE 1 Possible Causes of Nerve Injury Symptoms

Symptom Present	Compartment Syndrome	Arterial Injury	Nerve Injury
Increased compartment pressure	+	−	−
Pain with stretch	+	−	−
Paresthesia or anesthesia	+	+	+
Paresis or paralysis	+	+	+
Pulses intact	+	−	+

References

Mobarak SJ, Owen CA, Hargens AR, et al. Acute compartment syndrome: diagnosis and treatment with the aid of the wick catheter. J Bone Joint Surg 1978; 60-A:1091–1095.

Omer GE. Evaluation of the extremity with peripheral nerve injury and timing for nerve suture. AAOS Instructional Course Lectures 1984; 33:463–484.

Szabo RM, Madison M. Principle of nerve repair. In: Chapman M, ed. Operative orthopaedics. Vol. 2. Philadelphia: JB Lippincott, 1988:1337.

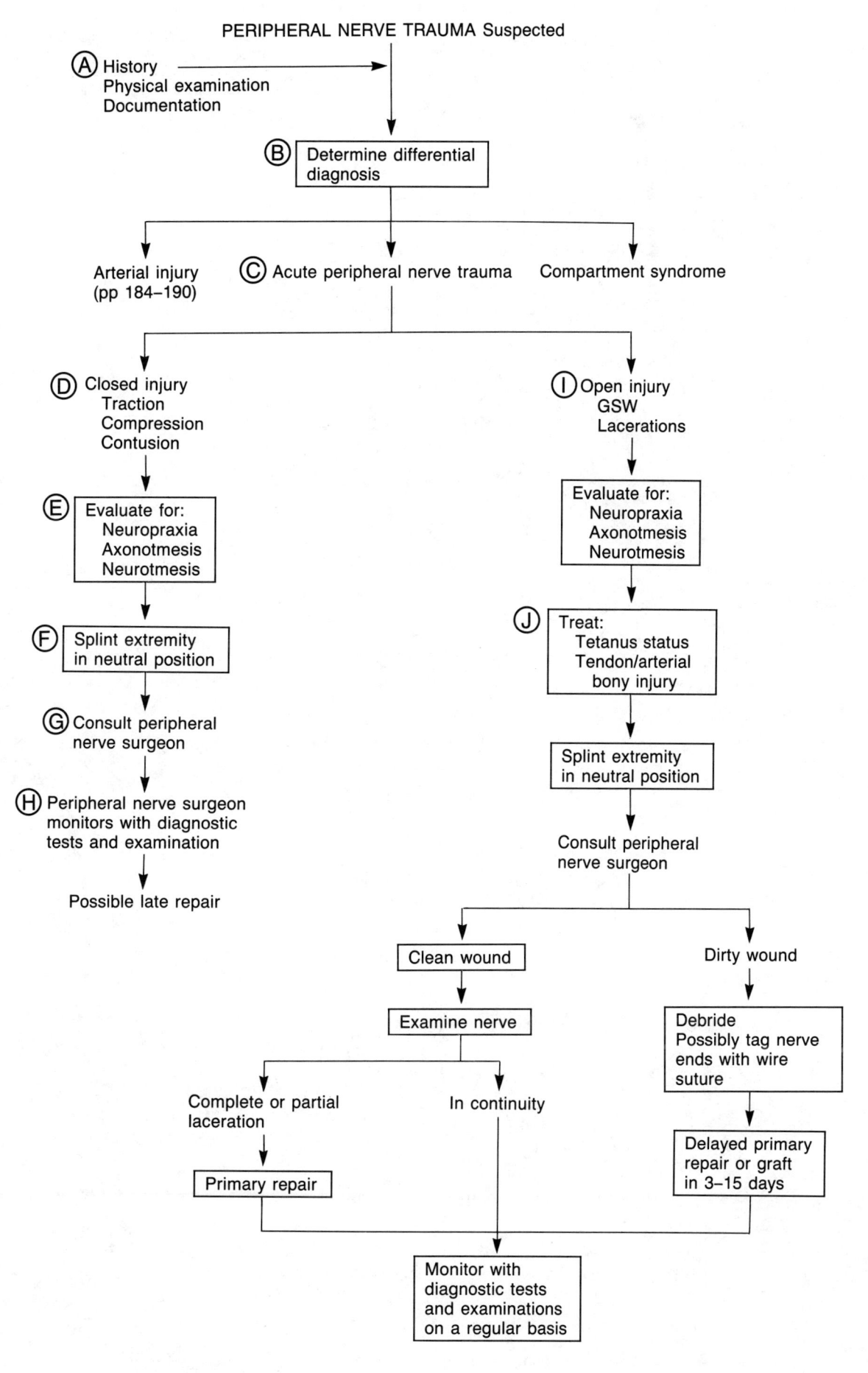

PERIPHERAL NERVE TRAUMA Suspected

- **A** History
  Physical examination
  Documentation

- **B** Determine differential diagnosis
  - Arterial injury (pp 184–190)
  - **C** Acute peripheral nerve trauma
  - Compartment syndrome

Acute peripheral nerve trauma

- **D** Closed injury
  - Traction
  - Compression
  - Contusion

- **E** Evaluate for:
  - Neuropraxia
  - Axonotmesis
  - Neurotmesis

- **F** Splint extremity in neutral position

- **G** Consult peripheral nerve surgeon

- **H** Peripheral nerve surgeon monitors with diagnostic tests and examination

  Possible late repair

- **I** Open injury
  - GSW
  - Lacerations

  Evaluate for:
  - Neuropraxia
  - Axonotmesis
  - Neurotmesis

- **J** Treat:
  - Tetanus status
  - Tendon/arterial bony injury

  Splint extremity in neutral position

  Consult peripheral nerve surgeon

  - Clean wound
    - Examine nerve
      - Complete or partial laceration → Primary repair
      - In continuity
  - Dirty wound
    - Debride
      Possibly tag nerve ends with wire suture
    - Delayed primary repair or graft in 3–15 days

  Monitor with diagnostic tests and examinations on a regular basis

179

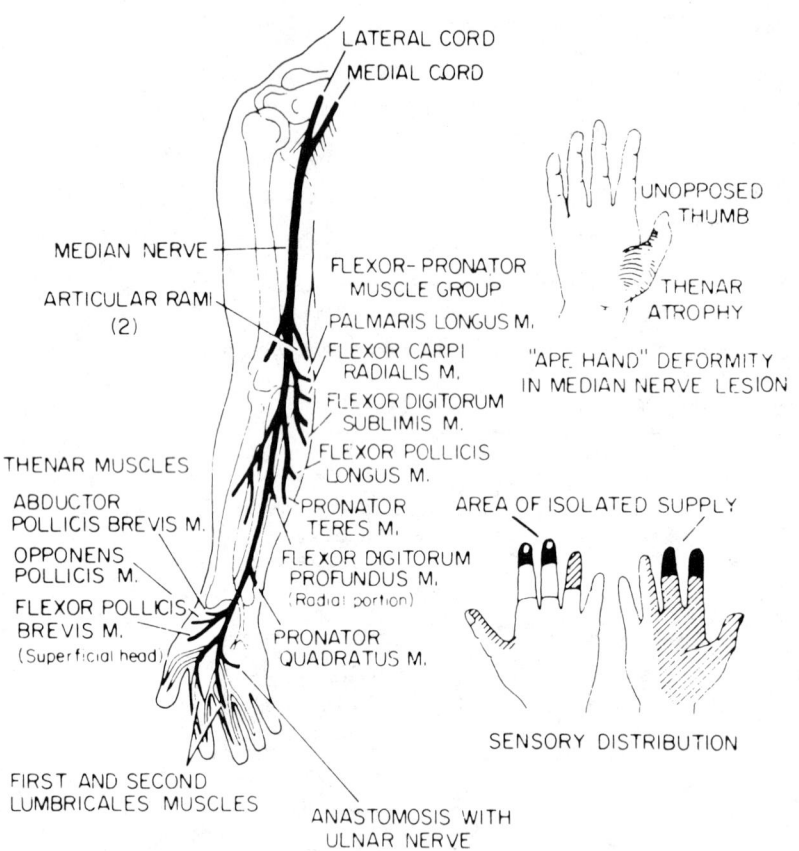

Figure 1 Median nerve distribution. (Figures 1 through 6 reprinted with permission from Omer G. Physical diagnosis of peripheral nerve injuries. Orthop Clin North Am 1981; 12(2):207–228.)

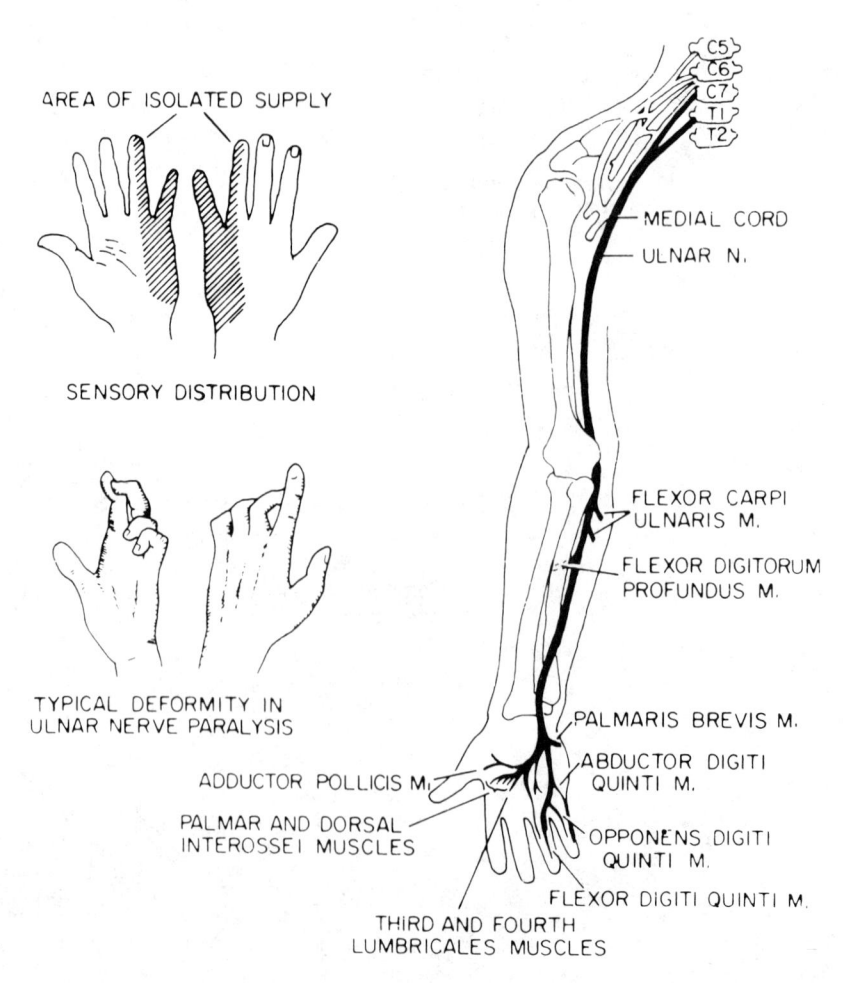

Figure 2 Ulnar nerve distribution.

Figure 3 Radial nerve distribution.

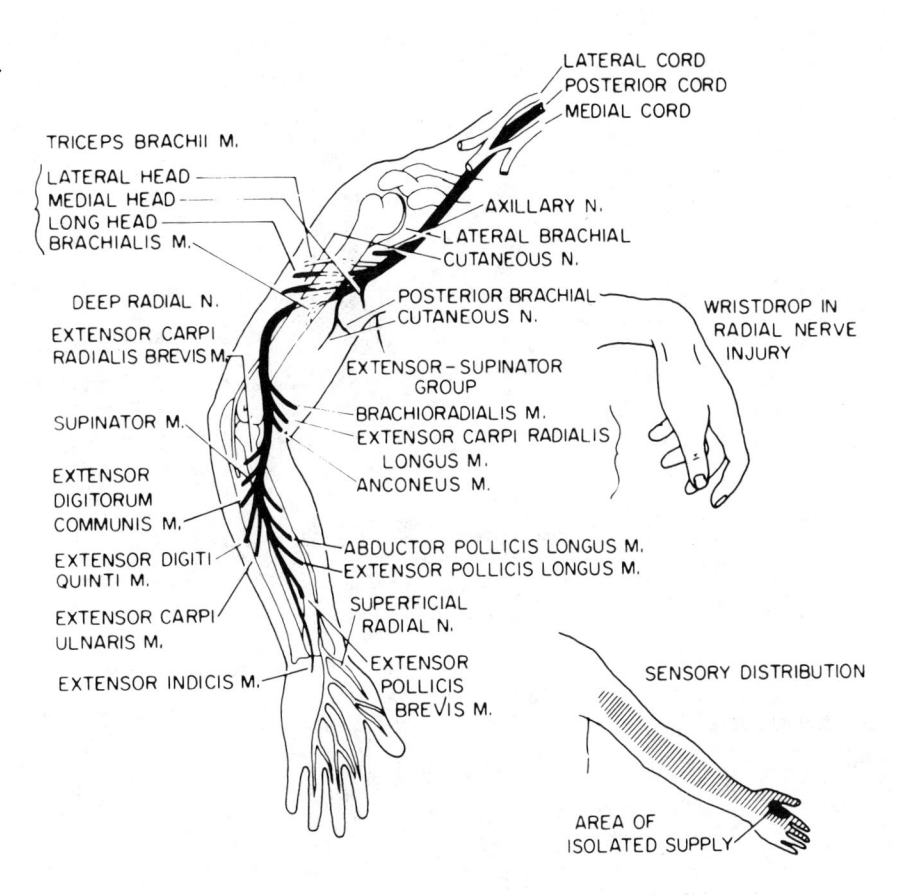

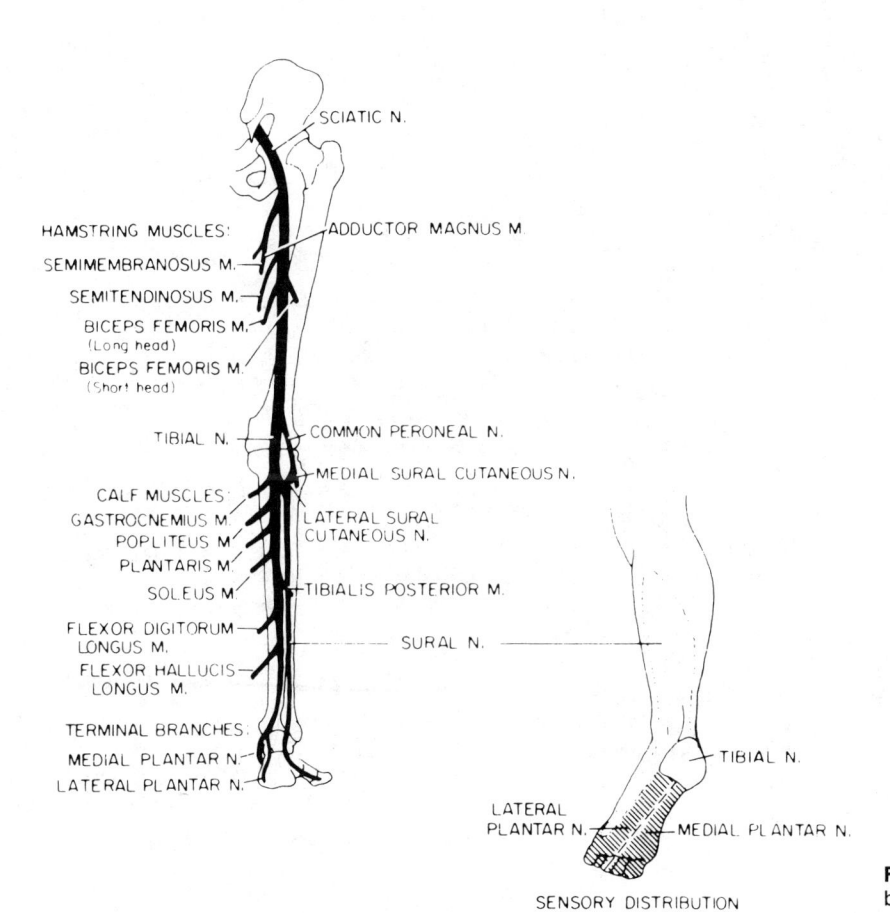

Figure 4 Sciatic and tibial nerve distribution.

Figure 5 Femoral and obturator nerve distribution.

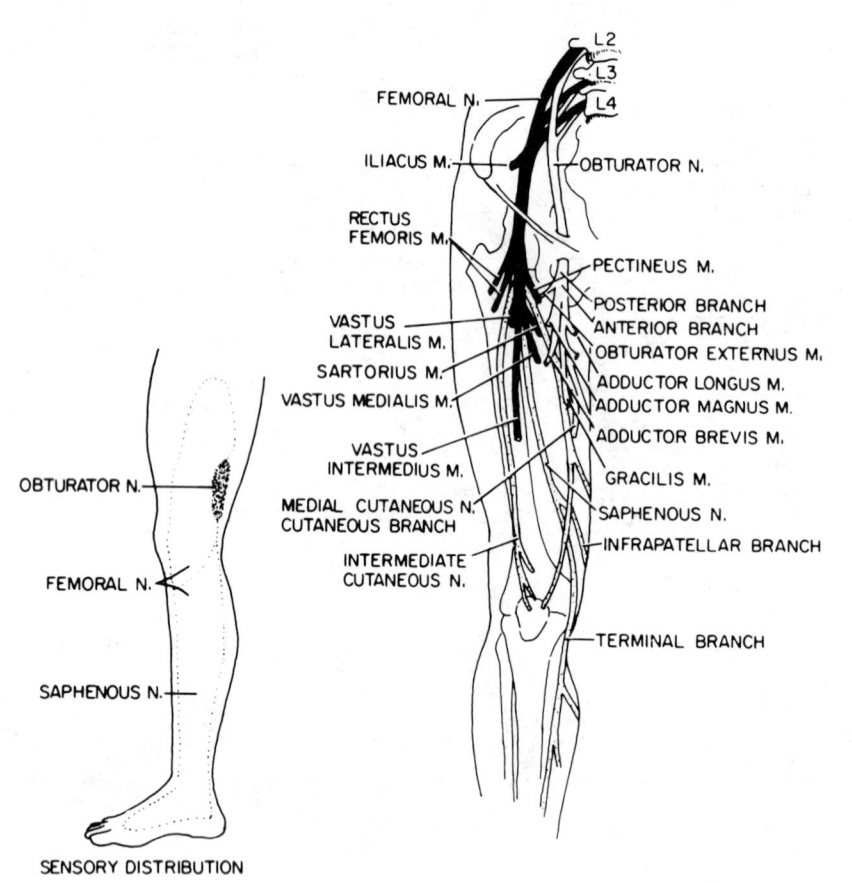

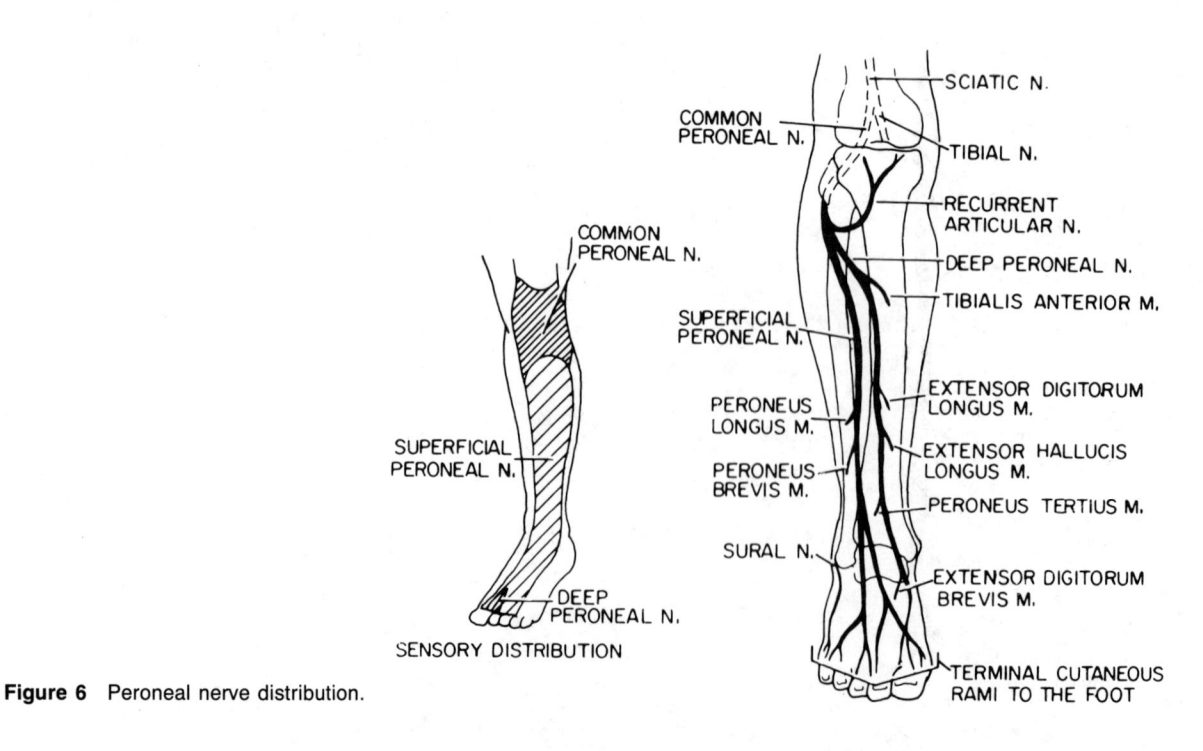

Figure 6 Peroneal nerve distribution.

VASCULAR TRAUMA

Carotid Artery Trauma
Subclavian, Axillary, and Brachial Artery
  Trauma
Iliofemoral Vascular Trauma
Popliteal and Tibial Vascular Trauma

CAROTID ARTERY TRAUMA

Robert P. Winter

A. Most carotid artery injuries result from penetrating cervical wounds, with a majority occurring on the left side. A high index of suspicion is necessary to detect blunt injuries to the carotid arteries because many patients present without neurologic manifestations or with intermittent symptoms. Patients who sustain hyperextension injuries or blows to the neck should be considered for evaluation of the carotid arteries.

B. Patency of the airway and maintenance of breathing are essential to patient survival. The neck should be immobilized to avoid neurologic damage from an associated spinal injury. Most patients can be managed expectantly or by orotracheal intubation using in-line cervical traction. Cricothyroidotomy should be reserved for patients in whom intubation is not possible or who have associated massive facial trauma. External hemorrhage can generally be controlled with manual compression. No effort should be made to clamp bleeding vessels through the wound.

C. Careful neurologic assessment provides important prognostic information and guidance in planning operative intervention. Morbidity and mortality are closely related to the neurologic condition of the patient on presentation.

D. Exsanguination or the inability to obtain an airway is an indication for immediate transfer to the operating room and surgical intervention.

E. Carotid artery dissection often extends to the skull base or beyond, thereby making surgical repair unfeasible. Such lesions are best managed initially by observation and anticoagulant medication.

F. Once an injury has been diagnosed, therapy should be based on the presence and severity of any neurologic deficit. Patients who present comatose or with a massive, fixed neurologic deficit risk progressive neurologic injury or death as a result of hemorrhagic infarction following vascular reconstruction. Under most circumstances, such patients are best treated by ligation of the injured vessel.

G. Patients with mild deficits or who are neurologically intact should undergo reconstruction of the carotid artery. The majority of injuries can be exposed through a standard incision along the anterior border of the sternocleidomastoid muscle. Injuries in Zone I may require median sternotomy for proximal control. Additional exposure of Zone III injuries can be obtained by subluxation of the mandible. In rare instances when the distal extent of the injury is at or beyond the base of the skull, consideration should be given to proximal ligation combined with extracranial-intracranial (EC-IC) bypass. Concomitant venous injuries and wounds of the aerodigestive tract must be managed appropriately during neck exploration.

References

Fry RE, Fry WJ. Extracranial carotid artery injuries. Surgery 1980; 88:581–586.

Perry MO. Extracranial carotid and vertebral arterial penetrating injury. In: Ernst CB, Stanley JC, eds. Current therapy in vascular surgery. Toronto: BC Decker, 1987:265–267.

Perry MO. Injuries of the brachiocephalic vessels. In: Rutherford RB, ed. Vascular surgery. 3rd ed. Philadelphia: WB Saunders, 1989:604–612.

Thal ER, Snyder WH, Hays RJ, et al. Management of carotid artery injuries. Surgery 1974; 76:955–962.

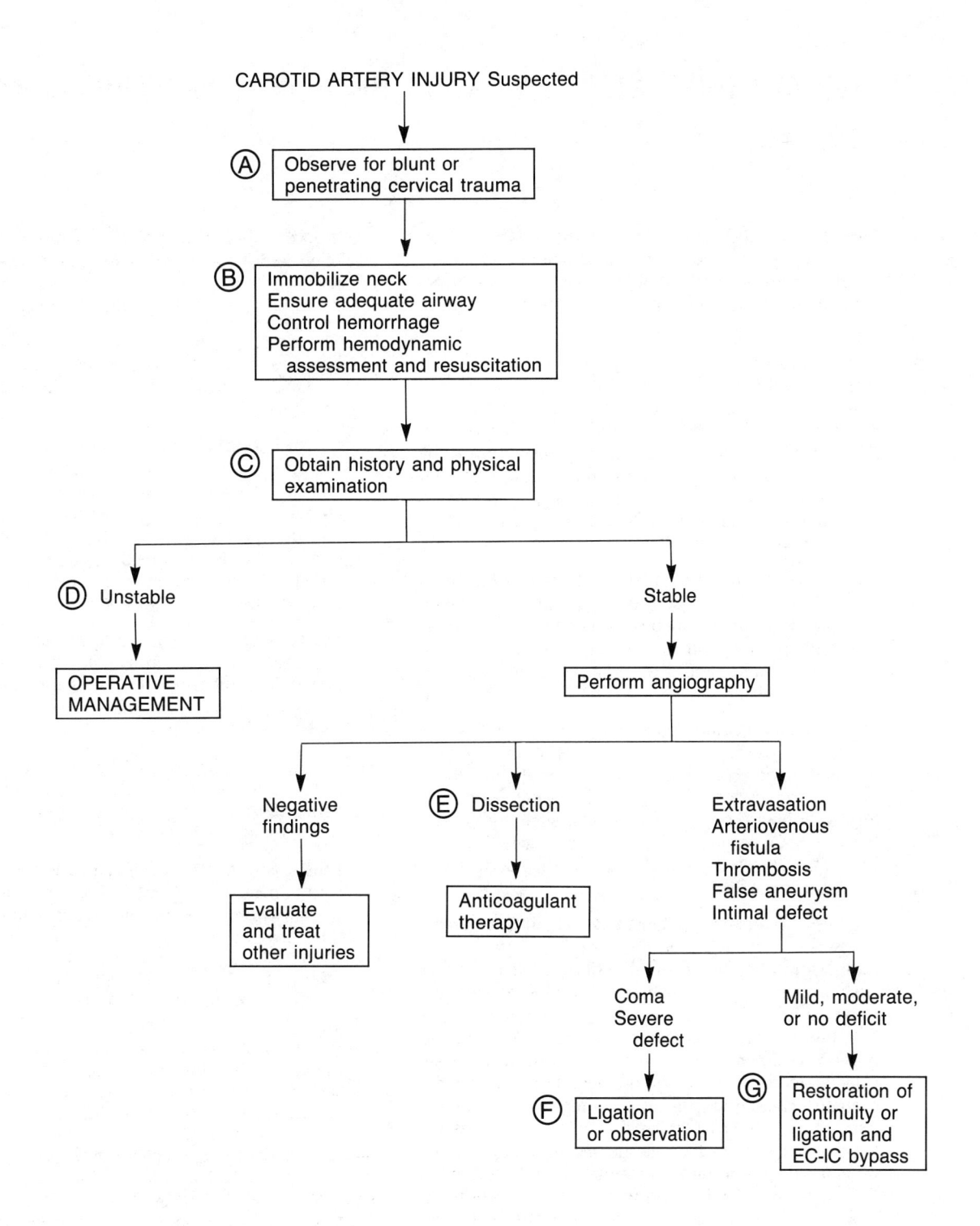

```
CAROTID ARTERY INJURY Suspected
                │
                ▼
  Ⓐ  Observe for blunt or
      penetrating cervical trauma
                │
                ▼
  Ⓑ  Immobilize neck
      Ensure adequate airway
      Control hemorrhage
      Perform hemodynamic
        assessment and resuscitation
                │
                ▼
  Ⓒ  Obtain history and physical
      examination
       ┌────────┴────────┐
       ▼                 ▼
  Ⓓ Unstable           Stable
       │                 │
       ▼                 ▼
  OPERATIVE       Perform angiography
  MANAGEMENT
            ┌────────────┼────────────┐
            ▼            ▼            ▼
         Negative     Ⓔ Dissection   Extravasation
         findings                    Arteriovenous
            │            │             fistula
            ▼            ▼           Thrombosis
         Evaluate    Anticoagulant   False aneurysm
         and treat   therapy         Intimal defect
         other injuries                    │
                                  ┌────────┴────────┐
                                  ▼                 ▼
                                Coma           Mild, moderate,
                                Severe         or no deficit
                                defect               │
                                  │                  ▼
                                  ▼          Ⓖ Restoration of
                              Ⓕ Ligation        continuity or
                                or observation   ligation and
                                                 EC-IC bypass
```

185

SUBCLAVIAN, AXILLARY, AND BRACHIAL ARTERY TRAUMA

Robert P. Winter

A. Over 90 percent of subclavian, axillary, and brachial arterial injuries result from penetrating wounds. However, injuries to these vessels should be searched for in patients with a history of contusion or stretch-traction of the arm and shoulder girdle.

B. Initial evaluation and resuscitation must proceed in a rapid and orderly fashion. The possibility of cardiac and pulmonary injuries coexistent with proximal subclavian artery injury should be considered. Thoracostomy tubes should be placed as dictated by chest films or by the clinical situation. Neurologic and orthopaedic injuries are frequently present in association with upper extremity trauma and should be investigated by careful examination and appropriate films.

C. Wounds of the thoracic inlet, superior mediastinum, supraclavicular region, and axilla can pose considerable diagnostic and therapeutic challenges. Such injuries can result in a spectrum of presentations, from immediate exsanguination and death to a stable, relatively innocuous appearance.

D. Patients suffering cardiopulmonary arrest secondary to cardiac or intrathoracic vascular injury should in most instances undergo emergency department thoracotomy. Repair, compression, or intrapleural packing can be performed, followed by transfer of the patient to the operating room. Cross-clamping of the descending thoracic aorta may preserve cerebral and coronary perfusion if the heart is contracting.

E. Patients who remain hypotensive despite initial attempts at resuscitation should be transferred to the operating room. Control of the proximal right subclavian artery is best obtained through a median sternotomy, whereas the proximal left subclavian artery is approached through a left anterolateral thoracotomy. Exposure of the second portion of either the right or the left subclavian artery is facilitated by resection of the medial one-third of the clavicle. The distal subclavian artery is approached through a supraclavicular incision. In rare instances, extensive exposure of the left subclavian artery may be provided by extending the anterolateral thoracotomy to the supraclavicular incision with a partial sternotomy, thereby creating a "book" thoracotomy. The axillary artery is exposed through an incision in the deltopectoral groove. Standard techniques of vascular repair are applied by using autologous tissue or, if necessary, prosthetic grafts. Concomitant venous injuries should be repaired if at all feasible, but ligation is generally well tolerated.

F. The stable patient with a suspected subclavian or axillary artery injury should undergo angiography to confirm the diagnosis and to aid in planning the operative approach.

G. Isolated upper extremity trauma that results in an obvious arterial injury and either active hemorrhage or limb ischemia should be explored without delay. Similarly, an obvious arterial injury in an adequately perfused limb may be repaired without further diagnostic studies. Fasciotomy should be considered as an adjunct to arterial repair if there is prolonged ischemia or compartmental hypertension.

H. Signs of vascular injury include hematoma, arterial bleeding, loss of pulses, bruit, pain, and distal neurologic deficit. In the absence of obvious arterial injury, the finding of any or all of these signs should raise suspicion that such an injury is present.

I. Angiographic signs of injury include obstruction, extravasation, filling defect, pseudoaneurysm, and arteriovenous fistula. Positive angiography should be followed by prompt surgical exploration.

J. Satisfactory vascular repair can be achieved in the majority of upper extremity arterial injuries. Long-term morbidity results from associated neurologic injuries. Amputation rates are in the range of 1 to 3 percent.

References

Borman KR, Snyder WH, Weigelt JA. Civilian arterial trauma of the upper extremity. Am J Surg 1984; 148:796–799.

Feliciano DV, Burch JM, Graham JM. Vascular injuries of the chest and abdomen. In: Rutherford RB, ed. Vascular surgery. 3rd ed. Philadelphia: WB Saunders, 1989:588–603.

Graham JM, Mattox KL, Feliciano DV, DeBakey ME. Vascular injuries of the axilla. Ann Surg 1982; 195:232–238.

Snyder WH, Thal ER, Perry MO. Vascular injuries of the extremities. In: Rutherford RB, ed. Vascular surgery. 3rd ed. Philadelphia: WB Saunders, 1989:613–637.

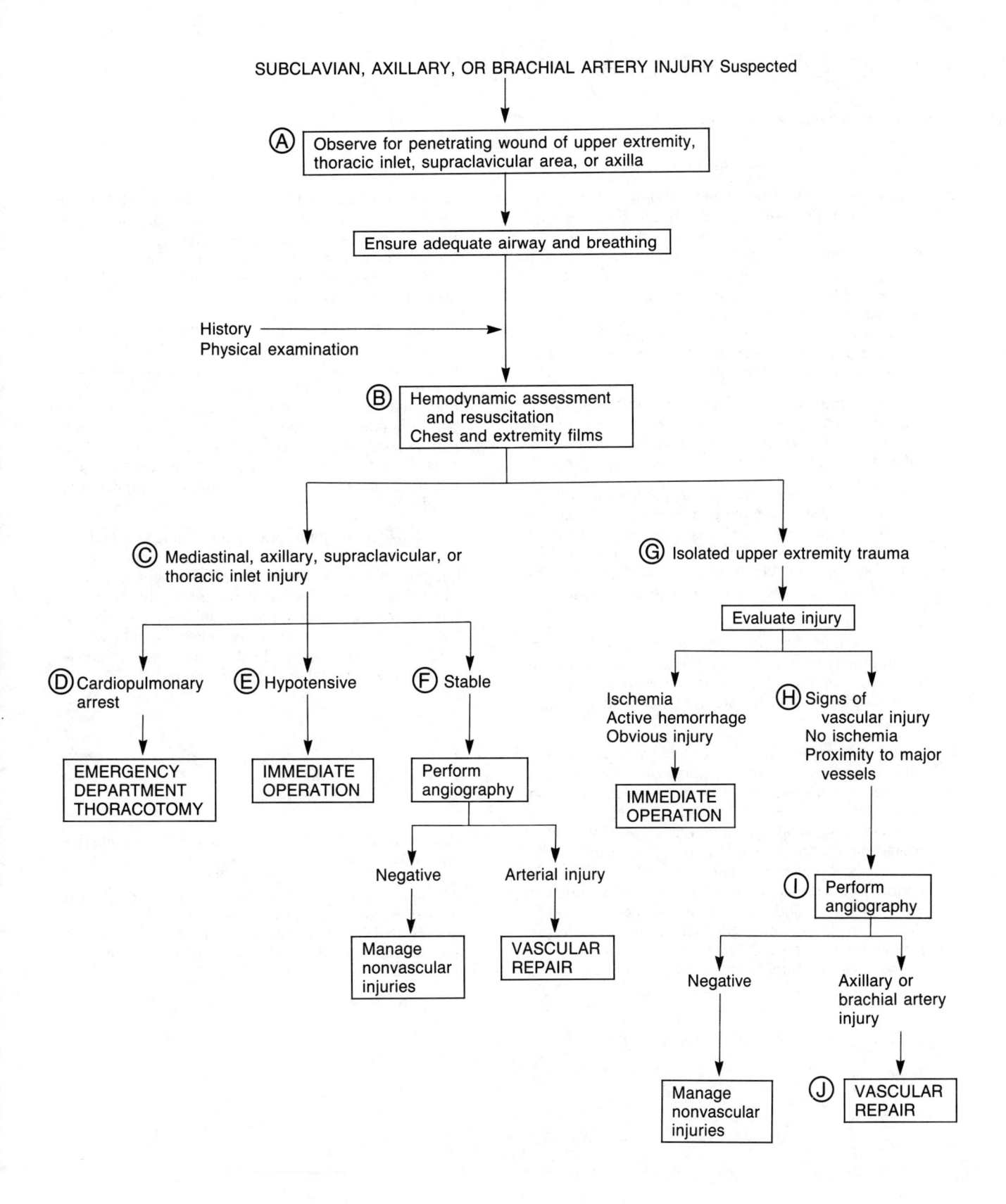

SUBCLAVIAN, AXILLARY, OR BRACHIAL ARTERY INJURY Suspected

(A) Observe for penetrating wound of upper extremity, thoracic inlet, supraclavicular area, or axilla

↓

Ensure adequate airway and breathing

History / Physical examination →

(B) Hemodynamic assessment and resuscitation
Chest and extremity films

(C) Mediastinal, axillary, supraclavicular, or thoracic inlet injury

- **(D) Cardiopulmonary arrest** → EMERGENCY DEPARTMENT THORACOTOMY
- **(E) Hypotensive** → IMMEDIATE OPERATION
- **(F) Stable** → Perform angiography
  - Negative → Manage nonvascular injuries
  - Arterial injury → VASCULAR REPAIR

(G) Isolated upper extremity trauma

Evaluate injury

- Ischemia / Active hemorrhage / Obvious injury → IMMEDIATE OPERATION
- **(H) Signs of vascular injury / No ischemia / Proximity to major vessels**
  - **(I)** Perform angiography
    - Negative → Manage nonvascular injuries
    - Axillary or brachial artery injury → **(J)** VASCULAR REPAIR

187

ILIOFEMORAL VASCULAR TRAUMA

Robert P. Winter

A. Any patient with a penetrating abdominal or pelvic wound and hypotension must be presumed to have a vascular injury. Iliac vessel injuries comprise approximately 10 percent of vascular trauma and are often fatal. Prompt recognition and control of such injuries are essential to patient survival. Femoral artery injuries make up roughly one-fourth of all peripheral arterial wounds. Although the majority are caused by penetrating injuries, approximately 15 percent of iliac vessel injuries are associated with blunt trauma.

B. Orderly, simultaneous evaluation and resuscitation are typically performed. External hemorrhage can generally be controlled with manual pressure. Care must be taken to identify all wounds and potential injuries.

C. Penetrating injuries above the inguinal ligament in a hypotensive patient warrant prompt abdominal exploration. The likelihood of iliac vessel injury in a patient with an abdominal wound below the umbilicus, with abdominal tenderness, and with hypotension is 40 percent. Distal limb ischemia also mandates urgent operation.

D. Penetrating abdominal wounds in stable patients may be evaluated more thoroughly, including evaluation of the genitourinary tract when appropriate. Patients with gunshot wounds should undergo mandatory celiotomy, whereas those with stab wounds may be managed selectively.

E. Control of hemorrhage from iliac artery injuries can be difficult and may require clamping of the distal aorta. Manual pressure using sponge sticks is helpful in controlling venous bleeding. Venous injuries should be repaired rather than ligated whenever possible. When replacement of the injured artery is necessary, autologous tissue is preferred—particularly if there is contamination from associated bowel injury. Ligation combined with fasciotomy and extra-anatomic bypass may be indicated in cases with significant fecal spill. Despite prompt recognition and treatment, iliac vascular injury is associated with mortality in 25 percent of patients.

F. Blunt or penetrating injuries to the groin or thigh that result in distal limb ischemia or uncontrollable hemorrhage should be evaluated and treated in the operating room. When the presence or location of an arterial injury is unknown, single injection angiography can be performed on the operating table.

G. Despite adequate distal perfusion, an arterial injury may be present. The presence of any of the five "P"s (pain, pallor, loss of pulse, paralysis or paresthesia) should arouse suspicion of an arterial injury. Similarly, expanding hematoma, pulsatile bleeding, a thrill or bruit, certain orthopaedic injuries, and proximity of a wound to major vessels should alert the examiner to the possibility of arterial trauma. Angiography is the best available means to define the location, extent, and number of arterial injuries.

H. Femoral arterial injuries are repaired using standard vascular techniques. Every effort should be made to use autologous tissue for repair. Saphenous vein is usually suitable for interposition grafting, should this be necessary. Associated venous injuries should be repaired rather than ligated in most instances. Fasciotomy should be considered in cases associated with prolonged ischemia or in combined arterial and venous injuries.

References

Feliciano DV, Burch JM, Graham JM. Vascular injuries of the chest and abdomen. In: Rutherford RB, ed. Vascular surgery. 3rd ed. Philadelphia: WB Saunders, 1989:588–603.

Ryan W, Snyder W, Bell T, Hunt J. Penetrating injuries of the iliac vessels. Am J Surg 1982; 144:642–645.

Snyder WH, Thal ER, Perry MO. Vascular injuries of the extremities. In: Rutherford RB, ed. Vascular surgery. 3rd ed. Philadelphia: WB Saunders, 1989:613–637.

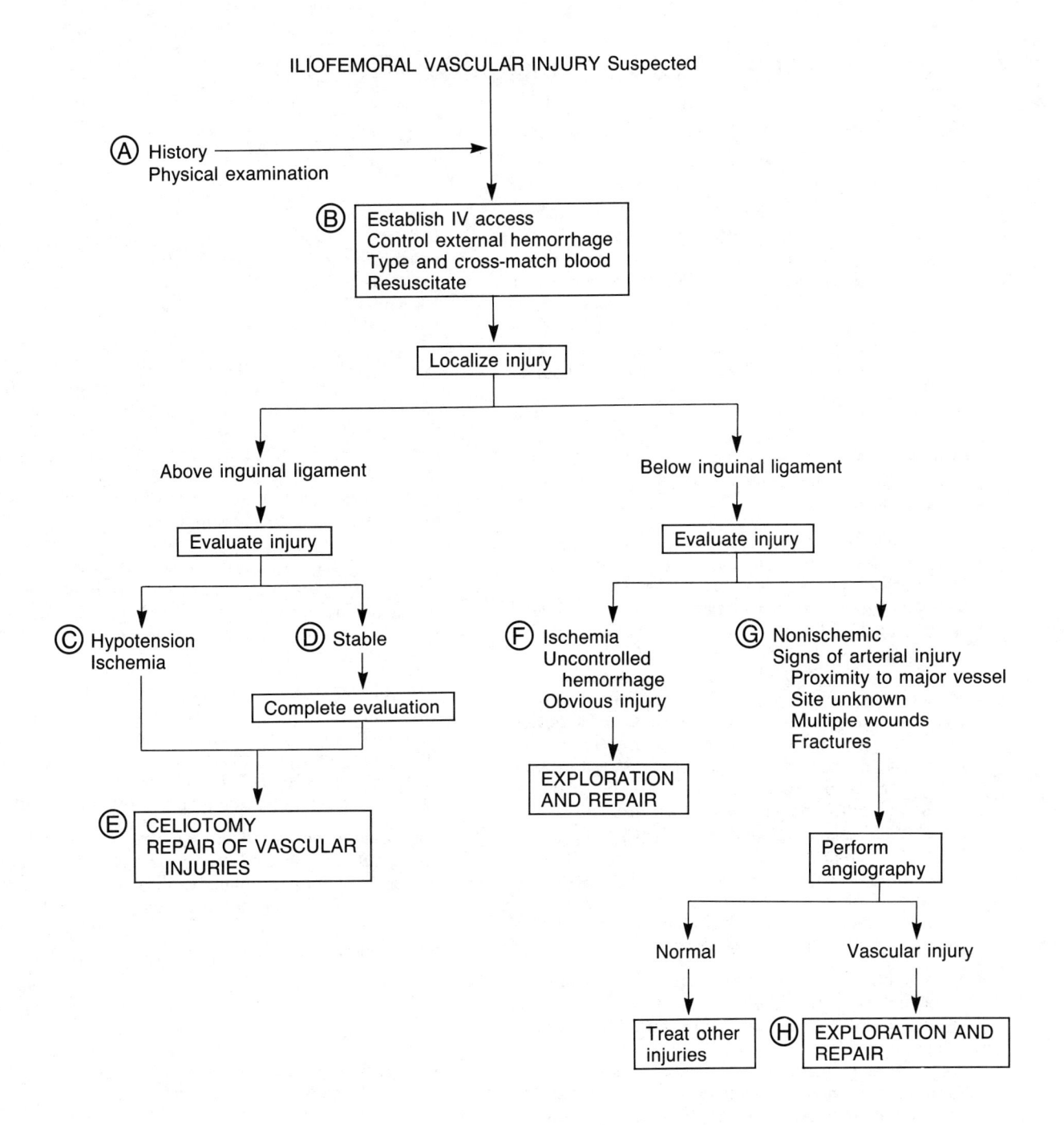

ILIOFEMORAL VASCULAR INJURY Suspected

- (A) History
- Physical examination

(B) Establish IV access
Control external hemorrhage
Type and cross-match blood
Resuscitate

Localize injury

Above inguinal ligament

Evaluate injury

- (C) Hypotension
- Ischemia

- (D) Stable

Complete evaluation

(E) **CELIOTOMY REPAIR OF VASCULAR INJURIES**

Below inguinal ligament

Evaluate injury

- (F) Ischemia
- Uncontrolled hemorrhage
- Obvious injury

EXPLORATION AND REPAIR

- (G) Nonischemic
- Signs of arterial injury
- Proximity to major vessel
- Site unknown
- Multiple wounds
- Fractures

Perform angiography

- Normal → Treat other injuries
- Vascular injury → (H) **EXPLORATION AND REPAIR**

POPLITEAL AND TIBIAL VASCULAR TRAUMA

David H. Wisner

A. Vascular injuries can result from either blunt or penetrating trauma. Fractures and dislocations associated with blunt mechanism of injury can lead to disruption of the vasculature by fracture or stretch injuries of the vessel with concomitant creation of an intimal flap and thrombosis. Some injuries, such as posterior dislocation of the knees and comminuted distal femur fracture, are particularly likely to cause vascular trauma. Gunshot wounds can cause both direct injury to blood vessels as well as stretch injuries from cavitation that occurs when the bullet passes close to a vessel. Both gunshot and stab wounds can lead to injury of adjacent arteries and veins, with the subsequent development of a traumatic arteriovenous fistula.

B. The vascular examination of the extremity consists of an assessment of temperature, capillary refill, and pulses. Temperature is assessed by feeling the great toe and comparing it with the contralateral side. Capillary refill is tested by using digital pressure to blanch the plantar surface of the great toe and by timing the return of color to the area. Capillary refill should be under 2 seconds and can be compared with that of the other foot. Femoral, popliteal, posterior tibial, and dorsalis pedis pulses should be palpated and graded as follows: 2, normal; 1, diminished; and 0, absent. Again, the contralateral lower extremity can be used for comparison. Popliteal pulses can be difficult to palpate even when normal. Lack of palpable pulses is a sign of vascular injury until proved otherwise. Pulse signals obtained with a Doppler in the absence of palpable pulses do not rule out vascular injury and should not be relied on. A neurologic examination of the extremity should always be done in conjunction with the vascular examination.

C. Angiography should be performed in all cases of knee dislocation because of the high incidence of associated vascular injury. The vascular examination can be surprisingly normal in the presence of severe disruption of the popliteal artery after knee dislocation. Unless associated injuries and hemodynamic or neurologic instability preclude angiography, angiography should be done in all cases of dislocation regardless of the physical examination.

D. The presence of a warm, well perfused extremity in the presence of diminished or absent pulses may be caused by a partial vascular interruption or abundant collateral flow around an injured vessel. On occasion, an abnormal vascular examination improves markedly on realignment of fracture fragments by distal traction. Vascular injury should be searched for in such instances. A viable extremity with suspected vascular injury allows for angiography in the radiology suite.

E. Angiography can be done in either the radiology department or the operating room. The quality and detail of the films are better when formal angiography is done in the angiography suite, but such studies take longer to arrange and complete than does intraoperative angiography. Obviously ischemic extremities require revascularization as quickly as possible, and delays to obtain high quality films are not warranted. As opposed to its usefulness in cases of penetrating injury, intraoperative angiography is useful even in obvious cases of blunt vascular compromise to outline the location and extent of injury. Angiography of viable extremities may reveal small, subtle injuries of the vasculature, some of which can be treated with observation alone.

F. Physical examination of the extremity should include all of the components of the vascular and neurologic examination outlined in paragraph B. Further signs of vascular injury are a large, expanding hematoma or pulsatile bleeding from wounds. A bruit in the area of injury suggests the presence of a traumatic arteriovenous fistula.

G. The location of entrance and exit wounds should be noted. When the course of the wounding knife or bullet is in close proximity to a major vascular structure, angiography should be performed to rule out occult injury. These angiograms can be done in the radiology department and are not emergent.

References

American College of Surgeons. The early care of the injured patient. Philadelphia: WB Saunders, 1972.

Bishara RA, et al. Improved results in the treatment of civilian vascular injuries associated with fractures and dislocations. J Vasc Surg 1986; 3:707.

Blaisdell FW, Trunkey DD. Trauma to extremities: general principles. Sci Am 1988; 5:1–14.

Perry MO. The management of acute vascular injuries. Baltimore: Williams & Wilkins, 1981.

LOWER EXTREMITY VASCULAR INJURY Suspected

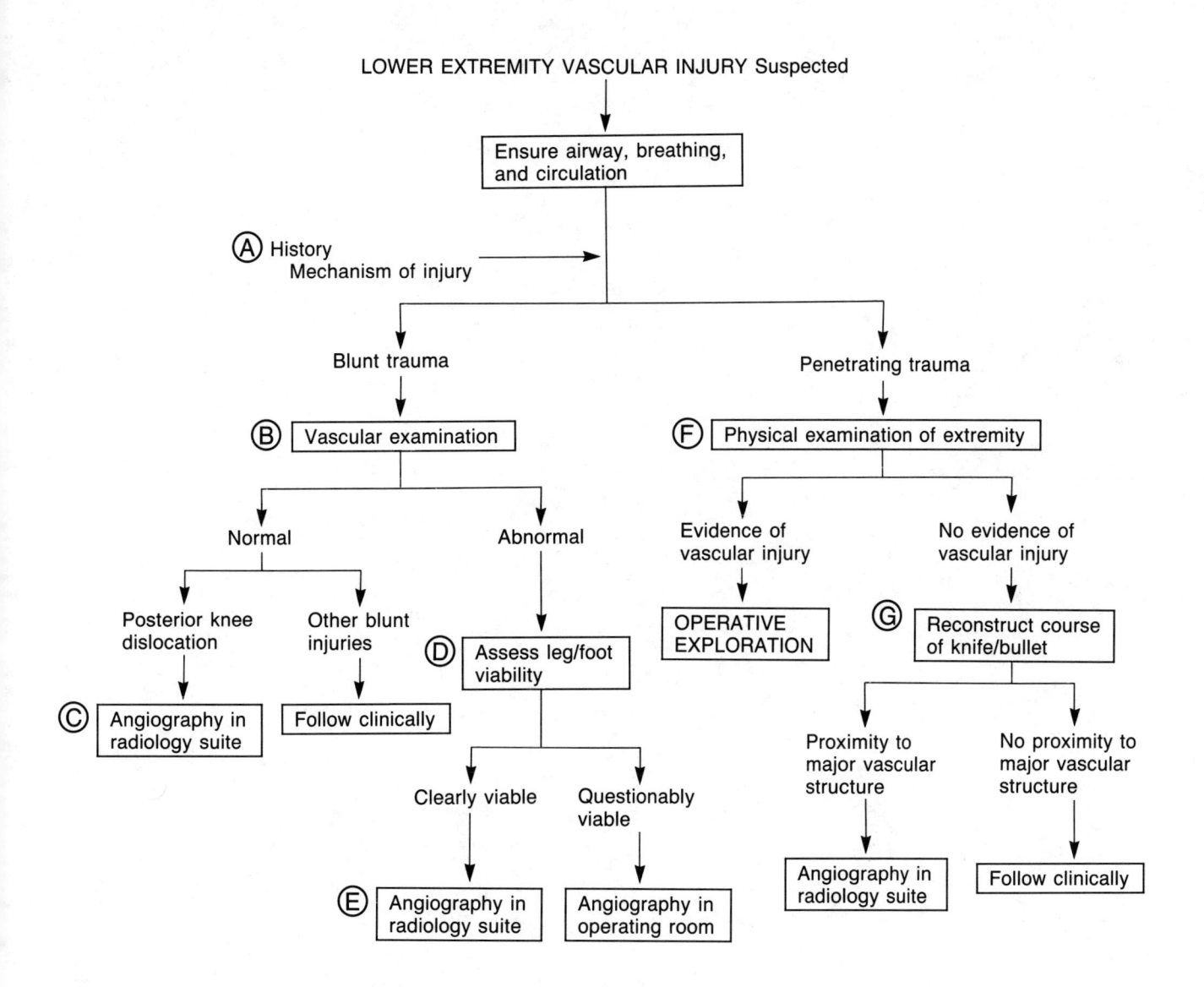

```
                    Ensure airway, breathing,
                    and circulation
                              │
    (A) History ──────────────┤
        Mechanism of injury   │
                ┌─────────────┴─────────────┐
            Blunt trauma              Penetrating trauma
                │                             │
        (B) Vascular examination      (F) Physical examination of extremity
            ┌───┴───┐                         ┌───────┴────────┐
          Normal  Abnormal              Evidence of      No evidence of
            │       │                   vascular injury  vascular injury
    ┌───────┴───┐   │                        │                │
Posterior   Other   │                    OPERATIVE    (G) Reconstruct course
knee        blunt   │                    EXPLORATION      of knife/bullet
dislocation injuries│                                       ┌────┴─────┐
    │         │  (D) Assess leg/foot                    Proximity to  No proximity to
(C) Angiography  viability                              major vascular major vascular
    in        Follow  ┌────┴──────┐                     structure     structure
    radiology clinically          │                         │             │
    suite   Clearly   Questionably                      Angiography   Follow
            viable    viable                            in radiology  clinically
              │          │                              suite
        (E) Angiography  Angiography
            in radiology in operating
            suite        room
```

191

ENVIRONMENTAL TRAUMA

Thermal Burn
Electrical Burn
Chemical Burn
Hypothermia and Frostbite
Escharotomy and Fasciotomy
Smoke Inhalation

THERMAL BURN

Gary F. Purdue
John L. Hunt

A. The mechanism of injury is important in determining treatment plan. Electrical, chemical, and facial burns; burns occurring in closed spaces, and those with traumatic injuries have special significance.

B. Patients with burns of the face and neck are at risk for sudden airway obstruction. Continual re-evaluation of the upper airway is necessary with endotracheal intubation as appropriate, preferably nasally with a low pressure cuff tube.

C. Initial nursing assessment incudes determining whether the injury occurred in a closed space and the presence of facial and neck burns or associated traumatic injuries, which require immediate evaluation and treatment.

D. Diagnosis and treatment of nearly all traumatic injuries takes precedence over the burn itself except with respect to airway management and fluid resuscitation.

E. All clothes must be removed and the patient *accurately* weighed (preferably in kilograms).

F. Burn size is expressed as a percentage of total body surface area (TBSA). This percentage includes areas of second-degree and third-degree burn but not of first-degree burn. Initial assessment of burn size may be via the "rule of nines" (Fig. 1). This does not apply to children, whose head and trunk proportions are larger than extremity sizes. For children and for more accurate determination of burn size, Lund-Browder or Berkow charts should be used. Burn depth may be expressed as first, second, or third degree or as partial thickness or full thickness. A first-degree burn is erythematous, with intact skin and without blisters. This injury (typified by sunburn) has minimal morbidity and no mortality, and is not included in measurements of burn size. A second-degree burn has blisters with pink moist tissue beneath and is analogous to a partial-thickness burn. The third-degree burn is dry, leathery, white, and insensate. This is the same as a full-thickness injury.

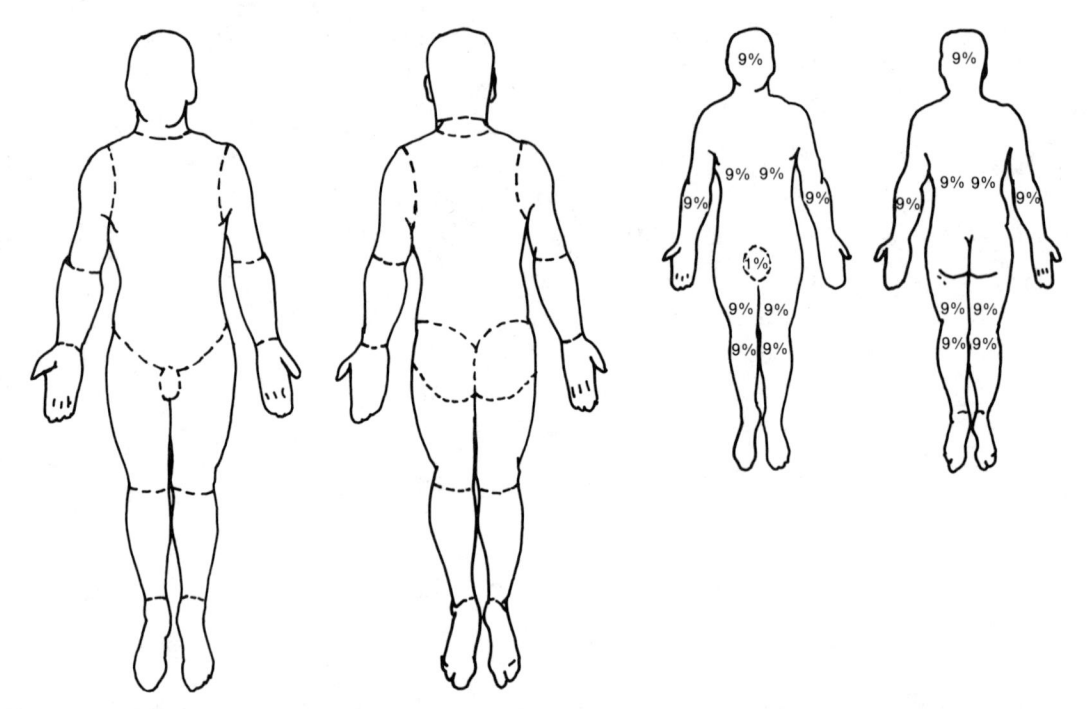

Figure 1 Initial assessment of burn size may employ the "rule of nines." (From Barton CW. Chemical and thermal burns. In: Callaham ML, et al, eds. Decision making in emergency medicine. Philadelphia: BC Decker, 1990:488.)

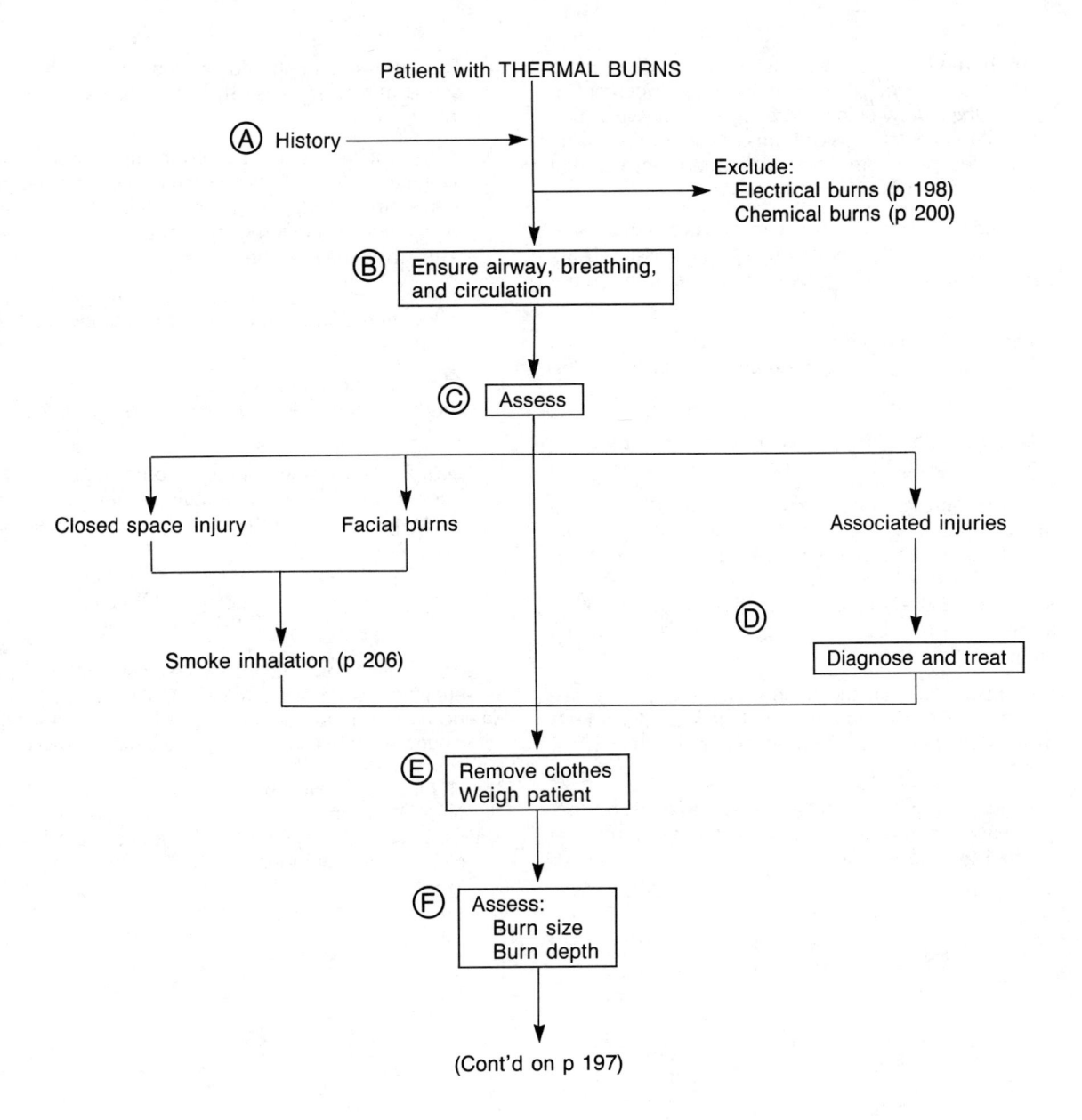

```
                    Patient with THERMAL BURNS
                              │
        Ⓐ  History ──────────▶│
                              │────▶ Exclude:
                              │         Electrical burns (p 198)
                              │         Chemical burns (p 200)
                              ▼
        Ⓑ  ┌─────────────────────────┐
           │ Ensure airway, breathing,│
           │ and circulation          │
           └─────────────────────────┘
                              │
                              ▼
        Ⓒ  ┌────────┐
           │ Assess │
           └────────┘
              │
   ┌──────────┼──────────┬──────────────────┐
   ▼          ▼          │                  ▼
Closed    Facial burns   │           Associated injuries
space                    │                  │
injury                   │         Ⓓ        ▼
   │                     │           ┌──────────────────┐
   ▼                     │           │ Diagnose and treat│
Smoke inhalation (p 206) │           └──────────────────┘
   │                     │                  │
   └─────────────────────┼──────────────────┘
                         ▼
        Ⓔ  ┌──────────────────┐
           │ Remove clothes   │
           │ Weigh patient    │
           └──────────────────┘
                         │
                         ▼
        Ⓕ  ┌──────────────────┐
           │ Assess:          │
           │    Burn size     │
           │    Burn depth    │
           └──────────────────┘
                         │
                         ▼
                 (Cont'd on p 197)
```

195

G. Major burn victims are those whose burns cover more than 20 percent of TBSA (or more than 10 percent of TBSA in the elderly or in children); who have over 5 percent full-thickness burns or burns of major joints, face, hands, feet, perineum, or genitalia; and those having multiple trauma or inhalation injury.

H. Intravenous access by a percutaneous peripheral route is preferred. This may be through burned tissue. Large bore catheters (14 to 16 gauge) should be used. Suture securely in place.

I. A nasogastric tube prevents acute gastric dilation with subsequent respiratory compromise and risk of aspiration.

J. A Foley catheter attached to a urimeter is necessary for the hourly evaluation of urinary output.

K. The Parkland formula is the most commonly used method of calculating fluid resuscitation (Ringer's lactate, 4 ml/kg per percentage TBSA burned in the first 24 hours). One-half is given in the first 8 hours, one-quarter in the next 8, and one-quarter in the last 8. Many other formulas are in use and may be selected by referral facilities.

L. Burn resuscitation mandates hourly evaluation of sensorium, vital signs, and urinary output with adjustments made to maintain a urine output of 1 ml/kg up to 50 ml per hour.

M. A major burn with full thickness that involves the special body components listed in paragraph G should be referred to a burn center.

N. The burn wound should be debrided of all clothing, debris, and burn tissue. Blisters on the palm may be left intact.

O. Partial-thickness burns are best treated by application of a natural biologic dressing such as porcine xenograft or a biosynthetic material such as Biobrane. Deeper wounds or wounds of indeterminate depth are usually treated with silver sulfadiazine.

P. Burns are tetanus prone wounds. Immunization should follow the recommendations of the American College of Surgeons.

Q. Circumferential full-thickness burns of the extremity should be evaluated hourly for neurovascular status (see p 202).

R. Disposition is determined by burn size, body parts burned, patient's age, and ability of the patient and/or the family to care for the burn. Each case should be individualized.

References

American College of Surgeons. Assessment and initial care of burn patients. Chicago: American College of Surgeons, 1979.

American College of Surgeons. Prophylaxis against tetanus in wound management. Chicago: American College of Surgeons, 1987.

Arts CP, Moncrief JA, Pruitt BA. Burns, a team approach. Philadelphia: WB Saunders, 1979.

Nebraska Burn Institute. Advanced life support course. Lincoln, NB: Nebraska Burn Institute, 1987.

(Cont'd from p 195)

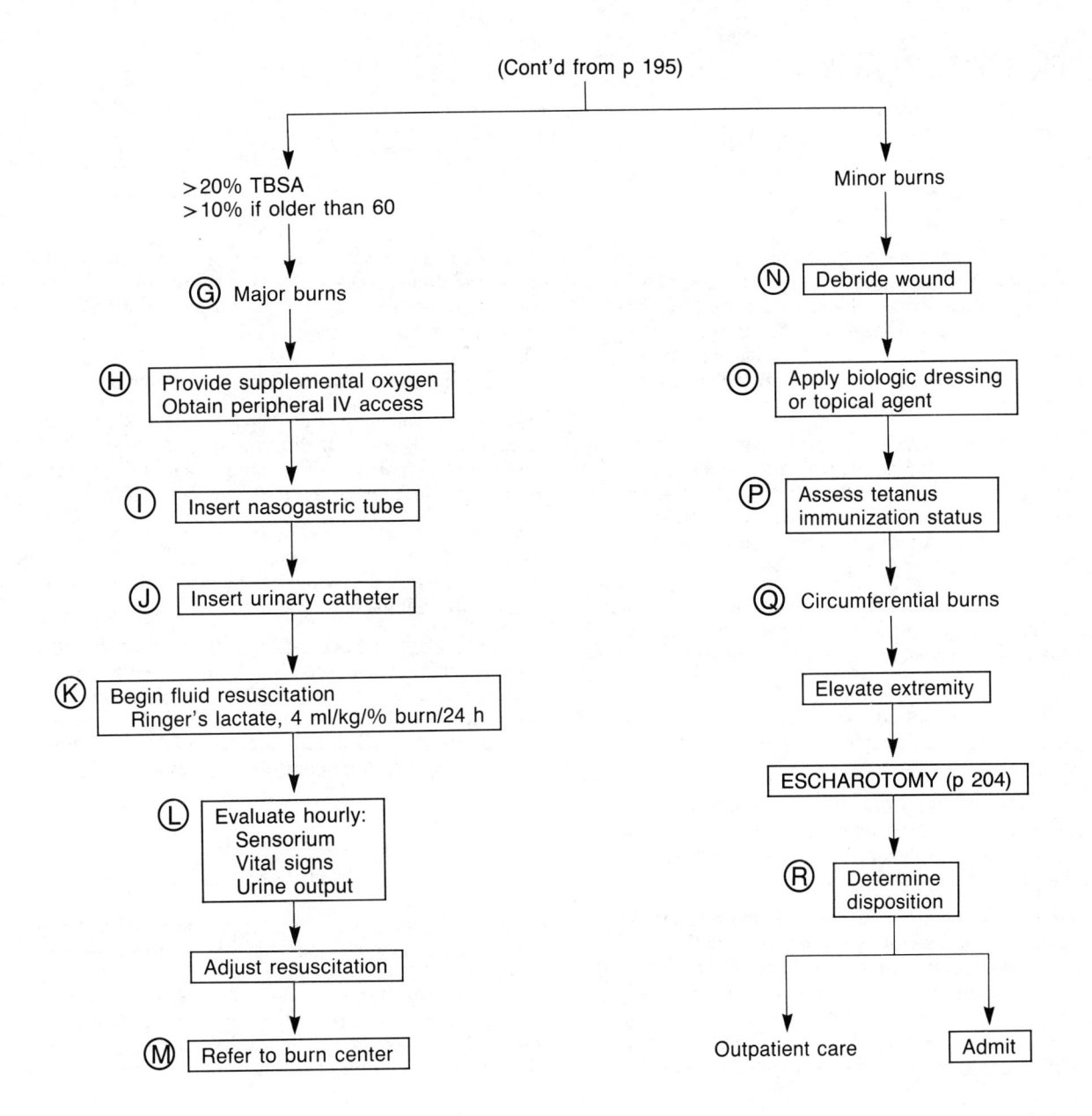

- >20% TBSA
- >10% if older than 60

Ⓖ Major burns

Ⓗ Provide supplemental oxygen
Obtain peripheral IV access

Ⓘ Insert nasogastric tube

Ⓙ Insert urinary catheter

Ⓚ Begin fluid resuscitation
Ringer's lactate, 4 ml/kg/% burn/24 h

Ⓛ Evaluate hourly:
Sensorium
Vital signs
Urine output

Adjust resuscitation

Ⓜ Refer to burn center

Minor burns

Ⓝ Debride wound

Ⓞ Apply biologic dressing or topical agent

Ⓟ Assess tetanus immunization status

Ⓠ Circumferential burns

Elevate extremity

ESCHAROTOMY (p 204)

Ⓡ Determine disposition

Outpatient care | Admit

197

ELECTRICAL BURN

Gary F. Purdue
John L. Hunt

A. When possible, determine voltage and type of current and whether the patient lost consciousness, had a documented cardiac arrest, or had an abnormal ECG during transport. Ascertain whether the patient sustained associated trauma, e.g., a fall. High voltage injuries are those caused by more than 1,000 volts. At lower voltages deep soft tissue injury is unlikely.

B. Establish whether the patient actually sustained an electrical burn with contact points (i.e., assess presence of deep demarcated burns). Evaluation of airway, breathing, and circulation (ABCs) and physical examination are performed the same as for any other burn patient with a high risk of traumatic injury.

C. If the patient sustained a thermal injury from an electrical arc rather than an actual current injury, treatment is the same as for thermal burns (p 194). This injury is a flash and/or flame burn.

D. A 12-lead ECG is performed and the patient placed on continuous cardiac monitoring. Arrhythmias are treated appropriately.

E. A Foley catheter with a urimeter is inserted. Urine is evaluated for gross urinary pigments (myoglobin and/or hemoglobin). If the evaluation is negative, re-evaluate after initial bladder emptying.

F. Gross urinary pigmentation (darker than pale red) should be treated to minimize pigment precipitation in the renal tubules. Intravenous (IV) access with large bore peripheral catheters should be performed with immediate administration of 25 g of mannitol (IV push) followed by 44 mEq of sodium bicarbonate ($NaHCO_3$) This is then followed immediately by administration of Ringer's lactate at a rate that will achieve urine output sufficient to clear the urine grossly (75 to 100 ml per hour). This is done to establish immediate urinary diuresis and alkalinize initial urinary output to minimize precipitation. Output is then maintained with Ringer's lactate. Further use of diuretics and bicarbonate is seldom necessary.

G. Neuromuscular status of all extremities should be evaluated hourly. Paresthesia, absent pulse, paralysis, swelling, and deep pain on active or passive motion are indications for immediate decompression (p 204).

H. Thermal burns are treated with silver sulfadiazine or biologic dressings as appropriate. The deep eschar of the contact points is treated with mafenide acetate because of its excellent eschar penetration.

I. In the absence of ECG abnormalities and arrhythmias during cardiac monitoring, the patient is either admitted or discharged, based on burn size or location. Patients who exhibit either rhythm or ECG abnormalities should be admitted and monitored for at least 24 hours with appropriate treatment of arrhythmias.

References

Hunt JL, Sato RM, Baxter CR. Acute electric burns: current diagnostic and therapeutic approaches to management. Arch Surg 1980; 115:434–438.

Purdue GF, Hunt JL. Electrocardiographic monitoring electrical injury: necessity or luxury. J Trauma 1986; 26:166–167.

Wilkinson C, MacDonald W. High voltage electric injury. Am J Surg 1978; 136:693–696.

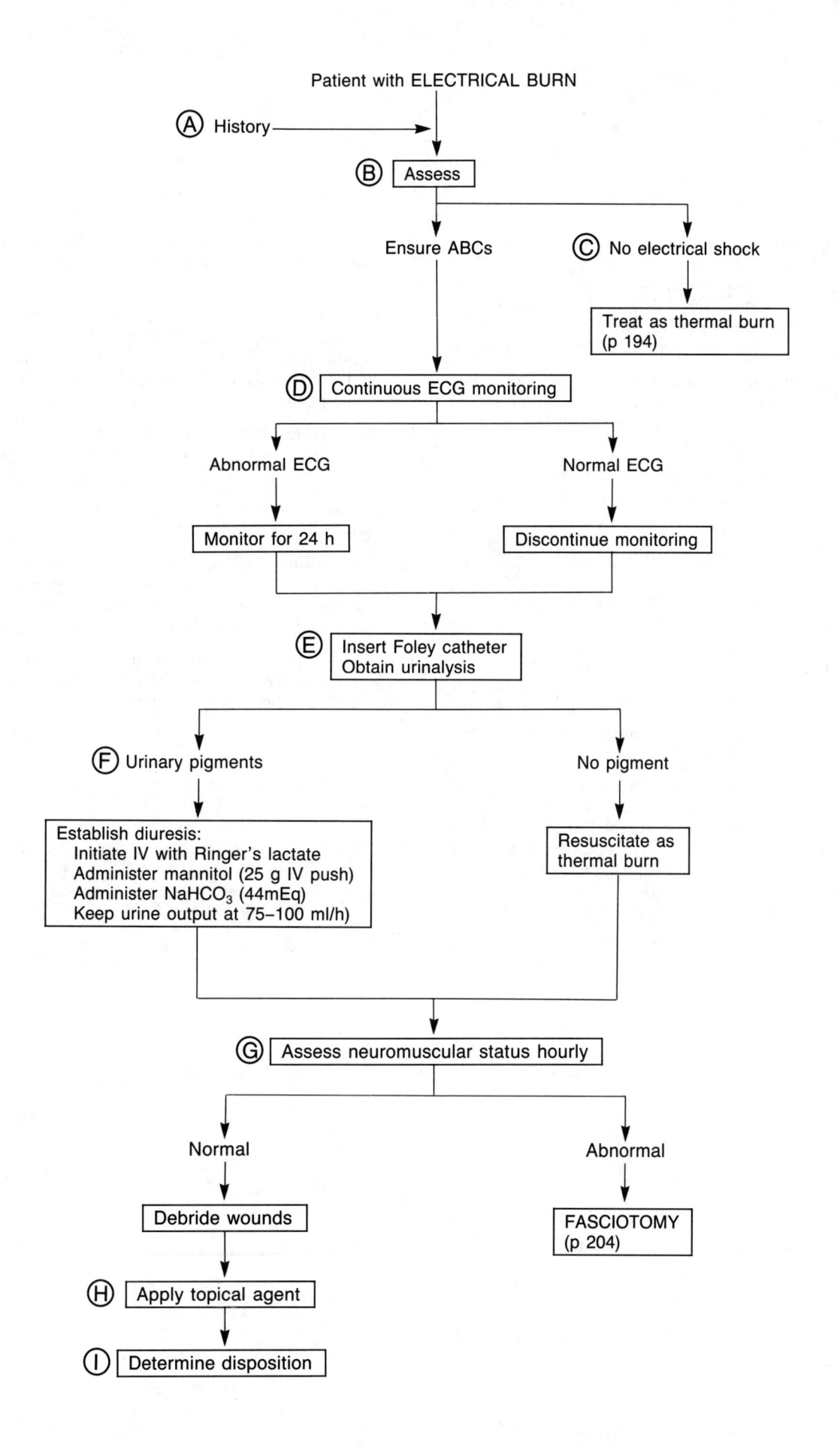

```
                    Patient with ELECTRICAL BURN
                                │
         Ⓐ History ─────────────▶│
                                 ▼
                          Ⓑ ┌─────────┐
                            │ Assess  │
                            └─────────┘
                              │       │
                              ▼       ▼
                       Ensure ABCs   Ⓒ No electrical shock
                              │              │
                              │              ▼
                              │       ┌──────────────────┐
                              │       │ Treat as thermal │
                              │       │ burn (p 194)     │
                              │       └──────────────────┘
                              ▼
                    Ⓓ ┌──────────────────────────┐
                      │ Continuous ECG monitoring │
                      └──────────────────────────┘
                          │                  │
                          ▼                  ▼
                    Abnormal ECG         Normal ECG
                          │                  │
                          ▼                  ▼
                  ┌───────────────┐   ┌──────────────────────┐
                  │ Monitor for 24 h│ │ Discontinue monitoring│
                  └───────────────┘   └──────────────────────┘
                          │                  │
                          └────────┬─────────┘
                                   ▼
                      Ⓔ ┌───────────────────────┐
                        │ Insert Foley catheter │
                        │ Obtain urinalysis     │
                        └───────────────────────┘
                           │                │
                           ▼                ▼
                   Ⓕ Urinary pigments    No pigment
                           │                │
                           ▼                ▼
         ┌──────────────────────────────────┐  ┌──────────────┐
         │ Establish diuresis:              │  │ Resuscitate as│
         │   Initiate IV with Ringer's lactate│ │ thermal burn │
         │   Administer mannitol (25 g IV push)│└──────────────┘
         │   Administer NaHCO₃ (44mEq)      │         │
         │   Keep urine output at 75–100 ml/h│        │
         └──────────────────────────────────┘         │
                           │                          │
                           └─────────────┬────────────┘
                                         ▼
                      Ⓖ ┌────────────────────────────────┐
                        │ Assess neuromuscular status hourly│
                        └────────────────────────────────┘
                              │                    │
                              ▼                    ▼
                           Normal               Abnormal
                              │                    │
                              ▼                    ▼
                     ┌──────────────┐      ┌──────────────┐
                     │ Debride wounds│     │ FASCIOTOMY   │
                     └──────────────┘      │ (p 204)      │
                              │            └──────────────┘
                              ▼
                     Ⓗ ┌──────────────────┐
                       │ Apply topical agent│
                       └──────────────────┘
                              │
                              ▼
                     Ⓘ ┌────────────────────┐
                       │ Determine disposition│
                       └────────────────────┘
```

CHEMICAL BURN

Gary F. Purdue
John L. Hunt

A. History to be obtained includes the exact type of agent involved, its concentration if appropriate, duration of exposure, and previous treatment. If possible, the patient, family, or Emergency Medical Services personnel should bring exact documentation of the agent, e.g., a label, a container, or literature, to the emergency department.

B. Copious tap water irrigation is begun immediately either in a shower or by utilizing a shower head. All personnel must take care to prevent exposure to chemical agents by using protective gloves and clothing.

C. *All* of the patient's clothing is removed to eliminate trapping of chemicals within the interstices of fabric.

D. The severity of a chemical burn is often grossly underestimated. Assessment should include careful examination of the eye.

E. Ocular irrigation is begun with normal saline, using either a commercial eye irrigator or a 21-gauge needle broken off at the hub, thereby creating a small nozzle. Irrigation begins medially to laterally for the initial wash away from the lacrimal ducts, then laterally to medially to wash through the lacrimal ducts. One liter of solution is used per eye, and an immediate ophthalmologic consultation should be obtained.

F. Exact determination of the burning agent is made and contact established with a poison control facility, the hazardous materials division of the fire department, or the chemical manufacturer to determine specific treatment modalities to be used in addition to irrigation. Under no circumstances should any attempt be made to neutralize an acid with a base or a base with an acid.

G. Specific treatment for agents such as hydrofluoric acid, phenol, and phosphorus should be immediately initiated.

H. Tap water irrigation is continued for 1 to 2 hours. This is facilitated by placing a chair in a shower stall and allowing the patient to sit. Liberal use of soap and a washcloth for mechanical removal of residual chemical is recommended.

I. The chemical burn is now treated in the same manner as a thermal burn, with debridement of all loose skin.

J. Tar is best removed by dissolving it. Application of a specific solvent, ointment, or mineral oil often makes mechanical removal unnecessary.

K. Application of the appropriate topical antimicrobial, usually silver sulfadiazine, is performed. Biologic dressings should not be used on chemical burns because of the danger of entrapping residual chemicals.

L. Most patients with chemical burns should be admitted to the hospital because of the high risk that the burn severity has been underestimated.

References

Mozingo DW, Smith AA, McManus WF, et al. Chemical burns. J Trauma 1988; 38:642–647.

Saydjari R, Abston S, Desai MH, et al. Chemical burns. J Burn Care Rehab 1986; 7:404–408.

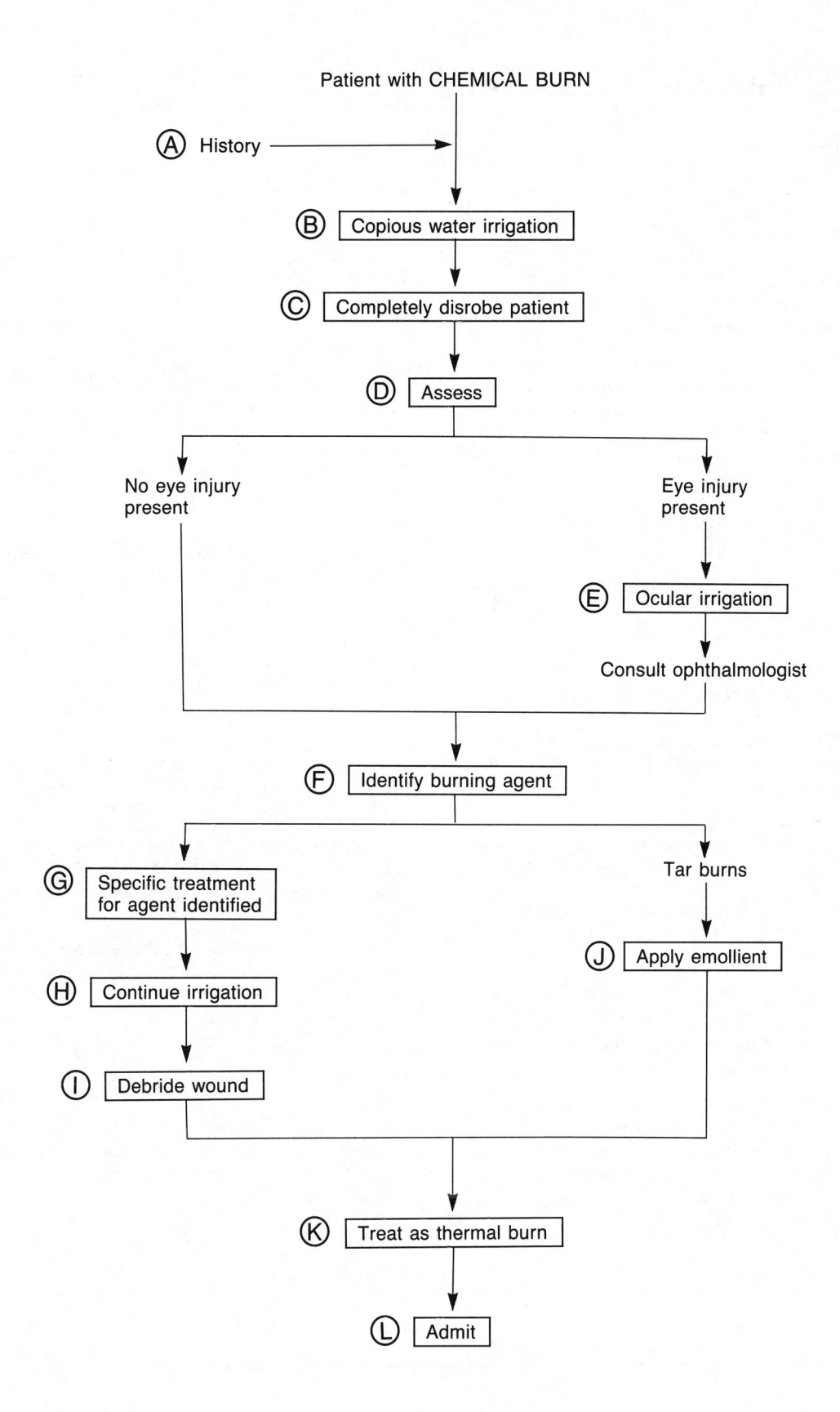

Patient with CHEMICAL BURN

- (A) History
- (B) Copious water irrigation
- (C) Completely disrobe patient
- (D) Assess
  - No eye injury present
  - Eye injury present
    - (E) Ocular irrigation
    - Consult ophthalmologist
- (F) Identify burning agent
  - (G) Specific treatment for agent identified
    - (H) Continue irrigation
    - (I) Debride wound
  - Tar burns
    - (J) Apply emollient
- (K) Treat as thermal burn
- (L) Admit

HYPOTHERMIA AND FROSTBITE

Gary F. Purdue
John L. Hunt

A. The history of the injury should be established, including the rapidity of cooling, the duration of exposure, and predisposing factors (e.g., drug usage, psychiatric or cardiac history, and ethanol use and/or abuse).

B. The airway, breathing, and circulation (ABCs) must be ensured. Vital signs in hypothermic patients are often imperceptible because they are motionless, flaccid, and pulseless and have fixed, dilated pupils. Cardiopulmonary resuscitation (CPR) may be performed for prolonged periods without neurologic deficit. *Note*: Hypothermic patients should *not* be pronounced dead until they are warmed (i.e., to a body temperature of greater than 35°C) and then clinically re-evaluated.

C. Body temperature is determined with a low range thermometer capable of recording temperatures below 34°C. Ideally, a rectal thermistor is used for continuous monitoring.

D. When the patient is conscious, hypothermia may be treated passively by covering and placing the patient in a warm room. This method may take up to 24 hours and is best suited for elderly patients and those with long-standing hypothermia.

E. Because of their mental confusion, patients should be carefully observed in a quiet setting. Stimulation that may precipitate ventricular fibrillation is thereby avoided.

F. Unconscious patients and those with unstable or unmeasurable vital signs are treated aggressively in an intensive care unit.

G. The electrocardiogram (ECG) is continuously monitored. The characteristic finding is a J or Osborn wave following the QRS complex. Patients are at special risk for ventricular arrhythmias during rewarming.

H. Measurement of arterial blood gases (corrected for temperature) and determinations of electrolytes, acid-base balance, and glucose are made. Correction of hyperglycemia and metabolic acidosis must proceed very carefully. Large quantities of potassium may be required to replace urinary losses.

I. Intravenous (IV) access and the insertion of a nasogastric (NG) tube and urinary catheter are necessary for fluid replacement and monitoring. The patient is resuscitated with Ringer's lactate, often administered in volumes similar to those given to a burn patient.

J. Controversy exists as to the best method of rewarming. External heating is readily available but risks rewarming shock. Core or internal warming using heated fluids minimizes rewarming shock but may be impractical because of logistics. Fluids should be no warmer than 40 to 42°C to achieve warming rates of greater than 0.55°C per hour.

K. Following treatment for hypothermia, extremities are evaluated for frostbite (i.e., note white, dry, or mottled skin).

L. If frostbite is suspected, the affected part(s) should be placed in a water bath at 38 to 42°C for 15 to 20 minutes. Rapid rewarming is associated with less tissue necrosis than is slow thawing. Narcotics are usually required for pain relief.

M. Frostbite is a tetanus prone wound. Prophylaxis should be given according to guidelines set by the American College of Surgeons.

N. Frostbite is usually treated conservatively with bed rest, elevation of the affected extremities, and avoidance of trauma. In most cases, admission to the hospital is required.

O. Most frostbite patients are admitted to the hospital. Patients without tissue damage may be admitted or discharged, depending on the presence of hypothermia at the time of admission.

References

American College of Surgeons. Prophylaxis against tetanus in wound management. Chicago: American College of Surgeons, 1987.

Purdue GF, Hunt JL. Cold injury: a collective review. J Burn Care Rehab 1986; 7:331–336.

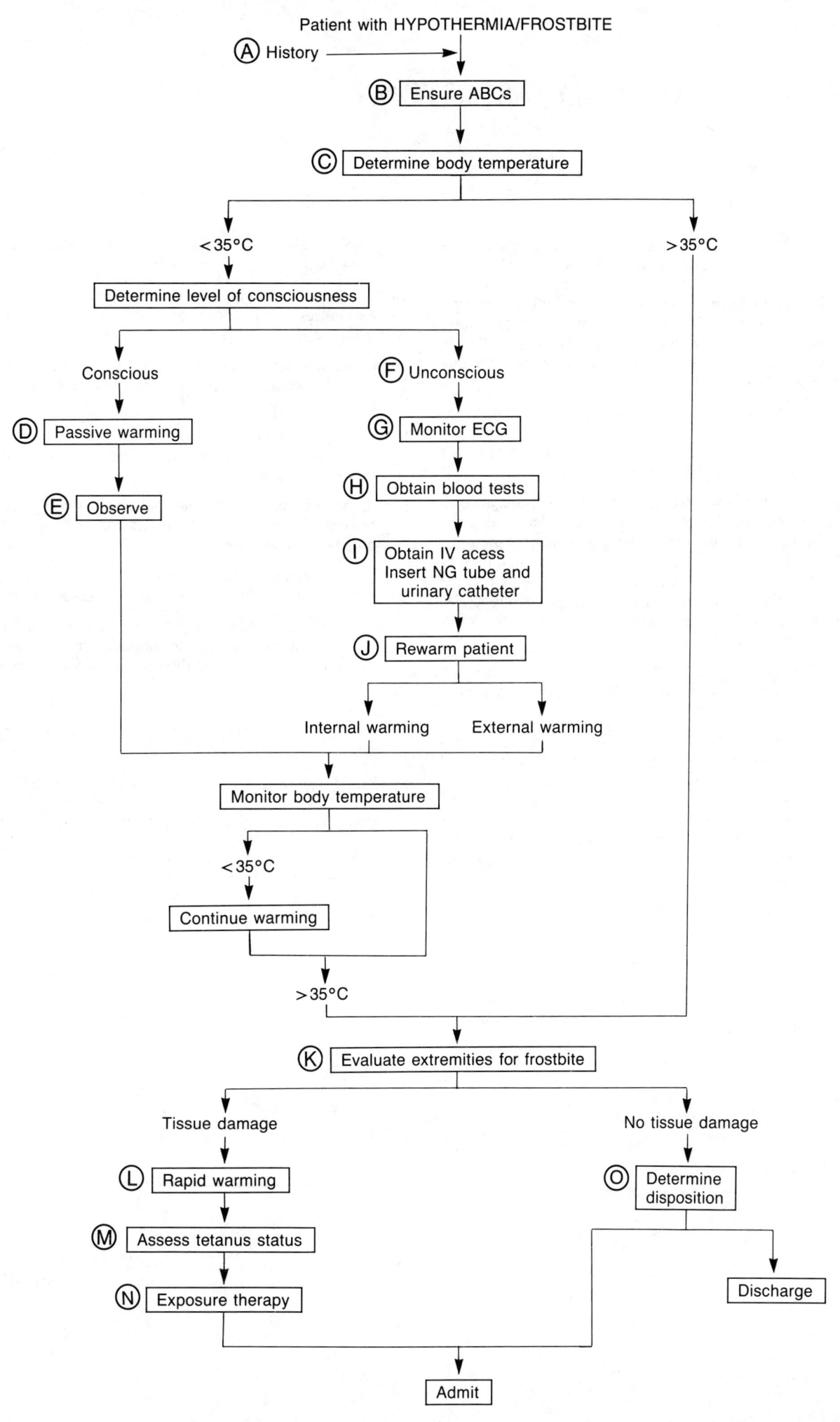

Patient with HYPOTHERMIA/FROSTBITE

- (A) History
- (B) Ensure ABCs
- (C) Determine body temperature

< 35°C:
- Determine level of consciousness
  - Conscious:
    - (D) Passive warming
    - (E) Observe
  - (F) Unconscious:
    - (G) Monitor ECG
    - (H) Obtain blood tests
    - (I) Obtain IV acess, Insert NG tube and urinary catheter
    - (J) Rewarm patient
      - Internal warming
      - External warming
    - Monitor body temperature
      - < 35°C: Continue warming
      - > 35°C

> 35°C:
- (K) Evaluate extremities for frostbite
  - Tissue damage:
    - (L) Rapid warming
    - (M) Assess tetanus status
    - (N) Exposure therapy
    - Admit
  - No tissue damage:
    - (O) Determine disposition
      - Discharge
      - Admit

ESCHAROTOMY AND FASCIOTOMY

Gary F. Purdue
John L. Hunt

A. Extremities with circumferential burns are at risk for vascular compromise. Although the patient usually has a circumferential full thickness burn, a partial thickness circumferential burn in a child or in a patient with a large burn (i.e., greater than 50 to 75 percent of total body surface are) is also at risk. Occasionally, a circumferential burn of the trunk restricts respiratory function, thereby necessitating escharotomies of the chest.

B. Patients with a history of high voltage electrical burn are more likely to require a fasciotomy than an escharotomy. Fasciotomy is often required in patients who present with or develop urinary pigmentation.

C. Elevation of the affected upper extremity is best accomplished by elevation of the head of the bed to 45 degrees followed by placing the arm in bias knit stockinette or in an elastic sleeve such as Surgifix or Elastonet, the upper end of which is secured to an intravenous pole or ceiling fixture. Elevation on pillows is not sufficient. Elevation of the lower extremities is performed by elevating the foot of the bed.

D. Active exercise performed for 5 minutes per hour helps to relieve venous obstruction and to maintain arterial flow.

E. Careful assessment is performed to evaluate vascular insufficiency. Cyanosis, impaired capillary filling, and progressive neurologic deterioration are good indicators of vascular insufficiency, whereas coolness and decreased motor function correlate poorly with need for escharotomy. Normal sensory response to pinprick and proprioception are the most reliable clinical signs for continued elevation and evaluation.

F. Signs of vascular insufficiency include paresthesia, cyanosis, poor capillary filling, and neurologic deterioration.

G. The presence of palpable radial and posterior tibial artery pulses usually indicates adequate peripheral perfusion. Notify the physician if the pulse decreases.

H. In the absence of palpable pulses, Doppler ultrasonography is used to evaluate the palmar arch and the posterior tibial artery.

I. When pulses are present, reassessment is performed hourly with continued elevation and exercise of the affected extremity.

J. In the absence of a Doppler pulse and in the presence of clinical signs of vascular insufficiency, the patient is prepared for escharotomy.

K. With the return of pulses following escharotomy, the affected limb is kept elevated and reassessed hourly.

L. If pulses remain absent and if the patient has continued signs of vascular insufficiency or pain disproportional to the injury, the patient is then prepared for fasciotomy.

References

Moylan JA, Inge WW, Pruitt BA. Circulatory changes following circumferential extremity burns evaluated by the ultrasonic flow meter: an analysis of sixty thermally injured limbs. J Trauma 1971; 11:763–770.

Pruitt BA, Dowling JA, Moncrief JA. Escharotomy in early burn care. Arch Surg 1968; 96:502–507.

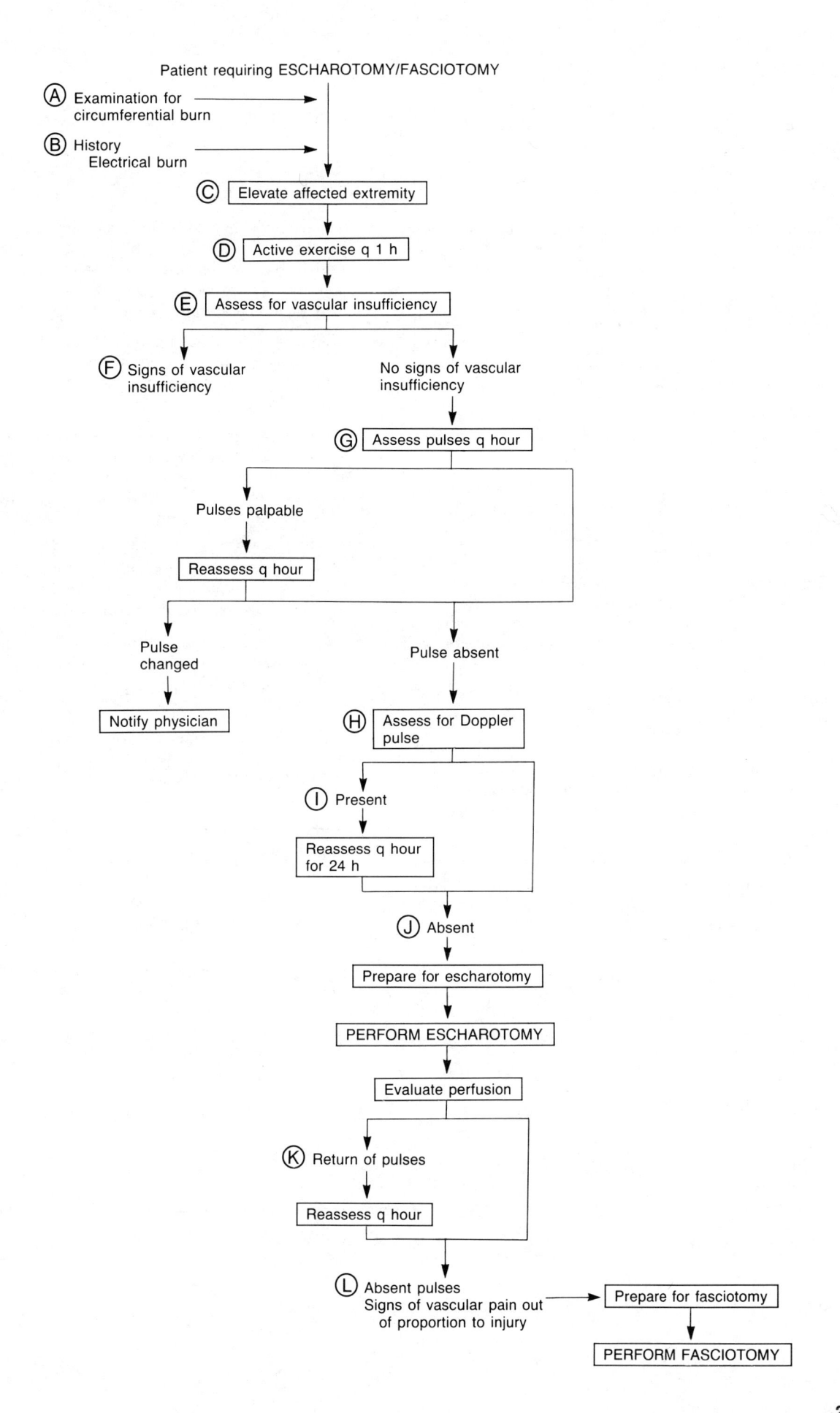

Patient requiring ESCHAROTOMY/FASCIOTOMY

(A) Examination for circumferential burn

(B) History Electrical burn

(C) Elevate affected extremity

(D) Active exercise q 1 h

(E) Assess for vascular insufficiency

(F) Signs of vascular insufficiency

No signs of vascular insufficiency

(G) Assess pulses q hour

Pulses palpable

Reassess q hour

Pulse changed

Notify physician

Pulse absent

(H) Assess for Doppler pulse

(I) Present

Reassess q hour for 24 h

(J) Absent

Prepare for escharotomy

PERFORM ESCHAROTOMY

Evaluate perfusion

(K) Return of pulses

Reassess q hour

(L) Absent pulses
Signs of vascular pain out of proportion to injury

Prepare for fasciotomy

PERFORM FASCIOTOMY

SMOKE INHALATION

Gary F. Purdue
John L. Hunt

A. Although a history of being trapped in a closed, smoke filled space is the sine qua non of smoke inhalation, exposure to extremely noxious gases may also produce inhalation injury, even outdoors.

B. All patients with suspected inhalation injury should receive supplemental oxygen. If the carboxyhemoglobin (COHb) level is greater than 20, then 100 percent oxygen should be given.

C. Assessment should be made for deep burns of the face and neck, presence of inhalation injury, or presence of both injuries.

D. Burns of the lower face and neck result in supraglottic and pharyngeal swelling. This injury is almost always above the vocal cords and has the risk of acute airway obstruction.

E. Burn edema is gravity dependent. Thus, facial swelling can be minimized by continuous elevation of the head of the bed at greater than 45 degrees for the first 48 hours after injury. Sitting in a chair and walking should be encouraged.

F. Upper airway evaluation is done hourly. Complaints of breathing difficulty, hoarseness, or swelling are significant.

G. If warning signs or symptoms are not present, the patient is observed closely. Evaluation may require direct or indirect laryngoscopy or bronchoscopy to ensure patency of the airway.

H. Swelling that threatens to compromise the airway is treated by endotracheal intubation, preferably nasally with a soft cuff tube. The tube must be well secured with umbilical tape and a safety pin through the tube to assure its safety.

I. True smoke inhalation occurs from exposure to noxious gases. The injury is similar to chemical pneumonitis and presents similar to adult respiratory distress syndrome.

J. Serial arterial blood gases (ABGs), physical examinations, and evaluation of work of breathing are performed.

K. The patient with a severe inhalation injury often requires mechanical ventilation with high tidal volumes (15 ml per kilogram) and possibly positive-end expiratory pressure. Ventilator management is guided by serial ABGs. This patient is admitted to the intensive care unit.

L. Pulmonary toilet (i.e., humidified inspired gases, frequent suctioning, chest physiotherapy, and possibly bronchodilators) minimizes complications associated with inhalation injuries.

M. Swelling of the upper airway generally increases for the first 24 hours with a gradual decrease over the next 48 to 72 hours, thereby permitting extubation. The primary complications of this injury are failure to intubate or accidental extubation with catastrophic results.

N. Additional diagnostic studies, including fiberoptic bronchoscopy and xenon ventilation isotope scans, may be performed to evaluate the extent of injury. When these studies are negative, inhalation injury is unlikely.

O. When diagnostic studies are positive, the patient should be continually observed with serial blood gases and physical examination. This patient is admitted to hospital.

P. The course of smoke inhalation injury is difficult to predict. Ventilatory care is based on clinical parameters. The use of antibiotics—either parenterally or nebulized—and steroids is contraindicated in the presence of a burn.

Q. Some patients have both upper airway and lower airway smoke inhalation injuries and are treated appropriately.

References

Arts CP, Moncrief JA, Pruitt BA, Burns A. Team approach. Philadelphia: WB Saunders, 1979:95–107.

Herndon DN, Thompson PB, Linares HA, Traber DL. Postgraduate course: respiratory injury. I: Incidence, mortality pathogenesis and treatment of pulmonary injury. J Burn Care Rehab 1986; 7(2):184–195.

```
Patient with SMOKE INHALATION
                │
   Ⓐ History ───┤
                ▼
            Ⓑ Administer oxygen
              If COHB >20,
              administer 100%
              oxygen
                │
                ▼
            Ⓒ Assess
   ┌────────────┼────────────────┐
   ▼            ▼                ▼
Ⓓ Facial/    Ⓘ Smoke         Ⓠ Upper and lower
  neck burns   inhalation        airway smoke
   │            │                inhalation injuries
   ▼            ▼                │
Ⓔ Elevate    Obtain chest        ▼
  head of    film             Treat appropriately
  bed >45      │
  degrees      ▼
   │        Ⓙ Perform serial ABCs
   ▼           and physical examination
Ⓕ Evaluate     │
  airway    ┌──┴──────┐
  q hour    ▼         ▼
   │     Inadequate  Adequate
 ┌─┴──┐  findings    findings
 Normal Swelling        │
   │     │              ▼
   ▼    Ⓗ Intubate   Pulmonary
Ⓖ Observe  │         toilet
  closely  │            │
   │       │            ▼
   ▼       │         Ⓝ Diagnostic studies
Treat burn │            │
   │       │       ┌────┴────┐
   ▼       │       ▼         ▼
Admit      │    Ⓞ Positive  Negative
           │      studies   studies
         Ⓚ Ventilate │         │
           │       ▼         ▼
           ▼    Ⓟ Observe  Treat burn
         Ⓛ Pulmonary │
           toilet   ▼
           │      Admit
           ▼
         Ⓜ Admit to
           intensive
           care unit
```

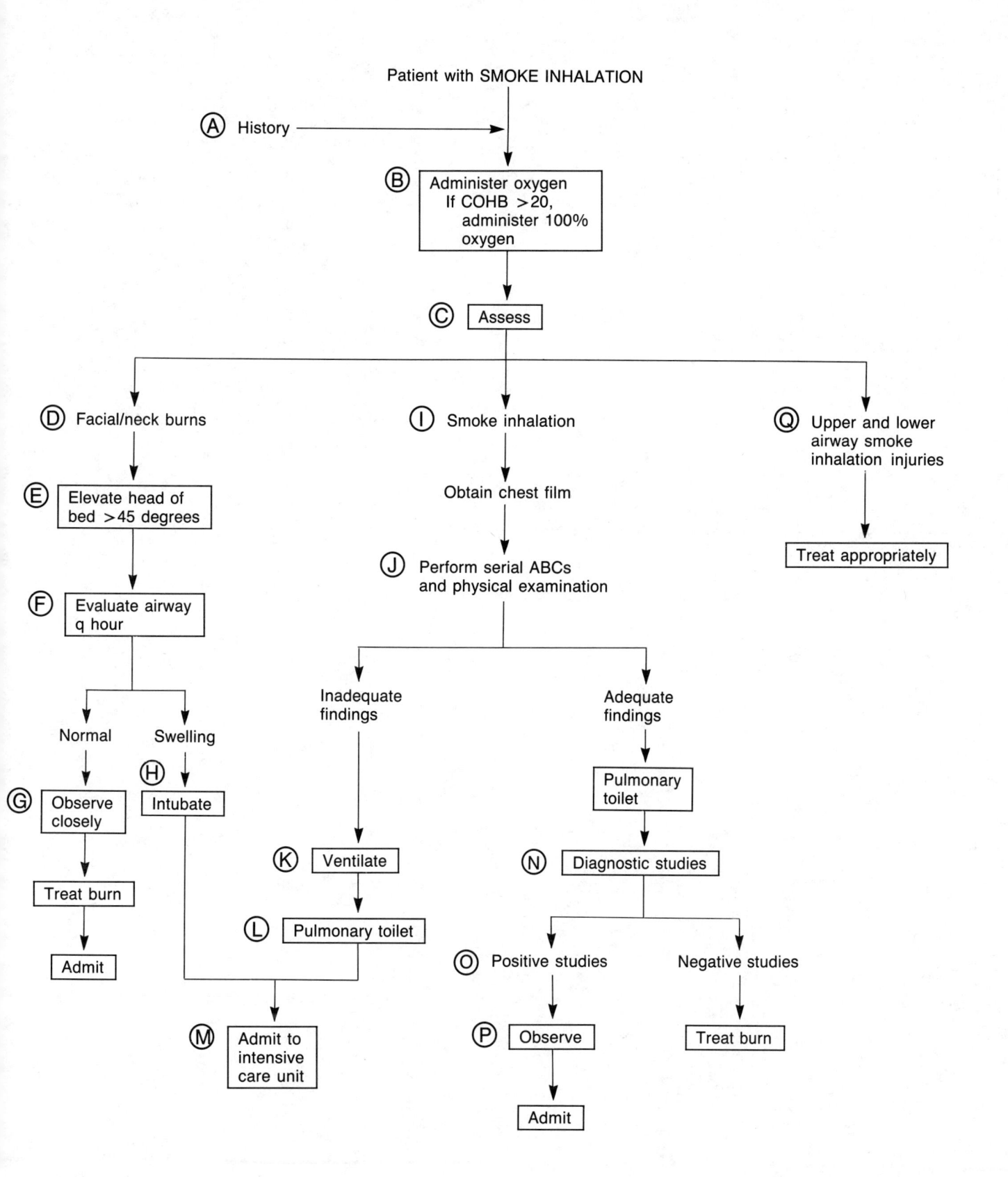

PEDIATRIC TRAUMA

Pediatric Trauma Triage
Resuscitation
Pediatric Head Trauma
Pediatric Thoracic Trauma

Pediatric Abdominal Trauma
Pediatric Extremity Trauma
Pediatric Burn Trauma
Child Abuse

PEDIATRIC TRAUMA TRIAGE

Louise Haubner
Louann Kitchen

A. The pediatric trauma center (PTC) candidate has been defined as any child who appears to be 14 years of age or younger. Children differ in the type of mechanism of injury they sustain and in their physiologic response to injury. A child's response to shock is often delayed as compared with that of an adult. Blood pressure may remain within normal limits until late in the clinical course. Therefore, a tool dependent on physiologic decompensation (i.e., drop in blood pressure) may not accurately depict the severity of the injury. At times the only overt sign of internal bleeding may be sustained tachycardia. In most cases it is difficult to discern the origin of the tachycardia because it may also be attributed to fear or anxiety.

B. The Children's Trauma Tool has been found to be an effective tool for evaluating pediatric trauma victims (Table 1). It incorporates mechanism of injury, physiologic presentation, and anatomic factors. It has been amended (October 1989) to include abdominal pain or discomfort. Children who sustain airway control problems that cannot be corrected by emergency care providers should be transported to the closest emergency receiving facility, regardless of the hospital's trauma or nontrauma status.

C. After the decision has been made regarding the patient's destination (i.e., to transport either to a PTC or to a nontrauma facility), the appropriate mode of transport must be decided. A patient being transported to a nontrauma facility should be stable for ground transport. An acute status or seriously injured child should be transported by the quickest and most advanced mode available.

D. When a pediatric trauma victim is admitted to a nontrauma facility, there may be sufficient time for the injured child to exhibit signs of physiologic decompensation. In this case a tool that incorporates physiologic parameters, such as the Pediatric Trauma Score, may be useful in identifying the patients who need transport to the PTC (Table 2).*

TABLE 1 Children's Trauma Tool*

Pedestrian struck (significant force on the body)
  Damage to car or truck (fender, hood, windshield)
  Child thrown or found more than 5 to 6 feet from car
  Child dragged by moving vehicle (abrasion, road rash)
  Child run over (tire marks)
  Hit at speed of >10 mph as per witness
 	
Motor vehicle accidents (with major vehicle damage)
  Rollover, unrestrained
  Passenger space intrusion and/or extrication
  Death of another passenger in same car
  Ejection from vehicle
 	
Falls
  Greater than 15 feet (second-story window)
	In addition, the following anatomic factors should alert emergency health care providers to the pediatric victim's need for evaluation by a pediatric trauma care specialist.
	
	Head injury
	  Loss of consciousness for more than 1 minute
	  Altered level of consciousness (disoriented, etc.)
	  Seizure activity after head injury
	
	Penetrating injuries
	  Above the midthigh or elbow
	
	Other anatomic injuries
	  Pelvic tenderness (on "rocking" or "stressing")
	  Suspected femur fracture
	  Unequal chest expansion or lung sounds
	  Abdominal pain or discomfort

*Developed by Kaufman IA, Stonecipher J, Kitchen L, Haubner LM, Jacobs S. (Reprinted with permission from Price D, Stonecipher J, Viglotti J. Prehospital assessment, intervention, and triage of the critically injured child. Top Emerg Med 1987; 9(3):29–30.)

---

*Personal communication with Maureen McArdle, Trauma Services Coordinator for Emergency Medical Services, San Diego, CA, 1989.

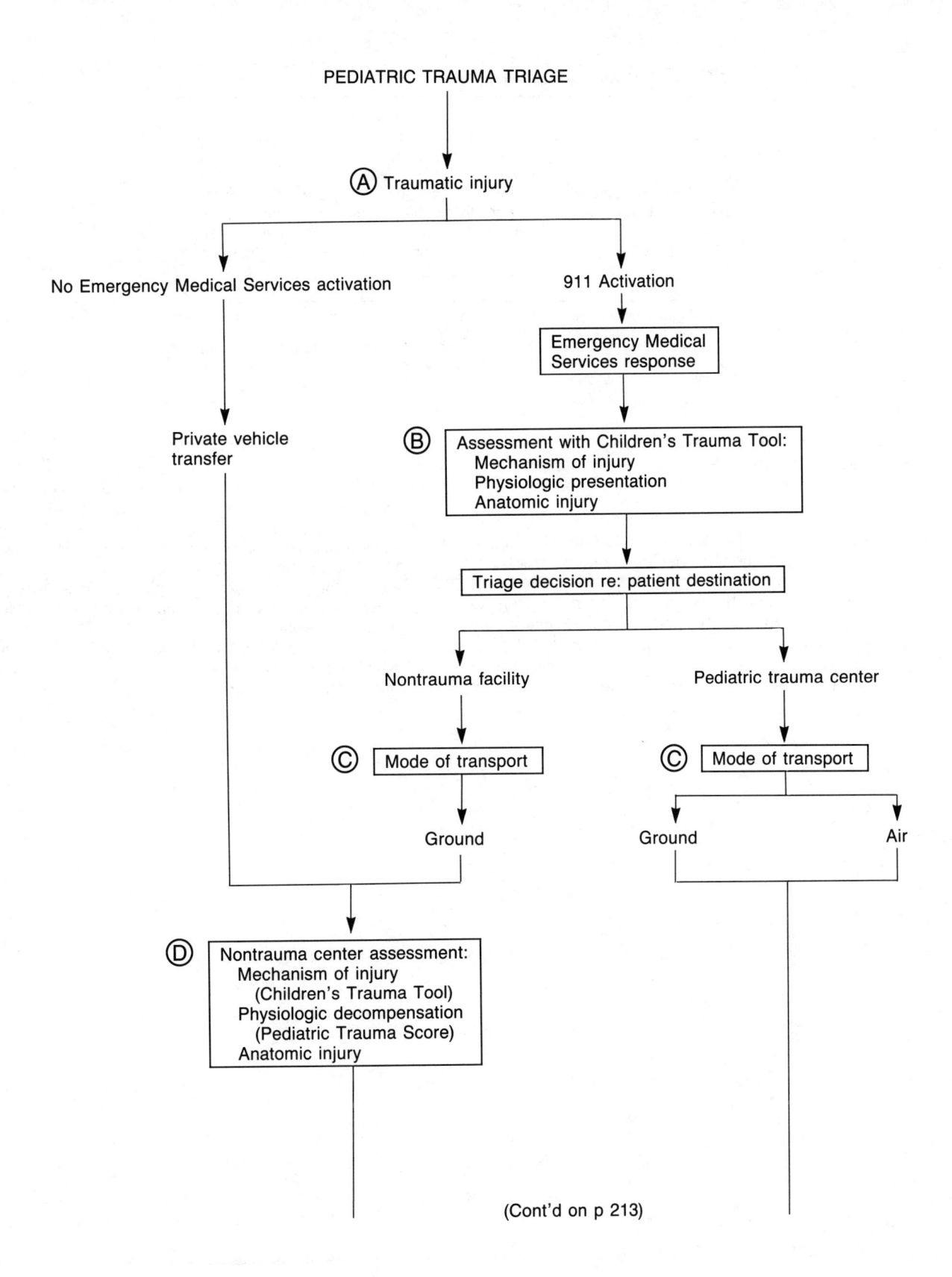

PEDIATRIC TRAUMA TRIAGE

```
                    PEDIATRIC TRAUMA TRIAGE
                              │
                              ▼
                      (A) Traumatic injury
                     /              \
                    ▼                ▼
   No Emergency Medical          911 Activation
   Services activation                │
           │                          ▼
           │                   Emergency Medical
           │                   Services response
           ▼                          │
   Private vehicle                    ▼
   transfer              (B) Assessment with Children's Trauma Tool:
           │                    Mechanism of injury
           │                    Physiologic presentation
           │                    Anatomic injury
           │                          │
           │                          ▼
           │              Triage decision re: patient destination
           │                     /              \
           │                    ▼                ▼
           │            Nontrauma facility   Pediatric trauma center
           │                    │                │
           │                    ▼                ▼
           │            (C) Mode of transport  (C) Mode of transport
           │                    │               /        \
           │                    ▼              ▼          ▼
           │                  Ground         Ground       Air
           │                    │              │
           ▼                    ▼              │
   (D) Nontrauma center assessment:            │
       Mechanism of injury                     │
         (Children's Trauma Tool)              │
       Physiologic decompensation              │
         (Pediatric Trauma Score)              │
       Anatomic injury                         │
                                               │
                    (Cont'd on p 213)
```

211

TABLE 2 Pediatric Trauma Score*

Component	+2	+1	−1
Size	>20 kg	10–20 kg	<10 kg
Airway	Normal	Maintainable	Unmaintainable
Central nervous system	Awake	Obtunded	Coma/decerebrate
Systolic blood pressure†	>90 mm Hg	90–50 mm Hg	<50 mm Hg
Open wound	None	Minor	Major/penetrating
Skeletal integrity	None	Closed fracture	Open/multiple fractures

Sum ___ PTS

*Check one category for each component. Children whose pediatric trauma scores are 8 or below require triage to the pediatric trauma center.
†If proper sized blood pressure cuff not available, blood pressure can be assessed by assigning +2, pulse palpable at wrist; +1, pulse palpable at groin; −1, no pulse palpable.
Reprinted with permission from Tepas JJ.

E. When deciding whether to admit a patient to a nontrauma facility or to transport to a PTC, consultation with pediatric trauma care specialists should occur.

F. Once the decision has been made to transport the patient to the PTC, one must decide the method of transport. This should be decided based on the patient's treatment needs and the length of transport time. Intrafacility transport of the stable pediatric patient may be accomplished by basic ambulance transport, whereas advanced life support and assessment may be provided by aeromedical or critical care transport.

References

Kitchen L, Haubner L. Guidelines for the triage of pediatric trauma patients. Emerg Nursing 1989; 15(5):414–415.

Price D, Stonecipher J, Viglotti J. Prehospital assessment, intervention, and triage of the critically injured child. Top Emerg Med 1987; 9(3):21–31.

Tepas JJ. Pediatric Trauma score: a rapid assessment and triage tool for the injured child. Jacksonville, FL: University Hospital of Jacksonville, 1986.

Tepas JJ, Ramenofsky ML, Mollit DL, et al. The Pediatric Trauma Score as a predictor of injury severity: an objective assessment. Trauma 1986; 26(7):685.

(Cont'd from p 211)

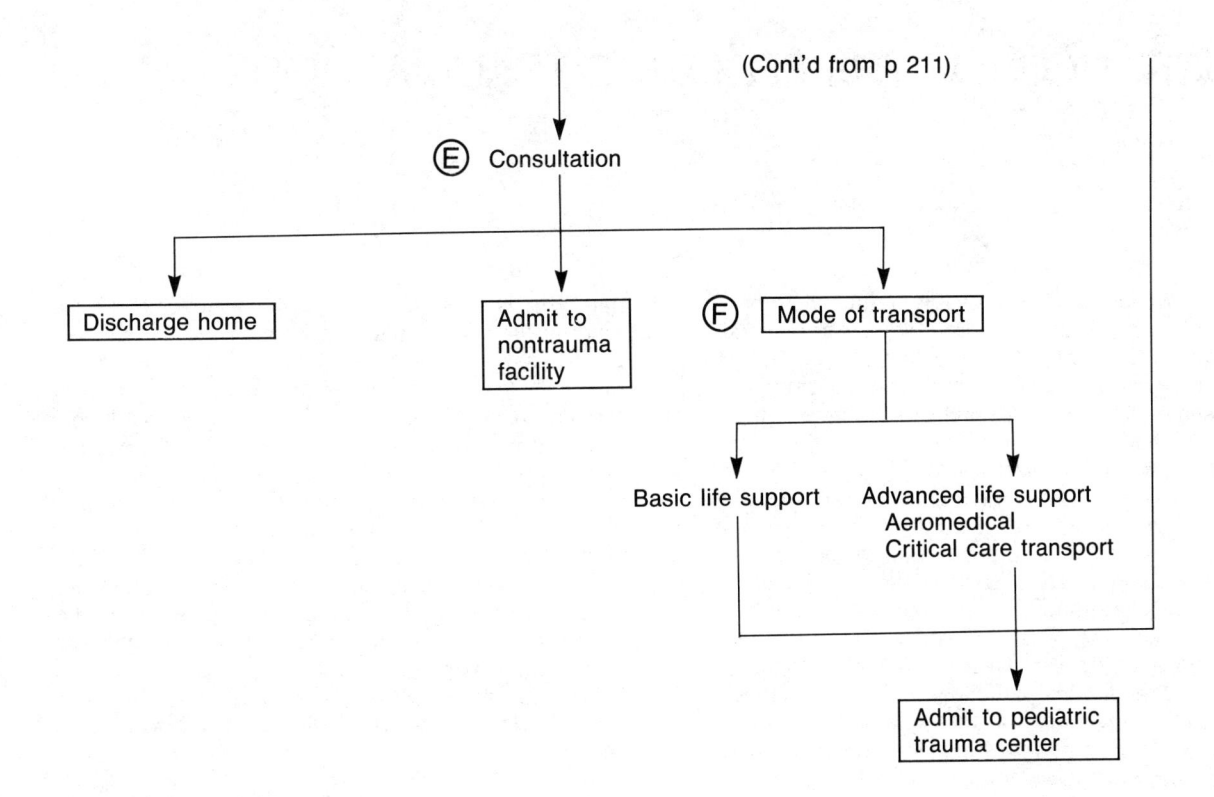

Ⓔ Consultation

- Discharge home
- Admit to nontrauma facility
- Ⓕ Mode of transport
  - Basic life support
  - Advanced life support
    Aeromedical
    Critical care transport

Admit to pediatric trauma center

RESUSCITATION OF THE PEDIATRIC TRAUMA VICTIM

Steven L. Moulton
Frank P. Lynch
Bradley Peterson

The resuscitation algorithm for pediatric trauma victims is similar to that for adult resuscitation. Airway, breathing, and circulation are the initial priorities. The differences between these two algorithms lie in their methods of establishing life support measures. The pediatric algorithm is meant to instruct the clinician on how to tailor instrumentation and therapy in accordance with variable patient size, injury severity, and psychological make-up. The present chapter discusses the liberal use of elective intubation and details an efficient approach to intravenous (IV) access and fluid therapy during rapid primary evaluation. The secondary survey of the pediatric resuscitation algorithm is broken down into its component parts in the chapters that immediately follow. These chapters present and discuss the resuscitation algorithms for pediatric thoracic, abdominal, extremity, and central nervous system trauma. Throughout all of these chapters there is a much greater reliance on noninvasive means to evaluate and treat the pediatric trauma patient.

A. The pediatric multiple trauma victim (MTV) is usually a young male pedestrian or bicyclist who has been struck by an automobile or injured as a passenger in a motor vehicle accident. Information regarding field evaluation of the victim and resuscitation measures instituted by prehospital care providers is transmitted to the receiving hospital by two way radio (p 14). This prehospital information includes mechanism of injury, current vital signs, level of consciousness, and transport time. Early transmission of this information to the receiving hospital provides an opportunity to anticipate the patient's arrival and to assemble the trauma team.

The ideal pediatric trauma team includes a board certified pediatric surgeon and a board certified intensivist; the latter is trained in anesthesia, pediatrics, and critical care. Both physicians must be comfortable with airway management as well as proficient in vascular access and invasive procedures; either may assume the role of "team captain." Other team members include two registered nurses, one to monitor vital signs and intravenous fluids and the other to record vital signs and coordinate the flow of medications and specimens; one respiratory therapist to monitor the airway and ventilation; a radiology technician to shoot and process films; a circulator to run specimens to the laboratory; and a social worker. The social worker acts as a temporary liaison; he or she must be informed of the child's injuries in order to provide appropriate information and emotional support to the family.

The clinician's ability to communicate with the injured child is usually reflected in how well the child cooperates during the resuscitation. A calm, friendly approach provides comfort and emotional support in the setting of pain and unfamiliar surroundings. It also provides a sense of caring and understanding, often by simply holding the child's hand or a gentle tousling of the hair. This is especially true of the younger child, for whom actions may allay fear more effectively than verbal reassurance. The older child tends to focus on the physical aspects of his or her injuries; there is concern about disfiguring lacerations, fractures, and the additional pain that may be caused by diagnostic or therapeutic maneuvers. To overcome these concerns and relieve anxiety before painful procedures, the clinician must use simple explanations and a firm but gentle tact. There are times, however, when explanations fail and the child displays physical or emotional agitation. To overcome these interruptions in the flow of the resuscitation, it may be necessary to impose physical restraint and/or sedation. If the child is particularly disruptive or experiences an inordinate amount of pain or emotional trauma, elective intubation under anesthesia is the procedure of choice.

B. As the child is brought into the resuscitation area, one makes an immediate visual assessment of injury severity and level of consciousness. Following this initial assessment, one physician must focus on establishing an adequate airway while the other confirms or establishes IV access.

C. Any child with severe respiratory difficulty or a Glasgow Coma Score (GCS) of eight or less requires intubation. This prevents airway obstruction, improves oxygenation and ventilation, decreases the risk of aspiration, and provides complete control of ventilation should hyperventilation be necessary. To prepare for intubation, the cervical spine must be immobilized by an assistant using in-line traction. The oropharynx should be visualized and cleared with a finger or suction as needed. If the child is breathing spontaneously with a good airway and effective ventilation, he or she may be preoxygenated by simply holding a clear mask with high flow oxygen over the face. An oral airway may be necessary in the obtunded or unconscious child, but it can also stimulate a gag reflex and lead to further problems. If the child's ventilations are ineffective, preoxygenate using bag-and-mask technique. Cuffed endotracheal tubes (ETTs) are generally not used in small children and infants because of the potential for airway damage, even with a low pressure cuff. There is added concern that an overinflated cuff could constrict the small lumen of a pediatric ETT. Nonetheless, a cuffed ETT is the airway of choice in the presence of major oropharyngeal bleeding and in children 4 years of age and older. The size of the ETT can be approximated by the diameter of the child's fifth finger. The following formula may also be used:

$$16 + \text{age of child in years} \div 4 = \text{internal diameter of ETT in millimeters}$$

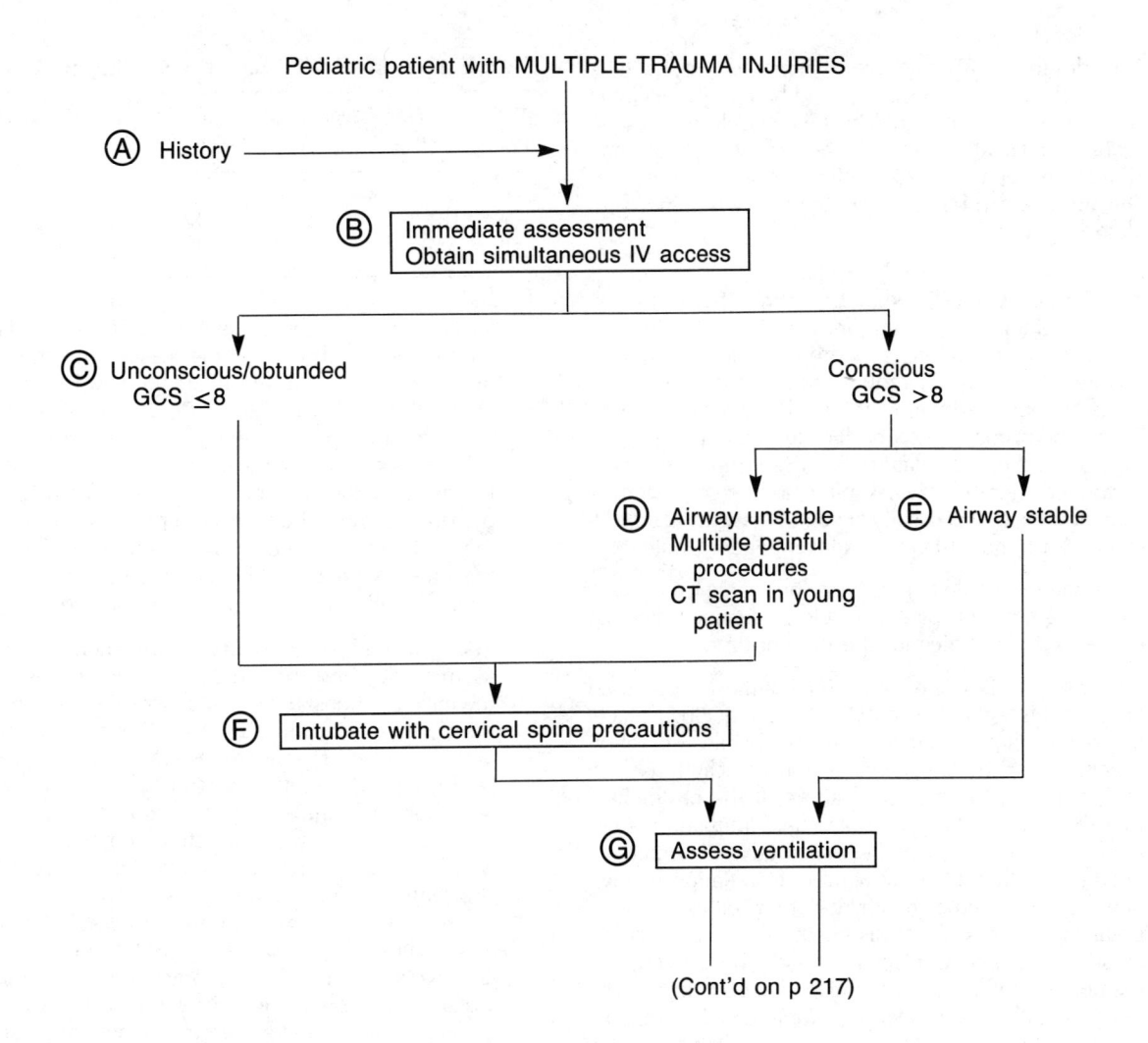

Pediatric patient with MULTIPLE TRAUMA INJURIES

Ⓐ History

Ⓑ Immediate assessment
Obtain simultaneous IV access

Ⓒ Unconscious/obtunded
GCS ≤8

Conscious
GCS >8

Ⓓ Airway unstable
Multiple painful
procedures
CT scan in young
patient

Ⓔ Airway stable

Ⓕ Intubate with cervical spine precautions

Ⓖ Assess ventilation

(Cont'd on p 217)

215

Two additional ETTs, one size smaller and one size larger than the calculated size, should be readily available at the time of intubation. The tube should easily pass beyond the vocal cords and be accompanied by a small air leak between 20 to 40 centimeters of water pressure. This air leak can be compensated for by a higher ventilatory flow rate.

D. If the child has a slowly deteriorating respiratory status or a Glasgow Coma Score that is falling—but still greater than eight—it is often prudent to institute early prophylactic intubation. Early prophylactic intubation is also helpful if the child requires multiple painful procedures or computed tomography (CT). This can be done during the primary or secondary survey, depending on the flow of the resuscitation. Elective intubation is best performed after the cervical spine has been radiographically evaluated. It is usually accomplished using a sedative and a nondepolarizing relaxing agent (Table 1).

E. If the patient is able to give his or her name or to speak easily, the airway is patent, and low flow supplemental oxygen should suffice for the present time.

F. The orotracheal route of intubation is almost always used because it is technically easy and fast and allows placement of the largest diameter ETT permissible. Intubation is accomplished using cervical spine precautions with in-line traction as described above. If the orotracheal route is unavailable and nasotracheal intubation is not a viable option, the next best alternative is immediate needle cricothyroidotomy with jet insufflation or high flow oxygen. Needle cricothyroidotomy provides a temporary airway. It is accomplished using a 12- or 14-gauge angiocath, which is placed through the cricothyroid membrane or trachea below the level of obstruction. The plastic sheath is connected to a commercially available jet ventilator system or, if this is unavailable, to a Y-connector and oxygen source flowing at 15 L per minute. Intermittent ventilation is achieved with high flow oxygen by blocking the side hole of the Y-connector for 1 of every 5 seconds. Needle cricothyroidotomy is a life saving maneuver that allows 30 to 45 minutes for urgent intubation or tracheostomy; it is rarely used.

G. After the airway is established, attention is directed toward ensuring adequate ventilation. The intubated infant requires 20 to 30 breaths per minute and the school aged child 15 breaths per minute. These ventilatory rates are lower than those listed in Table 2 for the spontaneously breathing child because the tidal volume of a ventilated breath is greater. During brief bilateral auscultation, the chest is exposed and palpated and its movements are observed. If the chest examination is symmetric and the child is intubated, it is still important to check the position of the ETT. This can be done by visualizing the position of the ETT in relation to the vocal cords or by noting the length of the ETT at the alveolar ridge or nares (Table 3). Other methods include palpation of the ETT cuff in the suprasternal notch, checking the end-tidal carbon dioxide, and/or confirming ETT placement with a chest film. Lastly, it is important to secure the tube firmly in the proper position.

H. The intubated patient with poor lung compliance or an asymmetric chest examination has one of the four following conditions: (1) the endotracheal tube is misdirected; (2) there is an obstruction within the lumen of the tube or trachea; (3) massive aspiration has occurred; or (4) there is volume constraint in one or both hemithoraces. If the endotracheal tube is properly placed and there is no airway obstruction or material in the airway, one must search for immediately life threatening chest injuries. These include tension pneumothorax and massive hemothorax; both are discussed in detail on p 224. The initial management of a tension pneumothorax involves insertion of a large bore (14- gauge) angiocatheter through the second intercostal space in the midclavicular line of the involved hemithorax. This helps relieve pressure within the hemithorax but does not allow complete re-expansion of the lung. Thus, a chest tube of approximately the same width as the fourth or fifth interspace is immediately placed and connected to suction. The amount of suction varies according to the size of the patient; use a 10-cm water column if the child weighs 10 kg or less; otherwise use 15 to 20 cm of water.

I. If the child is not intubated but is tachypneic or has evidence of diminished unilateral or bilateral breath sounds, the child may have a life threatening chest injury. The need for intubation and the present oxygen flow rate should be re- evaluated. If there is no immediate danger, the child can be further assessed with a chest film at the completion of the primary survey. In the meantime, the child can be connected to an oxygen saturation monitor for continuous evaluation.

TABLE 1 Rapid Sequence Induction: Most Frequent Pharmacology

Preoxygenation
Thiopental sodium, 3–6 mg/kg IV
Vecuronium, 0.3 mg/kg IV
Cricoid pressure
Intubation with cervical spine control

TABLE 2 Normal Vital Signs According to Age

Age (yr)	Respirations (breaths/min)	Heart Rate (beats/min)	Blood Pressure (mm Hg)
0–1	40	140	80/40
1–5	30	120	90/60
5–10	20	100	100/80

TABLE 3 Length of Endotracheal Tube by Route

Route	Location	Measurement
Oral	Alveolar ridge	Age + 10 cm
Nasal	Nares	Age + 15 cm

(Cont'd from p 215)

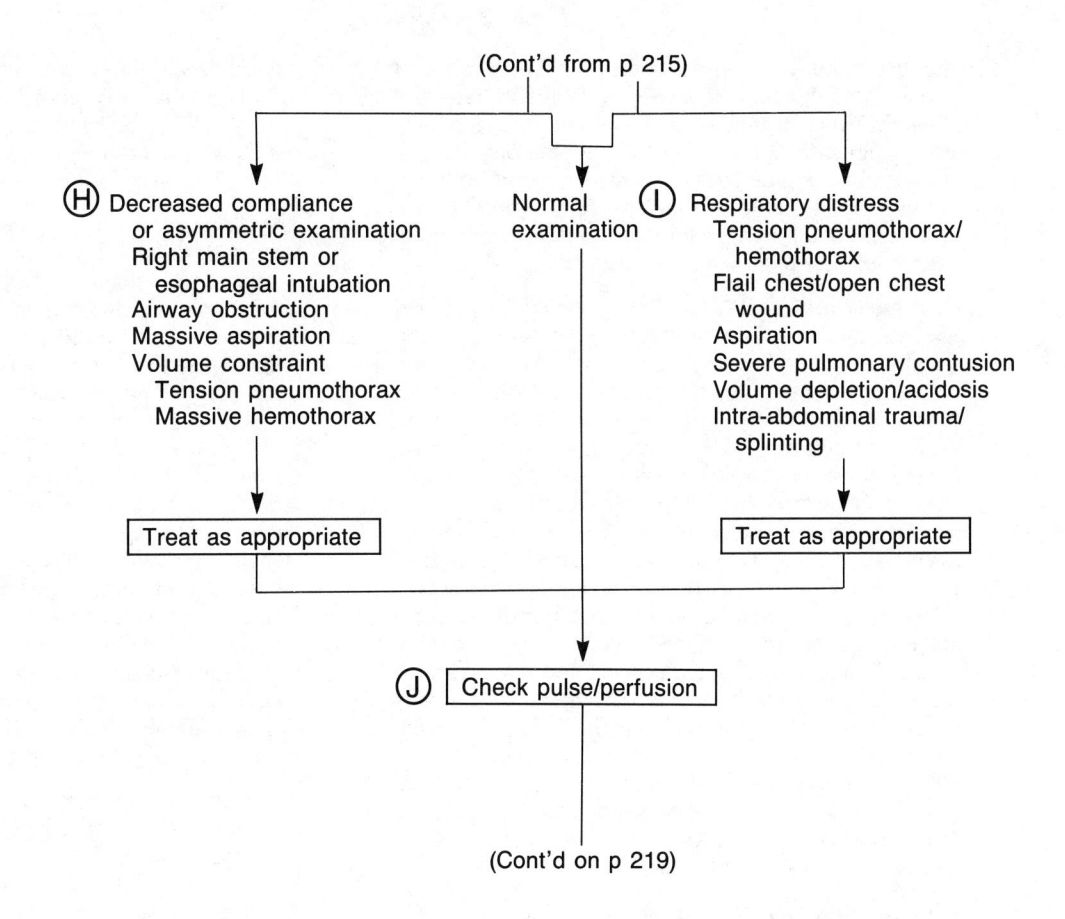

Ⓗ Decreased compliance or asymmetric examination
Right main stem or esophageal intubation
Airway obstruction
Massive aspiration
Volume constraint
  Tension pneumothorax
  Massive hemothorax

↓

[Treat as appropriate]

Normal examination

Ⓘ Respiratory distress
Tension pneumothorax/hemothorax
Flail chest/open chest wound
Aspiration
Severe pulmonary contusion
Volume depletion/acidosis
Intra-abdominal trauma/splinting

↓

[Treat as appropriate]

Ⓙ [Check pulse/perfusion]

(Cont'd on p 219)

J. The first maneuver to assess a child's circulatory status is to feel for a femoral pulse, noting its quality, rate, and regularity. Since tachycardia is a relative term in the pediatric population, it is helpful to know the upper limits of normal heart rate over a selected range of different age groups (see Table 2). One should also note the patient's skin color, temperature, and capillary refill time; pale, cool skin is a marker of hemorrhagic shock.

K. If a pulse is not detectable or if the patient is profoundly bradycardiac, cardiopulmonary resuscitation (CPR) should be initiated in accordance with advanced cardiac life support (ACLS) measures. One must then rule out the presence of respiratory failure attributable to a cervical spine or severe head injury. Other considerations include airway obstruction, tension pneumothorax, cardiac tamponade, and severe hypovolemia. Airway obstruction and tension pneumothorax should have already been diagnosed and initial treatment provided. Cardiac tamponade and severe hypovolemia require immediate, temporizing volume replacement. In penetrating trauma an emergency thoracotomy allows access to the pericardium for relief of tamponade and direct cardiac massage. It also provides access to the descending thoracic aorta, which can be cross-clamped or compressed with the hand to control massive hemorrhage below the diaphragm. Aggressive fluid resuscitation can then continue while the patient is transported to the operating room. Most centers have found emergency thoracotomy ineffective in blunt cardiac arrest.

L. If the patient has a pulse but shows evidence of shock, external hemorrhage must be identified and controlled while intravascular volume is repleted. Direct compression of an extremity artery in the axilla or groin is easily accomplished with digital pressure; hemorrhage from the scalp is best controlled with light packing and minimal pressure to avoid pressing fractured bone into the dura or underlying brain. Properly sized pediatric military antishock trousers (MAST) can minimize lower extremity and pelvic bleeding, thereby obviating the need for manual compression. One must be aware, however, of the MAST's potential to exacerbate respiratory distress by compressing the abdomen and raising both hemidiaphragms. Deflation of the MAST suit is accomplished one compartment at a time during the secondary survey, when fluid resuscitation is established and vital signs can be closely monitored.

M. Establishing dependable IV access in the pediatric MTV is made difficult by the small caliber of the peripheral veins and, in the presence of ongoing hemorrhage, a diminishing circulatory blood volume. The intravenous routes of greatest ease and utility include the hand and anticubital veins. If a 20-gauge or larger angiocatheter cannot be threaded into one of these vessels and bleeding is minimal, proceed to percutaneous access via one of the saphenous veins. If hemorrhage is severe, proceed to femoral and/or subclavian vein catheterization. Once a vein is catheterized, it is useful to draw off the necessary blood for type and cross-match, hemoglobin, hematocrit, platelets, and routine chemistries. If percutaneous access is not possible in the profoundly volume depleted child, one can perform an antecubital vein cutdown or a saphenous vein cutdown at the groin; however, this is almost never necessary. Preflushed infant feeding tubes or large bore introducers can then be passed toward the central venous system. Altogether, at least two reliable IV lines should be established. If the patient has pre-existing hypothermia or shock, warm blankets and in-line blood warmers may hasten the child's response to fluid resuscitation.

N. The blood volume in a child is about 8 percent of body weight, or 80 ml/kg. In the revised advanced trauma life support (ATLS) manual of the American College of Surgeons, bolus administration of Ringer's lactate solution is recommended in 20 ml/kg aliquots. The volume of balanced salt solution required to replace lost blood is three-to-one. Therefore, a total of three 20-ml/kg boluses are required to replace blood loss equivalent to one-fourth of the child's total blood volume. If the child requires a fourth 20-ml/kg bolus of Ringer's lactate before vital signs stabilize, the next two fluid boluses should each be 10 ml/kg of packed red blood cells. If the child remains hemodynamically unstable despite these fluid resuscitation efforts, there is substantial ongoing blood loss. At this point, consider the need to control cavitary bleeding in the operating room. As an important caveat to fluid resuscitation of the pediatric trauma patient, it should be remembered that the ATLS recommendations are only guidelines: the endpoint to fluid resuscitation is the restoration of adequate tissue perfusion.

O. Included in the primary survey is a brief neurologic examination. This is meant to establish the patient's level of consciousness, pupillary size and reactivity, and extremity movement in response to pain or command. This concise evaluation should alert the clinician to the presence or absence of central nervous system injury, so that early diagnostic studies can be performed during the secondary survey.

P. The final step in the primary survey is really the first step of the secondary survey; complete exposure of the patient is necessary for a thorough physical examination.

Q. The secondary survey consists of a careful head-to-toe physical examination with assessment of all injuries. The regions of the body are grouped as follows: head and neck, heart and lungs, abdomen, rectum and perineum, extremities, vascular system, central nervous system, and peripheral nervous system. Screening radiographs are obtained, including those of the lateral cervical spine, chest, abdomen, and pelvis if injury is suspected as well as any indicated long bone or craniofacial films. These radiographs complement physical examination findings, thereby allowing prioritization of all injuries in the context of planning for the next diagnostic procedure or therapeutic maneuver.

References

American College of Surgeons. Advanced trauma life support program. Chicago: American College of Surgeons, 1989.

Maier RV. Evaluation and resuscitation. In: Moore EE, ed. Early care of the injured patient. Philadelphia: BC Decker, 1990:56–73.

O'Neill JA. Emergency management of the injured child. In: Welch KJ, Randolph JG, Ravitch MM, O'Neill JA, Rowe MI, eds. Pediatric surgery. Chicago: Year Book, 1986:135–138.

Saletta JD, Geis WP. Initial assessment of trauma. In: Moylan JA, ed. Trauma surgery. Philadelphia: JB Lippincott, 1987:1–25.

(Cont'd from p 217)

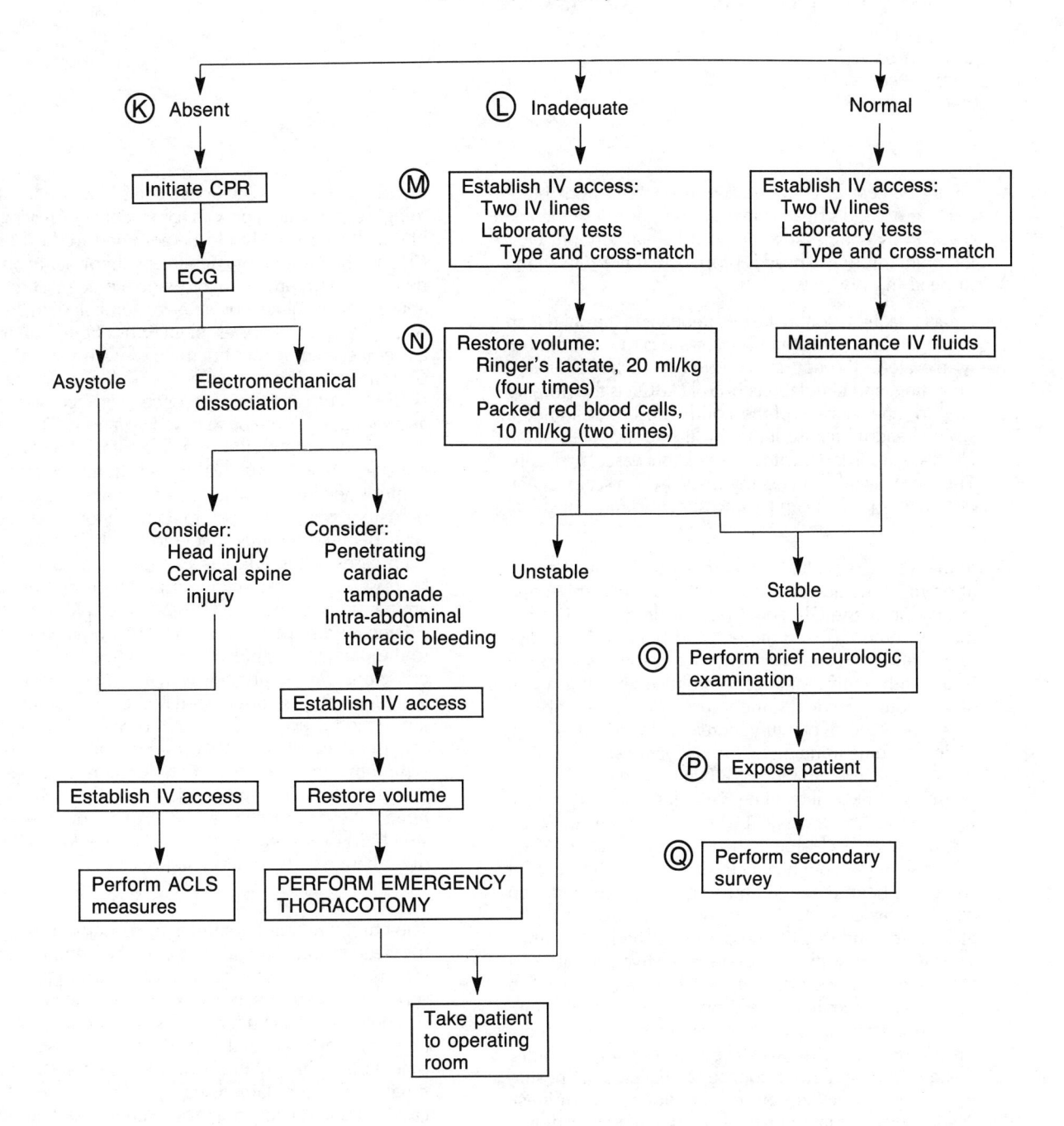

```
            ┌────────────────────┼────────────────────┐
        Ⓚ Absent             Ⓛ Inadequate         Normal
            │                    │                    │
      ┌──────────┐         Ⓜ ┌──────────────────┐  ┌──────────────────┐
      │Initiate  │           │Establish IV access:│  │Establish IV access:│
      │  CPR     │           │  Two IV lines      │  │  Two IV lines      │
      └──────────┘           │  Laboratory tests  │  │  Laboratory tests  │
            │                │  Type and cross-match│ │  Type and cross-match│
      ┌──────────┐           └──────────────────┘  └──────────────────┘
      │   ECG    │                   │                    │
      └──────────┘         Ⓝ ┌──────────────────┐  ┌──────────────────┐
         │     │              │Restore volume:     │  │Maintenance IV fluids│
         │     │              │  Ringer's lactate, │  └──────────────────┘
   Asystole   Electromechanical│  20 ml/kg          │
              dissociation    │  (four times)      │
                    │         │  Packed red blood  │
              ┌─────┴─────┐   │  cells, 10 ml/kg   │
          Consider:    Consider:│  (two times)      │
          Head injury  Penetrating└──────────────────┘
          Cervical     cardiac        │          │
          spine        tamponade   Unstable    Stable
          injury       Intra-abdominal │          │
                       thoracic bleeding│      Ⓞ ┌──────────────────┐
                           │            │        │Perform brief       │
                    ┌──────────────┐    │        │neurologic          │
                    │Establish IV  │    │        │examination         │
                    │access        │    │        └──────────────────┘
                    └──────────────┘    │                │
                           │            │        Ⓟ ┌──────────────────┐
                    ┌──────────────┐    │           │Expose patient    │
                    │Restore volume│    │           └──────────────────┘
                    └──────────────┘    │                │
    ┌──────────────┐       │            │        Ⓠ ┌──────────────────┐
    │Establish IV  │       │            │           │Perform secondary │
    │access        │       │            │           │survey            │
    └──────────────┘       │            │           └──────────────────┘
           │               │            │
    ┌──────────────┐ ┌──────────────────┐│
    │Perform ACLS  │ │PERFORM EMERGENCY ││
    │measures      │ │THORACOTOMY       ││
    └──────────────┘ └──────────────────┘│
                             │           │
                      ┌──────────────┐
                      │Take patient  │
                      │to operating  │
                      │room          │
                      └──────────────┘
```

PEDIATRIC HEAD TRAUMA

David Barba
Louann Kitchen
Brian Copeland

A. Eighty percent of childhood injuries result from blunt trauma. A child's head is large in proportion to the rest of the body and has less musculoskeletal support. During blunt injury, the head is propelled, thereby resulting in head injury.

B. Intracranial hematomas are less frequent in the child than in the adult, but intracranial pressure is more commonly elevated. Prompt intervention to achieve airway, breathing, and circulation control (ABCs) is the primary goal in management of the child who has sustained a severe head injury. Additionally, the surface area of the child's scalp is large with a remarkable vascular supply. Therefore, a child can exsanguinate from a scalp laceration, and an infant can go into shock from a subgaleal hematoma.

C. In the setting of pediatric head trauma, the initial evaluation must include attention to the cervical spine and evaluation of the Glasgow Coma Scale (GCS). The immature spine has well mineralized bone, healthy disk tissue, and increased elasticity of the soft tissue. Blunt injury with significant force to produce head injury can also produce cervical spine injury. An accurate history of the mechanism of injury increases the clinician's suspicion of spine injury in children. Diagnosis by clinical or radiologic examination is difficult in the crying or unconscious child. All children with blunt injury above the clavicle must have cervical spine precautions until the cervical spine is cleared in the resuscitation area. When the child is hemodynamically stable and the cervical spine has been assessed and stabilized, transportation may be initiated for further diagnostic evaluations. Evaluation of the child's GCS score is performed at this time. The GCS score is the sum of the objective evaluation of the response to eye opening, which is scored from 1 to 4: 1—no eye opening; 2—eye opening to painful stimuli; 3—eye opening to voice; 4—spontaneous eye opening. Motor response is scored from 1 to 6 points: 1—flaccid or no motor response; 2—decerebrate posturing (abnormal extension of the upper extremities); 3—decortication (abnormal flexion in the upper extremities); 4—withdrawal from painful stimuli; 5—localization to painful stimuli; 6—following commands. Verbal response score is scored from 1 to 5: 1—no verbal response or intubated; 2—simple noises; 3—single words; 4—confused speech; 5—oriented speech. The sum of the eye opening, motor response, and verbal scores serves to classify the level of the child's head injury as severe (GCS of 3 to 8), moderate (GCS of 9 to 12), or mild (GCS of 13 to 15).

D. The child who has been unconscious for more than 5 minutes, who has evidence of skull fractures, who vomits recurrently, who has evidence of a seizure or focal neurologic examination, or who has evidence of having been physically abused should be admitted to the hospital. Clearly, the presence of significant abnormality on computed tomography scan or evidence suggesting child abuse is an absolute indication for admission. In the child with minor head injuries, plain films of the skull remain a useful screening tool but in no way are a substitute for CT scanning. The presence of a skull fracture on plain skull films has a higher incidence of intracranial trauma and should therefore be followed by a head CT scan. The absence of abnormalities on skull films, however, does not rule out an intracranial mass lesion. Any child with a minor head injury who has a focal neurologic deficit, persistent vomiting, a full fontanel, and/or evidence of skull penetration must undergo head CT scanning. In such cases, if the CT scan is normal, the child should be observed. In the setting of a normal neurologic examination and a normal CT scan, the child may be considered for discharge home with appropriate instructions to the parents. A child who has suffered a brief loss of consciousness but presents with a normal neurologic examination may be discharged home (after initial assessment and observation) *only* if the parents or caretakers can demonstrate that they understand the signs and symptoms of neurologic deterioration and have the resources to assess the child frequently in the first 48 hours following discharge. Caretakers should receive instructions in writing that describe what to do in the case of a change in the child's status.

E. The child who has alterations in consciousness following head trauma should uniformly be admitted for observation. The presence of focal neurologic deficits, seizures, or skull fractures or any evidence of progressive deterioration in neurologic status should prompt immediate evaluation of the child by head CT scan. In the potentially critically ill child, it is essential that the optimal study be obtained with maximum safety for the child. This frequently requires an anesthesiologist for sedation and intubation of the child to allow good airway control and optimal CT scan quality. In the absence of ongoing pathology, a child's neurologic examination should remain stable and improve over the first 48 hours following head trauma. Any evidence of neurologic deterioration should be considered a neurologic emergency and may well herald the onset of worsening brain edema, increasing size of an intracranial mass lesion, or some other systemic problems (i.e., hypoxia, hypotension). Early recognition of these problems is critical, and the prompt recognition of an ongoing intracranial process or major systemic problem can be life saving.

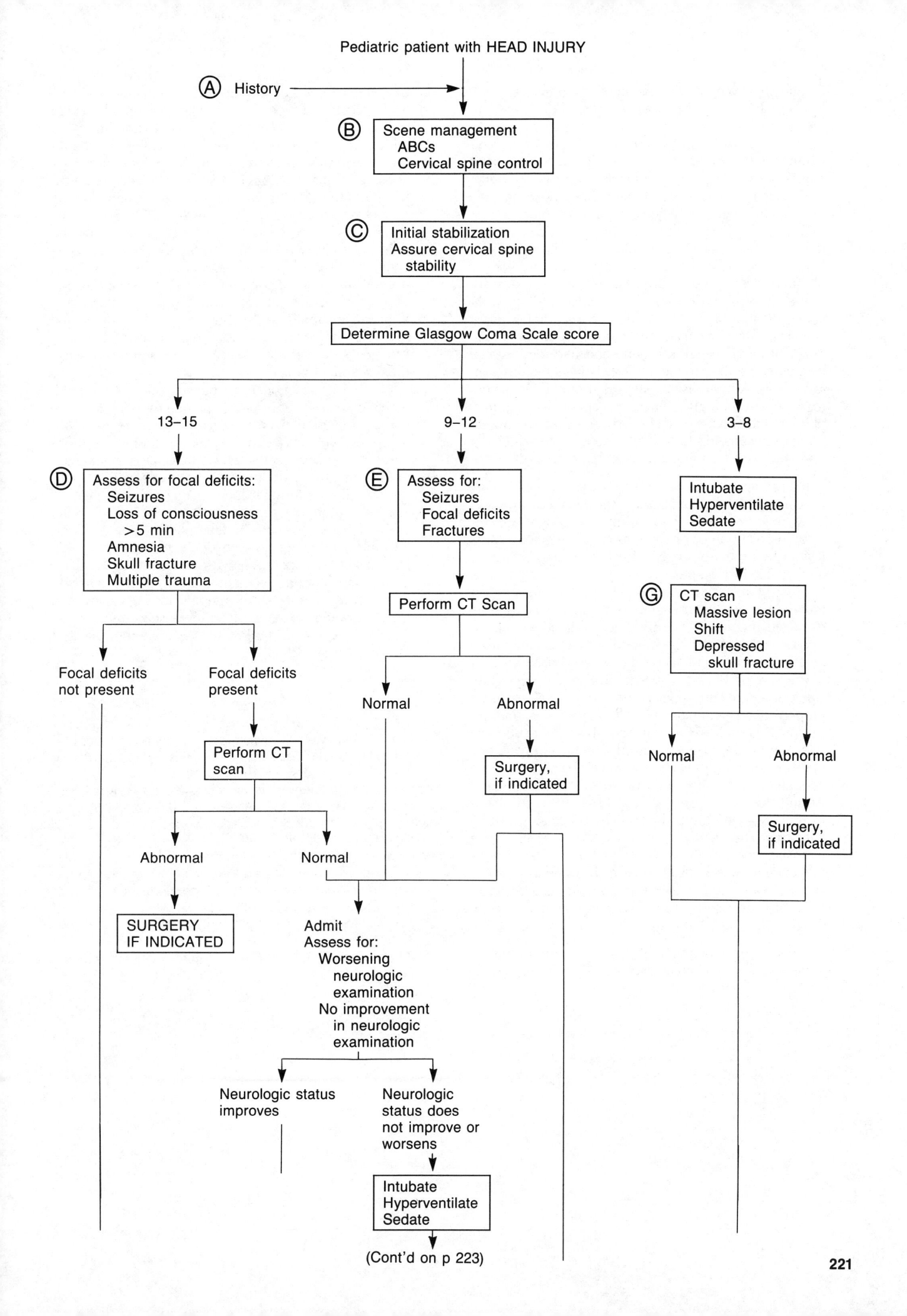

Pediatric patient with HEAD INJURY

- (A) History
- (B) Scene management
  - ABCs
  - Cervical spine control
- (C) Initial stabilization
  - Assure cervical spine stability

Determine Glasgow Coma Scale score

13–15
- (D) Assess for focal deficits:
  - Seizures
  - Loss of consciousness >5 min
  - Amnesia
  - Skull fracture
  - Multiple trauma
  - Focal deficits not present
  - Focal deficits present → Perform CT scan
    - Abnormal → SURGERY IF INDICATED
    - Normal → Admit, Assess for:
      - Worsening neurologic examination
      - No improvement in neurologic examination
      - Neurologic status improves
      - Neurologic status does not improve or worsens → Intubate, Hyperventilate, Sedate
      - (Cont'd on p 223)

9–12
- (E) Assess for:
  - Seizures
  - Focal deficits
  - Fractures
- Perform CT Scan
  - Normal
  - Abnormal → Surgery, if indicated

3–8
- Intubate, Hyperventilate, Sedate
- (G) CT scan
  - Massive lesion
  - Shift
  - Depressed skull fracture
  - Normal
  - Abnormal → Surgery, if indicated

221

F. Emotional, psychological, and intellectual problems following mild head injury have been well documented. These problems cannot always be anticipated based on clinical history or initial CT scan. Levin et al have documented a correlation between clinical sequelae and magnetic resonance imaging results, thereby confirming the suspicion that these changes are physiologically based. Although mortality for mild head injury is low, morbidity is significant and requires a multidisciplinary follow-up approach. This should begin with written instructions to the parents or caretakers that describe the physiologic and intellectual changes they may observe in the child in the first few weeks following injury. Instructions should include a clinic phone number and a contact person to facilitate a prompt follow-up clinic visit. This visit should begin with a questionnaire administered by a person skilled in identifying changes requiring intervention. A multidisciplinary team, including a neurologist, psychologist, nurse, occupational therapist, physical therapist, and social worker, should be available for consultation to facilitate recovery and return of the child to the family and school setting.

G. In the setting of pediatric head injury, the CT scan offers a clear anatomic picture of the intracranial contents and allows decision making regarding requirements for surgical intervention or ongoing medical treatment. Mass lesions that require surgical intervention and occasionally occult hydrocephalus can be recognized in this fashion, thereby prompting quick and specific surgical therapy. Lesions that do not require surgery can then be managed medically. The presence of large extra-axial masses with shift requires immediate surgical attention. Smaller lesions, particularly those based in the region of the temporal lobe, can frequently be considered lesions amenable to surgical therapy because of their propensity for peduncle herniation, even at normal intracranial pressures. Other lesions that require surgical intervention are open, depressed skull fractures and any open penetrating injury to the brain. These should be attended to surgically, allowing good debridement and wound closure to reduce the risk of seizures or CNS infections at a later time. The presence of small subdural hematomas frequently can be managed medically in the intensive care unit (ICU) while following the patient's intracranial pressure (ICP). This can be done using a variety of ICP monitoring devices that require surgical placement but can also be done under the same anesthetic required for the CT scan.

H. Medical management of pediatric head injury requires a specialized care team familiar with CNS pathophysiology and capable of monitoring intracranial pressure. Such monitoring should be undertaken in any child with a Glasgow Coma Scale score of 8 or less, in any child with a documented neurologic deterioration not requiring surgical intervention, and in some patients following surgical intervention. Following the placement of an ICP monitor, initial ICP control can be obtained using hyperventilation and a PCO_2 range of 27 to 30. During this time it is frequently necessary to paralyze and sedate the child to allow full respiratory control. Hyperventilation allows cerebral vasoconstriction, which will improve intracranial compliance and reduce intracranial pressure. Other initial strategies to control intracranial pressure should be the elevation of the head of the bed to 30 degrees and removal of all constrictive tapes or braces from the neck. This improves venous drainage, thereby reducing ICP.

Following sedation and hyperventilation of the child, other strategies to control ICP include further hyperventilation, the use of hyperosmolar therapy (i.e., mannitol, 0.5 g per kilogram per dose), and placement of an intraventricular catheter that allows drainage of spinal fluid or placement of a subdural bolt that allows ICP monitoring. When monitoring ICP in such a fashion, repeat CT scans are frequently required to monitor changes in the child's neurologic status. If deterioration is noted upon the child's neurologic examination (e.g., unilateral pupillary dilation) or if there is progressive rise in ICP, CT scans of the brain should be obtained again. Such studies allow documentation of new mass lesions or changes in the intracranial space, such as increased edema or infarction. Such studies allow further treatment plans to be initiated regarding the control of ICP.

References

Bruce DA. Cerebrovascular dynamics following brain insults. In: James H, et al, ed. Brain insults in infants and children. New York: Grune & Stratton, 1985:83–88.

Johnson DL. Head injury. In: Eichelberger MR, ed. Pediatric trauma care. Rockville, MD: Aspen Publishers, 1988:87.

Kitchen L, Lynch FP, Murphy P. Pediatric risks for injury. Emerg Care Q 1990; 5(4):82–86.

Levin HS, Amparo E, Eisenberg HM, et al. Magnetic resonance imaging and computerized tomography in relation to the neurobehavioral sequelae of mild and moderate head injuries. J Neurosurg 1987; 66(5):706–713.

Luerssen TG. Resuscitation of brain injured children: special considerations. Trauma Q 1985; 2(1):20–25.

Rimel R, Giordani MA, Barth J, et al. Disability caused by minor head injury. Neurosurg 1981; 9(3):221–228.

(Cont'd from p 221)

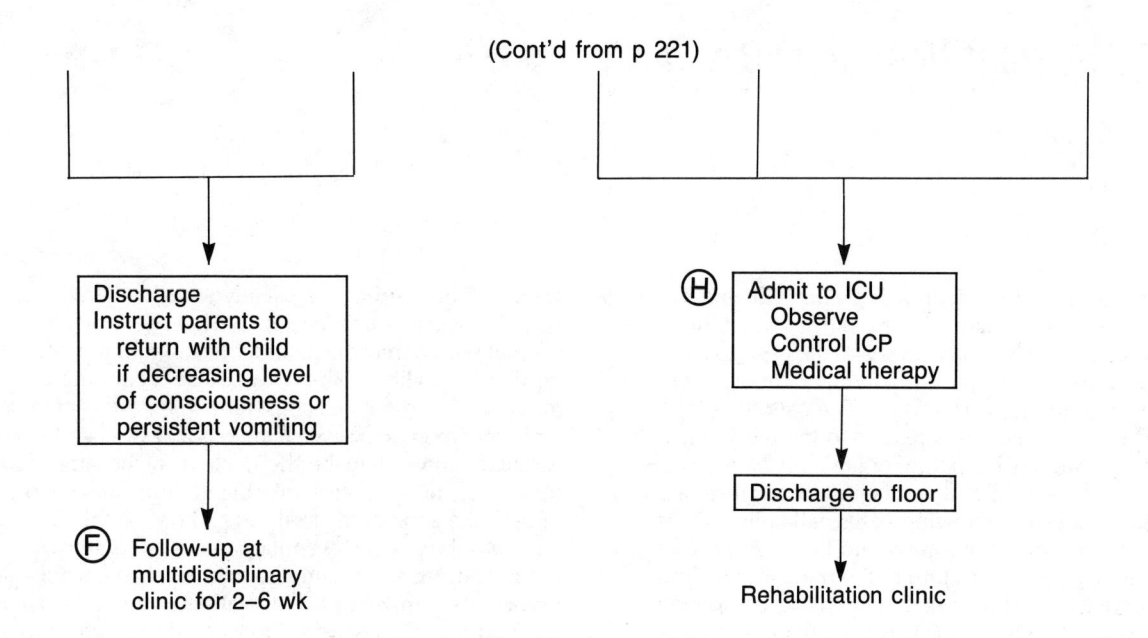

Discharge
Instruct parents to
return with child
if decreasing level
of consciousness or
persistent vomiting

Ⓕ Follow-up at
multidisciplinary
clinic for 2–6 wk

Ⓗ Admit to ICU
   Observe
   Control ICP
   Medical therapy

Discharge to floor

Rehabilitation clinic

PEDIATRIC THORACIC TRAUMA

Steven L. Moulton
Frank P. Lynch
Louann Kitchen

A. Several features of pediatric thoracic trauma distinguish it from the adult experience. These range from general considerations of small patient size and the need to tailor therapy accordingly to specific patterns of injury more common in children than in adults. The pattern of injury that is seen in children is related to the mechanism of injury and the flexible nature of the child's skeleton. Because a child's bony and cartilaginous structures are extremely pliable, compression of a small child's chest may cause major internal injury with little evidence of external injury and no fracture of the bony thorax. The greater mobility of a child's mediastinum may compound the degree of internal injury. This is particularly true of the infant, in whom wide shifts of the mediastinum can dislocate the heart or angulate and rupture the great vessels or major airways. The consequences of these pronounced cardiopulmonary derangements can be life threatening owing to major blood loss or air leak into one or both hemithoraces. Most chest injuries in children occur concomitantly with head or abdominal trauma. Thus, all children with significant trauma to the chest require a thorough neurologic examination with close follow-up and appropriate studies to rule out intra-abdominal injury. Treatment likely includes nasogastric decompression of the stomach to protect against aspiration and to decrease gastric dilation caused by aerophagia or bag-and-mask ventilation.

B. Because thoracic trauma can significantly compromise the cardiopulmonary status of the injured child, the diagnosis and management of thoracic trauma take high priority. The advanced trauma life support (ATLS) course of the American College of Surgeons continues to emphasize the ABCs of life support, as follows: Establishment and maintenance of an airway is the single most important immediate priority in the management of the multiple trauma victim. The next priority is to make sure that the patient is breathing or adequately ventilated if intubated under the guise of airway management. Circulatory status is quickly assessed and established, to complete the initial ABCs of life support.

C. Five thoracic conditions are *immediately* life threatening, and each must be excluded or corrected to ensure adequate ventilation and circulatory status. These include massive hemothorax, flail chest, tension pneumothorax, open chest wounds, and cardiac tamponade. All are relatively uncommon in children, with the exception of tension pneumothorax.

D. Massive hemothorax is uncommon in children and usually results from penetrating chest trauma, which may explain its frequent association with pneumothorax. The source of hemorrhage is usually a major intrathoracic vascular structure or a torn intercostal artery; either may present with hemorrhage under tension. In the event of tension hemothorax, the ATLS course recommends immediate placement of a chest tube to relieve ventilatory embarrassment. However, if there is an associated major vascular injury within the chest, release of the tamponade may result in uncontrollable bleeding or air embolus. Thus, if the appropriate facilities and personnel are available and the patient's ventilatory and circulatory status is adequate, massive hemothorax should be treated with immediate transfer to the operating room (OR). Then, if blood loss is massive on placement of a chest tube, an immediate thoracotomy can be performed.

E. Flail chest is rare in young children because the violent forces necessary to overcome chest wall pliability are usually fatal. If the child does survive, the diagnosis is clinically evident: the patient moves air poorly because of asymmetric and uncoordinated chest wall excursion. Although flail chest segments collapse on inspiration and impair ventilatory efficiency, instability of the chest wall is less important than pulmonary arteriovenous shunting through the underlying lung contusion. Hypoxemia is treated with supplemental oxygen, a limitation of crystalloid infusion, and frequently with intubation and ventilation. It is seldom necessary to stabilize the chest wall of a child.

F. Tension pneumothorax is the most common immediately life threatening thoracic injury in a child and can occur after any compressive injury to the chest. It usually results from pulmonary laceration, with or without fractured ribs. Tracheal and bronchial injuries may also result in tension pneumothorax and are more common in a child than in an adult. Respiratory distress is usually profound and may be associated with acute circulatory collapse, particularly if the child is intubated and on positive pressure ventilation. Treatment hinges on decompression of the affected hemithorax. This may be achieved with placement of an 18-gauge needle through the second or third intercostal space in the midclavicular line, without radiographic confirmation of the diagnosis. Initial decompression can be life saving and permits more controlled placement of a chest tube. Tube thoracostomy in the child is usually performed through the fourth or fifth intercostal space in the midaxillary line, with the tube directed posteriorly. Although it is usually impossible for the surgeon to place a finger through the narrow intercostal space of the child, the use of a trocar is ill-advised. Once the pneumothorax has been treated and circulation restored, a chest film is obtained to ascertain chest tube position and effectiveness.

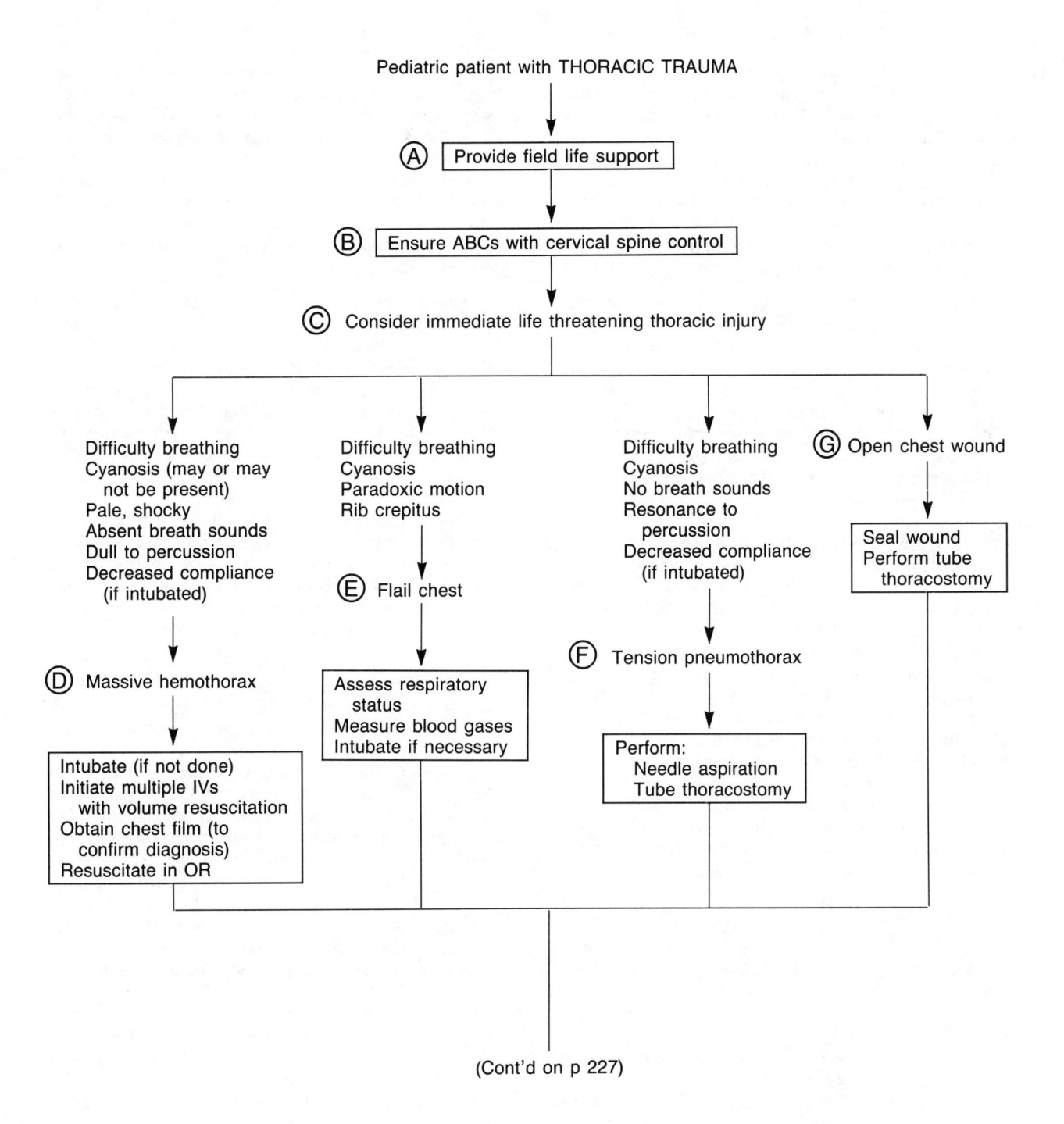

```
Pediatric patient with THORACIC TRAUMA
                │
                ▼
         (A) Provide field life support
                │
                ▼
         (B) Ensure ABCs with cervical spine control
                │
                ▼
         (C) Consider immediate life threatening thoracic injury
      ┌─────────────┬─────────────┬─────────────┐
      ▼             ▼             ▼             ▼
```

- Difficulty breathing
  Cyanosis (may or may not be present)
  Pale, shocky
  Absent breath sounds
  Dull to percussion
  Decreased compliance (if intubated)

  (D) Massive hemothorax

  Intubate (if not done)
  Initiate multiple IVs with volume resuscitation
  Obtain chest film (to confirm diagnosis)
  Resuscitate in OR

- Difficulty breathing
  Cyanosis
  Paradoxic motion
  Rib crepitus

  (E) Flail chest

  Assess respiratory status
  Measure blood gases
  Intubate if necessary

- Difficulty breathing
  Cyanosis
  No breath sounds
  Resonance to percussion
  Decreased compliance (if intubated)

  (F) Tension pneumothorax

  Perform:
    Needle aspiration
    Tube thoracostomy

- (G) Open chest wound

  Seal wound
  Perform tube thoracostomy

(Cont'd on p 227)

225

G. Open chest wounds are usually the result of penetrating chest injuries. However, they can occur as the result of blunt trauma, particularly with large avulsion injuries. If the chest wall opening has a larger diameter than the airway, air will preferentially pass in and out of the chest wall defect, nullifying ventilatory effort. The treatment of an open chest wound in a child is exactly the same as in an adult. The wound is sealed with a sterile occlusive dressing, and a chest tube is inserted to avoid development of a tension pneumothorax.

H. After the child's ability to ventilate has been restored, next in the order of importance is the restoration of circulation with volume resuscitation. Two large bore intravenous (IV) lines, preferably in the upper extremities, comprise the method of choice. In the severely hypovolemic child in whom percutaneous IVs are difficult to start, access may be obtained via the saphenous vein at the ankle or in the groin. The Seldinger technique is particularly useful for percutaneous femoral vein access in the small child. Fluid administration is well outlined in the pediatric section of the ATLS manual. A child's blood volume is approximately 80 ml/kg. If there is evidence of shock, the child has lost at least one-fourth of total blood volume. Therefore, it is recommended that the child with signs of hypovolemia receive an initial 20 ml/kg of Ringer's lactate as a fluid bolus. The volume of balanced salt solution required to replace lost blood is three-to-one. This fluid bolus regimen can be repeated four times. At this point, packed red blood cells with a volume of 10 ml/kg should be administered and may be repeated. It must be remembered that these are guidelines and that the endpoint is restoration of peripheral perfusion. If adequate volume has been provided and there is no response, one of two situations exists. Most commonly there is rapid, ongoing blood loss. Occasionally there is pump failure secondary to cardiac tamponade or severe myocardial injury. Evaluation of the cardiac status is indicated at this point, particularly if there is evidence of high central venous pressure, such as distended neck veins.

I. Cardiac tamponade caused by a penetrating injury is rare in children and frequently fatal. Blunt cardiac injury and major vessel disruption are other potential causes of cardiac tamponade. The patient usually presents with hypotension, a narrow pulse pressure, and muffled heart tones. Distended neck veins may be present on admission or after volume resuscitation. Cardiac tamponade must also be considered if bilateral chest tubes and fluid resuscitation do not result in a restoration of vital signs. Pericardiocentesis is both diagnostic and therapeutic; if any doubt remains, ultrasonographic examination confirms the diagnosis. Despite rapid diagnosis and immediate exploration, the mortality rate for blunt cardiac injury remains very high. Once the airway is secured, adequate ventilation has been obtained, and the circulation restored, the remainder of the primary survey is completed by performing a quick neurologic examination and exposing the patient.

J. The secondary survey consists of a careful head-to-toe physical examination with assessment of all injuries. Screening radiographs are obtained, including those of the lateral cervical spine, chest, abdomen, pelvis, and any indicated long bone views. During the secondary survey, *potentially* life threatening thoracic injuries are diagnosed. These include pulmonary parenchymal injury, airway disruption, diaphragmatic rupture, esophageal disruption, myocardial contusion with or without myocardial failure, and aortic disruption. Although all of these injuries result from compression or rupture of intrathoracic structures, and each may be overlooked during the initial examination, careful review of the chest film may suggest or confirm their diagnosis. Trivial injuries are also identified and treated. These include pneumothorax without tension, small hemothorax, and rib fractures.

K. Pulmonary parenchymal injury is the most common thoracic injury in a child. Clinical signs include subcutaneous emphysema, hemoptysis, or persistent air leak following chest tube placement. Types of pulmonary parenchymal injury include contusion, laceration, and hematoma, none of which can be differentiated with certainty on a chest film. Computed tomography (CT) is a sensitive means to diagnose different types of pulmonary parenchymal injury and can thereby guide appropriate therapy. The treatment of pulmonary contusion depends on the child's respiratory status. If shunting is minimal and oxygenation maintained, no real treatment is indicated. If pulmonary laceration produces a hemopneumothorax, a chest tube may be adequate treatment. If the child has a severe pulmonary contusion or laceration with significant alteration in oxygen delivery, intubation and ventilation are necessary. Pulmonary contusion and lung hematoma may be difficult to differentiate at the time of presentation. However, the hematoma may later cavitate, liquefy, and become an occult source of infection.

(Cont'd from p 225)

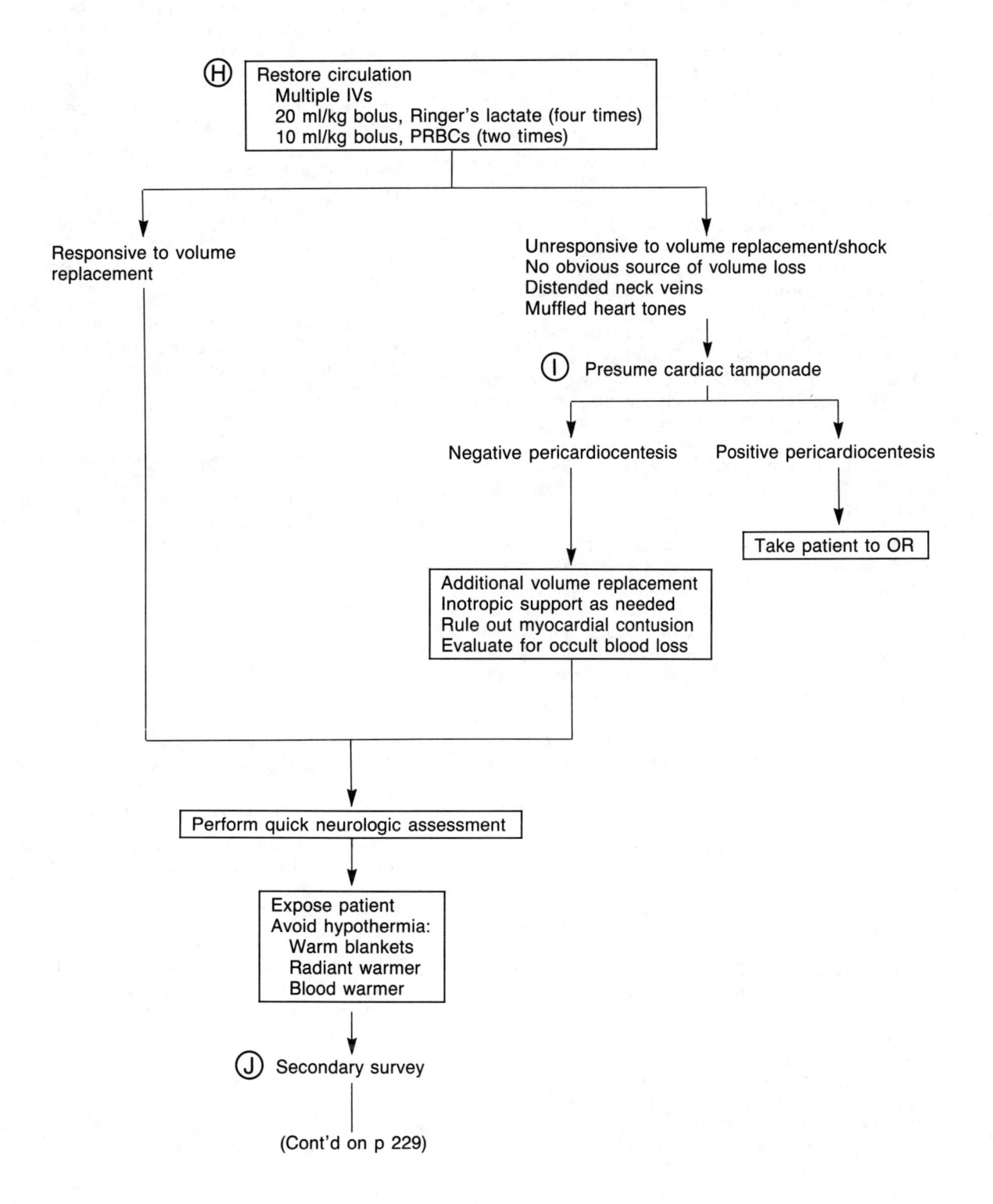

H — Restore circulation
- Multiple IVs
- 20 ml/kg bolus, Ringer's lactate (four times)
- 10 ml/kg bolus, PRBCs (two times)

Responsive to volume replacement

Unresponsive to volume replacement/shock
No obvious source of volume loss
Distended neck veins
Muffled heart tones

I — Presume cardiac tamponade

Negative pericardiocentesis

Positive pericardiocentesis → Take patient to OR

Additional volume replacement
Inotropic support as needed
Rule out myocardial contusion
Evaluate for occult blood loss

Perform quick neurologic assessment

Expose patient
Avoid hypothermia:
- Warm blankets
- Radiant warmer
- Blood warmer

J — Secondary survey

(Cont'd on p 229)

L. Airway disruption often presents as a tension pneumothorax. The tension pneumothorax should have been recognized and treated in the primary survey. The possibility of airway disruption is recognized in this situation by a large, continuous air leak from the chest tube. A chest film may reveal pneumomediastinum and perhaps a persistent pneumothorax with or without tension. Occasionally airway disruption occurs without a tension pneumothorax and presents with subcutaneous emphysema and pneumomediastinum. When airway disruption is suspected, the child should be taken to the operating room, where endoscopic evaluation of the respiratory tree will confirm the diagnosis. Airway disruption in a child is more common than in an adult, probably as a result of greater chest wall compliance and mediastinal mobility. Airway disruption usually consists of disruption of the membranous portion of the trachea, although bronchial tears are also well described. Definitive treatment is obviously determined by the anatomy of the injury. Repair of the membranous portion of the trachea can usually be performed by direct suture. If bronchial anastomosis of the small child's airway cannot be accomplished, pulmonary resection is indicated to avoid stricture formation and postobstruction atelectasis.

M. Diaphragmatic rupture nearly always occurs on the left side. It usually results from a severe compressive force to the abdomen with herniation of the abdominal contents into the left chest. The diagnosis is usually made on a chest or abdominal film. Findings include the presence of a nasogastric (NG) tube and/or the stomach in the left chest or a pneumothorax that has not been drained by a well placed chest tube; the diaphragm may be obscured or appear elevated. We have seen children on positive pressure ventilation with an initial chest film that was normal. In this instance the hernia was reduced by positive pressure ventilation, only to recur when the child was extubated. Treatment of diaphragmatic rupture in a child is the same as in an adult. It is best accomplished by direct suture repair through the abdomen because of the likelihood of associated intra-abdominal injuries.

N. Esophageal disruption or injury in a child is exceedingly rare and usually results from penetrating injury. Occasionally a child suffers esophageal rupture secondary to a severe compressive force on the abdomen against a closed glottis. The diagnosis of esophageal disruption should be considered in any patient with a pneumomediastinum or a left pneumothorax or hemothorax. The patient may have received a severe blow to the lower sternum or epigastrium and be in pain or shock out of proportion to the apparent injury. Particulate matter draining from a chest tube is a particularly ominous sign. Water-soluble contrast identifies most leaks. If the child is going immediately to the operating room for another more urgent condition, esophagoscopy by a competent observer will usually identify esophageal injury. The techniques of repair parallel those in the adult.

O. Children who sustain significant blunt injury to the myocardium usually demonstrate ECG changes, arrhythmias, elevation of cardiac enzymes, and/or evidence of myocardial injury on two-dimensional echocardiogram. These children should be appropriately monitored in the intensive care unit. Children who have elevation of cardiac enzymes without apparent functional defect should be monitored for arrhythmias during their early hospital course. Most children with myocardial contusion recover without sequelae.

P. Aortic disruption in a child is very uncommon and almost uniformly fatal. There are several reasons for this. A child's aorta is small and resilient, the mediastinum is mobile, and the sternum is rarely subjected to a direct blow (such as the steering wheel injury in an adult). Most children are either struck by a car, which results in dispersion of the compressive force over the entire body, or they are passengers, either restrained or unrestrained, within the confines of a car. Recent evidence suggests that when aortic rupture occurs in a child, it is usually the result of ejection from an automobile. The fact that aortic rupture is rare in children does not obviate its consideration. The signs of aortic rupture in a child are the same as in an adult. Radiographic findings may include a widened mediastinum, first or second rib fractures, apical cap, and deviation of the trachea to the right side. If there is any suspicion of aortic disruption, aortography should be immediately obtained. It is usually stated that only one in 10 adult aortograms will be positive; this figure should be lower in children. The treatment of aortic rupture consists of immediate repair through the left chest by a competent cardiac team. Recent evidence suggests that survival in a child requires more expeditious repair and is therefore more time dependent than in an adult.

Q. Trivial injuries, such as minimal pneumothorax, hemothorax, and rib fractures, can be diagnosed on chest film.

R. If a pneumothorax is small, and the child is not going to be intubated for any reason, it can often be followed clinically and radiographically. If the child will be undergoing general anesthesia for another reason, a pneumothorax is best treated with a prophylactic chest tube.

S. Blood in the thorax is best treated by removal. This is true in a child as well as in an adult. Although chest tubes can be placed in the resuscitation area, we have found that in the child it is helpful to insert them under anesthesia.

T. Rib fractures in a child usually require no treatment. Intercostal blocks can be used to lessen pain, as can epidural catheters. In most children, neither of these modalities is necessary.

References

Besson A, Saegesser F, eds. Color atlas of chest trauma and associated injuries. Oradell, NJ: Medical Economics Books, 1983.

Buntain WL, Lynch FP, Ramenofsky ML. Management of the acutely injured child. In: Maull KI, ed. Advances in trauma. Chicago: Year Book, 1987:43–86.

Eichelberger MR, Pratsch GL, eds. Pediatric trauma care. Rockville, MD: Aspen, 1988.

Eichelberger MR, Randolph JG. Thoracic trauma in children: symposium on pediatric surgery. Surg Clin North Am 1981; 61(5):1181–1197.

Haller JA. Thoracic injuries. In: Welch KJ, Randolph JG, Ravitch MM, O'Neill JA, Rowe MI, eds. Pediatric surgery. Chicago: Year Book, 1986:143–154.

(Cont'd from p 227)

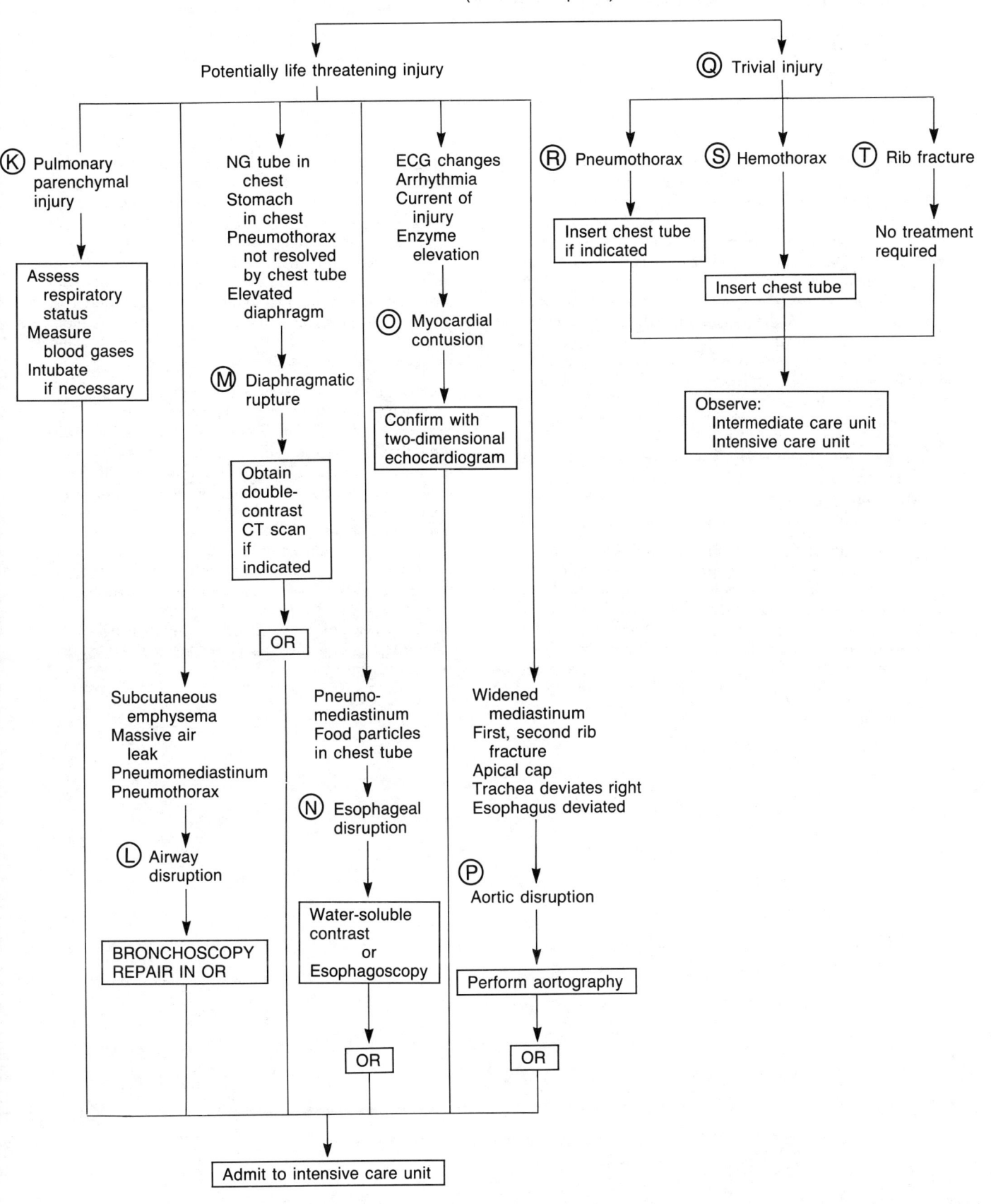

Potentially life threatening injury

(K) Pulmonary parenchymal injury
→ Assess respiratory status
Measure blood gases
Intubate if necessary

NG tube in chest
Stomach in chest
Pneumothorax not resolved by chest tube
Elevated diaphragm
→ **(M) Diaphragmatic rupture**
→ Obtain double-contrast CT scan if indicated
→ OR

ECG changes
Arrhythmia
Current of injury
Enzyme elevation
→ **(O) Myocardial contusion**
→ Confirm with two-dimensional echocardiogram

Subcutaneous emphysema
Massive air leak
Pneumomediastinum
Pneumothorax
→ **(L) Airway disruption**
→ BRONCHOSCOPY REPAIR IN OR

Pneumomediastinum
Food particles in chest tube
→ **(N) Esophageal disruption**
→ Water-soluble contrast or Esophagoscopy
→ OR

Widened mediastinum
First, second rib fracture
Apical cap
Trachea deviates right
Esophagus deviated
→ **(P) Aortic disruption**
→ Perform aortography
→ OR

→ Admit to intensive care unit

(Q) Trivial injury

(R) Pneumothorax
→ Insert chest tube if indicated

(S) Hemothorax
→ Insert chest tube

(T) Rib fracture
→ No treatment required

→ Observe:
Intermediate care unit
Intensive care unit

PEDIATRIC ABDOMINAL TRAUMA

Steven L. Moulton
Frank P. Lynch
Louann Kitchen

One of the principal differences between pediatric and adult abdominal trauma is the greater reliance on noninvasive means for evaluating children with suspected injury. This noninvasive strategy has extended into treatment practices, thereby allowing hemodynamically stable children with documented solid organ injury to be managed without operation. The guideline for this nonoperative approach is a high index of suspicion for abdominal injury because unique anatomic characteristics of the pediatric patient can lead to significant internal derangement with little evidence of external injury. One reason for this is the child's resilient skeleton, which is incompletely calcified and readily transmits kinetic energy to underlying structures. In addition, the child's smaller size causes linear forces from fenders, bumpers, or falls to be concentrated and absorbed over a smaller target area. Diminished body fat and the close proximity of multiple organs prevent these forces from being widely dissipated, thereby resulting in intense energy transfer to one or more intra-abdominal organs.

A. The majority of children who suffer multisystem trauma present with head injury, followed in decreasing frequency by limb fracture and torso trauma. Torso trauma includes thoracic and abdominal injury, which often occur together. The diagnosis and management of life threatening thoracic injuries occur during the primary survey, which is discussed on p 210. Evaluation of the abdomen is performed during the secondary survey. Significant intra-abdominal injury occurs in 25 percent of children who sustain multisystem trauma. The overwhelming cause is motor vehicle accidents, wherein children are either struck by a moving vehicle or are passengers within a vehicle. In fact, blunt injury accounts for 90 percent of pediatric abdominal trauma. The immediate treatment of abdominal trauma is primarily determined by the amount and rate of ongoing blood loss. Late complications are usually heralded by the development of peritonitis, which is caused by an unsuspected or delayed hollow viscus perforation.

B. During the secondary survey life support measures continue while a thorough examination is performed. This requires careful examination of the abdomen; keep in mind that injury to adjacent areas may confuse physical findings. For example, broken ribs in the lower thoracic region, contusions, pelvic fractures, and abrasions may manifest themselves as abdominal tenderness. In a traumatic situation many children are unable to localize pain within the abdomen, yet they can often confirm or deny its presence. Physical examination of the child may be further hampered by fear, apprehension, or regression to emotional lability. The examiner must therefore gain the child's confidence early and remember that physical findings are the most important key to the diagnosis of visceral injury.

Pediatric patient with ABDOMINAL TRAUMA

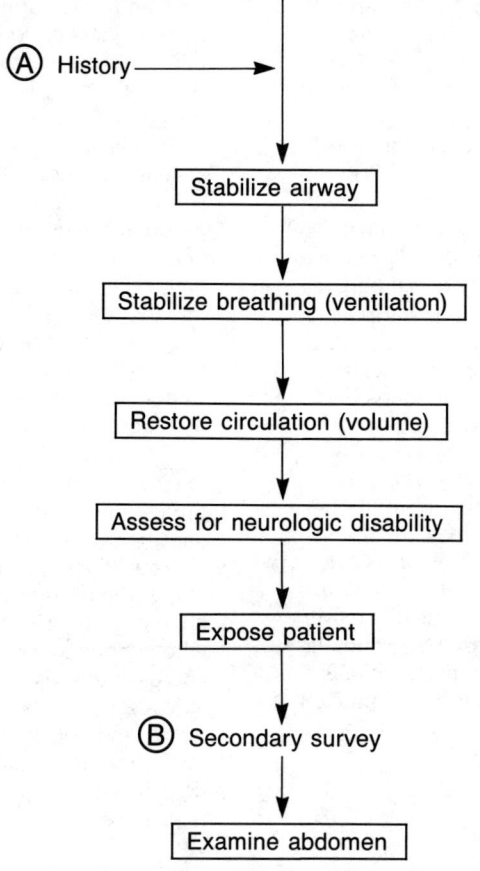

Ⓐ History ⟶

↓

Stabilize airway

↓

Stabilize breathing (ventilation)

↓

Restore circulation (volume)

↓

Assess for neurologic disability

↓

Expose patient

↓

Ⓑ Secondary survey

↓

Examine abdomen

(Cont'd on p 235)

C. It is easiest to classify patients based on their ability to respond. The child who can respond may be able to assist the examiner in determining whether a seemingly minor abdominal injury is getting better or worse. The child who is unconscious on admission must be assumed to have a significant intra-abdominal injury until proved otherwise. In either instance, findings such as contusions, abrasions, or tire marks may be evidence of solid or hollow organ injury. Volume status is reassessed along with the presence or absence of bowel sounds, abdominal distention, tenderness, and peritoneal signs. The presence of bowel sounds is highly suggestive of normal peristalsis, whereas their absence may be caused by aerophagia, ileus, or a primary intraperitoneal process. A careful rectal examination evaluates the status of the anal sphincter and the overall status of the intrapelvic structures and checks for the presence of blood in the rectal ampulla.

D. If there is no evidence of intra-abdominal injury, the conscious child may be followed with frequent, serial physical examinations. We typically obtain liver enzymes in these patients as a routine screening procedure. One of the most frequently missed significant injuries in our experience is a stellate laceration in the dome of the liver. We regard aspartate amino transaminase (AST) and alanine amino transaminase (ALT) levels of greater than 200 and 100 IU, respectively, to be markers of significant hepatic injury, which is easily confirmed by computed tomography (CT) scan.

E. In the child who is stable, yet suspected or assumed to have an intra-abdominal injury, a CT scan of the abdomen is relatively quick, noninvasive, and reliable. It is particularly useful for splenic, hepatic, and genitourinary system trauma because it provides a three-dimensional image of solid organ injury. Retroperitoneal structures, including the duodenum and major vessels, are well visualized; the one exception is the pancreas. The volume of blood loss into the peritoneal cavity or retroperitoneum can be estimated to assess the degree of injury further. Before leaving the resuscitation area and proceeding to the CT scanner, contrast should be instilled into the stomach by swallowing or through a nasogastric tube. In the absence of pelvic, perineal, or urethral injuries, a Foley catheter can be inserted and clamped to document extravasation from the bladder following the injection of intravenous contrast. If one depends on a CT scanner for the evaluation of intra-abdominal trauma, the scanner must be set up so that optimal care continues throughout the procedure. This requires an anesthesia machine, an oxygen saturation monitor, pressure transducers, and the appropriate readout equipment, along with resuscitative equipment and medications. The child must be accompanied in the CT scanner by those who performed the resuscitation; i.e., a pediatric surgeon and/or intensivist, pediatric trauma nurses, and a pediatric respiratory therapist. If these commitments to equipment and personnel are not possible within an institution, it is best to manage the child with diagnostic peritoneal lavage, followed by laparotomy if the lavage is positive.

F. A hollow viscus injury is difficult to diagnose with an abdominal CT scan. It should be suspected in any child who has free intraperitoneal fluid and no solid viscus injury. In this case peritoneal lavage may confirm the diagnosis. Occasionally free air or extravasated contrast material is present on the CT scan, but these are uncommon findings. Children who have lap belt injuries should be suspected of having hollow viscus injury until proved otherwise. In selected cases this may entail exploratory laparotomy in the presence of a negative CT scan and peritoneal lavage, particularly if a lumbosacral spine injury is present.

G. If the CT scan documents a solid organ injury that will require operative intervention for ongoing blood loss, or if there is a severe retroperitoneal injury such as a transected pancreas, the child obviously needs to go to the operating room. If, however, the child is stable and has a solid organ injury that can be easily managed with reasonable volume replacement, he or she can be transferred to the intensive care unit (ICU) for further management. This may include placement of invasive monitoring devices such as an arterial catheter or intracranial pressure transducer. The patient's hematocrit level should be checked approximately every 4 hours, depending on the rate of ongoing blood loss; keep typed and crossmatched blood readily available for transfusion. The importance of serial abdominal examinations by the same examiner cannot be overemphasized.

H. Diagnostic peritoneal lavage (DPL) is ideally suited for rapid evaluation of the abdomen; it is fast, inexpensive, and highly sensitive in detecting intraperitoneal bleeding. It is particularly useful in the neurologically impaired or hemodynamically unstable patient, the latter demonstrating a systolic blood pressure of less than 60 mm Hg, a heart rate of greater than 160 beats per minute, or a pulse pressure of less than 20 mm Hg in the presence of ongoing fluid resuscitation. The sensitivity of peritoneal lavage is the primary reasons that its use is relegated to the unstable patient. By comparison, routine peritoneal lavage for the evaluation of abdominal trauma leads to nontherapeutic laparotomy in greater than 20 percent of pediatric patients. This limitation in specificity, combined with the invasiveness of the procedure, illustrates the drawbacks of peritoneal lavage in the stable child. Before insertion of the lavage catheter a nasogastric tube should be passed to decompress the stomach, aspirate gastric contents, and assess for the presence of blood. The bladder should be decompressed with a Foley catheter if pelvic, perineal, and direct urethral injuries have been excluded.

I. A positive DPL may be indicated by initial aspiration of 10 ml of gross blood, an effluent red blood cell count of greater than 100,000, or an effluent white blood cell count of greater than 500. The effluent may also be evaluated for bile, bacteria, stool, or an elevated amylase level. If the peritoneal lavage is positive for a hemoperitoneum and the child is unstable, plans should be made for emergency transfer to the operating room. If, however, the patient's pulse and blood pressure stabilize in response to fluid resuscitation, the decision must be made as to whether this child requires a laparotomy. In some centers a hemoperitoneum in a stabilized child is used as an indication to obtain a CT scan. The CT scan allows the child's fluid requirements to be assessed in parallel with known intra-abdominal injuries, so that the need for operation can be more readily anticipated. The CT scan does not, however, accurately assess the amount and location of the child's hemoperitoneum, which is a combination of blood and lavage fluid. The danger in obtaining a CT scan after a positive peritoneal lavage lies in transporting the once unstable child to an area in the hospital ill-equipped to continue and perhaps reinstitute aggressive resuscitation. This risk can be reduced by setting up the CT scanner in such a way that the child's care is not jeopardized during the procedure. This requires the ready availability of appropriate monitoring devices, resuscitative equipment, and personnel. Any stabilized child with a hemoperitoneum who cannot be adequately monitored in the CT scanner should be taken to the operating room for an exploratory laparotomy. This is especially true of the head injured patient, whose neurologic outcome could be jeopardized by an episode of hypotension. A significant fall in blood pressure can occur 1 or more hours after injury, when the circulating volume diminishes to a point below which increased peripheral resistance can maintain arterial pressure.

J. Peritoneal lavage is performed in a child in much the same fashion as in an adult, except that the volume infused is 15 ml/kg. The subumbilical open technique is preferred, with the lavage catheter gently directed into the pelvis. If the peritoneal lavage is negative and the child remains in hemorrhagic shock, potential sources of extra-abdominal hemorrhage, such as pelvic or long bone fractures, should be investigated. If the peritoneal lavage is negative and the child is stabilized, further observation and monitoring are performed in the ICU. One should remember, however, that, if the peritoneal lavage is done shortly after injury, it may miss a subtle or delayed hollow viscus injury. Therefore, serial abdominal examinations are important even after a negative peritoneal lavage.

K. A child is deemed to have failed nonoperative management of an intra-abdominal solid organ injury if the amount of blood transfused in a 24-hour period exceeds 50 percent of the child's blood volume (assuming a normal blood volume of 80 ml per kg). Similarly, any child who develops peritoneal signs must be taken expeditiously to the operating room.

L. The intraoperative management of both solid and hollow organ injuries in children is similar to the adult experience. Splenorrhaphy should be attempted whenever possible to minimize the risk of postsplenectomy sepsis. Yet the amount of time required to complete splenorrhaphy must be titrated against the potential threat of prolonged operative intervention and evolving or poorly controlled hypovolemic shock. Hepatic injuries are best treated by simple debridement of devitalized tissue and direct vascular ligation. A duodenal hematoma is best managed without operation by employing hyperalimentation and nasogastric decompression.

M. If the child has a penetrating abdominal injury, an open wound with evisceration, or evidence of pneumoperitoneum, it is best to proceed directly to the operating room (OR). Moreover, if the patient has an extra-abdominal injury that requires emergent operative intervention, further evaluation of the abdomen can be performed in the operating room with DPL.

References

Buntain WL, Lynch FP, Ramenofsky ML. Management of the acutely injured child. In: Maull KI, ed. Advances in trauma. Chicago: Year Book, 1987:43–86.

Newman KD, Eichelberger MR, Randolph JG. Abdominal Injury. In: Pratsch G, ed. Pediatric trauma care. Rockville, MD: Aspen, 1988:101.

Peckham L, Kitchen L. Abdominal and genitourinary trauma. In: Connie J, ed. Pediatric trauma nursing. Rockville, MD: Aspen, 1989:102–118.

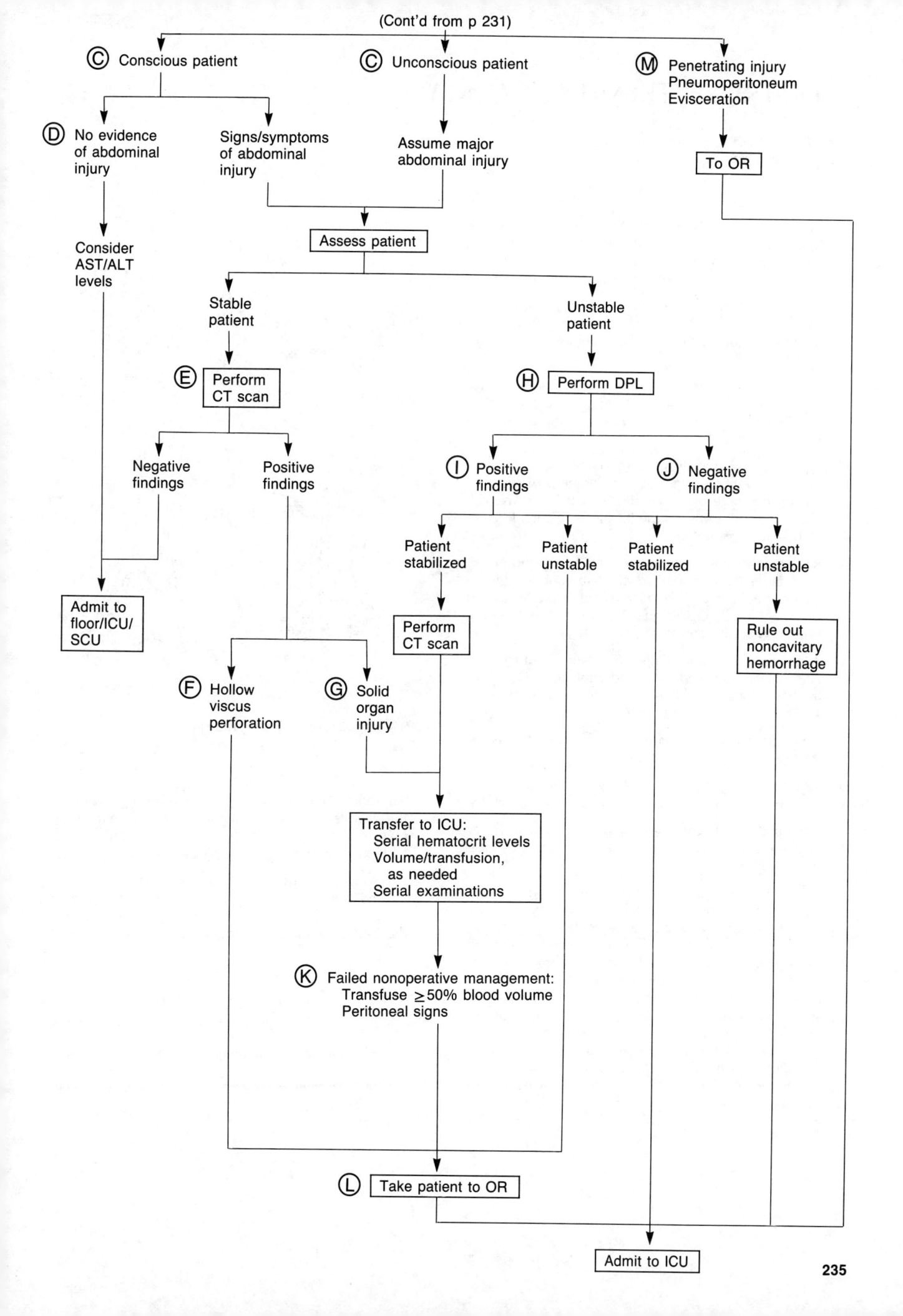

```
(Cont'd from p 231)
                    │
    ┌───────────────┼────────────────────┐
    │               │                    │
Ⓒ Conscious    Ⓒ Unconscious      Ⓜ Penetrating injury
   patient         patient              Pneumoperitoneum
    │               │                    Evisceration
    │               │                    │
┌───┴────┐          │                  ┌─┴──┐
│        │          │                  │ To OR │
Ⓓ No    Signs/    Assume major
evidence symptoms  abdominal injury
of       of
abdominal abdominal
injury   injury
│        │          │
│        └──────────┤
│                   │
Consider        ┌───┴────┐
AST/ALT         │ Assess │
levels          │patient │
│               └───┬────┘
│           ┌───────┴────────┐
│          Stable          Unstable
│          patient         patient
│           │                │
│         Ⓔ Perform       Ⓗ Perform
│           CT scan          DPL
│           │                │
│       ┌───┴───┐         ┌──┴────┐
│    Negative Positive  Ⓘ Positive  Ⓙ Negative
│    findings findings    findings     findings
│      │        │          │              │
│      │        │     ┌────┼────┐    ┌────┴────┐
│      │        │  Patient Patient Patient  Patient
│      │        │ stabilized unstable stabilized unstable
│      │        │    │                │
│      │        │  Perform             Rule out
│      │        │  CT scan             noncavitary
│      │        │    │                 hemorrhage
└──────┤        │    │
   Admit to    │    │
   floor/ICU/  │    │
   SCU        ┌┴───┐│
          Ⓕ Hollow Ⓖ Solid
            viscus   organ
            perforation injury
              │       │
              │       │
              │    Transfer to ICU:
              │      Serial hematocrit levels
              │      Volume/transfusion,
              │        as needed
              │      Serial examinations
              │       │
              │    Ⓚ Failed nonoperative management:
              │      Transfuse ≥50% blood volume
              │      Peritoneal signs
              │       │
              └───┬───┘
              Ⓛ Take patient to OR
                        │
                    Admit to ICU
```

PEDIATRIC EXTREMITY TRAUMA

Sally A. Knauer
John Tompkins

A. Information obtained from the patient, family or bystanders should include mechanism of injury, characteristics of the injury site including potential contamination, and previous medical illness or injury.

B. Assess extremities for deformity, swelling, wounds, perfusion, tenderness, sensation, crepitation (especially in the unconscious patient), active mobility, and range of motion.

C. Alignment or splinting of limbs should take place prior to transfer of the patient for any further diagnostic testing. The elbow should be stabilized in the position in which it is found.

D. Open wound management must include control of bleeding, antibiotic therapy, tetanus prophylaxis, and wound coverage until definitive surgical care may be accomplished. Consider the diagnosis of open fracture or traumatic arthrotomy.

E. Radiographs must include the joints above and below the established fracture. Growth plate injury should be clearly identified and classified regarding prognosis and treatment (Fig 1). Obtain an anteroposterior pelvis film, especially in the comatose patient.

F. A common and potentially devastating injury to the elbow is the displaced supracondylar fracture. Definitive treatment usually includes manipulation under anesthesia and percutaneous pinning.

G. Femur fractures are common and are usually treated by traction and subsequent casting.

H. Pelvic fractures may result in significant blood loss, retroperitoneal hematoma, or associated urologic injury.

I. Most pediatric fractures are managed satisfactorily by closed reduction and appropriate stabilization by casting or splinting.

J. Compartment syndrome occurs when tissue pressure rises above that of the capillary bed, thereby resulting in ischemia of muscle and nerve. Permanent paralysis or contractures may occur. Prompt recognition followed by loosening of any constrictive dressing or cast is critical. Fasciotomy may be necessary. Signs and symptoms include pain that is commonly increased by passive stretching of involved muscles, tense swelling of the involved region, and late signs of decreased sensation or weakness of involved muscles. Status of distal pulses or capillary filling does not identify compartment syndromes reliably. Compartmental pressure measurement may assist in diagnosis.

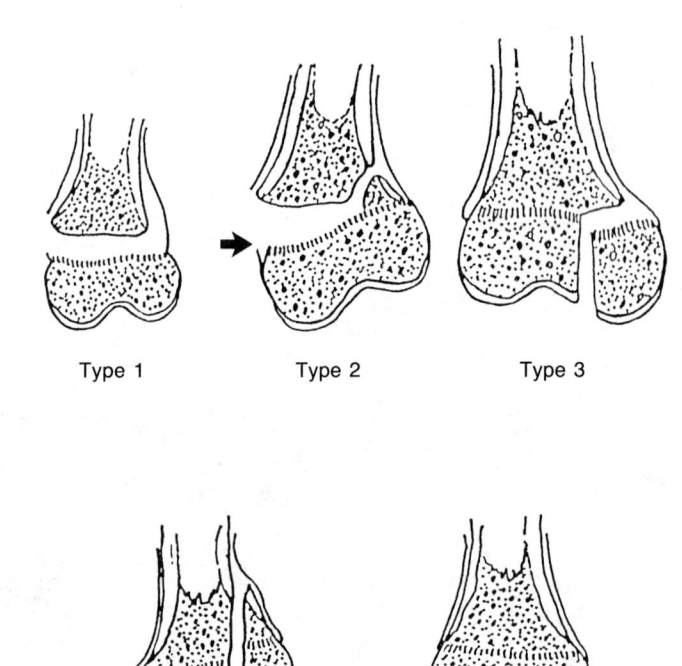

Figure 1 Classification of growth plate injuries.

K. Appropriate counseling of parents regarding severity of injuries and prognosis is an integral part of the management of orthopaedic injuries in the pediatric patient. Note growth plate injury implications.

L. Vascular status must be assessed and arteriography considered in suspected injury. Obtain appropriate vascular surgery consultation. Assess previously applied splint or dressing for possible tourniquet effect (see paragraph J).

References

Eichelberger MR. Pediatric trauma care. Rockville, MD: Aspen, 1988:133–144.
Marcus RE. Trauma in children. Rockville, MD: Aspen, 1986:32–35; 99–141.
Rockwood CA. Fractures in children. Philadelphia: JB Lippincott, 1984:117–138.

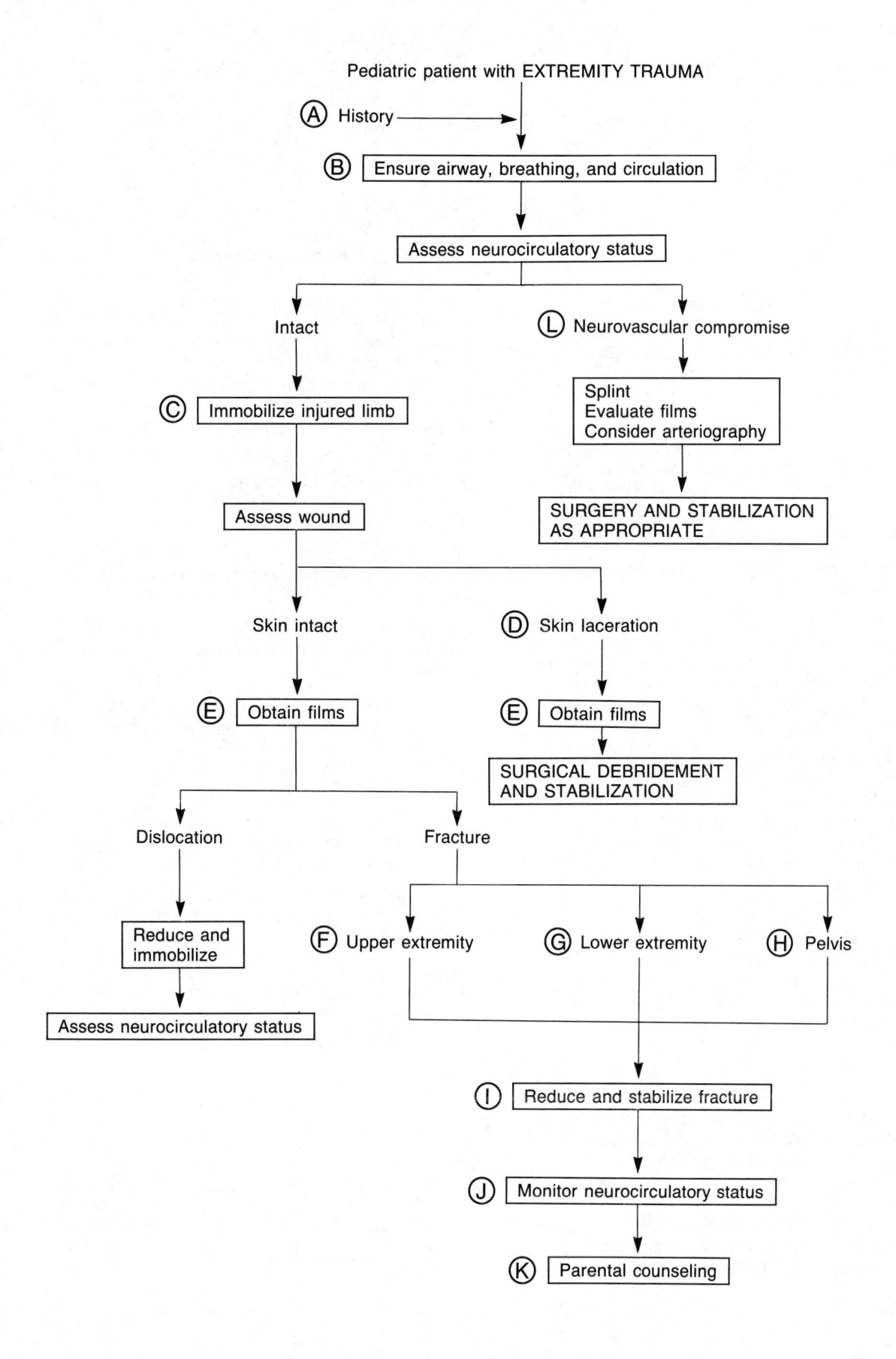

```
                    Pediatric patient with EXTREMITY TRAUMA
              Ⓐ  History ─────────→
                              ↓
              Ⓑ  │ Ensure airway, breathing, and circulation │
                              ↓
                  │ Assess neurocirculatory status │
                     ↓                         ↓
                  Intact              Ⓛ  Neurovascular compromise
                     ↓                         ↓
                                          │ Splint            │
              Ⓒ  │ Immobilize injured limb │   │ Evaluate films    │
                                          │ Consider arteriography │
                     ↓                         ↓
                  │ Assess wound │         │ SURGERY AND STABILIZATION │
                                          │ AS APPROPRIATE            │
                  ↓         ↓
             Skin intact   Ⓓ Skin laceration
                  ↓              ↓
              Ⓔ │ Obtain films │  Ⓔ │ Obtain films │
                                       ↓
                                  │ SURGICAL DEBRIDEMENT │
                                  │ AND STABILIZATION    │
              ↓           ↓
          Dislocation   Fracture
              ↓             ↓         ↓          ↓
        │ Reduce and │  Ⓕ Upper    Ⓖ Lower     Ⓗ Pelvis
        │ immobilize │   extremity   extremity
              ↓
        │ Assess neurocirculatory status │
                                      ↓
                              Ⓘ │ Reduce and stabilize fracture │
                                      ↓
                              Ⓙ │ Monitor neurocirculatory status │
                                      ↓
                              Ⓚ │ Parental counseling │
```

237

PEDIATRIC BURN TRAUMA

Gary F. Purdue
John L. Hunt

The pediatric patient with a burn has special problems not encountered in the adult.

A. The first consideration is to maintain airway, breathing, and circulation (ABCs). The very small airway of a child is at greater risk for sudden airway obstruction. Endotracheal intubation is often performed earlier than in the adult. Extreme care should be used in fixing the tube in place.

B. Initial assessment includes determining whether the injury occurred in a closed space, discovering the presence of facial and neck burns and associated traumatic injuries, and suspecting child abuse. If findings are positive for any of the above, immediate evaluation and treatment are required.

C. All clothes must be removed and the patient *accurately* weighed, preferably in kilograms.

D. Temperature maintenance is a critical part of pediatric burn care. Temperature should be closely monitored and maintained above 37°C. Adjunctives include keeping the patient continually wrapped in blankets, avoidance of fluids applied to the wound, heating of intravenous (IV) fluids, and use of heat shields over the bed.

E. The rule of nines does not apply to children, whose head and trunk sizes are relatively larger than extremity size. Lund-Browder or Berkow charts should be used. Estimation of burn depth is more difficult in children because of the thinness of skin. Scald burns that have a cherry red appearance beneath the blisters are usually full-thickness burns. Major and minor burns are differentiated in the same way as for adults.

F. Intravenous access is preferably done by a percutaneous peripheral route, which may be through burned tissue. All catheters are sutured securely in place. A nasogastric tube prevents acute gastric dilatation with subsequent respiratory compromise and risk of aspiration. A Foley catheter attached to a urimeter is necessary for the hourly evaluation of urinary output in all age groups. Diaper weights are insufficient for this evaluation.

G. Fluid resuscitation with nonburn maintenance fluids is calculated via the Parkland formula. It is necessary to maintain urine output at a rate of 1 ml/kg per hour. In children, especially those younger than 2 years of age, nonburn maintenance fluids are administered in five to 10 times larger doses than those for an adult. Endogenous glucose production is limited in children; therefore frequent serum glucose determinations (i.e., with Dextrostix) and the use of sugar containing intravenous fluids are required. Children are also sensitive to changes in sodium concentration and especially to hyponatremia; seizure activity may occur at levels below 130 meq/dl. Thus, daily maintenance is with 5 percent dextrose/0.25 normal saline, 1 ml per kilogram per percentage of total body surface area (TBSA) burned, plus nonburn maintenance. Evaluation of oral intake must be made and appropriate restrictions applied. Many other formulas are in use and may be selected by referral facilities.

H. Burn resuscitation mandates hourly or half-hourly evaluation of sensory and vital signs and urinary output with adjustments made to maintain the urine output at a rate of 1 ml/kg per hour.

I. The major burn—of full thickness and involving special body components (face, feet, hands, genitalia, or major joints)— should be referred to a burn center.

J. The burn should be debrided of all clothing, debris, and burn tissue. Burns of the palm or sole may have blisters left intact.

K. Partial-thickness burns are best treated by the application of a biologic dressing such as porcine xenograft or a biosynthetic material such as Biobrane. Deeper wounds or wounds of indeterminate depth are treated with silver sulfadiazine.

L. Burns are tetanus prone wounds. Immunization should follow the recommendations of the American College of Surgeons. Incomplete immunization is not protective.

M. Disposition of the patient is determined by burn size, body parts burned, patient age, and ability of the family to care for the burn. Each case should be individualized.

N. Children are more likely to develop neurovascular compromise in a circumferential burn than is an adult, and as a result, they may require escharotomy for circumferential deep partial-thickness burns.

References

Advanced Life Support Course. Lincoln, NB: Nebraska Burn Institute, 1987.

Hummel RP, ed. Clinical burn therapy: a management and prevention guide. Boston: John Wright, 1982:429–475.

O'Neill JA. Burns in children. In: Artz CP, Moncrief JA, Pruitt BA, eds. Burns, a team approach. Philadelphia: WB Saunders, 1979:341–351.

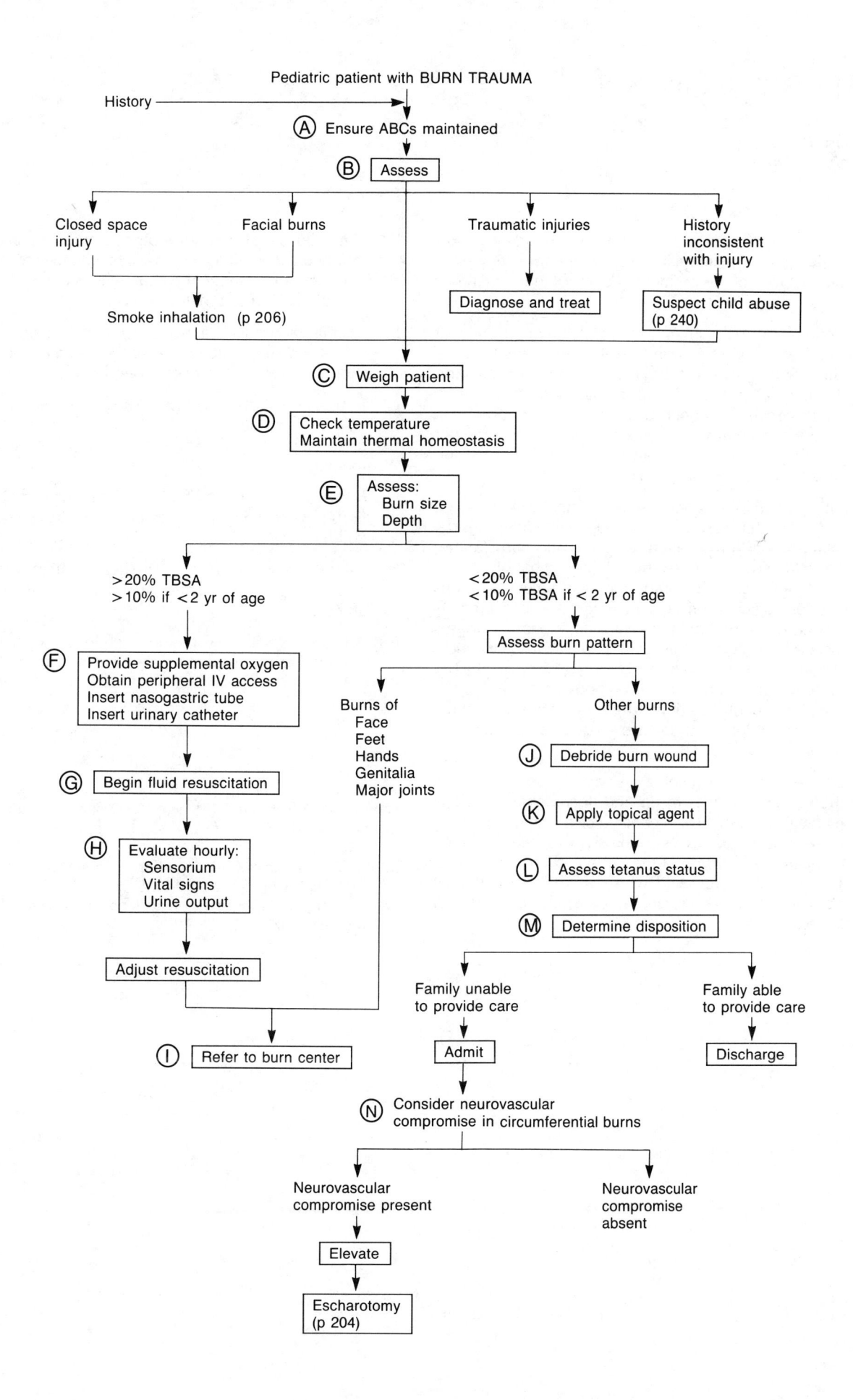

```
                    Pediatric patient with BURN TRAUMA
History ─────────────────────►
                         Ⓐ Ensure ABCs maintained
                              │
                         Ⓑ [Assess]
          ┌──────────────┬────┴────┬──────────────┐
    Closed space     Facial burns  Traumatic    History
    injury                         injuries     inconsistent
                                                with injury
          │              │            │            │
          └──────┬───────┘            ▼            ▼
                 ▼                 Diagnose    Suspect child
          Smoke inhalation (p 206)  and treat   abuse (p 240)
                 │
                 ▼
           Ⓒ [Weigh patient]
                 │
                 ▼
           Ⓓ [Check temperature
              Maintain thermal homeostasis]
                 │
                 ▼
           Ⓔ [Assess:
              Burn size
              Depth]
        ┌────────┴─────────┐
   >20% TBSA           <20% TBSA
   >10% if <2 yr of age <10% TBSA if <2 yr of age
        │                   │
        ▼                   ▼
                     [Assess burn pattern]
                     ┌────────┴─────────┐
                Burns of            Other burns
                 Face                    │
                 Feet                    ▼
                 Hands           Ⓙ [Debride burn wound]
                 Genitalia               │
                 Major joints            ▼
                                Ⓚ [Apply topical agent]
                                         │
                                         ▼
                                Ⓛ [Assess tetanus status]
                                         │
                                         ▼
                                Ⓜ [Determine disposition]
                                  ┌──────┴──────┐
                             Family unable   Family able
                             to provide care to provide care
                                  │              │
                                  ▼              ▼
                               [Admit]      [Discharge]
```

Ⓕ Provide supplemental oxygen
   Obtain peripheral IV access
   Insert nasogastric tube
   Insert urinary catheter

Ⓖ Begin fluid resuscitation

Ⓗ Evaluate hourly:
   Sensorium
   Vital signs
   Urine output

Adjust resuscitation

Ⓘ Refer to burn center

Ⓝ Consider neurovascular compromise in circumferential burns

Neurovascular compromise present → Elevate → Escharotomy (p 204)

Neurovascular compromise absent

239

CHILD ABUSE

Gary F. Purdue
John L. Hunt

A. History of the injury is an extremely important part of evaluation of the traumatized child. A completely plausible history of the accident is one of the hallmarks of an accidental injury.

B. An injury for which there is no explanation or one that varies with telling or with the teller is extremely suspicious. Self injury in a child under 6 months of age, inordinate delay in seeking appropriate medical attention, injuries occurring under suspicious circumstances, or a history of repetitive accidents (i.e., more than three per year that require medical attention) should raise suspicion of nonaccidental injury.

C. Although an injury completely consistent with the given history is rarely suspicious for abuse, certain injuries demand further investigation. Fractures and burns, either unexplained by mechanism of injury or out of proportion to mechanism of injury, and multiple or suspicious injuries suggest nonaccidental injury. The cutaneous aspects of injury should be evaluated, especially bruises that have characteristic linear or loop patterns that denote striking with a hard flat object, belt, or cord. The presence of multiple bruises on body parts that are seldom injured, bruises of varying ages, or bruises that occur on multiple body planes all suggest suspicion of nonaccidental injury.

D. Evaluation of the psychological reactions of the child and the child's family is made and documented. Lack of parental concern, lack of concern by the child for parental separation, and excessive passivity for age should be compared with those of the normal child in an emergency setting. The child who tells the examiner that abuse has occurred presents an imperative indication of abuse.

E. The child is evaluated for motor development and neuromuscular coordination consistent with the mechanism of injury. For example, the child who is unable to stand cannot climb into a bathtub.

F. A radiographic skeletal survey (i.e., "babygram") is performed on all children with suspected child abuse and should include skull, chest, long bones, and pelvis.

G. If suspicion exists and films are negative, then the skeletal survey can be repeated in 2 weeks. At this time, evidence of periosteal changes consistent with healing are looked for.

H. Meticulous recording of all conversations and observations is a necessity in the appropriate care of the abused child.

I. All states have laws that require health care providers to report suspicion of child abuse to the appropriate authorities.

J. All patients with a suspicion of child abuse should be admitted to the hospital unless cleared by the appropriate authorities.

References

Kempe CH, Silverman FN, Steele BF, Droegemueller W, Silver HK. The battered child syndrome. JAMA 1962; 181:17–24.

Reece RM, Grodin MA. Recognition of non-accidental injury. Pediatr Clin North Am 1985; 32:41–60.

Weller CMR. Assessing the non-accident, non-accidental injury. JEN 1977; 3:17–26.

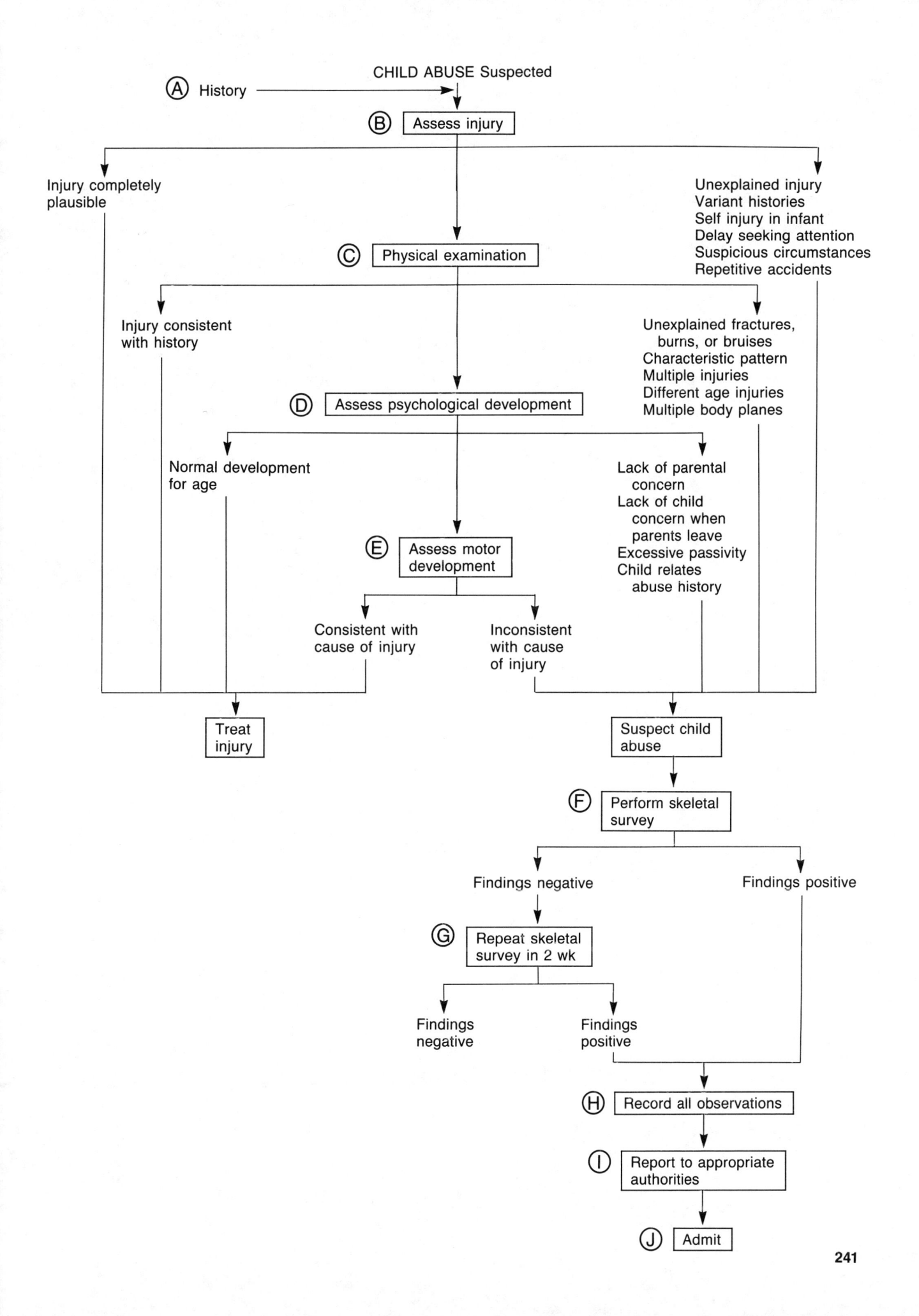

CHILD ABUSE Suspected

Ⓐ History →

Ⓑ Assess injury

- Injury completely plausible
- Unexplained injury
  Variant histories
  Self injury in infant
  Delay seeking attention
  Suspicious circumstances
  Repetitive accidents

Ⓒ Physical examination

- Injury consistent with history
- Unexplained fractures, burns, or bruises
  Characteristic pattern
  Multiple injuries
  Different age injuries
  Multiple body planes

Ⓓ Assess psychological development

- Normal development for age
- Lack of parental concern
  Lack of child concern when parents leave
  Excessive passivity
  Child relates abuse history

Ⓔ Assess motor development

- Consistent with cause of injury
- Inconsistent with cause of injury

Treat injury

Suspect child abuse

Ⓕ Perform skeletal survey

- Findings negative
- Findings positive

Ⓖ Repeat skeletal survey in 2 wk

- Findings negative
- Findings positive

Ⓗ Record all observations

Ⓘ Report to appropriate authorities

Ⓙ Admit

241

SPECIAL CONSIDERATIONS IN EVALUATION OF TRAUMA PATIENTS

Dog Bite
Animal Bite
Spider Bite
Snake Bite

Alleged Criminal Assault
Trauma in Pregnancy
Trauma in the Elderly
Trauma in the Homeless
Drowning and Near Drowning
Evidence Collection

DOG BITE

John A. Weigelt

A. The first decision that needs to be made is whether the dog bite was provoked or unprovoked. A provoked attack is most common. A careful history is often necessary to decide whether the attack was provoked. Despite the best history, it is often unclear whether the bite victim gave the animal cause to bite, and the episode must be considered an unprovoked attack.

B. If the bite is considered to be provoked, the wound should be cleaned as any laceration or puncture, and no rabies prophylaxis is given. Treatment of dog bites must emphasize debridement, irrigation, and appropriate antibiotic use. Debridement is the first step in reducing the infectious complications of dog bites. A reduction in infection from 17 percent to 7 percent was noted when adequate debridement was practiced. Irrigation of the wound after adequate local anesthesia can help in this debridement. However, puncture wounds are not easily treated in this fashion, and infection rates are higher.

Infection is a major risk of dog bite. An incidence of 6 to 13 percent is reported in bites that penetrate the skin. A dog's jaws exert a pressure of 200 to 450 psi, which results in a laceration and crush injury with devitalized tissue. The dog's mouth harbors numerous bacteria; all wounds are considered contaminated. *Pasteurella multocida* is commonly reported as a pathogen in 20 to 50 percent of infected dog bites. *Staphylococcus aureus* is isolated in 15 percent and *Pseudomonas* is isolated in 10 percent of infections.

Antibiotics remain controversial in the treatment of dog bites. Because so many bacteria are isolated from the bite wound, selection of an appropriate antibiotic is difficult. Suggestions include penicillin, penicillinase-resistant penicillin, cephalexin, erythromycin, tetracycline, and drugs containing beta-lactamase inhibitors. Our approach is to use penicillin for a maximum of 3 days.

Lacerations are closed whenever possible. A drain is often used and the wound loosely closed if swelling is excessive or if the wound penetrates deeply. All attempts are made to immobilize the wound with a bulky bandage or splint. Inspection of the wound is done at 24 to 72 hours. Puncture wounds are managed in the same manner. If the wound shows progression of swelling or inflammation at the first wound check, hospitalization, wound exploration, and intravenous antibiotics are added.

C. If the dog has a history of receiving rabies vaccine, no rabies prophylaxis is required. The dog should nevertheless be observed for a minimum of 10 days. If the dog's vaccination history is not known, the dog *must* be observed for 10 days and a decision made regarding rabies prophylaxis.

D. Major determinants for rabies prophylaxis after dog bites include whether the bite was provoked or unprovoked, the vaccination status of the dog, and the prevalence of rabies in the canine population in the immediate area. The latter two criteria are usually easily obtained. The decision regarding whether the attack was provoked or unprovoked requires a careful and thoughtful history. The territorial rights of dogs must be considered as well as what a dog may view as threatening. Thus, the biting of a deliveryman on the dog's back porch is unfortunate but is unlikely to be an unprovoked attack. Similarly, the toddler bitten when approaching the family dog's food is, in fact, a provoked attack. Unfortunately, these rational approaches are often forgotten when the decision to administer rabies prophylaxis is made.

It is believed that fewer than 20 percent of the 30,000 to 40,000 treatment courses for rabies given annually in the United States are necessary. The reasons for this incidence of treatment include the following: (1) rabies is always fatal, (2) physicians are unfamiliar with the recommendations for prophylaxis, (3) medicolegal considerations, (4) demand by patient or family, and (5) perception of the vaccine as more innocuous than the disease.

Human diploid cell vaccine (HDCV) is the vaccine of choice. It is superior to the duck embryo vaccine in potency, thereby causing fewer reactions and requiring fewer injections. The vaccine is given as a 1-ml dose on days 1, 3, 7, 14, and 28. Human rabies immune globulin (HRIG) can be given with the first dose (20 IU per kilogram of body weight). Serum is drawn to test for rabies antibody at the time of the last dose and then 2 to 3 weeks later. A titer of at least 1:16 is expected and considered protective.

E. If the animal is destroyed, the brain or parotid glands should be examined for Negri bodies. This examination is available through most Department of Health agencies.

References

American College of Surgeons. A guide to prophylaxis against rabies in exposed persons. Chicago: American College of Surgeons, 1982.

Anderson LJ, Winkler WG, Hafkin B, et al. Clinical experience with a human diploid cell rabies vaccine. JAMA 1980; 244(8):781–784.

Callaham M. Dog bite wounds. JAMA 1980; 244(20):2327–2328.

Greenberg JH. The new rabies vaccine. Texas Med 1981; 77:46–47.

Ordog GJ. The bacteriology of dog bite wounds on initial presentation. Ann Emerg Med 1986; 15:1324–1329.

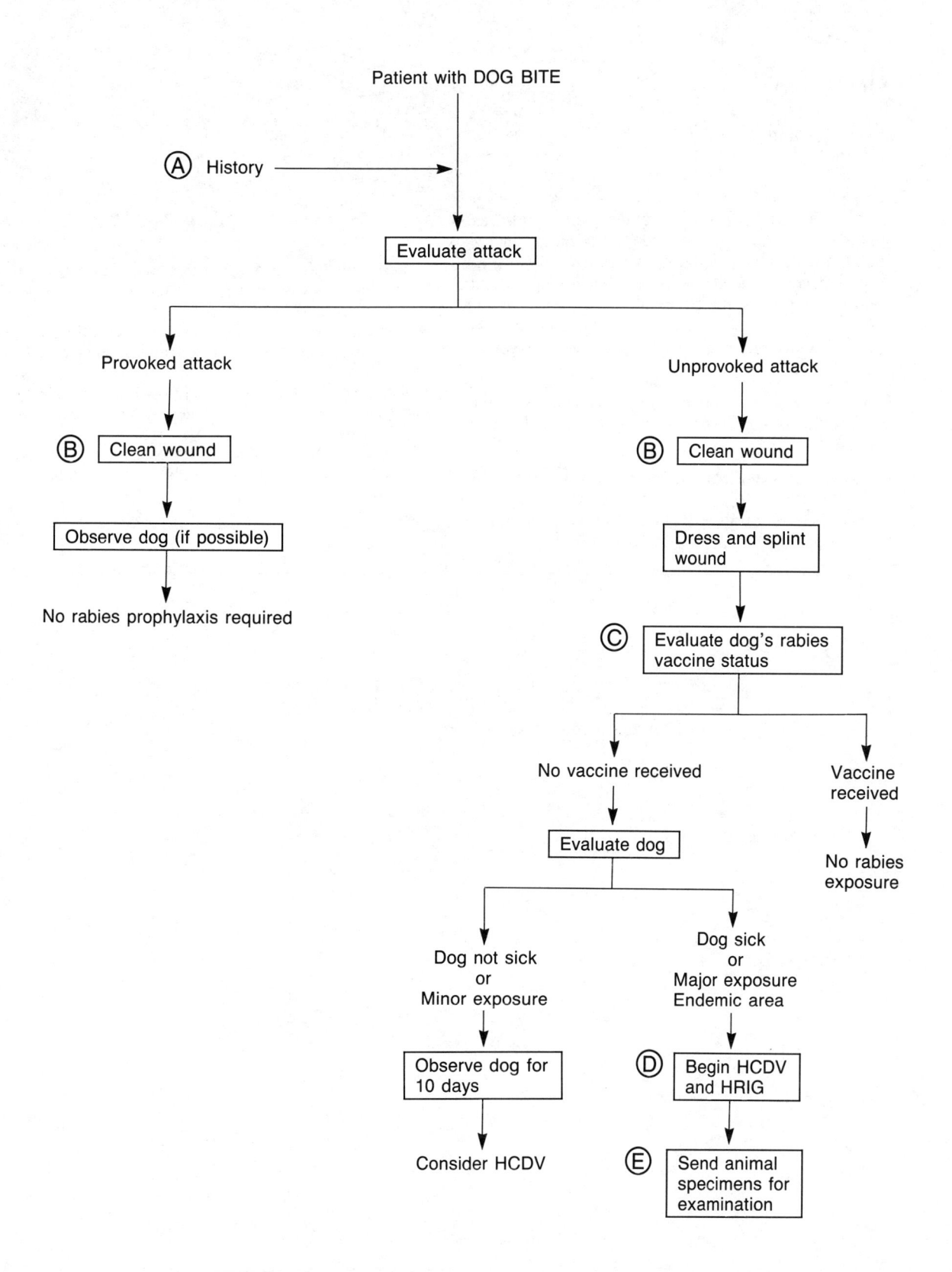

```
                    Patient with DOG BITE
                             │
          (A) History ──────→│
                             ▼
                      ┌─────────────┐
                      │Evaluate attack│
                      └─────────────┘
                       │           │
              Provoked attack   Unprovoked attack
                       │           │
                       ▼           ▼
                 (B)┌─────────┐ (B)┌─────────┐
                    │Clean wound│  │Clean wound│
                    └─────────┘    └─────────┘
                       │              │
                       ▼              ▼
              ┌──────────────────┐  ┌──────────────┐
              │Observe dog (if   │  │Dress and splint│
              │possible)         │  │wound          │
              └──────────────────┘  └──────────────┘
                       │              │
                       ▼              ▼
              No rabies prophylaxis (C)┌──────────────┐
              required                 │Evaluate dog's│
                                       │rabies vaccine│
                                       │status        │
                                       └──────────────┘
                                        │          │
                                  No vaccine    Vaccine
                                  received      received
                                        │          │
                                        ▼          ▼
                                 ┌───────────┐  No rabies
                                 │Evaluate dog│  exposure
                                 └───────────┘
                                   │        │
                              Dog not sick  Dog sick
                              or            or
                              Minor exposure Major exposure
                                            Endemic area
                                   │        │
                                   ▼        ▼
                            ┌──────────┐ (D)┌──────────┐
                            │Observe dog│   │Begin HCDV │
                            │for 10 days│   │and HRIG   │
                            └──────────┘    └──────────┘
                                   │            │
                                   ▼            ▼
                            Consider HCDV  (E)┌──────────┐
                                              │Send animal│
                                              │specimens  │
                                              │for        │
                                              │examination│
                                              └──────────┘
```

245

ANIMAL BITE

John A. Weigelt

A. If the animal is known to carry rabies, rabies prophylaxis should be offered. The most common animal bites associated with rabies include those of bats, skunks, foxes, and raccoons. Smaller animals, such as squirrels, rats, and rabbits, may be infected with rabies; however, they are not usually considered vectors of the disease. Other animal vectors include cows, horses, and wolves.

B. If the animal is considered to be a vector for rabies, human cell diploid vaccine (HCDV) should be used for rabies prophylaxis. HCDV is given on days 1, 3, 7, 14, and 28.

C. If the animal is available, tissue should be sent for examination for Negri bodies. The best tissue to send for analysis is brain or parotid gland. The tissue should be sent frozen and not placed in formalin.

References

American College of Surgeons. A guide to prophylaxis against rabies in exposed persons. Chicago: American College of Surgeons, 1982.

Anderson LJ, Winkler WG, Hafkin B, et al. Clinical experience with a human diploid cell rabies vaccine. JAMA 1980; 244(8):781–784.

Callaham M. Dog bite wounds. JAMA 1980; 244(20):2327–2328.

Greenberg JH. The new rabies vaccine. Texas Med 1981; 77:46–47.

Ordog GJ. The bacteriology of dog bite wounds on initial presentation. Ann Emerg Med 1986; 15:1324–1329.

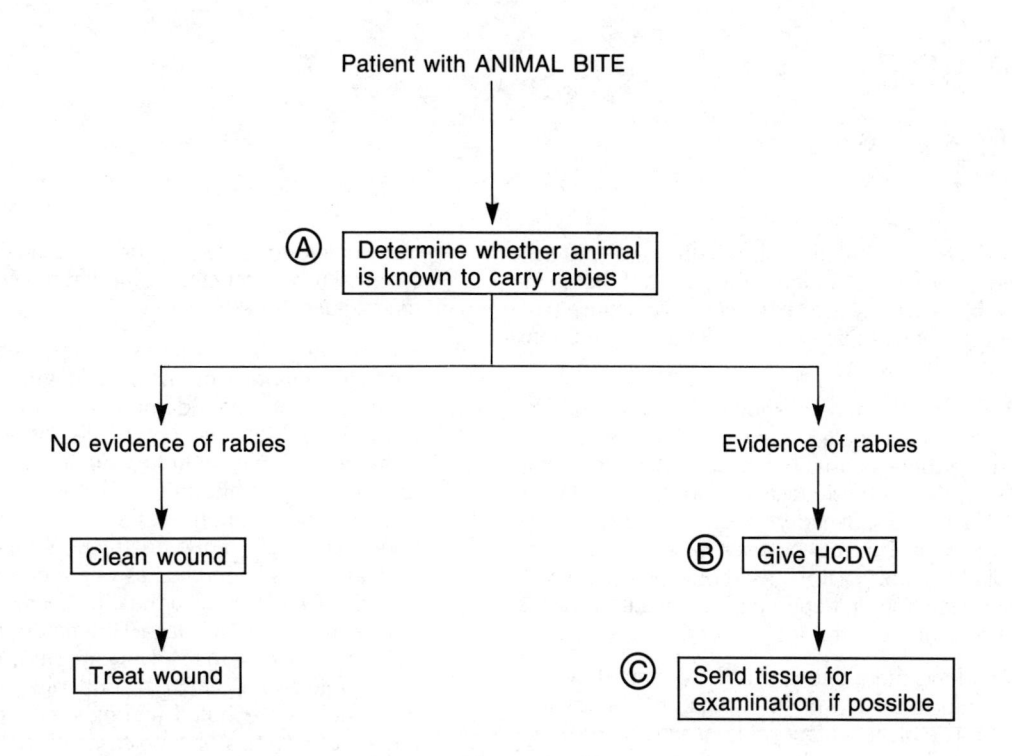

```
                    Patient with ANIMAL BITE
                              │
                              ▼
                    Ⓐ ┌─────────────────────────┐
                      │ Determine whether animal │
                      │  is known to carry rabies│
                      └─────────────────────────┘
                              │
              ┌───────────────┴───────────────┐
              ▼                               ▼
     No evidence of rabies           Evidence of rabies
              │                               │
              ▼                               ▼
        ┌───────────┐                 Ⓑ ┌──────────┐
        │Clean wound│                   │Give HCDV │
        └───────────┘                   └──────────┘
              │                               │
              ▼                               ▼
        ┌───────────┐                 Ⓒ ┌──────────────────┐
        │Treat wound│                   │Send tissue for    │
        └───────────┘                   │examination if possible│
                                        └──────────────────┘
```

SPIDER BITE

John A. Weigelt

A. The first decision to be made is whether the spider is venomous. Venomous spiders in the United States include the black widow (Fig. 1A) and brown recluse (Fig. 1B). Nonvenomous spiders may produce systemic signs consistent with anaphylaxis.

B. Patients bitten by spiders should be observed for anaphylaxis. An adequate history regarding previous insect or spider bites is usually present, although it may not be available. For severe local reactions, diphenhydramine hydrochloride (Benadryl), 50 mg parenterally, is usually sufficient. This may be given intravenously or intramuscularly. Anaphylactic shock should be treated with fluid administration and epinephrine. Injections at the site of the wound are not recommended.

C. A black widow spider bite is usually identified by having the spider available or by the patient's signs and symptoms. The black widow spider (*Lactrodectus mactans*) bite produces paresthesia, abdominal pain, and hypertension. Treatment is usually supportive. Intravenous fluids, muscle relaxants, and calcium gluconate are suggested. Antivenom is usually not required and has the complication of serum sickness.

D. The brown reclusive spider, *Loxosceles reclusa*, is a common inhabitant of the central and southern United States. The spider is 10 to 15 mm in length, light tan to brown in color, and has a species specific dark violin shaped band over the dorsal cephalothorax. The venom causes necrosis and hemolysis and contains a spreading factor that is probably hyaluronidase. Most bites are not noted by the patient. Several hours after the bite, a painful red area appears with a pale mottled cyanotic center that may blister. A hemorrhagic zone is present around the center, which is indurated and surrounded by a large area of erythema. Pain is severe at this time. Within 6 to 7 days, the center forms a black eschar that may slough and leave a central ulcer encircled by induration. Necrosis may extend under the skin edges.

E. Patients with brown recluse spider bites often do not seek medical attention until necrosis begins to occur. Surgical excision and debridement is often necessary at this time. When bites are seen earlier, other treatment options are available, including surgical excision, antibiotics, steroids, antihistamines, dapsone, antivenom, and expectant observation. All these treatments have proponents, although no one treatment is superior. The time to healing has been used as one measure of treatment success. The duration of healing averages 40 days and ranges from 1 to 360 days. The majority of wounds require 2 to 6 weeks to resolve. One study compared dapsone, antivenom, and dapsone plus antivenom. No differences were noted among these three groups in degree of necrosis or time to healing.

Surgical excision is attractive, although it can be hazardous. The most difficult aspect is judging the extent of tissue involvement. Often an adequate debridement is thought to have occurred, only to have the skin edges die and the wound ulcerate. This result is no better than the expected natural history of the bite. Additionally, some bites do not lend themselves to surgical excision and primary closure. Specific antivenom treatment seems most appropriate. Animal experiments demonstrate decreased lesion size when antivenom is used. However, antivenom is not commercially available at this time.

F. Occasionally, the bite undergoes necrosis or most commonly becomes secondarily infected. At this time, surgical debridement and antibiotic therapy are required. The necrosis can become severe, and tissue loss can occur. Initial wound care has been our most successful tech-

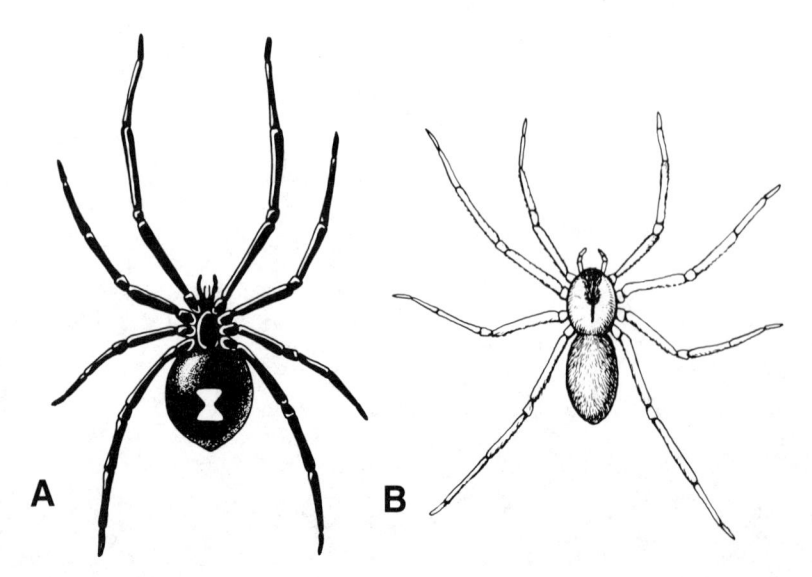

Figure 1 *A*, Ventral view of the black widow spider; *B*, dorsal view of the brown recluse spider. (Reprinted with permission from Gorzeman JA. Spider bite. In: Mancini ME, ed. Decision making in emergency nursing. Toronto: BC Decker, 1987:68.)

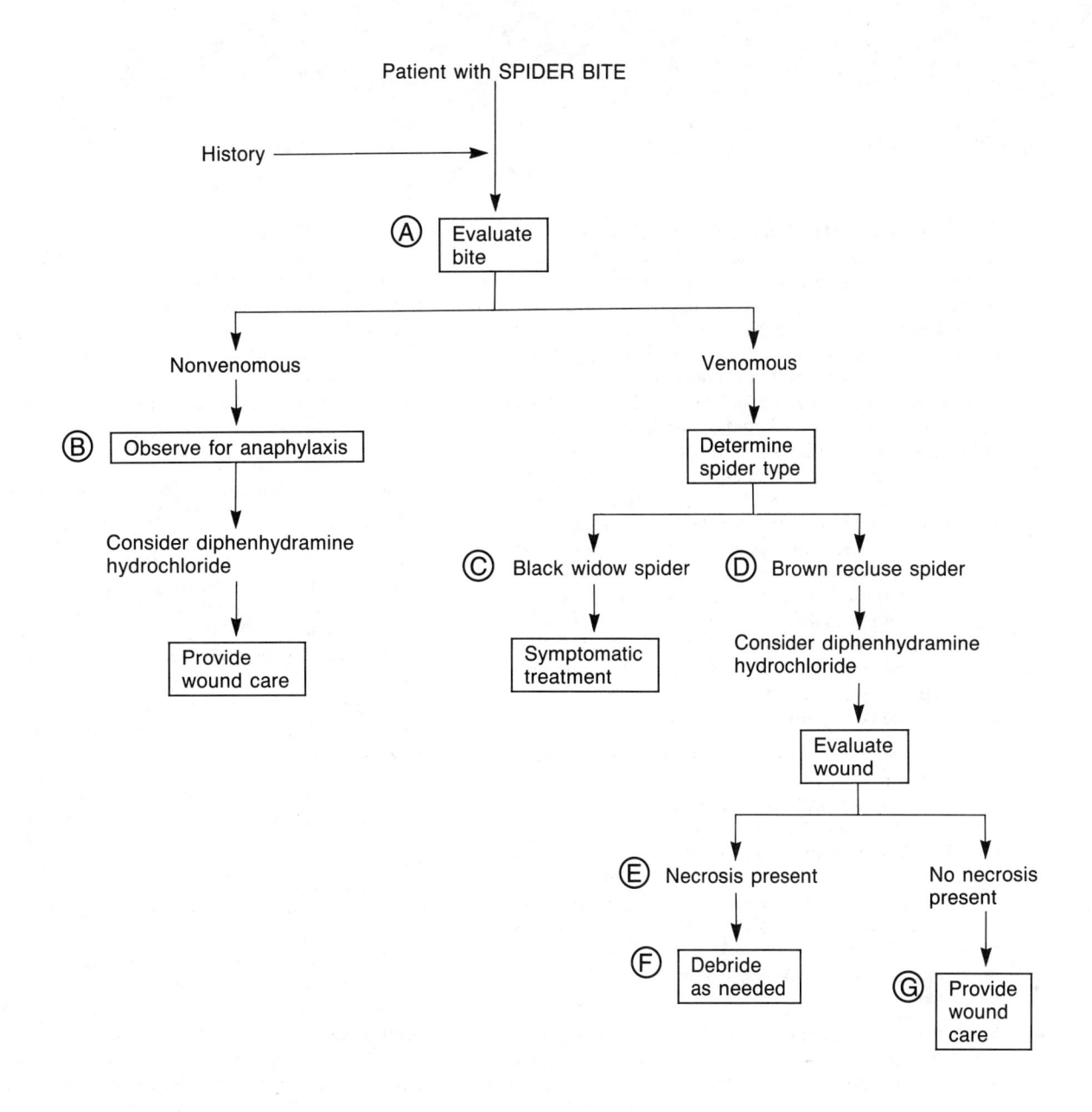

```
                    Patient with SPIDER BITE
                              │
        History ──────────────▶
                              │
                              ▼
                         Ⓐ ┌─────────┐
                           │Evaluate │
                           │  bite   │
                           └─────────┘
                    ┌──────────┴──────────┐
                    ▼                     ▼
               Nonvenomous            Venomous
                    │                     │
                    ▼                     ▼
              Ⓑ ┌──────────────┐     ┌──────────┐
                │Observe for   │     │Determine │
                │anaphylaxis   │     │spider type│
                └──────────────┘     └──────────┘
                    │              ┌──────┴──────┐
                    ▼              ▼             ▼
            Consider         Ⓒ Black widow   Ⓓ Brown recluse
            diphenhydramine    spider           spider
            hydrochloride        │                │
                    │            ▼           Consider
                    ▼       ┌──────────┐    diphenhydramine
               ┌────────┐   │Symptomatic│   hydrochloride
               │Provide │   │treatment │         │
               │wound   │   └──────────┘         ▼
               │care    │                   ┌─────────┐
               └────────┘                   │Evaluate │
                                            │ wound   │
                                            └─────────┘
                                         ┌──────┴──────┐
                                         ▼             ▼
                                   Ⓔ Necrosis    No necrosis
                                      present       present
                                         │             │
                                         ▼             ▼
                                   Ⓕ ┌────────┐  Ⓖ ┌────────┐
                                     │Debride │    │Provide │
                                     │as      │    │wound   │
                                     │needed  │    │care    │
                                     └────────┘    └────────┘
```

nique in avoiding tissue loss. Adjunctive therapy, except for administration of antihistamines, has not been helpful.

G. At present, management of brown recluse spider bites is best described as "do no harm." Management is also dictated by the time when the patient arrives for care. When the bite is seen early, a course of antihistamines and wound care are prescribed. This includes keeping the wound dry and clean. Topical antibiotic ointment can be used, although it is probably most useful as a way to ensure that the patient cares for the wound. The wound ideally progresses to a firm eschar, which heals in 2 to 6 weeks. If secondary infection is prevented, operative debridement is often not necessary.

References

King LE, Rees RS. Dapsone treatment of a brown recluse bite. JAMA 1983; 250(5):648.

Moss HS, Binder LS. A retrospective review of black widow spider envenomation. Ann Emerg Med 1987; 16:188–192.

Rees RS, Altenbern P, Lynch JB, King LE. Brown recluse spider bites. A comparison of early surgical excision versus dapsone and delayed surgical excision. Ann Surg 1985; 202(5):659–663.

Rees R, Campbell D, Rieger E, King LE. The diagnosis and treatment of brown recluse spider bites. Ann Emerg Med 1987; 16:945–959.

Rees RS, O'Leary JP, King LE. The pathogenesis of systemic loxoscelism following brown recluse spider bites. J Surg Res 1983; 35:1–10.

SNAKE BITE

John A. Weigelt

A. Most poisonous snakes in the United States are pit vipers, members of the family *Crotalidae*. Pit vipers include rattlesnakes, copperheads, and cottonmouths and account for 95 percent of all venomous bites. Coral snakes, of the family *Elapidae*, account for about 2 percent and exotic snakes for the remaining three percent. Identification of the snake is helpful but unfortunately not always possible. Care must be taken in handling suspected poisonous snakes, even when they are dead, because accidental inoculation by the fangs can occur. In general it is best to depend on the patient's history and symptoms to aid in deciding whether the injury is secondary to a poisonous snakebite. It is important to remember that at least 25 percent of pit viper bites result in no envenomation. Envenomation results in immediate pain and the rapid onset of swelling and edema, with ecchymosis of the area. Other systemic symptoms include nausea, vomiting, weakness, and hypotension. The degree of local and systemic symptoms helps to determine the presence of envenomation and its severity. A number of grading systems are used.

B. Grade 0 is equal to no envenomation and is identified by the absence of local or systemic symptoms. Grade I has local swelling and no systemic signs. Grade II has swelling that progresses beyond the area of the bite but no systemic symptoms. Progression is defined as being 10 cm or more above the bite. Grade III is characterized by systemic symptoms. This grading system helps to decide whether antivenom is administered. Antivenom is usually not required for Grade 0 and Grade I bites, whereas it may be needed for Grade II bites and is indicated in Grade III bites.

C. First aid measures include immobilization, limiting physical activity, placing a lymphatic tourniquet 5 to 10 cm above the bite, and incising and suctioning. Two mistakes include placing the tourniquet too tightly and making too vigorous an incision. The tourniquet should easily allow space for two fingers, and the incision should be single and placed over the puncture wound. The patient should be transported to a medical facility as soon as possible.

Hospital treatment should start with ensuring airway, breathing, and circulation (ABCs). Intravenous access is begun and the wound graded. In any Grade II or III bite, the following laboratory tests should be drawn: complete blood cell count, platelet count, prothrombin time, partial thromboplastin time, bleeding time, fibrinogen level, fibrin split products, creatinine level, serum electrolyte level, and urinalysis. If antivenom use is contemplated, a skin test should be performed immediately. Inject 0.02 ml intradermally of a 1:10 dilution of antivenom. A positive reaction shows a wheal and erythema.

If the patient is not in shock, the tourniquet may be released after the skin test is performed. If shock is present, the tourniquet can be left in place. Local excision of the bite and underlying tissue is occasionally helpful. The debridement should not sacrifice vital structures and should be limited to necrotic and ecchymotic tissue.

D. Antivenom should not be used routinely, because at least 25 percent of bites have no venom injected. The polyvalent antivenin is produced by Wyeth Laboratories. It is prepared from horse serum, and given as an intravenous drip. Antivenom is given until the symptoms subside. Pain is often the best symptom to follow. Antivenom may be given to allergic patients, if necessary. Patients should receive 50 to 100 mg of diphenhydramine and 100 mg of hydrocortisone intravenously. An infusion of 100 mg hydrocortisone can be titrated with the antivenom to control allergic symptoms. The most common allergic reaction is a pulmonary reaction manifested by wheezing.

E. Wound care is important. Necrotic tissue must be debrided; simple puncture wounds are kept clean. Patients are given penicillin for 3 to 5 days. Compartment pressures must be monitored and fasciotomies performed if pressures are elevated. Putting the bitten area at rest and beginning early physical therapy are important for a smooth recovery period.

Antivenom therapy can cause serum sickness. The incidence is directly related to the number of vials of antivenom administered. A 22 percent incidence is reported after 5 vials. Patients should be monitored for at least 7 to 10 days after antivenom administration. Joint pain, muscle pain, pruritus, rash, wheals, lymphadenopathy, and hematuria should be considered presumptive evidence of serum sickness. Most cases are mild and can be treated with antihistamines and steroids. Treatment with diphenhydramine, 25 to 50 mg three times a day, at the time of antivenom use and for 7 to 10 days afterward may block antibody formation and decrease the incidence of serum sickness.

Snake bite is a rare occurrence. Emergency departments should have a protocol established before the patient arrives. General knowledge of snake species and their habits in the community that the hospital serves is important. A resource for information should also be known. This might be a local medical facility or the local zoo. The Oklahoma City Zoo has long been a resource concerning poisonous snakebites.

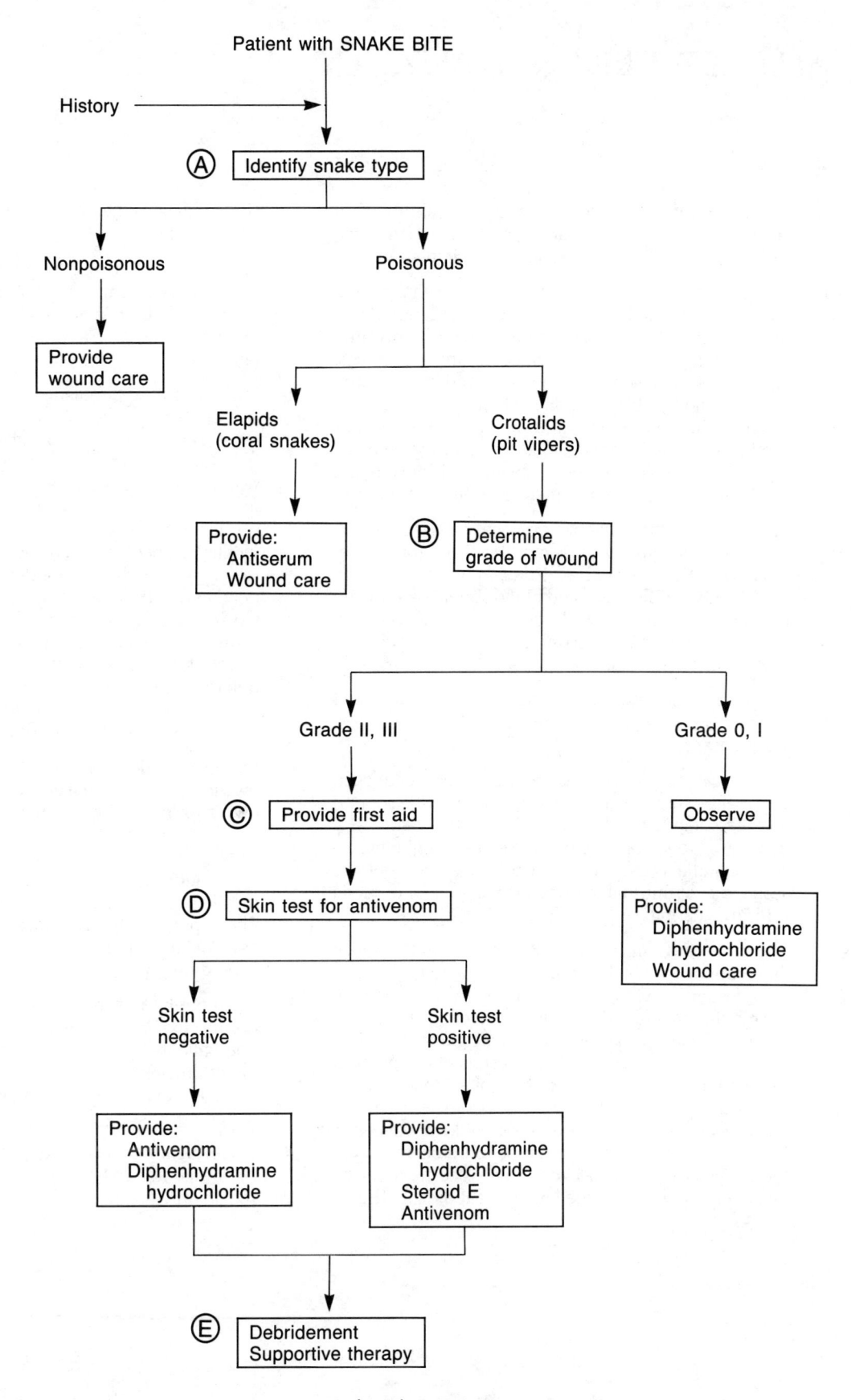

```
                Patient with SNAKE BITE
                         │
History ─────────────────▶
                         ▼
                  Ⓐ Identify snake type
                    ┌────┴────┐
              Nonpoisonous  Poisonous
                   │        ┌────┴────┐
                   ▼     Elapids    Crotalids
              Provide   (coral      (pit vipers)
              wound care snakes)        │
                          │             ▼
                          ▼         Ⓑ Determine
                      Provide:         grade of wound
                      Antiserum       ┌────┴────┐
                      Wound care   Grade II,III  Grade 0,I
                                      │           │
                                      ▼           ▼
                                  Ⓒ Provide    Observe
                                    first aid     │
                                      │           ▼
                                      ▼        Provide:
                                  Ⓓ Skin test  Diphenhydramine
                                    for        hydrochloride
                                    antivenom  Wound care
                                   ┌───┴───┐
                              Skin test  Skin test
                              negative   positive
                                 │          │
                                 ▼          ▼
                            Provide:    Provide:
                            Antivenom   Diphenhydramine
                            Diphen-     hydrochloride
                            hydramine   Steroid E
                            hydro-      Antivenom
                            chloride
                                 └────┬─────┘
                                      ▼
                                  Ⓔ Debridement
                                    Supportive therapy
```

References

Buntain WL. Successful venomous snakebites neutralization with massive antivenin infusion in a child. J Trauma 1983; 23(11):1012–1014.

Huang TT, Lynch JB, Larson DL, Lewis SR. The use of excisional therapy in the management of snakebite. Ann Surg 1974; 179(5):598–607.

Jurkovich GJ, Luterman A, McCullar K, et al. Complications of *Crotalidae* and antivenin therapy. J Trauma 1988; 28(7):1032–1037.

Pennell TC, Babu SS, Meredith JW. The management of snake and spider bites in the southeastern United States. Am Surg 1987; 53(4):198–204.

Russell FE. Snake venom poisoning. Philadelphia: JB Lippincott, 1980.

ALLEGED CRIMINAL ASSAULT

Patti Willis

A. Establish priorities based on injuries, the stability of vital signs, and on the mechanism of the traumatic incident. Maintain airway, breathing, and circulation.

B. The patient identified with an alleged criminal assault may present multiple problems. The aftermath of the assault becomes a personal crisis for the patient and family. Obtaining a history assists in determining priorities. The date of the last menstrual period and birth control status should be obtained from all female victims. Many patients will suffer associated traumatic injuries, such as attempted strangulation, aggravated assault, and penetrating trauma. It is imperative to obtain the history of the mechanism of injury to facilitate the evaluation process.

C. Management of the patient's oxygenation is reassessed. Shock management and hemorrhage control are re-evaluated. Replacement of lost vascular fluids with warmed crystalloid fluids and blood should be initiated if indicated. Precautions should be taken to preserve potential evidence when possible (e.g., cutting of clothes, placing of Foley catheter).

D. Priorities of care and definitive treatment are established on the basis of ongoing monitoring and continuous reassessment.

E. There are no age limits or gender restrictions for alleged criminal assaults. The trauma team must provide support and reassurance to all trauma victims. The victim may be too frightened or too embarrassed to describe the assault on initial presentation. The trauma team should be suspicious of unusual injuries such as vaginal or rectal bruising, tearing, or lacerations.

F. The victim must make a formal complaint to the Police Department for legal action to be initiated. A police record number will be given to the hospital for use on the medical records and evidence collection kit. The latter comprises a special kit with specific forms to be used for documenting the history and results of the physical examination. Be aware of the chain of evidence collection protocols. Once the examination process is initiated, the examiner should never let the evidence collection kit out of sight. When the examination process is over, the examiner will complete the forms, place the collected evidence specimens in the kit, and seal the kit. The kit should be taken by the examiner and given to the investigating officer or to the identified place.

G. The patient may be experiencing a wide range of emotions, ranging from hysteria and terror to apathy, shame, and/or guilt. Obtain and make use of appropriate emotional support, such as rape crisis or psychiatric consultation.

H. In the pediatric population, criminal assault is usually perpetrated by a person well known to the child. The most common form of assault is incest. Alleged criminal assault should be considered when a child presents with vaginal or rectal bleeding, lacerations, tearing, bruising, or foreign bodies in the vagina or rectum. There are two major types of sexual assault in children, as follows: fondling (either fondling of the child's genitals by an adult or forcing the child to fondle the adult's genitals) and penetration. Penetration may involve nonassaultive sexual intercourse or sodomy with the minor. The team should encourage the patient to provide a detailed account of the alleged incident. An anatomically correct doll may be helpful for the younger child to demonstrate actions that the child cannot describe. Be aware of specific regulations related to notifying child welfare.

I. Special consideration should be given to the male sodomy victim. Male sexual abuse is frequently not reported owing to the victim's embarrassment or unwillingness to admit the act took place. Special equipment may be necessary in examining the pediatric male with rectal penetration. The anal and rectal area must be evaluated to rule out mucosal tears, lacerations, and contusions. The appropriately sized anascope and proctoscope are essential in identifying injury. Support groups exist and should be contacted if the patient agrees.

J. Examine the patient as soon as possible on arrival to hospital to minimize physical and psychological injuries. The patient should be cautioned regarding the potential destruction of evidence, such as self-cleaning when going to the bathroom. Hand washing may remove evidence from nailbeds.

K. The evidence collection kit provides a consistent format by which to collect all necessary information and specimens.

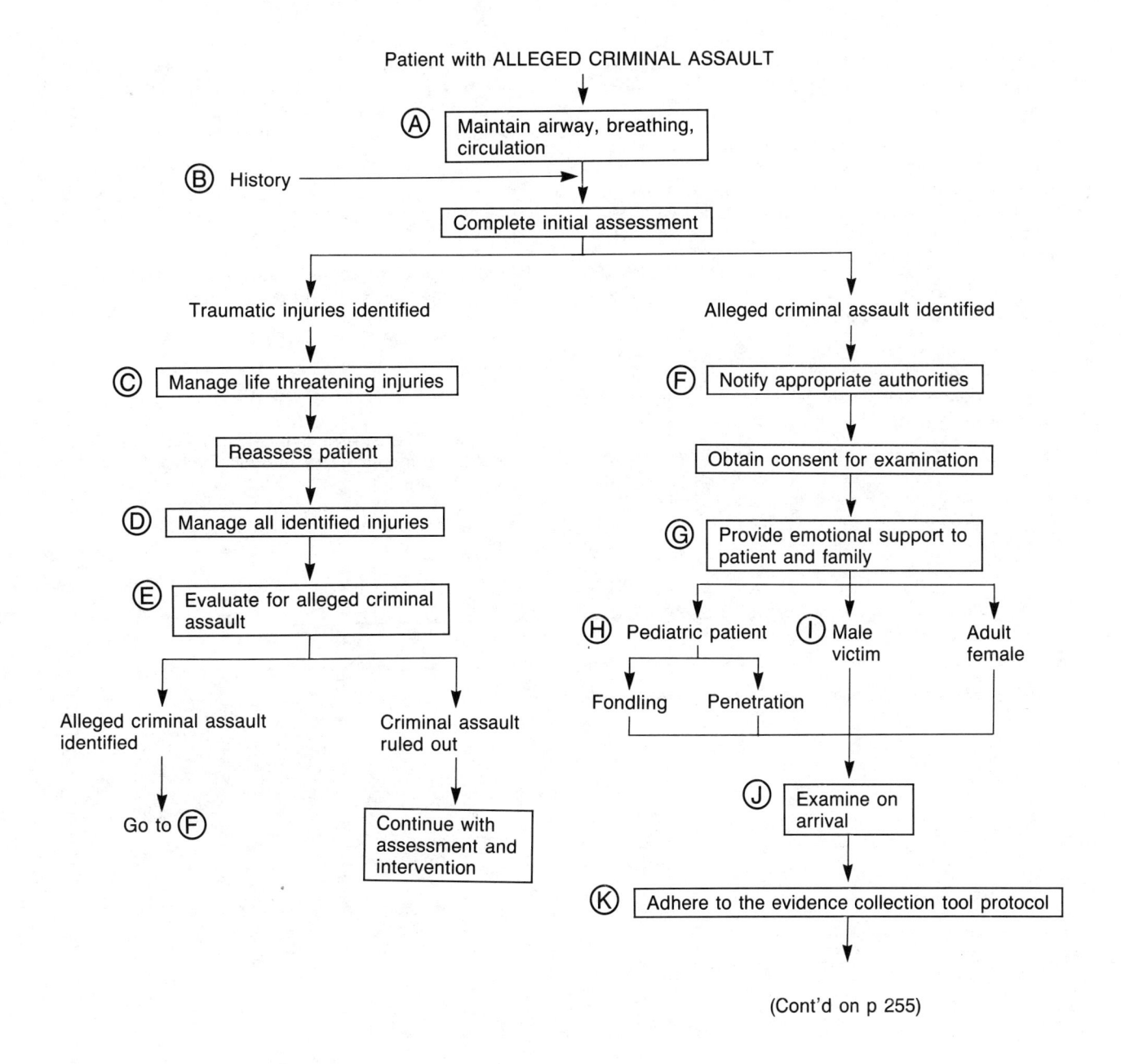

```
Patient with ALLEGED CRIMINAL ASSAULT
                    │
                    ▼
          Ⓐ  Maintain airway, breathing,
              circulation
Ⓑ History ─────────────►│
                    ▼
          Complete initial assessment
          ┌─────────┴─────────┐
          ▼                   ▼
Traumatic injuries    Alleged criminal assault
    identified              identified
          ▼                   ▼
Ⓒ Manage life         Ⓕ Notify appropriate
  threatening injuries    authorities
          ▼                   ▼
  Reassess patient     Obtain consent for examination
          ▼                   ▼
Ⓓ Manage all          Ⓖ Provide emotional support to
  identified injuries     patient and family
          ▼              ┌────┼────┐
Ⓔ Evaluate for         ▼    ▼    ▼
  alleged criminal   Ⓗ Pediatric  Ⓘ Male   Adult
  assault              patient     victim   female
     ┌────┴────┐     ┌───┴───┐
     ▼         ▼     ▼       ▼
Alleged     Criminal Fondling Penetration
criminal    assault
assault     ruled out
identified       ▼
     ▼      Continue with          ▼
   Go to Ⓕ assessment and    Ⓙ Examine on
            intervention         arrival
                                  ▼
                          Ⓚ Adhere to the evidence collection tool protocol
                                  ▼
                             (Cont'd on p 255)
```

L. It is helpful for the patient to undress while standing on a piece of clean white paper to identify hair, soil, or fibers that may be important evidence.

M. Place items in a paper bag. Do not use plastic, which encourages mildew formation. Steps should be taken to maintain the legal chain of evidence. The team should document in the legal and medical records what evidence was turned over to the authorities and who received the evidence.

N. The patient should be asked for permission to take photographs of any significant findings.

O. The examination should be done by a person experienced and trained in criminal examinations. Some facilities identify specific physicians or specially trained nurses for this role.

P. The specimens required are determined by the circumstances of the assault. They may include an aspirate or scraped specimen from any of the patient's orifices that may contain sperm of seminal fluid, any debris combed from the victim's pubic hair, or a cut specimen of the victim's pubic hair. Laboratory specimens should also be obtained for gonorrhea cultures, Venereal Disease Research Laboratories test, and blood types.

Q. The completed document and all specimens should be placed in the kit, sealed, and given to the investigating officer or carried by hand to the proper place by the examiner.

R. Prophylactic medications for sexually transmitted disease and for pregnancy should be administered.

References

Mancini ME. Sexual assault. In: Mancini ME, ed. Decision making in emergency nursing. Toronto: BC Decker, 1987:200–201.

Rund DA. Essentials of emergency medicine. Norwalk, CT: Appleton-Century-Crofts, 1982:405–406.

(Cont'd from p 253)

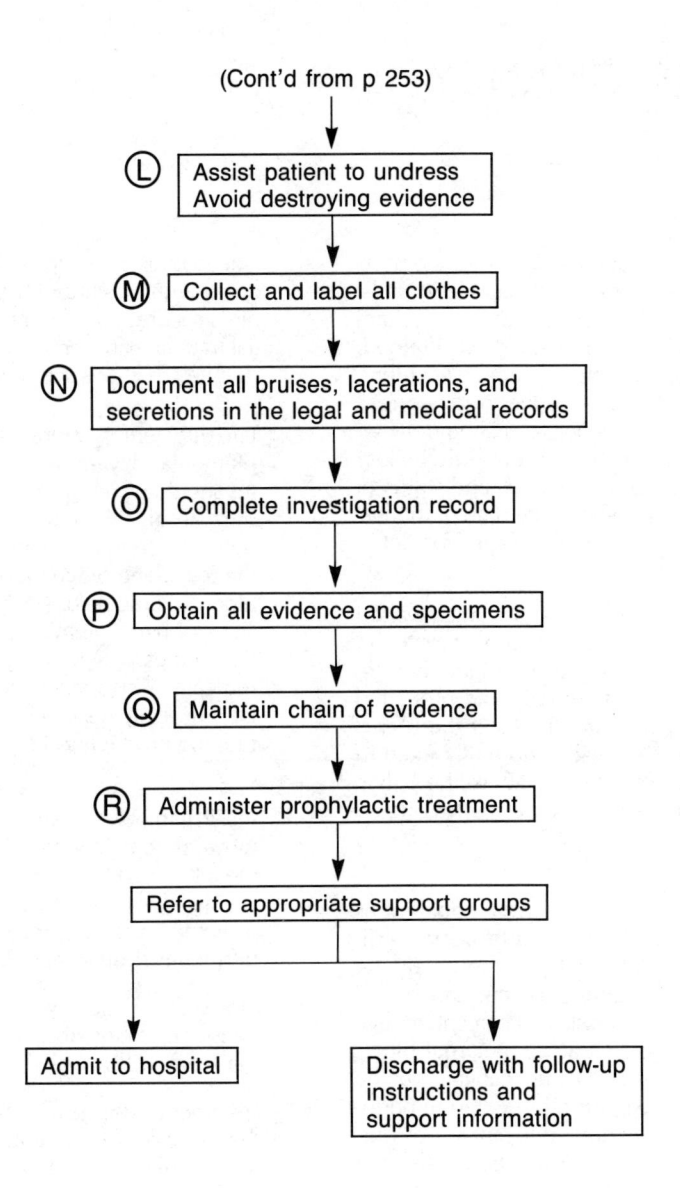

- Ⓛ Assist patient to undress
  Avoid destroying evidence
- Ⓜ Collect and label all clothes
- Ⓝ Document all bruises, lacerations, and secretions in the legal and medical records
- Ⓞ Complete investigation record
- Ⓟ Obtain all evidence and specimens
- Ⓠ Maintain chain of evidence
- Ⓡ Administer prophylactic treatment

Refer to appropriate support groups

- Admit to hospital
- Discharge with follow-up instructions and support information

TRAUMA IN PREGNANCY

Patti Willis

A. The most common cause of traumatic injury for the pregnant population includes motor vehicle accidents, falls, burns, and firearm injuries. The history of the mechanism of injury and preceding events should be obtained. In the mechanism of injury is a motor vehicle accident, identify whether the patient was a driver or passenger, whether she was wearing a seatbelt and shoulder harness, and the severity of the crash. An obstetric history including the gestational age of the fetus and status of the pregnancy must be established. The date of the last menstrual period is the most accurate factor for determining gestational age.

B. During the first trimester, the uterus is a thick-walled structure, confined in the bony pelvis. During the second trimester, the uterus leaves its protected intrapelvic location. The small fetus is freely mobile and protected by the amniotic fluid. By the third trimester the uterus is large and thin walled. The head is normally fixed in the pelvis, and the body of the fetus is above the pelvic rim. The placental vasculature is normally dilated throughout gestation and is extremely sensitive to catecholamine stimulation.

C. Physiologic changes during pregnancy are apparent as early as 10-weeks gestation. After the tenth week, cardiac output is increased by 1.0 to 1.5 L per minute. By the thirty-fourth week, the circulatory volume can be increased by 50 percent and can mask a 30 percent gradual blood loss or a 10 to 15 percent acute maternal blood loss. Maternal vital signs may remain unchanged, but the fetus may be at risk because of decreased uterine perfusion. The white blood cell count (WBC) increases during pregnancy to a high of 20,000. Serum fibrinogen and clotting factors are elevated. Prothrombin and partial thromboplastin times may be shortened, but bleeding and clotting times are unchanged. The serum albumin level falls to 2.2 to 2.8 meq per deciliter, thereby causing a drop in serum protein levels. Serum osmolarity remains 280 mOsm per liter. The respiratory system is also altered during pregnancy. Upper respiratory passages become engorged by capillaries. The respiratory rate may remain unchanged or increase by 15 percent. Tidal volume increases by 40 percent, and the residual volume falls. The hyperventilation state of pregnancy produces arterial blood gas alterations. $PaCO_2$ levels drop to 25 to 30 mm Hg and PaO_2 increases to 101 to 104 mm Hg. A normal pH level is maintained by the excretion of bicarbonate via the kidneys. The respiratory changes predispose the patient to hypoxia. Gastric emptying is greatly prolonged during pregnancy. There is an increase in the glomerular filtration rate and in the renal plasma blood flow. Creatinine and blood, urea, nitrogen levels may fall to 50 percent of the normal level. Eclampsia may mimic a head injury. Eclampsia should be considered if seizures occur with or without hypertension, especially if hyperplexia is present. The trauma team must understand initial trauma management and intervention and the normal changes that occur during pregnancy.

D. Life threatening injuries are managed as identified. Supplemental oxygen is administered. The circulatory status should be monitored closely because of the increased intravascular volume and the rapid contraction of the uteroplacental circulation that shunts blood away from the fetus. The pregnant patient may loose 35 percent of blood volume before tachycardia, hypotension, and other signs of hypovolemia occur. Crystalloid fluid resuscitation and early type-specific blood administration may be indicated. Vasopressor administration should be avoided. These agents can further reduce uterine blood flow, thereby producing fetal hypoxia.

E. The evaluation includes vital signs, an assessment of uterine irritability, fundal height and tenderness, and fetal movement. A Doppler device should be used to assess the fetal heart tones (FHTs) for 2 full minutes to identify any decelerations. The uterus should be monitored closely for the presence of contractions. Evaluation of the perineum should include a formal pelvic examination.

F. The stable patient with no significant trauma may be transferred to the obstetric floor for monitoring. The trauma team will act as the consulting service.

G. Treatment priorities for an injured pregnant patient are the same as for any trauma patient. Airway, breathing, and circulation must be quickly assessed and managed appropriately. If intubation is indicated, the use of nasal airways or endotracheal tubes should be avoided to prevent nasal bleeding. Intubation should be done with a smaller (6.0 mm to 6.5 mm) well lubricated endotracheal tube. Monitoring the central venous pressure (CVP) response to shock management is valuable in maintaining the relative hypervolemia required for fetal perfusion.

H. Supine hypotension may be misleading. The vena cava syndrome reduces venous return to the heart and decreases cardiac output, thereby aggravating the shock state. The pregnant patient should be evaluated and transported with the right hip elevated to displace the uterus to the left. Vena cava compression in the supine position may decrease cardiac output by 30 to 40 percent. If hypotension dissipates with changes in position, immediately reassess and evaluate for fluid resuscitation needs. If there is no hemodynamic change with position change, the team should proceed with shock therapy and ongoing assessment.

Patient with TRAUMA IN PREGNANCY

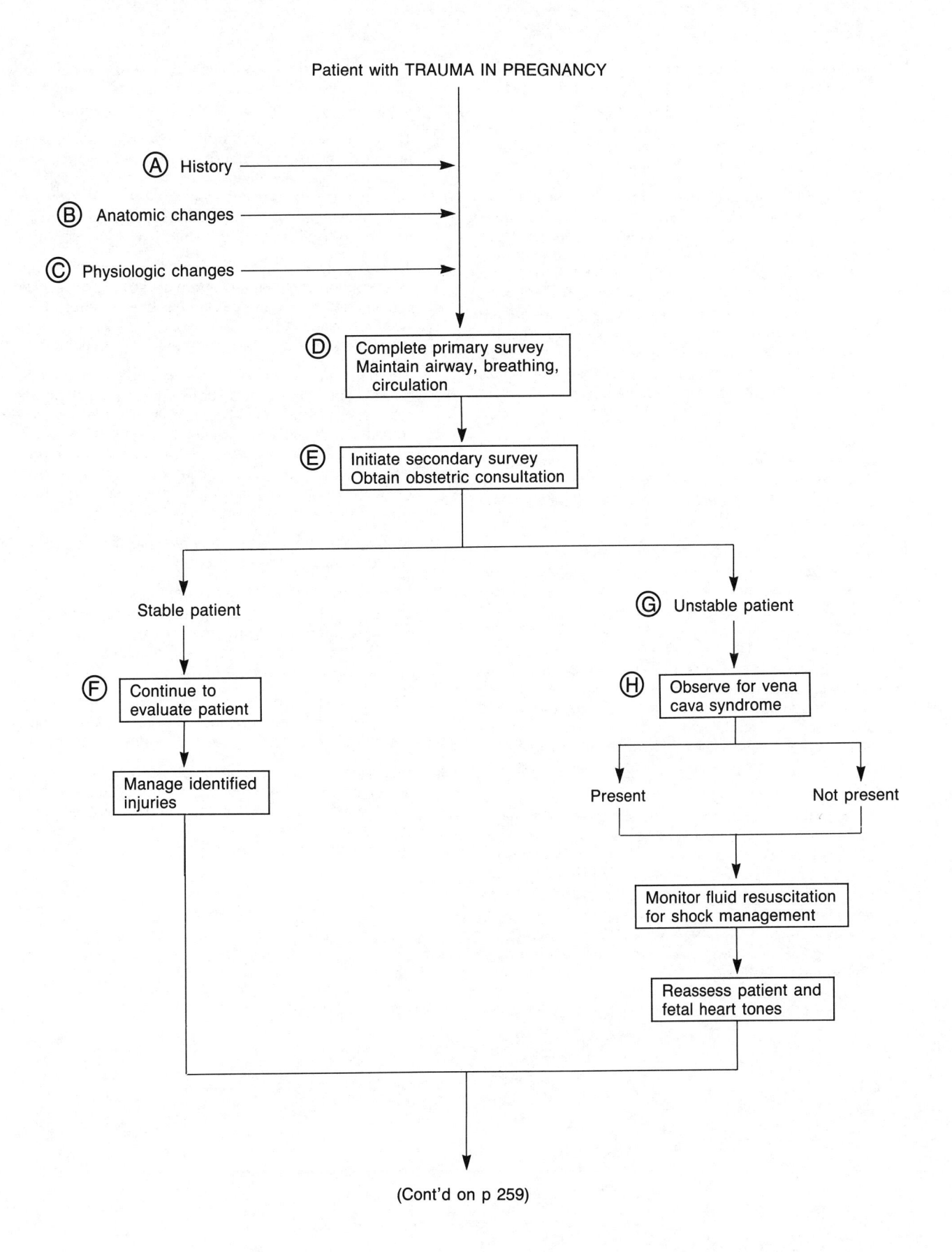

- Ⓐ History
- Ⓑ Anatomic changes
- Ⓒ Physiologic changes

Ⓓ Complete primary survey
Maintain airway, breathing, circulation

Ⓔ Initiate secondary survey
Obtain obstetric consultation

Stable patient

Ⓕ Continue to evaluate patient

Manage identified injuries

Ⓖ Unstable patient

Ⓗ Observe for vena cava syndrome

Present / Not present

Monitor fluid resuscitation for shock management

Reassess patient and fetal heart tones

(Cont'd on p 259)

I. Uterine damage may consist of lacerations, tears, or partial or complete rupture. If rupture has occurred, the uterus is usually tender to palpation. The abdomen may be distended, and vaginal bleeding is evident. If rupture is complete, two distinct masses may be palpable. Milder forms of uterine damage are more common.

J. The trauma/obstetric team should identify the status of the amniotic membrane if not previously done. Indications of labor must be noted. A history of sudden gush of fluid following the impact suggests a possible premature rupture of amniotic membranes. The fluid should be tested for pH level (normal pH for amniotic fluid is 7 to 7.5 and for urine is 4.8 to 6.0). Inspect the perineum and vagina. Immediate intervention is indicated if the umbilical cord is visible. Core temperature and WBC must be closely monitored for developing amnionitis, which is an indication for labor induction.

K. Determine whether the patient is in early labor. Contractions that cause dilation of the cervix indicate labor onset. Assess the duration and frequency of the contractions. Premature labor may indicate fetal or uterine injury. Injury must be ruled out before measures to inhibit the progression of labor are instituted.

L. Abruptio placentae is the second leading cause of fetal death. Signs and symptoms are vaginal bleeding, premature labor, abdominal pain, uterine tenderness to palpation, and uterine tetany. The expanding uterus or rising of the fundus height, maternal shock, and fetal distress or absence of FHTs may indicate—too late—that there was injury to the placenta. Placental abruption can occur more than 48 hours after the initial traumatic incident. Coagulation changes are rare following a mild abruption, but if fetal demise occurs, the patient may develop severe coagulopathy. Early detection of an abruption and appropriate action increase the chance of fetal survival.

M. Continuous fetal monitoring is ideal because uterine perfusion decreases as an initial response to maternal shock. FHTs should be assessed for 2 full minutes when the mother's vital signs are assessed to identify any fetal decelerations. Ultrasonography may be diagnostic in determining the extent of fetal injuries and in approximating gestational age. If distress is identified and the fetus is of viable age, an emergency cesarean section should be performed. If fetal death is identified, the fetus may be removed by a cesarean section or allowed to remain in utero for a vaginal delivery. In the critical trauma patient, a cesarean section to remove a dead fetus may be indicated to prevent disseminated intravascular coagulation. If no injury is identified, admit for observation.

N. The principles of resuscitation are the same as those for nonpregnant patients. Standard cardiopulmonary resuscitation combined with advanced trauma life support and advanced cardiac life support measures are instituted. A team member should be assigned to manually displace the uterus to allow venous return.

O. The two key factors in determining the appropriateness of a postmortem cesarean section are gestational age and the amount of time the patient has been in arrest. Neonatal resuscitation may be necessary after delivery. Emergency equipment must be immediately available.

P. The trauma/obstetric team must provide a comprehensive plan of care to detect subtle changes in patient and fetus status. The general goal is to provide aggresive maternal care while minimizing fetal stress. Care should focus on the immediate treatment of traumatic injuries and on prevention of complications. The potential for delayed presentation of abruptio placentae and premature labor should be assessed continuously.

Q. Monitor CVP, pulmonary artery pressure, and cardiac output to identify developing complications.

R. The pregnant immobilized patient is at risk for venous stasis and phlebitis resulting from normal physiologic changes. Intermittent pneumatic compression stocking devices are an effective treatment modality. It is important to mobilize the patient as soon as possible.

S. Pain can cause further stress for mother and fetus. The trauma/obstetric team should develop a pain management plan by consulting with a pharmacology expert.

T. The patient and family need psychosocial support. Encourage interaction with trauma support groups. Keep the family informed of the status of both mother and fetus. Patients with identified fetal death should be referred to the appropriate support group.

References

Jastremski MS, et al. The whole emergency medicine catalog. Philadelphia: WB Saunders, 1985.

Rund DA. Essentials of emergency medicine. New York: Appleton-Century-Crofts, 1982:405–406.

(Cont'd from p 257)

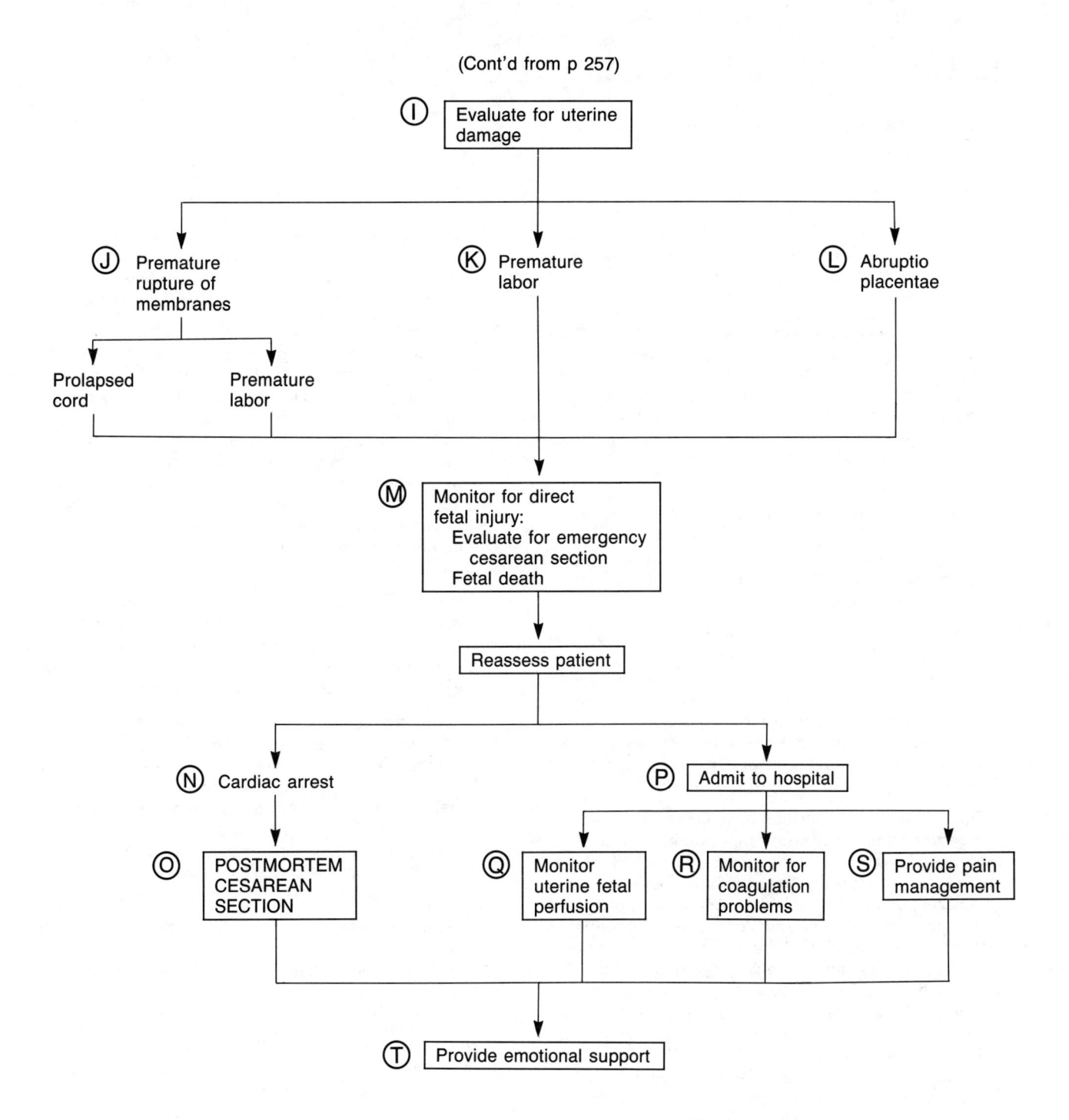

- **I** Evaluate for uterine damage
  - **J** Premature rupture of membranes
    - Prolapsed cord
    - Premature labor
  - **K** Premature labor
  - **L** Abruptio placentae
- **M** Monitor for direct fetal injury:
  - Evaluate for emergency cesarean section
  - Fetal death
- Reassess patient
  - **N** Cardiac arrest
    - **O** POSTMORTEM CESAREAN SECTION
  - **P** Admit to hospital
    - **Q** Monitor uterine fetal perfusion
    - **R** Monitor for coagulation problems
    - **S** Provide pain management
- **T** Provide emotional support

TRAUMA IN THE ELDERLY

Denise L. Stewart
Thomas Drury

Trauma in the elderly usually results in a higher mortality and morbidity rate, with a lower injury severity score, than does trauma in the young. Age alone, however, does not change trauma therapy protocols.

A. As with all trauma patients, the initial assessment must be completed. Ensure baseline blood studies, including complete blood cell count with differential, electrolytes, type and cross-match, alcohol level, and drug screen are complete. Insertion of two large bore (16 gauge or greater) intravenous (IV) lines, a Foley catheter, and a nasogastric tube is essential during resuscitation.

B. Trauma in the elderly is primarily caused by motor vehicle accidents, falls, and burns. Determination of the exact mechanism of injury can be difficult in the elderly. A complete and accurate report of events leading up to the injury must be elicited from prehospital personnel, family, and the patient.

C. A medical history, including pre-existing diseases, must be obtained. A complete list of medications that the patient currently takes must be determined. Widespread stereotypes of the elderly by the caregiver must be avoided. Not all elderly patients have impaired cardiovascular function or decreased senses. However, an increased amount of monitoring is needed because of the higher associated risk of mortality and morbidity.

D. There tends to be a decline in cardiovascular functioning and a diminished reserve for responding to stress in the elderly. The initial blood pressure may be high because of pre-existing hypertension; however, fluid replacement may be inadequate on the basis of this assumption. Assessment and continued monitoring of trends and of overall response to resuscitation are needed. Invasive monitoring should be considered for more accurate evaluation of fluid status, cardiac output, and other cardiovascular parameters. The presence of initial arrhythmias should not be assumed to be age related. Rather, an evaluation for the relationship to the trauma should be completed. Serial electrocardiograms (ECGs), cardiac enzymes, and isoenzymes should be obtained. Therefore, continuous monitoring is essential. The use of inotropic support may be necessary.

E. The process of aging can decrease such pulmonary functions as vital capacity, expansion of rib cage, and ability to clear the respiratory tract. A Swan-Ganz catheter may be indicated by the patient's status. The catheter assists in fluid resuscitation and maintenance. The elderly have a higher risk of pneumonia. Therefore, meticulous pulmonary care is a goal. Adequate pain relief for rib fractures, sterile suctioning techniques, and good basic nursing care are essential. Studies have shown that once an elderly patient is intubated, the incidence of pneumonia increases. Furthermore, the length of required ventilation time is longer. Careful evaluation before intubation is required.

F. An initial and complete assessment of baseline mental status is necessary. An examination for impairment of senses and alterations in cognitive processes must be documented. Remember, older patients with head injuries may have cerebral bleeding.

G. The elderly may have limitations in musculoskeletal activity as well. Patients who fall and sustain hip fractures must also be assessed for associated arm and skull fractures. A limitation in joint and muscle flexibility, muscle atrophy, and pre-existing arthritis must be considered by the caregiver. A major complication in the elderly is immobility following musculoskeletal injuries. The care is directed to maintaining mobility. Therefore, passive and active range of motion and turning are necessary when on bed rest. An elderly patient benefits from early activity.

H. Baseline laboratory tests assist in the assessment of renal functioning. There may be a need to adjust drug dosages with elderly patients. Therefore, careful monitoring of urinary output, specific gravity, creatinine, creatinine clearance, and blood urea nitrogen levels is essential.

I. The elderly patient may have short-term memory loss, confusion attributable to sensory overload, or pre-existing dementia. Continuing orientation to time and place may be necessary. The presence of family members and personal objects can assist in the recovery process. Speaking slowly, facing the patient, and identifying oneself assist the communication process. An assessment of the patient's daily activity and independence status is necessary. The appropriate referrals should be made.

J. As with all unstable trauma patients, the possibility of emergency surgery is great. The pre-existing disease process may necessitate the need for postoperative intensive care monitoring.

K. Stable trauma patients are admitted for observation and serial examinations. The elderly have higher incidence of infection and therefore catheter sites should be frequently assessed. IV and Foley catheters should be removed as soon as possible. Early mobilization, prevention of complications, and maintaining function as near to the preinjured level as possible are the goals of trauma care of the elderly.

References

Champion H. Major trauma in geriatric patients. Am J Publ Health 1989; 79:1278–1281.
Horst H. Factors influencing survival of elderly trauma patients. Crit Care Med 1986; 14:681–684.
Oreskovich M. Geriatric trauma: injury patterns and outcome. J Trauma 1984; 24:565–572.
Osler T. Trauma in the elderly. Am J Surg 1988; 156:537–542.

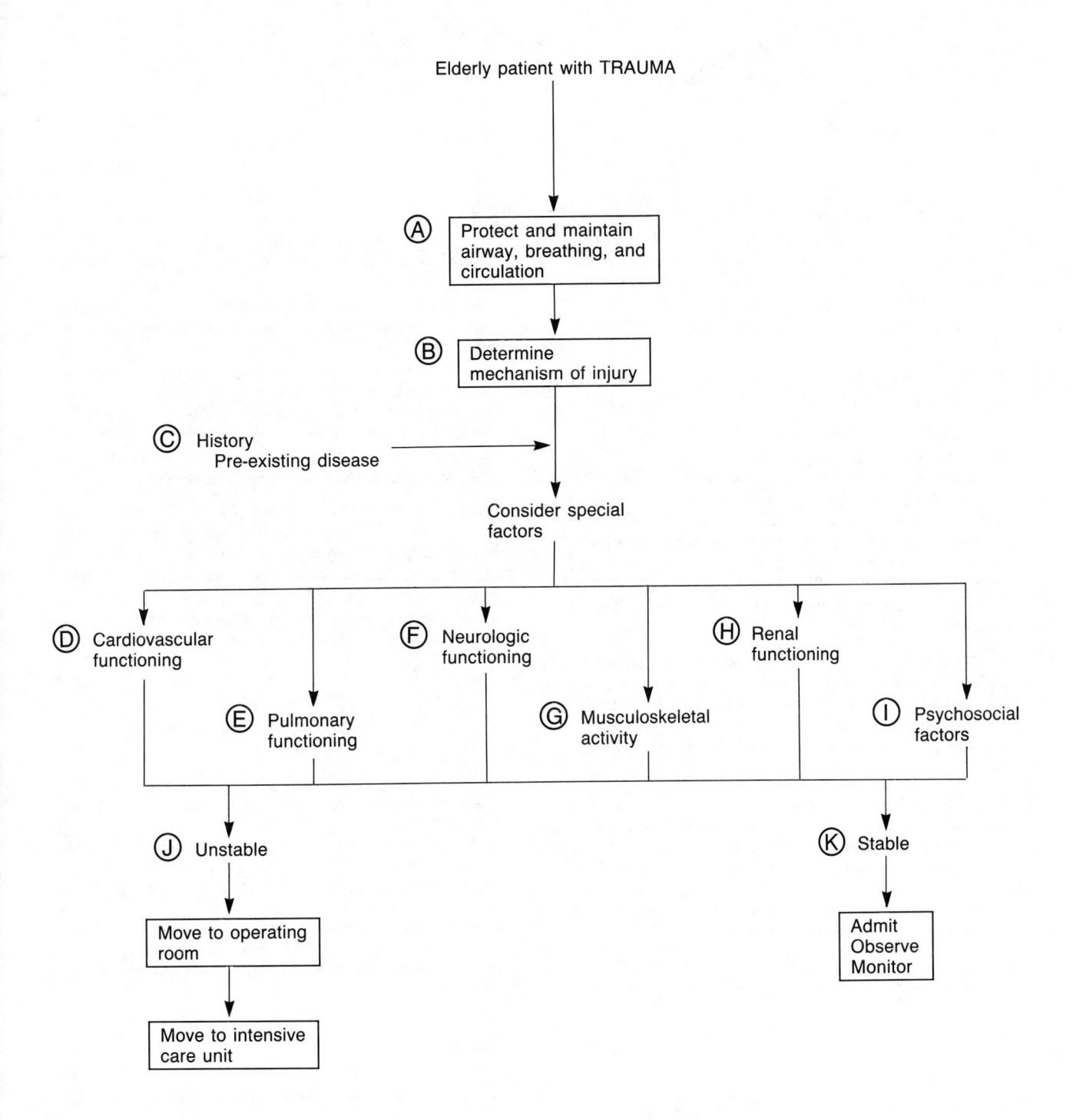

```
                    Elderly patient with TRAUMA
                                │
                                ▼
                    Ⓐ  Protect and maintain
                       airway, breathing, and
                       circulation
                                │
                                ▼
                    Ⓑ  Determine
                       mechanism of injury
                                │
    Ⓒ History                   │
       Pre-existing disease ──▶ │
                                ▼
                       Consider special
                          factors
```

- Ⓓ Cardiovascular functioning
- Ⓔ Pulmonary functioning
- Ⓕ Neurologic functioning
- Ⓖ Musculoskeletal activity
- Ⓗ Renal functioning
- Ⓘ Psychosocial factors

Ⓙ Unstable → Move to operating room → Move to intensive care unit

Ⓚ Stable → Admit / Observe / Monitor

261

TRAUMA IN THE HOMELESS

Eileen McMenemy

A. Trauma has a major impact on the homeless. The homeless are victims of all types of trauma, including vehicle/pedestrian accidents, stab wounds, gunshot wounds, aggravated assaults, fractures, criminal assaults, and child abuse. Alcohol and/or drugs are a major component of trauma; however, they are not necessarily used by the victim.

B. The homeless patient is assessed with primary and secondary evaluation and treated as any other patient.

C. Who are the homeless? This can be extremely difficult to determine. Does the patient "look homeless"? Not every patient lives on "skid row." Many families now live in shelter facilities. Patients are often reluctant to admit to their living conditions. If the staff has a high index of suspicion, they must use compassion and dignity in determining the patient's living arrangements. The staff should attempt to identify patients with special needs. When a homeless patient is identified, the chart should be clearly labeled.

D. When a homeless patient expires, involved agencies should be notified. Attempts should be made to notify the next-of-kin. Agencies that may be used include the medical examiner, the chaplin's office, community outreach coalitions, and the various shelter providers in the area.

E. The patient should be supported throughout his or her stay. Various services should be coordinated depending on individual needs. Activities may include informing the homeless health care team, social worker, or drug and alcohol counselor. Medical and nursing staff should be informed about the patient's social status so they can be sensitive to the patient's needs.

F. When the homeless patient is ready to be discharged, attempts should be made to find suitable accommodations. Several factors are considered, such as whether the shelter can meet the patient's medical needs. The patient must be mobile and capable of self-care. Many patients require convalescent care. Homeless people do not have family support to provide this, and shelters do not provide this environment. Therefore, hospitalization may be prolonged if there is no facility able to care for the patient. Medical statements might be required for the shelter providers so that the patient will be allowed to stay beyond the maximum stay limits. Consideration should be given to whether the homeless health care team has access to the facility so that the team can help with dressing changes and wound checks.

G. The patient should be informed of available support systems. These supports may include being followed by the homeless health care team and, if necessary, arrangements can be made for specific care such as dressing changes. Patients should also be informed about how to access specialty services and arrangements made for transporting the patient for clinic visits.

References

Baumann D, Grigsby C. Understanding the homeless: From research to action. Austin: Hogg foundation for Mental Health, 1988.

Kelly JT. Trauma: With the example of San Francisco's shelter programs. In: Brickner PW, Scharer LK, Conanan B, Elvy A, Savarese M, eds. Health care of homeless people. New York: Springer, 1985:77–92.

Wright JD. The national health care for the homeless program. In: Bingham RD, Green RE, White SB, eds. The homeless in contemporary society. Newbury Park: SAGE, 1987:150–169.

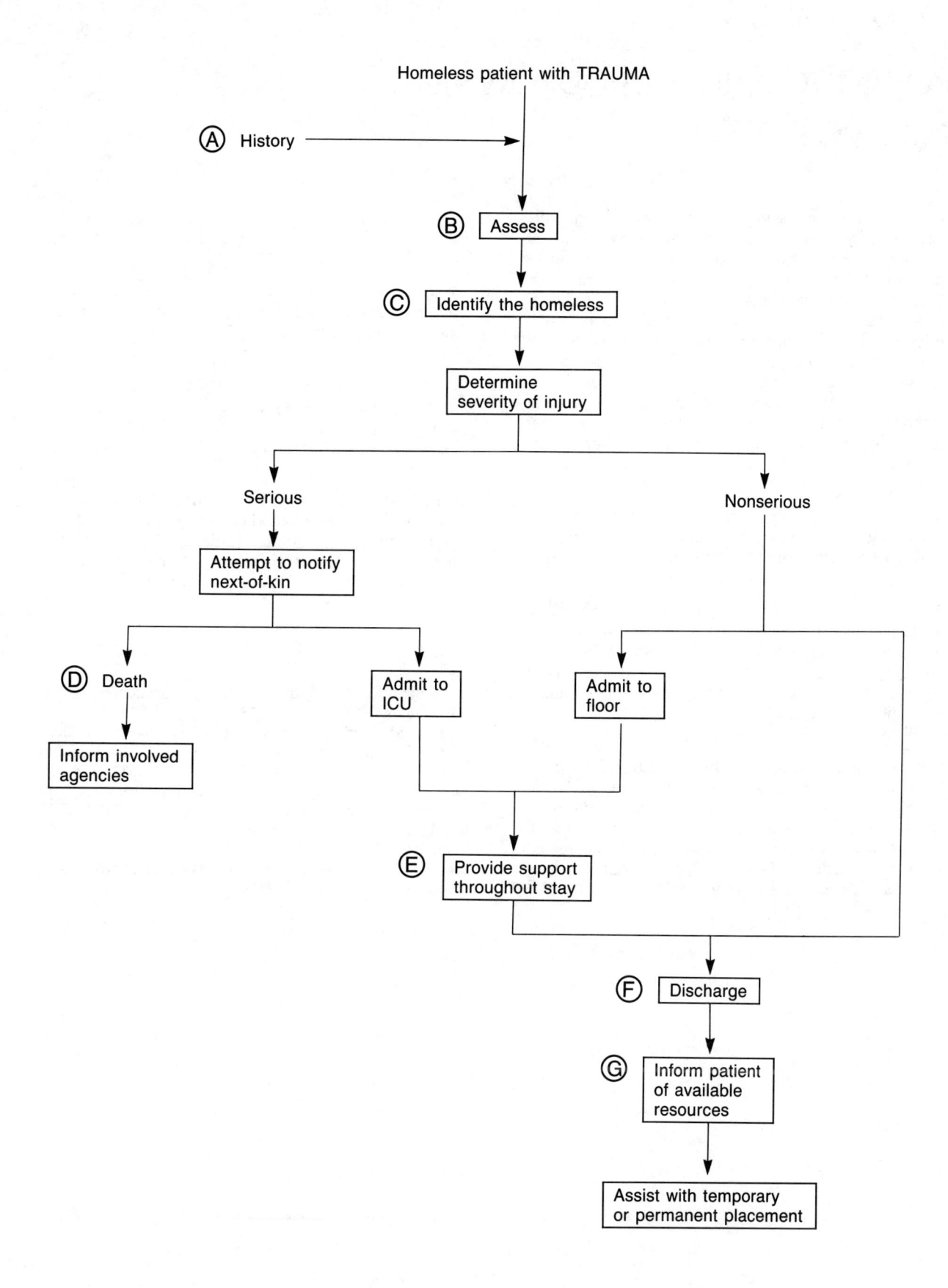

```
                    Homeless patient with TRAUMA
                                │
   Ⓐ History ───────────────────▶│
                                 ▼
                          Ⓑ  ┌─────────┐
                             │ Assess  │
                             └─────────┘
                                 │
                                 ▼
                      Ⓒ  ┌──────────────────┐
                         │ Identify the     │
                         │ homeless         │
                         └──────────────────┘
                                 │
                                 ▼
                         ┌──────────────────┐
                         │ Determine        │
                         │ severity of injury│
                         └──────────────────┘
                            │           │
                       Serious        Nonserious
                            │           │
                            ▼           │
                   ┌──────────────┐     │
                   │ Attempt to   │     │
                   │ notify       │     │
                   │ next-of-kin  │     │
                   └──────────────┘     │
                     │         │        │
                     ▼         ▼        ▼
              Ⓓ Death    ┌────────┐ ┌────────┐
                   │     │Admit to│ │Admit to│
                   ▼     │  ICU   │ │ floor  │
           ┌──────────┐  └────────┘ └────────┘
           │ Inform   │       │         │
           │ involved │       │         │
           │ agencies │       ▼         │
           └──────────┘  Ⓔ ┌──────────────┐
                            │ Provide support│
                            │ throughout stay│
                            └──────────────┘
                                   │
                                   ▼
                            Ⓕ  ┌──────────┐
                               │ Discharge│
                               └──────────┘
                                   │
                                   ▼
                            Ⓖ ┌──────────────┐
                              │ Inform patient│
                              │ of available  │
                              │ resources     │
                              └──────────────┘
                                   │
                                   ▼
                              ┌──────────────────┐
                              │ Assist with temporary│
                              │ or permanent placement│
                              └──────────────────┘
```

DROWNING AND NEAR DROWNING

William Gary Reed

A. Death from submersion in water is most frequently caused by hypoxia. Consequently, the re-establishment of adequate respiratory function is the most important aspect of the treatment of these patients. A small portion of deaths by submersion are attributable to laryngospasm or asystole secondary to intense vagal activation (diving reflex). It is not uncommon for foreign objects to be aspirated during a near drowning episode; careful consideration of this possibility is important. Traditional teaching emphasizes the need to drain the lungs of aspirated saltwater in near drowning; freshwater near drowning patients do not require this maneuver. Recent studies suggest that this procedure may not be necessary in either case.

B. Most cardiac arrhythmias seen with near drowning are caused by hypoxia. However, patients should be treated with conventional antiarrhythmic agents in addition to oxygen, if serious arrhythmias occur.

C. The general assessment of the patient is very important. Many patients suffer from hypothermia after submersion into cold water. Hypothermia can markedly increase the amount of time the patient can tolerate hypoxia without significant brain injury. In addition, evidence of trauma to the head and cervical spine should be carefully sought in all near drowning patients.

D. Patients with near drowning almost always have aspirated a significant amount of water, thereby causing a breakdown of surfactant with resultant noncardiogenic pulmonary edema. This results in severe hypoxia with a subsequent lactic acidosis. Hypoxia should be treated with oxygen administration and severe lactic acidosis with the judicious use of sodium bicarbonate.

E. The chest film is important in detecting early signs of noncardiogenic pulmonary edema and aspirated foreign objects.

F. Ventilatory support should include endotracheal intubation if respiratory failure exists. In general, mild to moderate hypoxia can be managed with oxygen by mask if hypoventilation is not present.

G. Cardiopulmonary resuscitation (CPR) should be performed by advanced cardiac life support standards in appropriate patients. Hypothermic patients should be aggressively warmed during CPR if cardiac arrest has occurred.

H. Laboratory tests upon admission should include at least the following: arterial blood gases, electrolytes, complete blood count, prothrombin time, and partial thromboplastin time. Other laboratory tests may be necessary in some patients, e.g., toxicology screen.

References

Fandel I, Bancalari E. Near drowning in children: clinical aspects. Pediatrics 1976; 58:573–578.

Giammona ST, Modell JH. Drowning by total immersion. Effects on pulmonary surfactant of distilled water, isotonic saline and sea water. Am J Dis Child 1967; 114:612–615.

Modell JH, Graves SA, Ketover A. Clinical course of 91 consecutive near-drowning victims. Chest 1976; 70:127–132.

Orlowski JP. Prognostic factors in pediatric cases of drowning and near-drowning. JACEP 1979; 8:176–181.

Segarra F, Redding RA. Modern concepts about drowning. Can Med Assoc J 1974; 110:1057–1061.

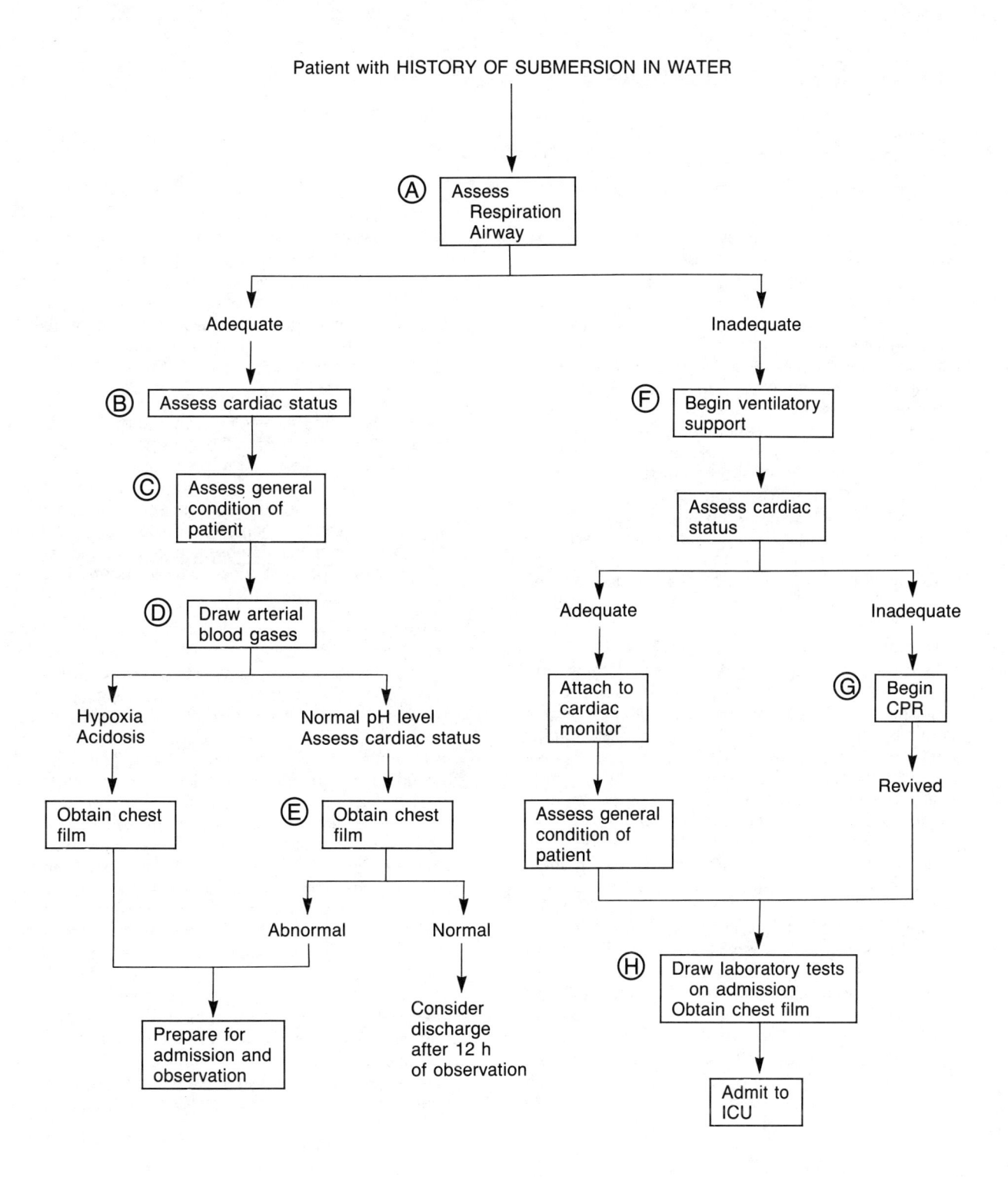

```
                    Patient with HISTORY OF SUBMERSION IN WATER
                                        │
                                        ▼
                               Ⓐ ┌─────────────┐
                                 │   Assess    │
                                 │ Respiration │
                                 │   Airway    │
                                 └─────────────┘
                          ┌─────────────┴─────────────┐
                          ▼                           ▼
                       Adequate                   Inadequate
                          │                           │
                          ▼                           ▼
                  Ⓑ ┌──────────────────┐      Ⓕ ┌──────────────────┐
                    │ Assess cardiac   │        │ Begin ventilatory│
                    │     status       │        │     support      │
                    └──────────────────┘        └──────────────────┘
                          │                           │
                          ▼                           ▼
                  Ⓒ ┌──────────────────┐        ┌──────────────────┐
                    │ Assess general   │        │ Assess cardiac   │
                    │ condition of     │        │     status       │
                    │ patient          │        └──────────────────┘
                    └──────────────────┘          ┌─────┴─────┐
                          │                       ▼           ▼
                          ▼                   Adequate     Inadequate
                  Ⓓ ┌──────────────┐              │           │
                    │ Draw arterial│              ▼           ▼
                    │ blood gases  │        ┌──────────┐  Ⓖ ┌──────┐
                    └──────────────┘        │ Attach to│    │Begin │
                     ┌────┴─────┐           │ cardiac  │    │ CPR  │
                     ▼          ▼           │ monitor  │    └──────┘
                 Hypoxia    Normal pH level └──────────┘        │
                 Acidosis   Assess cardiac       │              ▼
                     │      status               ▼           Revived
                     ▼          ▼           ┌──────────┐
                 ┌──────┐  Ⓔ┌──────┐        │Assess    │
                 │Obtain│    │Obtain│        │general   │
                 │chest │    │chest │        │condition │
                 │film  │    │film  │        │of patient│
                 └──────┘    └──────┘        └──────────┘
                     │       ┌──┴───┐             │
                     │       ▼      ▼             │
                     │   Abnormal  Normal         │
                     │       │      │             │
                     └───────┤      ▼             ▼
                             │  Consider     Ⓗ ┌──────────────┐
                             ▼  discharge       │Draw laboratory│
                         ┌────────┐ after 12 h  │tests on       │
                         │Prepare │ of          │admission      │
                         │for     │ observation │Obtain chest   │
                         │admission│            │film           │
                         │and     │             └──────────────┘
                         │observation│                │
                         └────────┘                   ▼
                                                 ┌────────┐
                                                 │Admit to│
                                                 │  ICU   │
                                                 └────────┘
```

EVIDENCE COLLECTION

Suzy Baulch
Gwen J. Hall

A. Trauma victims are frequently involved in events that result in adjudication. Attentive observation and proper documentation facilitate the investigation. Necessary treatments and medical care are of first priority; preservation of evidence is secondary. Personnel should make use of all senses (visual, tactile, auditory, and olfactory) when assessing the patient and environment (scene). Information to be given to the physician and/or recorder includes standard run sheet information, agency investigator, apparent events, scene description, weapon position, appearance of patient's injuries, and treatment at scene. Preparation for transport includes collecting *all* equipment and debris in a plastic bag and placing sharp objects in containers. Debris left behind only adds confusion to the investigative scene. Keep clothing with the patient while he or she is in transport. If the patient is pronounced dead at the scene, take care to leave the scene undisturbed. Thorough documentation of observations is essential.

B. If the patient requires treatment for which clothing must be removed, it is preferable to cut garments adjacent to their side seams to preserve defects in clothing that were caused by bullet wounds or stab wounds. Save clothing and property in a separately labeled paper bag. If clothing is wet, inform the officer who receives the evidence. At the time of drawing blood, it is highly desirable to obtain additional tubes of original blood (i.e., one gray-top, one yellow-top, and one purple-top) for the forensic laboratory and to store it in a well labeled manner with the patient's name and the time and date of accident. If at all possible, avoid altering wounds by therapeutic measures (e.g., do not incise wounds or insert chest tubes through wounds). Therapeutic features should be identified as such (e.g., circle therapeutic needle punctures with a ballpoint pen and mark "Rx" next to them).

C. If the patient is pronounced dead, clothing should remain on the body; leave the body as is and transport it wrapped in a sheet. A labeled paper bag should be used to transport other loose clothing and/or objects. Leave all therapeutic tubes in place. Any specimen obtained during life should be noted and samples sent with the body. If there is any indication that the victim's hands may contain evidence (e.g., gunshot residue or fibers), each hand should be enclosed in a small brown paper bag that is fastened around the wrist with rubber bands or adhesive tape.

D. If the patient survives, evidence should be saved, packaged, labeled, and retained for transport to the police. Clothing should never be released to the family until release is cleared by police. Meaningful information to be documented includes treatments, the patient's response to treatment, and final disposition. A simple sketch or diagram that demonstrates injuries and/or therapeutic endeavors is of great value to the medical examiners or legal authorities.

E. Items to be identified and preserved include physical evidence (e.g., bullets, bags of white powder, pills, weapons, or other foreign objects); trace evidence (e.g., loose hairs, paint chips, fibers); biologic evidence (e.g., patient's blood, body fluids, patient's pulled hair, or hair that is shaved to expose a gunshot wound); and clothing and its contents. Each must be individually packaged (preferably in paper), sealed, and labeled. Labels should note the date and time of trauma, patient's name, item description, where item was recovered, and your name or initials. Designate a person to set up a plastic bag with the patient's name and to collect *all* items taken from the patient. These should be inventoried, placed in paper containers, and documented in a timely fashion. Biologic evidence may also be placed in this bag. Do *not* remove contents from clothing other than items needed for identification. Clothing should never be released to the family; it is retained and safely placed in the hands of the investigating officer. Photographs and diagrams (an important form of documentation) should be labeled with the date, time, and location of trauma on the back. Document statements made by the patient in quotations and bring these to the attention of the law enforcement officer.

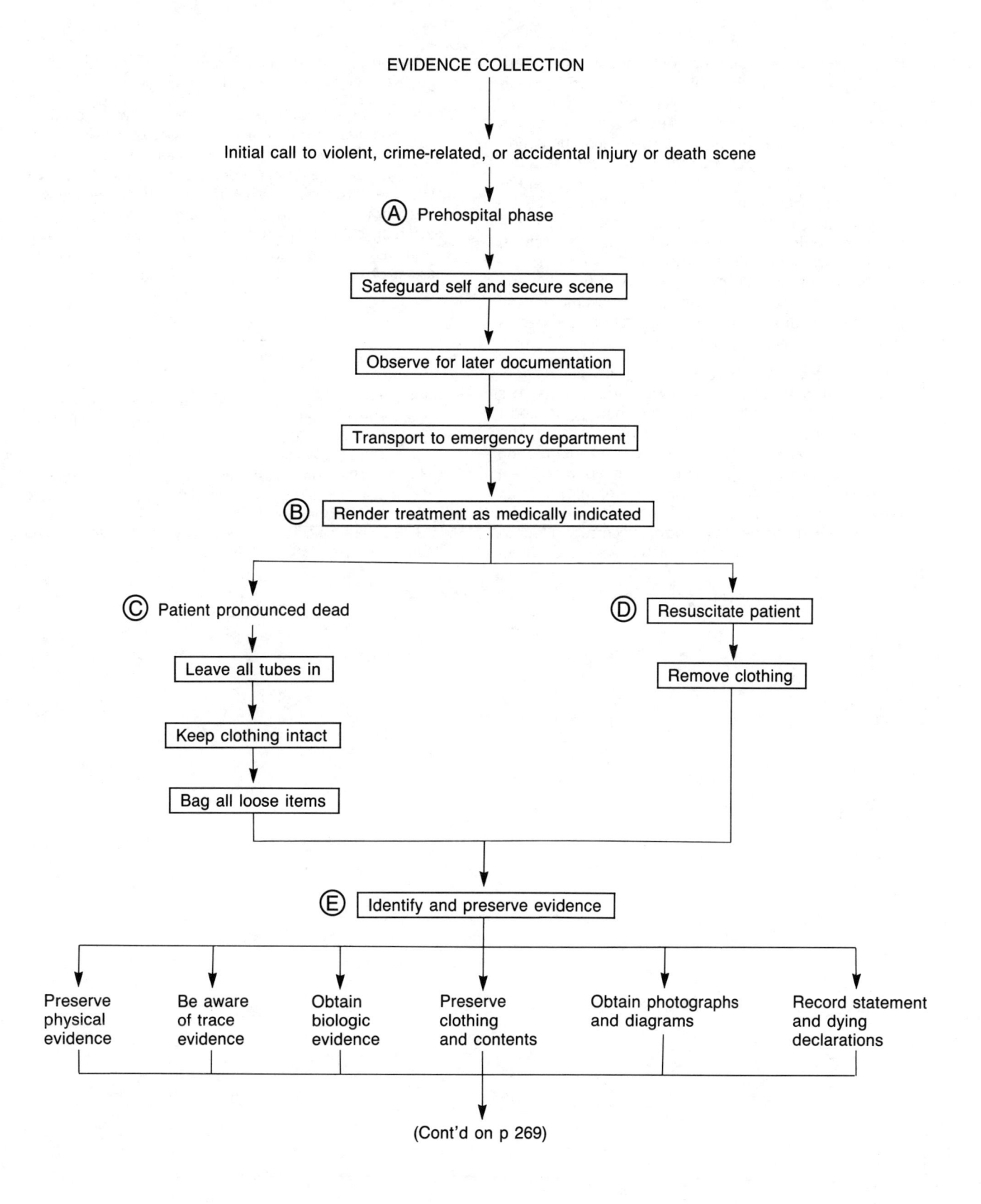

EVIDENCE COLLECTION

Initial call to violent, crime-related, or accidental injury or death scene

(A) Prehospital phase

→ Safeguard self and secure scene
→ Observe for later documentation
→ Transport to emergency department

(B) Render treatment as medically indicated

- **(C) Patient pronounced dead**
  - Leave all tubes in
  - Keep clothing intact
  - Bag all loose items

- **(D) Resuscitate patient**
  - Remove clothing

(E) Identify and preserve evidence

- Preserve physical evidence
- Be aware of trace evidence
- Obtain biologic evidence
- Preserve clothing and contents
- Obtain photographs and diagrams
- Record statement and dying declarations

(Cont'd on p 269)

F. Proper, accurate, and thorough documentation is essential. Reporting must be objective (e.g., small round wound) not subjective (e.g., entrance wound, exit wound). Include how and when the patient arrived, the mechanism of injury if known or suspected, the condition of the patient on arrival, and therapeutic measures taken and the times they were rendered. Document times of collection, handling, and disposition of evidence. Include in the charting the names of visitors and law enforcement officials (include badge number) present in the room with the patient. Transportation of the patient and his or her final disposition should be noted, along with times and dates. Final disposition must include the patient's condition, mode of transportation, and names of persons accompanying the patient.

G. Procedures for evidence collection may very slightly from jurisdiction to jurisdiction. However, evidence must pass through a documented, unbroken chain of custody. Failure to do so may alter its admissibility in court. The record to be kept with the evidence must include the name of the patient, hospital number, and other relative data and concludes with the date and time of transfer, the signature of the person receiving, and the reason for transfer. When storage of the body is necessary, a locked box, refrigerator, or freezer is preferable, with access limited to an identified few. Keep the chain simple and involve as few exchanges and persons as possible.

H. Preparation for court begins as soon as you are aware of a potential criminal or civil action. Attention to evidence and its accurate and proper documentation is essential. Accurate, concise documentation will serve as your memory, making you a more confident, reliable witness should the need arise. Be prepared to explain and teach the court but do not talk beyond the scope of questions asked. Offer no more information than you are asked or that is beyond your expertise.

References

Besant-Matthews PE. Evidence collection and protection. Emergency nursing symposium. Dallas: Parkland Hospital, 1987.

Carmona R, Prince K. Trauma and forensic medicine. J Trauma 1989; 29(9):1222–1225.

Chamberlain RT. Chain of custody: importance of requirements for clinical laboratory specimens. Hialeah, FL: Smith Kline Bioscience Laboratory, 1989.

Smialek JE. Forensic medicine in the emergency department. Med Clin North Am 1983; 1(3):693–704.

(Cont'd from p 267)

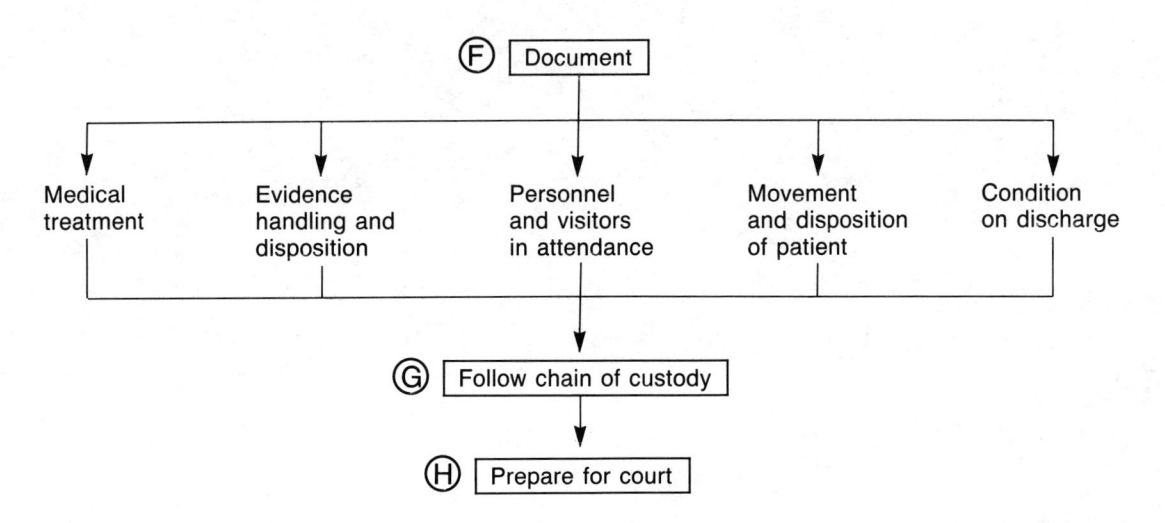

Ⓕ Document

- Medical treatment
- Evidence handling and disposition
- Personnel and visitors in attendance
- Movement and disposition of patient
- Condition on discharge

Ⓖ Follow chain of custody

Ⓗ Prepare for court

TRAUMA SCORING

Data Collection for Trauma Patients
E Codes
CRAMS Score
Trauma Score and Revised Trauma Score
Injury Severity Score

DATA COLLECTION FOR TRAUMA PATIENTS

Mary M. Lawnick
Maureen E. Flanagan

A. The prehospital and hospital records of the trauma patient contain information that can be used to assess the trauma system. Most trauma registries are hospital based because the hospital is the source of most data.

B. These prehospital and hospital data can be used for many purposes. Prehospital data can be used during triage to direct the patient to the appropriate facility or to evaluate prehospital care. Hospital data generate statistics for particular services (i.e., emergency department or trauma service), demographic information for trends, and various quality assurance purposes. Outcome assessments include mortality rate, morbidity rate, and evaluation of care. Data may also be used for research studies pertaining to a particular patient, service, injury, population, or region. Data collected for a hospital based registry may also be sent to a regional, state, or national registry. Determine how the data are to be used, and ensure that the necessary data are available in the records.

C. Before data collection begins, identify the patient population and data collection personnel and determine the frequency and methods for collection and computation. Consider the available resources, in terms of time and personnel, when making these decisions. To ensure data consistency, define precise operational definitions for each data element. A trial 2-week data collection period will identify any problems and allow for a revision of methods before data collection actually begins.

D. To ensure accuracy and completeness, the data and collection methods should be reviewed routinely. Ensure that data are collected for all patients who meet the criteria and that all data are complete.

E. Analyze the collected data and interpret the results. The following several chapters contain various scores that may be calculated using a minimum data set. The revised trauma score (RTS) and the injury severity score (ISS), with patient age, are used to calculate TRISS. The American College of Surgeons Committee on Trauma recommends the use of TRISS as well as approximately 12 other quality assurance audit filters. These quality assurance filters are being revised by the College in 1990. Each hospital should add audit filters pertinent to its particular setting. Important monthly statistics that can be obtained from collected data include numbers of admissions, discharges, types of injury, disposition from ED, mortality statistics, and transfer information.

F. Share your results with the appropriate persons through publications or presentations.

References

American College of Surgeons Committee on Trauma. Hospital and prehospital resources for optimal care of the injured patient. Appendices A through J. Chicago: American College of Surgeons, 1987.

Boyd CR, Tolson MA, Copes WS. Evaluating trauma care: the TRISS method. J Trauma 1987; 27:370–378.

Champion HR, Sacco WJ, Hunt TK. Trauma severity scoring to predict mortality. World J Surg 1983; 7:4–11.

National Research Council Committee on Trauma Research. Injury in America: a continuing health problem. Washington, DC: National Academy Press, 1985.

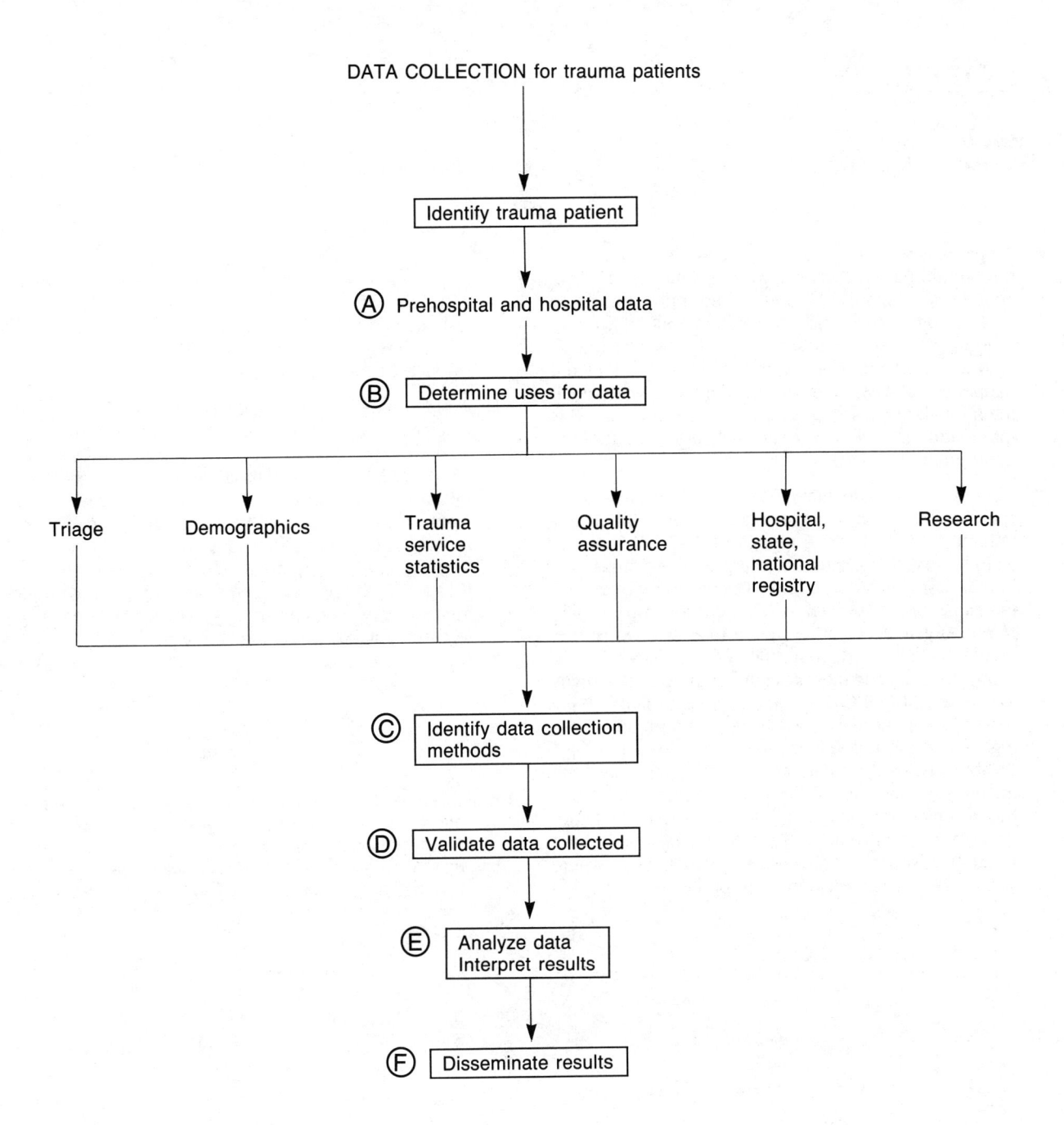

```
DATA COLLECTION for trauma patients
                │
                ▼
      ┌──────────────────────┐
      │ Identify trauma patient │
      └──────────────────────┘
                │
                ▼
   Ⓐ  Prehospital and hospital data
                │
                ▼
   Ⓑ  ┌──────────────────────┐
      │ Determine uses for data │
      └──────────────────────┘
                │
   ┌──────┬──────────┬──────────┬──────────┬──────────┬──────────┐
   ▼      ▼          ▼          ▼          ▼          ▼
 Triage  Demographics  Trauma    Quality   Hospital,   Research
                       service   assurance state,
                       statistics          national
                                           registry
                │
                ▼
   Ⓒ  ┌──────────────────────┐
      │ Identify data collection │
      │ methods                  │
      └──────────────────────┘
                │
                ▼
   Ⓓ  ┌──────────────────────┐
      │ Validate data collected │
      └──────────────────────┘
                │
                ▼
   Ⓔ  ┌──────────────────────┐
      │ Analyze data            │
      │ Interpret results       │
      └──────────────────────┘
                │
                ▼
   Ⓕ  ┌──────────────────────┐
      │ Disseminate results     │
      └──────────────────────┘
```

E CODES

Mary M. Lawnick
Maureen E. Flanagan

A. All patients with traumatic or suspected traumatic injuries should have a complete history obtained. The patient, witnesses, police, and rescue personnel should be asked to provide as much information about the injury event as possible, including the mechanism of injury; who was involved; where, when, and how the incident happened; and whether the incident was accidental, intentional, or caused by unknown circumstances. This information is necessary for accurate assignment of the appropriate E code(s).

B. E codes are supplementary ICD-9-CM codes developed specifically for coding the external cause of injury. Volume II of the Disease Index of ICD-9-CM includes an index to external causes of injury and poisonings (section 3). Use this index to find a key word that describes the cause of injury, such as fall, gunshot wound, stab, motor vehicle accident, or "pedestrian" struck. For example, the key word group "fall, falling" lists multiple causes for a fall and indicates the first three E code digits to review in ICD-9-CM, Volume I, Diseases Tabular List. Note that the index is cross-referenced for many headings, i.e., "gunshot wound" refers one to "shooting." "Stab" lists the three-digit code for stabbing, but if the incident was accidental the user is directed to "cut." Motor vehicle accident is not listed; one must look under "accident, motor vehicle." Similarly, "pedestrian" is not listed, but "struck by" directs the user to "hit by," where various pedestrian accidents can be located.

C. If a patient sustains more than one external cause of injury, secondary causes may also be coded. For example, a patient who sustains a blunt assault may also be stabbed, thereby resulting in two external causes of injury. The principal E code should reflect the cause that resulted in the most severe injury.

D. An important supplemental E code (E849) indicates the place of injury occurrence. ICD-9-CM guidelines indicate this code is to be used with E850-E869 and E888-E928, but many trauma registries use it to denote location for all traumatic events. The fourth digit assignment of E849 denotes the specific location, and examples for each are listed in the index under "Accident occurring (at) (in)" or under each fourth digit listing in ICD-9-CM, Volume I. E codes are important data elements and should be considered for inclusion in all research databases relating to injury.

References

Commission on Professional and Hospital Activities. The international classification of diseases. 9th revision. Ann Arbor, MI: Edwards Brothers, 1986.

McClain PW, Pollock DA. A microcomputer program for coding external cause of injury. J Trauma 1989; 29(1):55–58.

Assignment of E Codes to Patient with TRAUMA

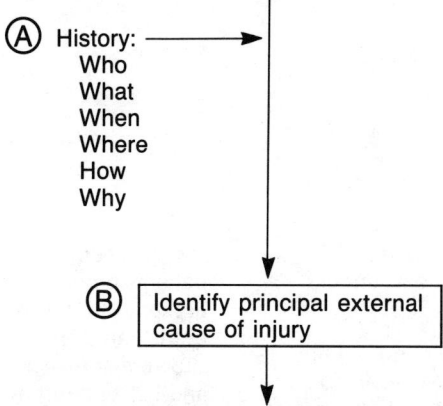

(A) History:
- Who
- What
- When
- Where
- How
- Why

(B) Identify principal external cause of injury

Categories for external cause of injury:
- Transport accidents
- Accidental poisoning
- Misadventures during surgical and medical care
- Surgical and medical procedures
- Accidental falls
- Accidents caused by fire and flames
- Accidents due to natural and environmental factors
- Accidents caused by submersion, suffocation, and foreign bodies.
- Other accidents
- Drugs, medicinal, and biological substances causing adverse effects in therapeutic use
- Suicide and self-inflicted injury
- Homicide and injury purposely inflicted by other persons
- Legal intervention
- Injured undetermined whether accidental or purposely inflicted
- Injury resulting from operation of war

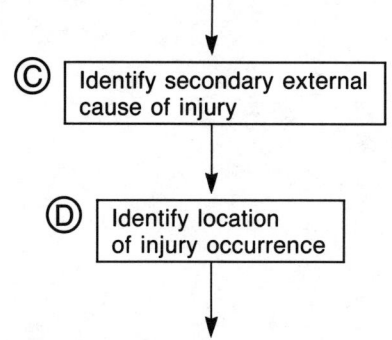

(C) Identify secondary external cause of injury

(D) Identify location of injury occurrence

Categories for location of injury occurence:
- Home
- Farm
- Mine and quarry
- Industrial place and premises
- Place for recreation and sport
- Street and highway
- Public building
- Residential institution
- Other specified places
- Unspecified places

CRAMS SCORE

Mary M. Lawnick
Maureen E. Flanagan

A. Complete the primary survey of the trauma patient. Ensure the integrity of the airway, breathing, and circulation (ABCs) of the patient.

B. As the secondary survey is completed, all components of the CRAMS scale are assessed. The CRAMS scale consists of the five following components: circulation, respiration, abdomen, motor function, and speech. The circulation component includes assessment of the patient's capillary refill (i.e., normal, delayed, or none) and blood pressure (BP). The respiratory component is an assessment of respirations; i.e., normal, abnormal (labored or shallow), or absent. The abdomen and thorax are assessed for tenderness and for the presence of penetrating wounds. The abdomen is also examined for rigidity and the chest for the presence of flail segment(s). The motor component is scored according to the presence of normal motor movement, response to pain only, or no response or decerebrate posturing to pain. The final assessment, speech, is scored as normal, confused, or no intelligible words spoken. The CRAMS score may then be calculated by adding the score for each component.

C. A score of eight or less is considered major trauma; these patients require trauma center care. A score of nine or higher indicates minor trauma; these patients do not require transportation to a trauma center. Studies have shown that the CRAMS scale is relatively easy to assess and calculate in the field. However, as a triage tool, it is more effective when combined with other triage guidelines.

References

Clemmer TP, Orme JF Jr, Thomas F, Brooks KA. Prospective evaluation of the CRAMS scale for triaging major trauma. J Trauma 1985; 25(3):188–191.

Gormican SP. CRAMS scale: field triage of trauma victims. Ann Emerg Med 1982; 11(3):132–135.

Knudson P, Frecceri CA, DeLateur SA. Improving the field triage of major trauma victims. J Trauma 1988; 28(5):602–606.

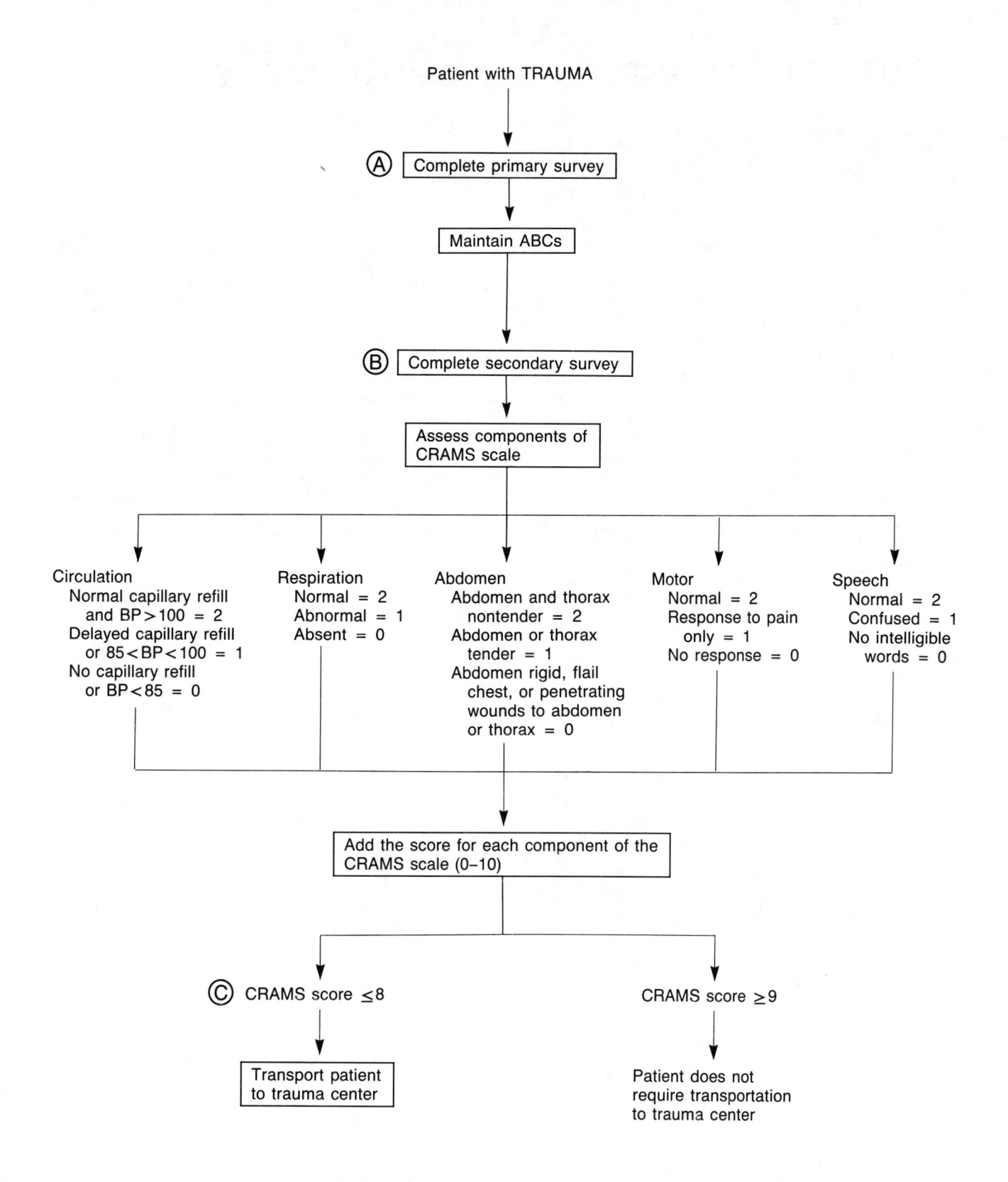

```
                        Patient with TRAUMA
                                │
                                ▼
                  (A) ┌─────────────────────────┐
                      │ Complete primary survey │
                      └─────────────────────────┘
                                │
                                ▼
                      ┌─────────────────┐
                      │ Maintain ABCs   │
                      └─────────────────┘
                                │
                                ▼
                  (B) ┌───────────────────────────┐
                      │ Complete secondary survey │
                      └───────────────────────────┘
                                │
                                ▼
                      ┌─────────────────────┐
                      │ Assess components of│
                      │    CRAMS scale      │
                      └─────────────────────┘
```

Circulation	Respiration	Abdomen	Motor	Speech
Normal capillary refill and BP>100 = 2	Normal = 2	Abdomen and thorax nontender = 2	Normal = 2	Normal = 2
Delayed capillary refill or 85<BP<100 = 1	Abnormal = 1	Abdomen or thorax tender = 1	Response to pain only = 1	Confused = 1
No capillary refill or BP<85 = 0	Absent = 0	Abdomen rigid, flail chest, or penetrating wounds to abdomen or thorax = 0	No response = 0	No intelligible words = 0

```
                      ┌─────────────────────────────────────┐
                      │ Add the score for each component of │
                      │      the CRAMS scale (0–10)         │
                      └─────────────────────────────────────┘
                           │                       │
                           ▼                       ▼
              (C)  CRAMS score ≤ 8           CRAMS score ≥ 9
                           │                       │
                           ▼                       ▼
                   ┌────────────────┐      Patient does not
                   │Transport patient│     require transportation
                   │to trauma center │     to trauma center
                   └────────────────┘
```

TRAUMA SCORE AND REVISED TRAUMA SCORE

Mary M. Lawnick
Maureen E. Flanagan

A. Complete the primary survey and ensure the patient's airway, breathing, and circulation (ABCs) are maintained.

B. As the nurse continues with the secondary survey, elements of the trauma score (TS) or revised trauma score (RTS) are easily obtained, usually in less than 1 minute.

C. After ensuring the airway, count the patient's spontaneous respiratory rate (RR) for 15 seconds and multiply that number by four. Respiratory effort (assessed for trauma score only) should be evaluated while the respiratory rate is counted. Effort is shallow or retractive if the chest movement or air exchange is markedly decreased, accessory muscles are used, or intercostal retraction is present. None of these symptoms indicates normal respiratory effort. The systolic blood pressure (SBP) may be obtained by auscultation or palpation in either arm. Capillary refill (assessed for trauma score only) is obtained by depressing the nailbed, forehead, or lip mucosa until it blanches and then releasing. If color returns within 2 seconds, refill is normal; if it takes more than 2 seconds, it is delayed. If color does not return, it is recorded as "none."

D. The three elements of the Glasgow Coma Scale (GCS) are then assessed. The first element, eye opening, is an assessment of the stimulus required to induce a patient to open his or her eyes. The second element is an assessment of the patient's best verbal response. The final element of the GCS is an assessment of the patient's best motor response. The GCS ranges from three to 15. The total score for the GCS is converted, using different conversion tables for the trauma score and revised trauma score. The converted score is added to the scores for the physiologic components.

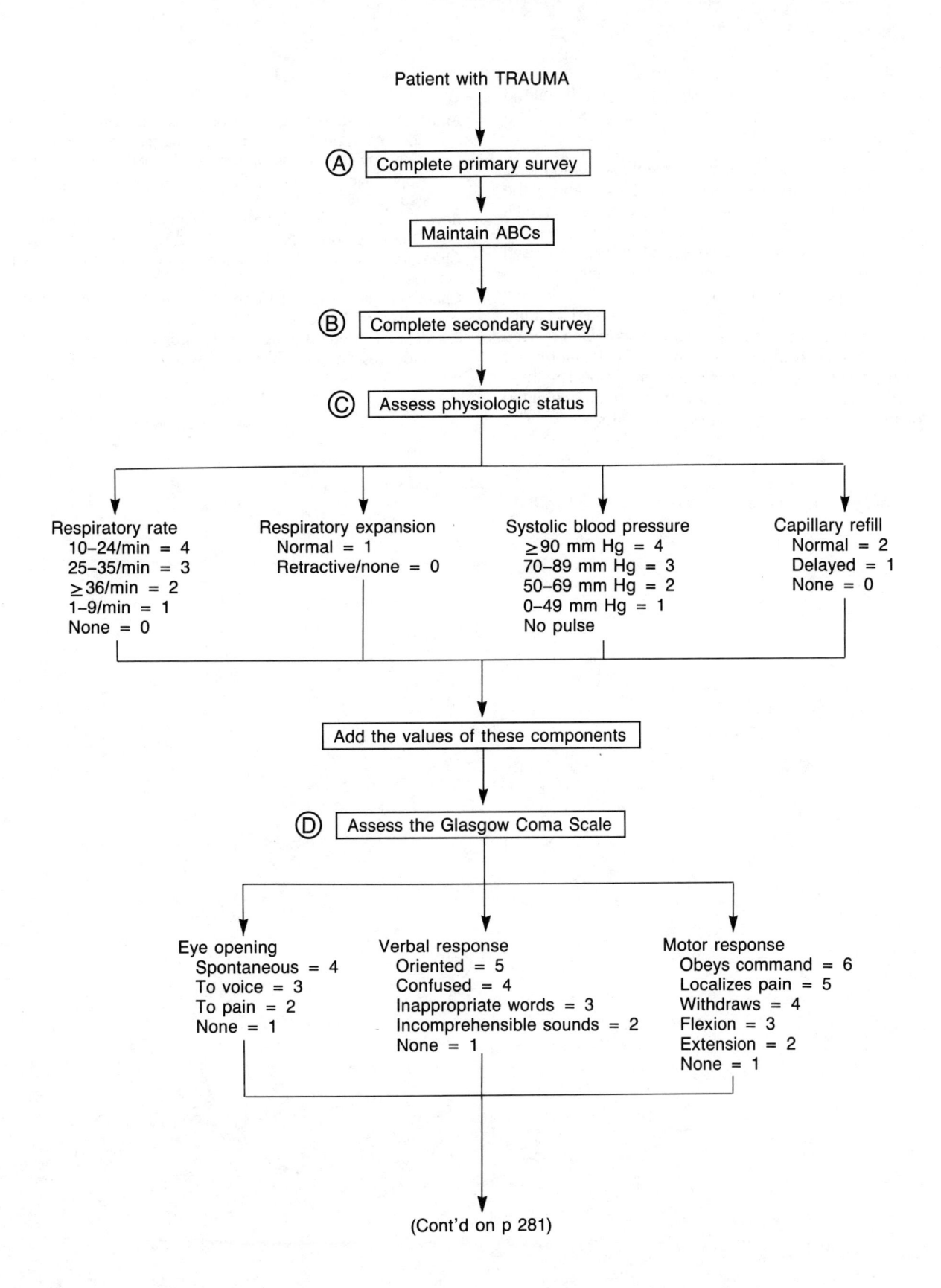

Patient with TRAUMA
↓
(A) Complete primary survey
↓
Maintain ABCs
↓
(B) Complete secondary survey
↓
(C) Assess physiologic status
↓

Respiratory rate	Respiratory expansion	Systolic blood pressure	Capillary refill
10–24/min = 4	Normal = 1	≥90 mm Hg = 4	Normal = 2
25–35/min = 3	Retractive/none = 0	70–89 mm Hg = 3	Delayed = 1
≥36/min = 2		50–69 mm Hg = 2	None = 0
1–9/min = 1		0–49 mm Hg = 1	
None = 0		No pulse	

↓
Add the values of these components
↓
(D) Assess the Glasgow Coma Scale
↓

Eye opening	Verbal response	Motor response
Spontaneous = 4	Oriented = 5	Obeys command = 6
To voice = 3	Confused = 4	Localizes pain = 5
To pain = 2	Inappropriate words = 3	Withdraws = 4
None = 1	Incomprehensible sounds = 2	Flexion = 3
	None = 1	Extension = 2
		None = 1

↓
(Cont'd on p 281)

E. Add the coded values of the four physiologic components (respiratory rate, respiratory expansion, systolic blood pressure, and capillary refill) and of the GCS to calculate the trauma score.

F. Add the coded values of the two physiologic components (respiratory rate and systolic blood pressure) and of the GCS to calculate the revised trauma score for triage (T-RTS). The T-RTS ranges from 0 to 12. The trauma score and the T-RTS (sum of the coded values) may be used as the physiologic component for triage using American College of Surgeons guidelines. Patients with a trauma score of 12 or less or a T-RTS of 11 or less should be transported to a trauma center. The trauma score and revised trauma score may also be used in TRISS calculations for quality assurance assessments of trauma care. The three coded values of the revised trauma score are weighted for use in TRISS. The equation is as follows:

$$RTS = 0.9368\ GCS_o + 0.7326\ SBP_o + 0.2908\ RR_o$$

The range of revised trauma score is from 0 to 7.841.

References

American College of Surgeons. Appendix G to hospital resources document: quality assurance in trauma care. Hospital and prehospital resources for optimal care of the injured patient. Appendices A through J. Chicago: American College of Surgeons, 1987.

Boyd CR, Tolson MA, Copes WS. Evaluating trauma care: the TRISS method. J Trauma 1987; 27:370–378.

Champion HR, Sacco WJ, Carnazzo AJ, et al. Trauma score. Crit Care Med 1981; 9:672–676.

Champion HR, Sacco WJ, Copes WS, et al. A revision of the trauma score. J Trauma 1989; 29:623–629.

Teasdale G, Jennett B. Assessment of coma and impaired consciousness: a practical scale. Lancet 1974; 2:81–84.

(Cont'd from p 279)

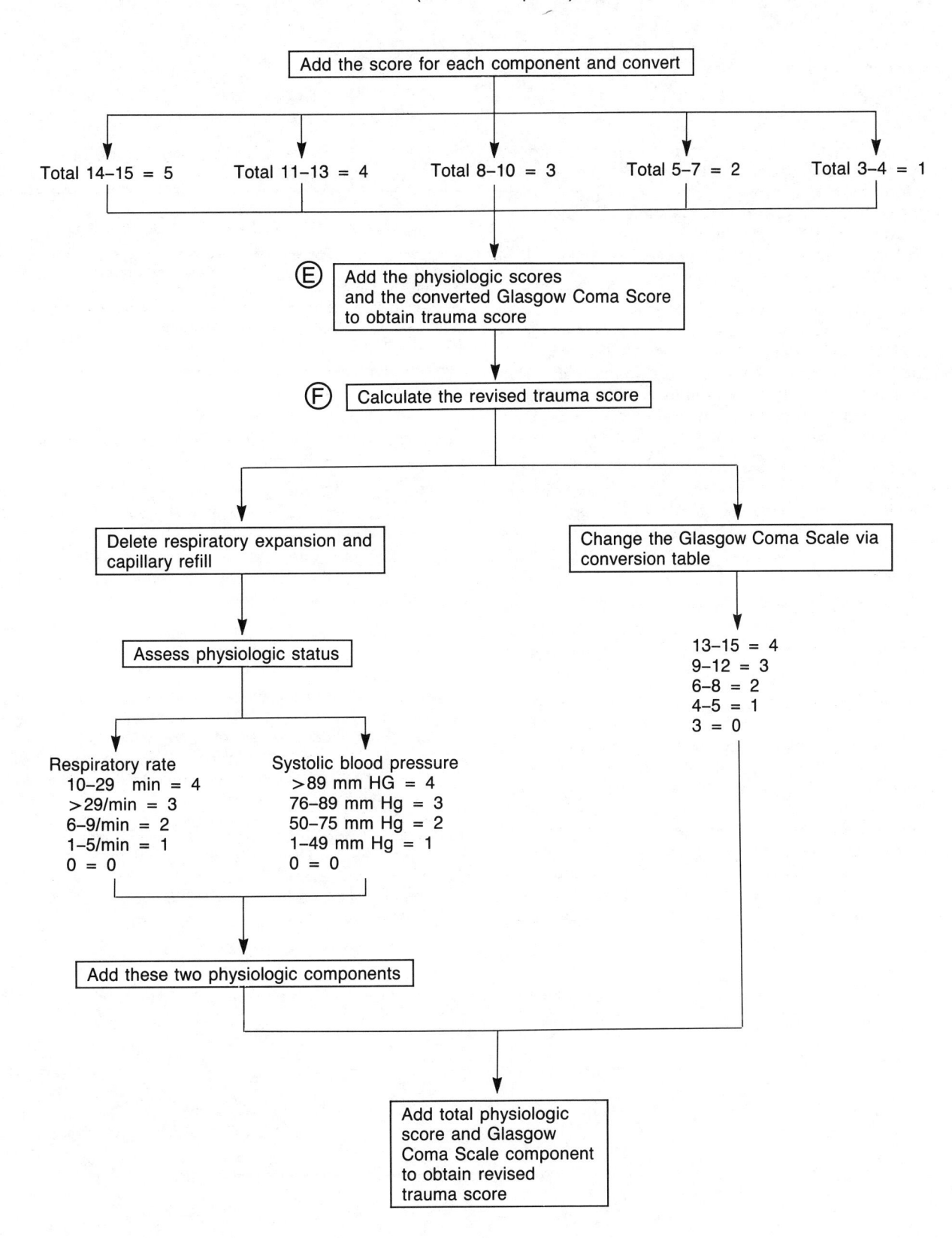

```
                    ┌─────────────────────────────────────────┐
                    │ Add the score for each component and convert │
                    └─────────────────────────────────────────┘
         ↓              ↓              ↓              ↓              ↓
   Total 14–15 = 5  Total 11–13 = 4  Total 8–10 = 3  Total 5–7 = 2  Total 3–4 = 1
                                      ↓
                    ┌─────────────────────────────────────────┐
                 (E)│ Add the physiologic scores              │
                    │ and the converted Glasgow Coma Score    │
                    │ to obtain trauma score                  │
                    └─────────────────────────────────────────┘
                                      ↓
                 (F)│ Calculate the revised trauma score │
```

Delete respiratory expansion and capillary refill

Change the Glasgow Coma Scale via conversion table

Assess physiologic status

13–15 = 4
9–12 = 3
6–8 = 2
4–5 = 1
3 = 0

Respiratory rate
10–29 min = 4
>29/min = 3
6–9/min = 2
1–5/min = 1
0 = 0

Systolic blood pressure
>89 mm HG = 4
76–89 mm Hg = 3
50–75 mm Hg = 2
1–49 mm Hg = 1
0 = 0

Add these two physiologic components

Add total physiologic score and Glasgow Coma Scale component to obtain revised trauma score

INJURY SEVERITY SCORE

Mary M. Lawnick
Maureen E. Flanagan

A. Injuries sustained by trauma patients must be confirmed by physical examination, radiographic studies, surgical intervention, or autopsy. Internal organ injuries should not be based on physical examination only; they must be confirmed by a diagnostic procedure. The nurse must abstract *all* injuries from a complete patient medical record.

B. The injury severity score (ISS) is an index of anatomic injury that takes values from one to 75. Higher scores generally indicate more severe injuries. Calculation of the ISS is based on the abbreviated injury scale (AIS), an integer scale that scores injury severity from one (minor injury) to six (virtually unsurvivable injury). An AIS score is assigned to each injury a patient sustains.

C. Each injury is also sorted into one of six ISS body regions, as follows: head and neck, face, chest, abdominal and pelvic contents, extremities and pelvic girdle, and external region. Be aware that body regions listed in the AIS manual do not always correspond to ISS body regions.

D. List the highest AIS score in each ISS body region. If injuries occur in only one region, regardless of how many injuries exist, only the highest AIS score in that region is listed.

E. Square the highest three AIS scores from the list in *D*. If injuries occur in more than three regions, the highest AIS scores in only three regions are used for calculation. There is one exception: If an AIS score of six is assigned to any injury, that patient's ISS is automatically 75. An AIS score of six may only be assigned to the specific injuries listed in the manual and may not be assigned based on the patient's outcome. An example of this scoring system is shown in Table 1. In the example, the highest AIS scores in three different body regions are three (chest), three (extremities), and two (head and neck). To square these three highest scores, one calculates as follows: $3^2 = 9$, $3^2 = 9$, and $2^2 = 4$.

F. To obtain the ISS, add the squares of the highest AIS scores in the three different body regions. In the example in Table 1, the ISS would be $9 + 9 + 4 = 22$. The ISS has been correlated with outcome. TRISS calculations for quality assurance assessments of trauma care utilize ISS in the analysis.

TABLE 1 AIS Score and ISS Body Region of Injured Patient

Injury	AIS Score	ISS Body Region
Concussion	2	Head and neck
Pulmonary contusion	3	Chest
Superficial liver laceration	2	Abdominal and pelvic contents
Fractured femur	3	Extremities
Scalp laceration	1	External

References

American Association for Automative Medicine. The abbreviated injury scale (AIS)—1990 revision. Des Plaines, IL: American Association for Automotive Medicine, 1990.

Baker SP, O'Neill B, Haddon W, Long WB. The injury severity score: a method for describing patients with multiple injuries and evaluating emergency care. J Trauma 1974; 14:187–196.

Copes WS, Champion HR, Sacco WJ, Lawnick MM, et al. The injury severity score revisited. J Trauma 1988; 28:69–77.

Copes WS, Lawnick MM, Champion HR, Sacco WJ. A comparison of abbreviated injury scale 1980 and 1985 versions. J Trauma 1988; 28:78–86.

Patient with TRAUMA

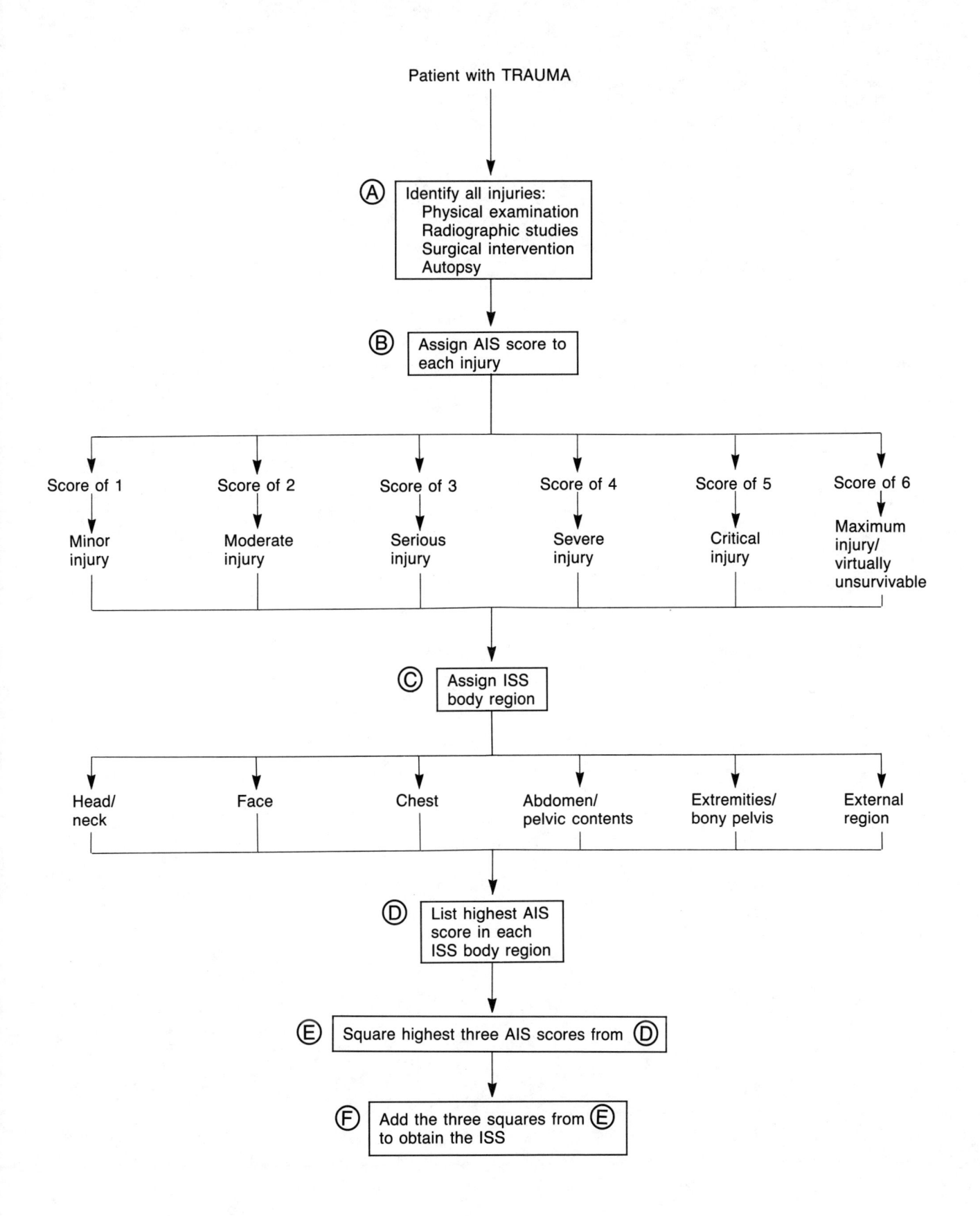

- **(A)** Identify all injuries:
  - Physical examination
  - Radiographic studies
  - Surgical intervention
  - Autopsy

- **(B)** Assign AIS score to each injury

Score of 1	Score of 2	Score of 3	Score of 4	Score of 5	Score of 6
Minor injury	Moderate injury	Serious injury	Severe injury	Critical injury	Maximum injury/ virtually unsurvivable

- **(C)** Assign ISS body region

| Head/neck | Face | Chest | Abdomen/pelvic contents | Extremities/bony pelvis | External region |

- **(D)** List highest AIS score in each ISS body region

- **(E)** Square highest three AIS scores from **(D)**

- **(F)** Add the three squares from **(E)** to obtain the ISS

STABILIZATION/SUPPORTIVE CARE

Anesthesia for the Trauma Patient
Nutritional Support
Fluid, Electrolyte and Acid-Base Imbalance
Operating Room Management
Open Wounds
Coagulation Problems
Febrile Syndromes
Acute Renal Failure
Gas Gangrene Infection
Hepatic Failure
Respiratory Failure
Mechanical Ventilation

Delayed Shock Management
Cardiogenic Shock
Neurogenic Shock
Septic Shock
Multiple Organ Failure
Stress Gastritis
Pulmonary Embolism
Deep Vein Thrombosis
Therapy for Infectious Processes
Organ Procurement
Crisis Intervention
Helicopter and Fixed-Wing Transportation

ANESTHESIA FOR THE TRAUMA PATIENT

Kevin W. Klein

A. A thorough evaluation of the trauma patient prior to surgery is the key to avoiding anesthetic mishaps. Of course the ABCs—airway, breathing, and circulation—should be checked first. Examination of the airway is crucial for an uneventful intubation. Auscultation of the heart and lungs helps detect airway obstruction or pneumothorax. Measurement of blood pressure, heart rate, and hemoglobin concentration allows estimation of the degree of blood loss and the adequacy of fluid replacement. The time of the last meal and evidence of intoxication should be noted, as should pre-existing disease and current drug therapy. The completeness of this examination is dictated by the urgency of surgery.

B. There are many factors that influence the choice of anesthetic technique, but immediately important are the extent and location of all injuries and the degree of hemorrhage and resuscitation. Minor procedures may be performed with intravenous or intramuscular ketamine. A potential danger with most parenteral sedatives, however, is loss of laryngeal reflexes and the risk of vomiting and aspiration. An intravenous regional block is useful for brief procedures such as closed reduction of hand and forearm fractures. Regional anesthesia may be used for selected cases, e.g., a brachial plexus block for hand and forearm procedures. Spinal and epidural anesthesias are generally to be avoided if there is any question about volume status or extent of injury. Most patients, especially those who are unstable, are best treated with general endotracheal anesthesia. Rapid sequence intubation with succinylcholine, cricoid pressure, and a cuffed endotracheal tube provides the best protection against aspiration.

C. The intraoperative period offers a unique setting for resuscitation. Ventilation can be judged by breath-to-breath end tidal carbon dioxide monitoring, and oxygenation can be assessed by pulse oximetry, both of which are now present in most operating rooms. Arterial blood gas measurements may provide additional information. Intravascular volume and perfusion may be assessed clinically by noninvasive measurement of blood pressure, pulse, and urine output. For the patient in shock, more invasive monitoring—including arterial pressure, central venous pressure, pulmonary artery pressure, thermodilution cardiac output, and saturation of mixed venous hemoglobin—may be warranted. Hemoglobin or hematocrit in the normovolemic patient should be kept at an adequate level to ensure oxygen delivery to all organs. Patients who are volume depleted and exposed are almost uniformly hypothermic. Warming measures should be taken to prevent cold induced coagulopathy. Metabolic disturbances are especially common in the shock trauma patient and should be assessed with arterial blood gas and base change measurement. Electrolytes can be measured and corrected with subsequent fluid therapy. The normal kidney takes care of most of these problems. The massively transfused patient also develops coagulation disturbances which should be aggressively treated. Measuring prothrombin time, partial thromboplastin time, platelets, fibrinogen, and fibrin split products helps guide blood product and drug therapy.

D. The anesthesiologist must provide the postanesthetic patient with a smooth transition of care. Recovery from anesthetic drugs must be complete. Ventilation and circulation should be stable. The patient should have an appropriate amount of analgesia so that the surgeon may reassess the extent of injury. Lastly, any complications should be assessed and addressed.

References

Barie PS, Shires GT. Initial trauma management of multiple injuries. In: Parrillo JE, ed. Current therapy in critical care medicine. Toronto: BC Decker, 1987: 306–314.

Donnan GB, Giesecke AH. Principles of trauma care. New York: McGraw-Hill, 1985: 62–84.

Giesecke AH, Grande CM, Whitten CW. Overview of trauma anesthesia and critical care. Crit Care Clin 1990; 6:61–71.

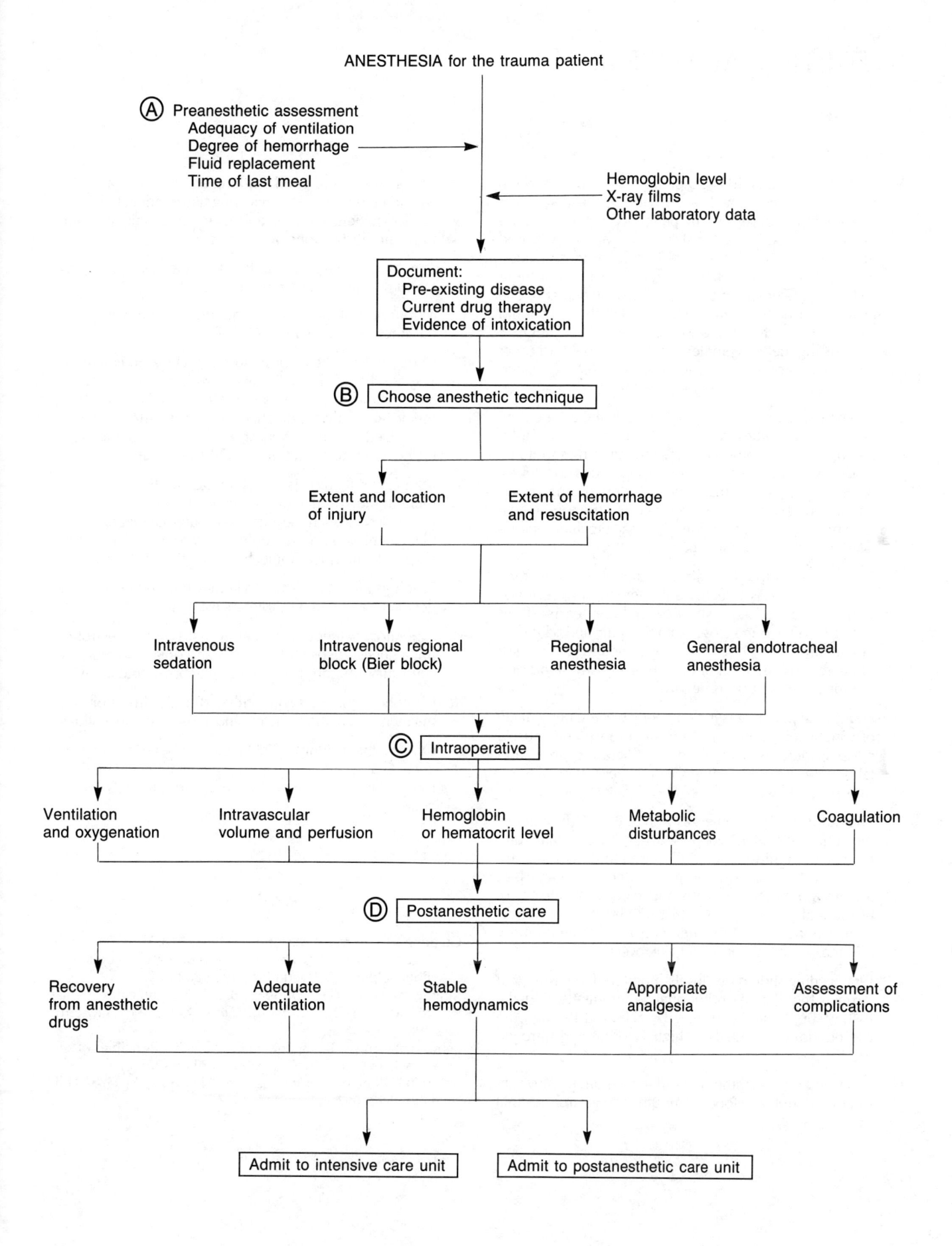

ANESTHESIA for the trauma patient

(A) Preanesthetic assessment
- Adequacy of ventilation
- Degree of hemorrhage
- Fluid replacement
- Time of last meal

- Hemoglobin level
- X-ray films
- Other laboratory data

Document:
- Pre-existing disease
- Current drug therapy
- Evidence of intoxication

(B) Choose anesthetic technique
- Extent and location of injury
- Extent of hemorrhage and resuscitation

- Intravenous sedation
- Intravenous regional block (Bier block)
- Regional anesthesia
- General endotracheal anesthesia

(C) Intraoperative
- Ventilation and oxygenation
- Intravascular volume and perfusion
- Hemoglobin or hematocrit level
- Metabolic disturbances
- Coagulation

(D) Postanesthetic care
- Recovery from anesthetic drugs
- Adequate ventilation
- Stable hemodynamics
- Appropriate analgesia
- Assessment of complications

- Admit to intensive care unit
- Admit to postanesthetic care unit

NUTRITIONAL SUPPORT

Jodi Luke

A. It is estimated that 40 to 50 percent of hospitalized patients are malnourished, even without the associated stress of injury or sepsis. The patient with multiple injuries is at a much greater risk because of the increased metabolic demands associated with injuries, wound healing, and complications such as sepsis. All of these result in long-term high calorie and protein demand. The history is usually obtained from the family and should include such factors as previous unexplained weight loss, pre-existing medical problems such as diabetes or other metabolic problems, previous gastrointestinal disturbances, and assessment of the preinjury nutritional state.

B. The patient's assessment should include the extent of injuries because nutritional deficits increase with multiple injuries. Gastrointestinal tract functioning should be assessed, including the presence of nasogastric tubes, bowel sounds, abdominal injuries, history of emesis, and elimination patterns. The presence of an endotracheal tube or massive facial injuries that may preclude oral intake should also be noted.

C. Early attention to the repair of injuries and the restoration of homeostasis decrease the length of hypermetabolic states. Goals should include early fluid resuscitation, wound closure, bone repair, and pain control, all of which reduce catecholamine levels and assist in decreasing the level of hypermetabolism found during the initial period of recovery.

D. Nutritional parameters include body weight; percentage of weight loss; anthropometry of adipose and muscle masses; measurement of immunologic response; and laboratory values including creatinine excretion, and serum protein levels.

E. The nutritional parameters as well as the nutritional history, physical evidence of pre-existing disease states, and the extent of injuries should be used to determine current nutritional needs. The patient should be assessed for nutritional requirements and means of delivery of nutritional support within 48 to 72 hours after admission. The nutritional requirements need to be continually reassessed as the patient recovers.

F. Oral feeding should be closely monitored to ensure that it meets the patient's nutritional requirements. If intake is low, supplementation may be achieved through the use of additional meals or high calorie, high nitrogen foods.

G. Tube feeding is commonly used in the patient who cannot or will not take food by mouth. The gastrointestinal tract should be in good working order, and a gag reflex should be present. Administering tube feeding to the obtunded patient with an endotracheal or tracheostomy tube should be done with great care.

H. The three primary types of tubes are the nasogastric, gastrostomy, and jejunostomy tubes.

I. Monitoring of electrolytes and glucose levels is essential because imbalances can occur.

J. Common complications include aspiration and diarrhea. The diarrhea can usually be controlled by adjusting the rate, volume, or concentration of the formula. Tube placement should always be checked prior to administration of the feeding. The patient should be placed in the head-up position, and suction should be available.

K. Intravenous feeding is used for total nutritional management in the absence of oral intake. Catheters are usually inserted through the external or internal jugular veins. Placement should be confirmed via chest film. Strict aseptic technique should be used to avoid sepsis.

L. Feedings are administered via infusion pumps, and the flow rates and patient's tolerance are closely monitored.

M. Laboratory values are frequently assessed for electrolyte imbalance, glucose intolerance, and organ function. Insulin may be administered for glucose intolerance.

N. Complications are usually related to the insertion and maintenance of the catheters and to septic complications.

O. Observe the patient's weight patterns and general appearance. Reassess nutritional supplementation and delivery route during recovery because the patient's needs change.

References

Cordona VD, Hurn PP, Mason PJ, Schlipp AM, Veise-Berry SW. Trauma nursing from resuscitation through rehabilitation. Philadelphia: WB Saunders, 1988:284–313.

Kinney MR, Packa DR, Dunbar SB. AACN's clinical reference for critical-care nursing. New York: McGraw-Hill, 1988:360–362.

Schwartz SI, Shires TG, Spencer FC, Storer EH. Principles of surgery. New York: McGraw-Hill, 1979:86–97.

Shires TG. Principles of trauma care. New York: McGraw-Hill, 1985:592–607.

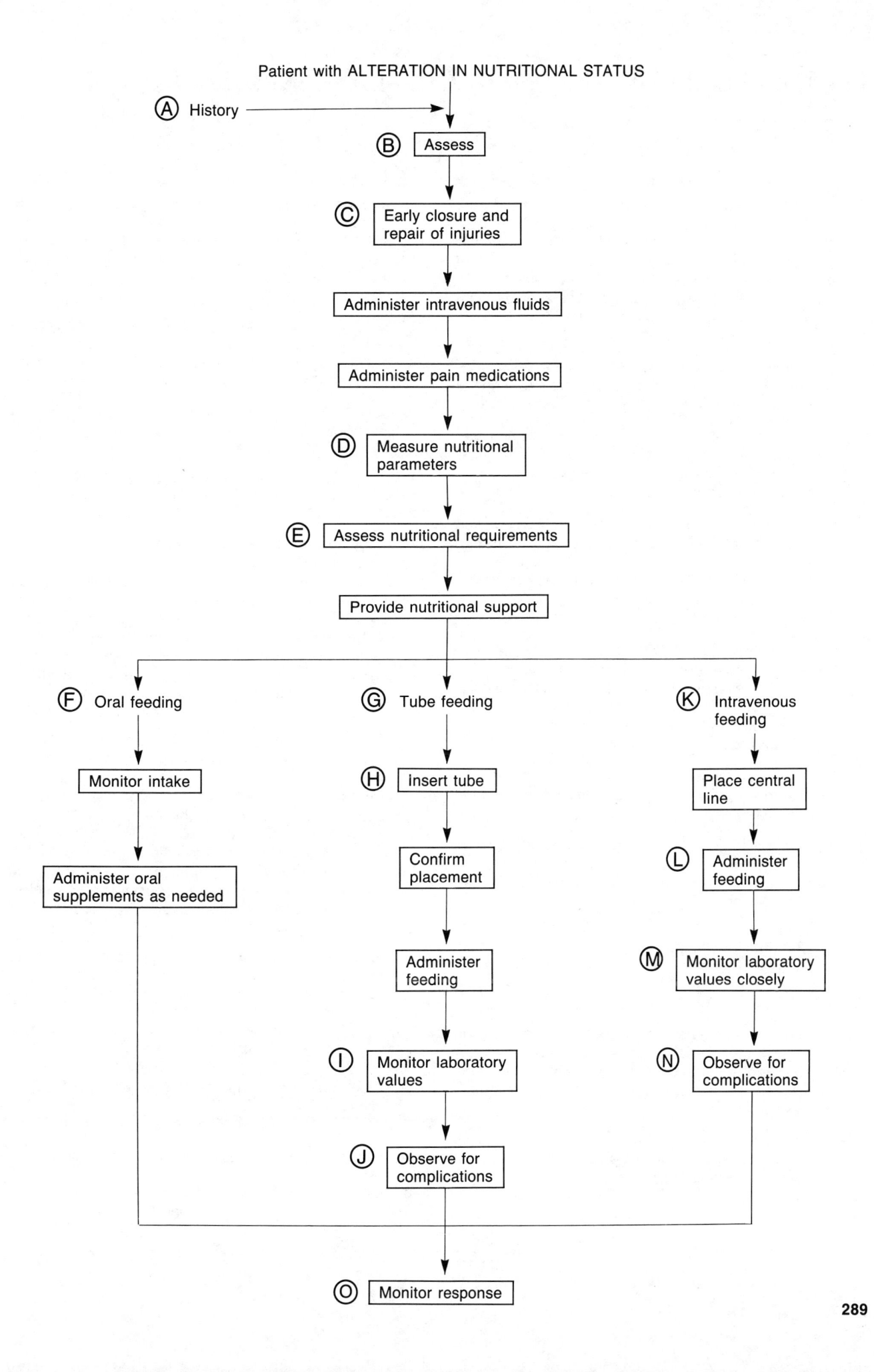

Patient with ALTERATION IN NUTRITIONAL STATUS

```
(A) History ──────────────→ ↓
                           (B) Assess
                                ↓
                    (C) Early closure and
                        repair of injuries
                                ↓
                    Administer intravenous fluids
                                ↓
                    Administer pain medications
                                ↓
                    (D) Measure nutritional
                        parameters
                                ↓
                    (E) Assess nutritional requirements
                                ↓
                    Provide nutritional support
         ┌──────────────────────┼──────────────────────┐
         ↓                      ↓                      ↓
   (F) Oral feeding       (G) Tube feeding       (K) Intravenous
         ↓                      ↓                     feeding
   Monitor intake         (H) Insert tube              ↓
         ↓                      ↓                Place central
   Administer oral         Confirm                  line
   supplements as needed   placement                  ↓
                                ↓                (L) Administer
                           Administer                feeding
                           feeding                    ↓
                                ↓                (M) Monitor laboratory
                           (I) Monitor laboratory    values closely
                               values                 ↓
                                ↓                (N) Observe for
                           (J) Observe for          complications
                               complications
         └──────────────────────┼──────────────────────┘
                                ↓
                        (O) Monitor response
```

289

FLUID, ELECTROLYTE, AND ACID–BASE IMBALANCE

Molly A. Seaman

A. Patient care begins with a careful history. The trauma patient with one injury or multisystem injury is susceptible to fluid and electrolyte imbalance. Additionally, the postsurgical patient continues to be at risk for fluid and electrolyte imbalance. Excessive nasogastric suctioning and massive transfusions are but a few of the treatments that can place the patient at risk.

B. Perform a thorough physical assessment. Carefully note any symptoms that might indicate a disturbance in fluids or electrolytes. The patient may have dry skin, edema, seizures, or rales. Record observations to plan care.

C. Baseline laboratory studies should be obtained and recorded. Although the patient may demonstrate signs or symptoms of imbalance, laboratory data gives specific direction for treatment.

D. Fluid choices depend on the degree of dehydration and the patient's overall circulatory status. Diuresis may be indicated for those who have purely a sodium gain. Treat hypernatremia caused by water loss by replacing with D_5W infusion. These patients must be monitored closely for fluid overload during and after treatment.

E. Those patients whose laboratory tests show hyponatremia may be physically dehydrated, edematous, or clinically nonsymptomatic. Those who have lost both sodium and water can be treated with normal saline bolus. Again, however, watch for fluid overload. Those who are edematous should have fluids restricted.

F. If the patient progresses to having seizures or to a decreased level of consciousness, treat more aggressively with diuretics.

G. The trauma patient is susceptible to a drop in potassium level caused not only by injury but also for overexcretion of potassium by the kidney or through prolonged nasogastric suctioning. Correct the potassium level by adding supplements to intravenous infusions.

H. Patients must be monitored closely for cardiac arrhythmias.

I. Monitor patients for a drop in calcium level.

J. Hypercalcemia can result from prolonged immobilization and/or use of thiazide diuretics. In most cases this can be corrected by forced hydration with normal saline. As with any patient receiving a fluid challenge, watch for overload.

K. More aggressive treatment may include diuretics such as furosemide (Lasix) to increase calcium excretion that is inhibited by thiazides.

L. For those who are hypocalcemic, possibly as a result of dialysis or massive transfusions, calcium supplements may be given. Intravenous calcium gluconate is given over a short period and followed by continued infusion if necessary.

M. Hypermagnesium often results from renal insufficiency. Agents are given intravenously to increase uptake of magnesium. These may include calcium chloride, glucose, and/or insulin infusions. Dialysis may need to be considered.

N. As with other electrolyte deficiencies, supplements can be given. Magnesium sulfate can be given parenterally to correct the problem of hyponagnesium.

O. Examine arterial blood gas results and determine whether acid-base imbalance is caused by respiratory, metabolic, or mixed component.

P. Respiratory acidosis occurs when carbon dioxide accumulates in the blood secondary to hypoventilation. In the trauma patient or postoperative patient, anything that restricts breathing or expansion can place the patient at risk. Treatment consists of correcting the restrictive problem if possible and/or increasing ventilations on the respirator if intubated. Metabolic acidosis can occur as a result of lactic acid buildup. This usually occurs in shock patients. Treat by correcting the underlying cause. The administration of sodium bicarbonate can also help. Monitor arterial blood gases closely.

Q. Respiratory alkalosis results from hyperventilation. Many factors may contribute to this condition, such as hypoxemia, sepsis, pain, or CNS lesions. Treat the underlying cause and use sedation or rebreathing devices to control hyperventilation. Metabolic alkalosis occurs when the bicarbonate level increases. In the trauma patient, this may be caused by vomiting, prolonged nasogastric suctioning, hypokalemia, or overcorrection of other electrolyte imbalances. Treatment is aimed at correcting the underlying cause.

R. When abnormalities have been stabilized, continue to monitor vital signs, intake and output, laboratory results, and the clinical appearance of the patient for changes.

References

Dubin HG. Calcium and magnesium metabolism: a review. Trauma Q 1986; 2:32–41.
Kemper SM. Hyponatremia and hypernatremia. Trauma Q 1986; 2:55–60.
Sullivan F. Hypokalemia and hyperkalemia. Trauma Q 1986; 2:61–73.

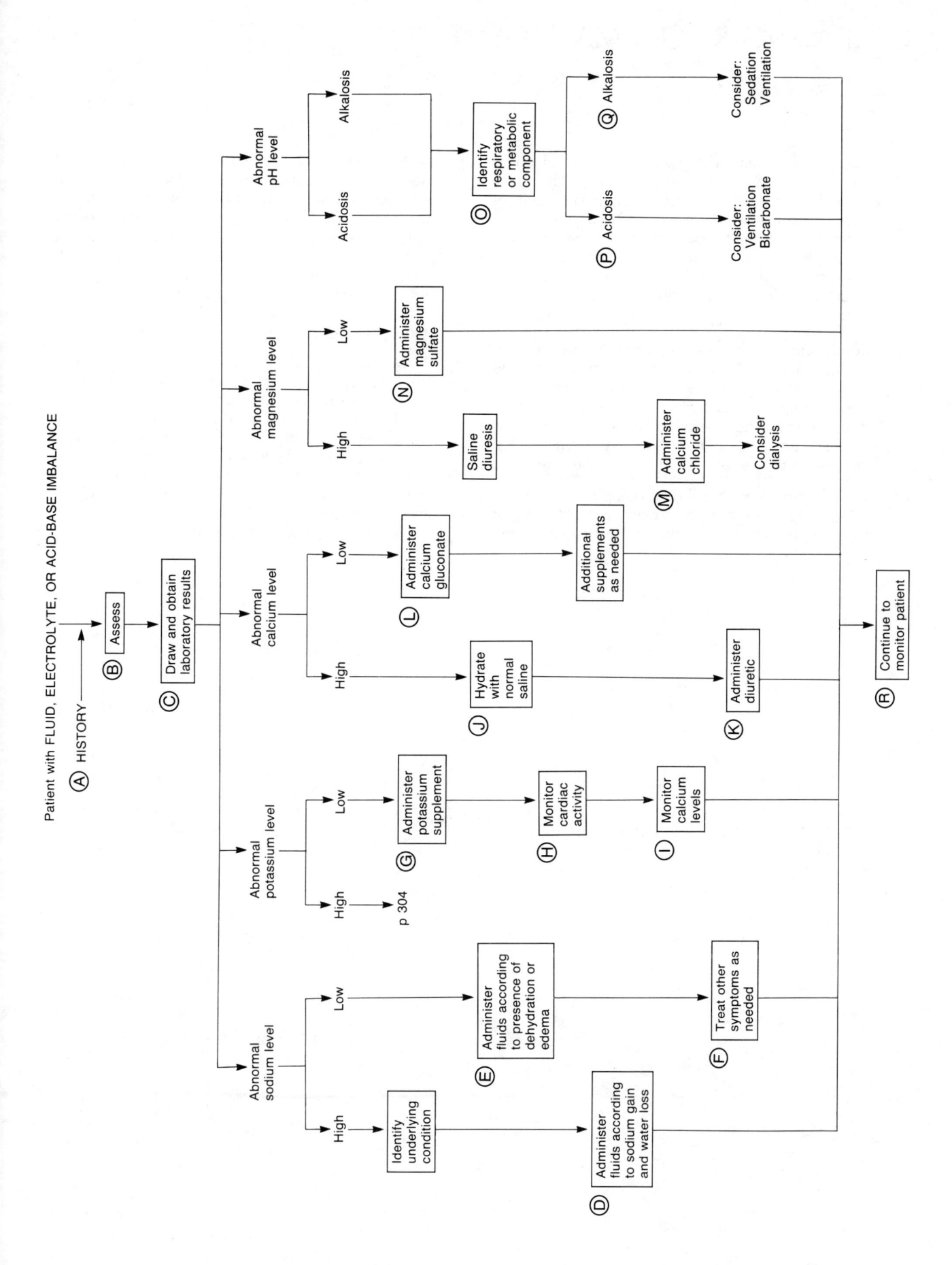

Patient with FLUID, ELECTROLYTE, OR ACID-BASE IMBALANCE

- **A** HISTORY
- **B** Assess
- **C** Draw and obtain laboratory results

Abnormal sodium level
- **High** → Identify underlying condition → **D** Administer fluids according to sodium gain and water loss
- **Low** → **E** Administer fluids according to presence of dehydration or edema
- **F** Treat other symptoms as needed

Abnormal potassium level
- **High** → p 304
- **Low** → **G** Administer potassium supplement → **H** Monitor cardiac activity → **I** Monitor calcium levels

Abnormal calcium level
- **High** → **J** Hydrate with normal saline → **K** Administer diuretic
- **Low** → **L** Administer calcium gluconate → Additional supplements as needed

Abnormal magnesium level
- **High** → Saline diuresis → **M** Administer calcium chloride → Consider dialysis
- **Low** → **N** Administer magnesium sulfate

Abnormal pH level
- Alkalosis
- Acidosis
- **O** Identify respiratory or metabolic component
  - **Q** Alkalosis → Consider: Sedation, Ventilation
  - **P** Acidosis → Consider: Ventilation, Bicarbonate

- **R** Continue to monitor patient

291

OPERATING ROOM MANAGEMENT

Doreen Reynolds

A. Multisystem trauma is defined as injuries sustained by two or more body systems. One or more may be life threatening. The predominant symptom that often requires immediate surgery is hypovolemic shock resulting from severe hemorrhage. Pulmonary parenchymal injuries, cardiac injuries, brain injury, and spinal cord injury may further complicate the clinical picture. Documentation of assessment and interventions is critical.

B. Priorities are established according to injuries that pose the gravest danger to the patient. Hemorrhage must be stopped, circulating volume returned to normal, and tissue oxygenation improved before other injuries are treated. In caring for the multisystem trauma patient, focus is on early intervention in the shock syndrome, on anticipation of problems, and on appropriate action.

C. Attention should be initially placed on controlling the environment, reassuring the patient, and planning for proper positioning and padding. It is extremely important to maintain body alignment when moving the patient onto the operating table. There may be undiagnosed fractured or dislocated vertebrae and other skeletal injuries. Cervical collars, sandbags, and splints should be left in place until radiographs rule out fractures. Decreased circulating volume, peripheral vasoconstriction, and subsequent diminished tissue oxygen supply increase the patient's risk of pressure ulcers and equipment burns; these complications require the use of proper padding. Proper grounding must also be assured.

D. Frequent checks and recording of peripheral circulation are important. Particular attention is paid to areas distal to known injuries (e.g., pedal and tibial pulses below a fractured tibia and fibula). It is also important that no equipment or operating room team member applies pressure to the patient's body. Improper positioning and pressure can cause brachial and ulnar nerve damage. The patient on a warming blanket must be adequately protected from burns; hyperthermia units and blood warmers should be properly monitored.

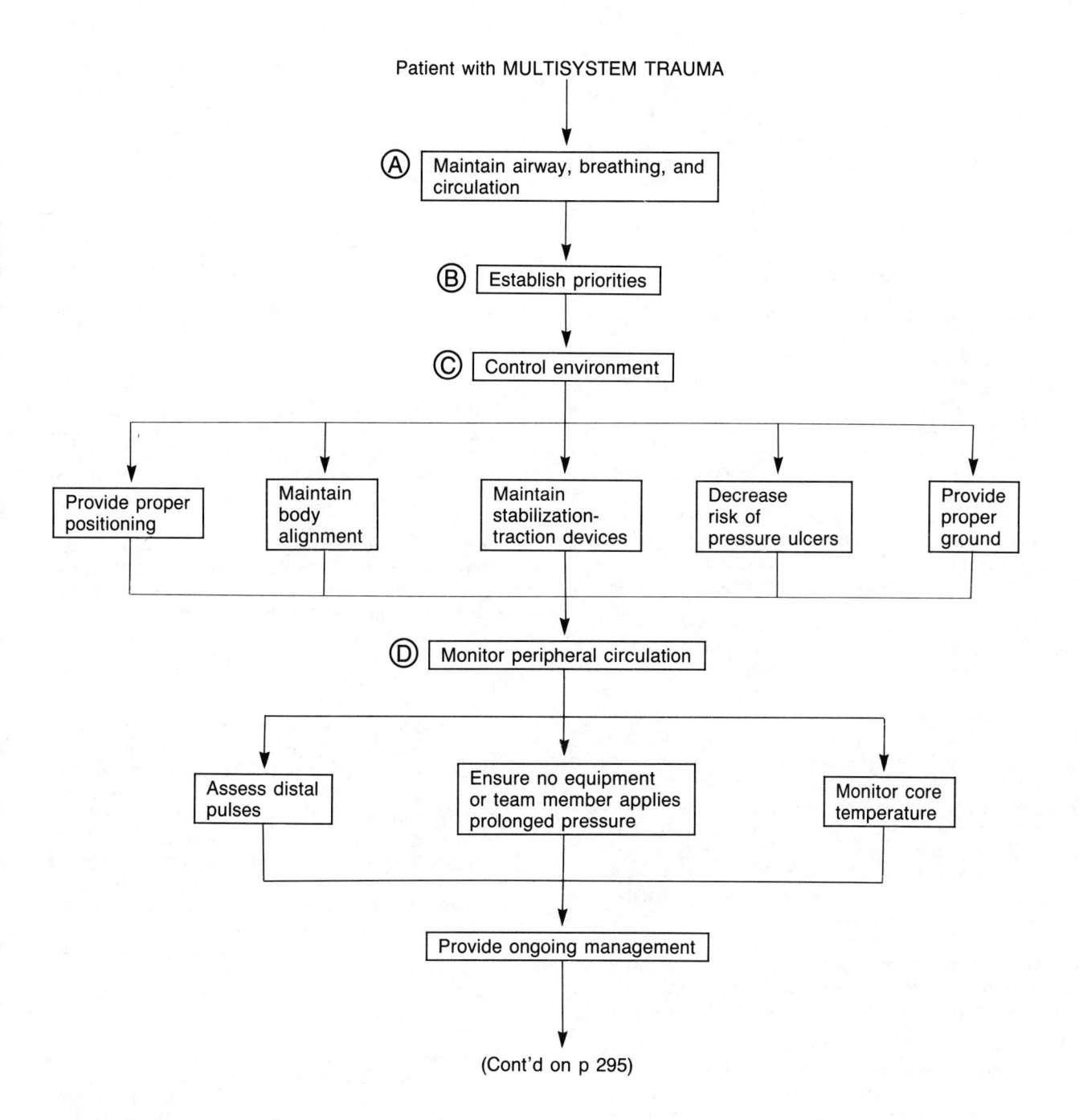

Patient with MULTISYSTEM TRAUMA
↓
(A) Maintain airway, breathing, and circulation
↓
(B) Establish priorities
↓
(C) Control environment
↓
- Provide proper positioning
- Maintain body alignment
- Maintain stabilization-traction devices
- Decrease risk of pressure ulcers
- Provide proper ground

↓
(D) Monitor peripheral circulation
↓
- Assess distal pulses
- Ensure no equipment or team member applies prolonged pressure
- Monitor core temperature

↓
Provide ongoing management
↓
(Cont'd on p 295)

E. Hypovolemic shock is treated by rapid infusion of volume expanders and by pneumatic antishock garment (PASG) or military antishock trousers. These inflatable trousers increase the blood circulating to the heart, brain, lungs, and kidneys. The trousers should not be removed until the surgeon is confident the hemorrhage is controlled. Surgery can be performed by deflating the abdominal section of the trousers. The legs are left inflated to improve circulation to the vital organs. Periodically the nurse should ask the surgeon about deflating the PASG.

F. Fluid resuscitation is the most critical phase of care for the multisystem trauma patient. This is begun at the scene and continued until the hemorrhage is surgically stopped and circulating volume is restored. Volume expanders are started initially; these are crystalloids (Ringer's lactate and normal saline) and colloids (albumin, Plasma-Lyte). Whole blood must be started immediately in the operating room. It may be necessary to give type O, Rh-negative (i.e., universal donor) blood. When type-specific or complete cross-matched blood is available, it should be administered rapidly. The patient's oxygen transport problems are not resolved until there is adequate hemoglobin to carry oxygen to the tissues.

G. Operating room teams may use autotransfusion to replace volume. Autologous blood is salvaged during surgery, filtered to remove debris, and reinfused through available intravenous lines. The advantages of autotransfusion include decreased risk of transfusion reaction compared with homologous blood and rapid blood replacement in the face of severe blood shortages. This method is valuable, particularly if the patient has a rare blood type. However the disadvantages of autotransfusion include the possibility that infected or malignant cells in the operative field may be returned to the systemic circulation. As well, coagulation abnormalities may develop from hemolysis of red blood cells. The additional step of washing the erythrocytes prior to reinfusion reduces the likelihood of coagulation disorders. Disseminated intravascular coagulation is seen less frequently because the technology and skill in treating hypovolemic shock have improved.

H. Intravenous intake, central venous pressure (CVP), urinary output, and output from other sources—such as suction, chest tubes, and the nasogastric tube—must be monitored throughout fluid resuscitation. CVP readings indicate the circulating volume returning to the heart and the cardiac pump action. A continuous low CVP reading indicates that further fluid resuscitation is necessary. A rapid increase in CVP could indicate pump failure. If this increase is coupled with sudden rales and rhonchi in the chest, fluid overload should be suspected.

I. Because hypovolemic shock is accompanied by metabolic acidosis, arterial blood gas samples should be taken frequently. The results determine the level of acidosis and compensation. Arterial blood gases also indicate how well therapy is working. Intravenous sodium bicarbonate may be given to reverse metabolic acidosis. Brain injured patients usually have vital signs that are the reverse of hypovolemic shock (i.e., high blood pressure and slow pulse). Hypovolemic shock is always treated first, since brain injury is usually not immediately life threatening.

J. Fluid resuscitation can lower the body's core temperature to the extent that severe hypothermia results. Hypothermia is also a late complication of shock. Because of the cool operating room environment, the patient can also experience losses in core temperature from open surgical wounds. All fluids given intravenously should be warmed. This can be rapidly accomplished with a fluid warmer. The patient should be on a warming blanket throughout the surgery. The patient may also be covered with Thermadrape. Untreated hypothermia causes circulatory collapse and death.

K. Because urinary output is an indication of improved circulation and perfusion, the amount of urine must be closely monitored. A Foley catheter must be inserted early. The collection system should be calibrated to measure small amounts of urine accurately. An accurate record must be kept of all output, including that from suction, chest tubes, and nasogastric tube, in order that the patient's volume output can be replaced. This also includes blood loss on sponges. Accurate intake and output records greatly improve fluid resuscitation. Serious, unnoticed fluid overload can increase intracranial pressure and adversely affect the injured brain. Pulmonary complications and acid-base disturbances develop following fluid overload. Excess fluid is absorbed into the interstitial spaces, and oxygen–carbon dioxide gas exchange is altered. Decreased circulating volume causes cellular hypoxia, which partially results from the loss of hemoglobin. The remaining blood has less oxygen carrying ability. Hyperventilation compensates for metabolic acidosis and increases the oxygen supply to the available hemoglobin. Trauma patients with associated pulmonary injuries can develop respiratory acidosis caused by decreased ventilation (oxygen–carbon dioxide exchange) at the alveolar level. The brain injured patient also has decreased ventilation, which is attributable to damage to respiratory drive centers. High flow oxygen and rapid manual or mechanical ventilation decrease carbon dioxide levels. This is the preferred treatment for respiratory acidosis.

L. After surgery, a report is called to the receiving unit. The report should include total fluid intake and output; present urinary output rate; and output from all sources, including chest tubes and nasogastric tube. Vital signs before, during, and after surgery as well as the most recent blood pressure, pulse, and CVP must be communicated. Medications given before and during surgery should be brought to the attention of the receiving team.

References

Shires GT. Principles of trauma care. New York: McGraw-Hill, 1985:3–41.

Lockwood B. Preparing for patients with multi-system trauma. AORN 1981; 34:829–837.

Toombs B. OR nursing care of trauma patients. AORN 1978; 28:227–231.

(Cont'd from p 293)

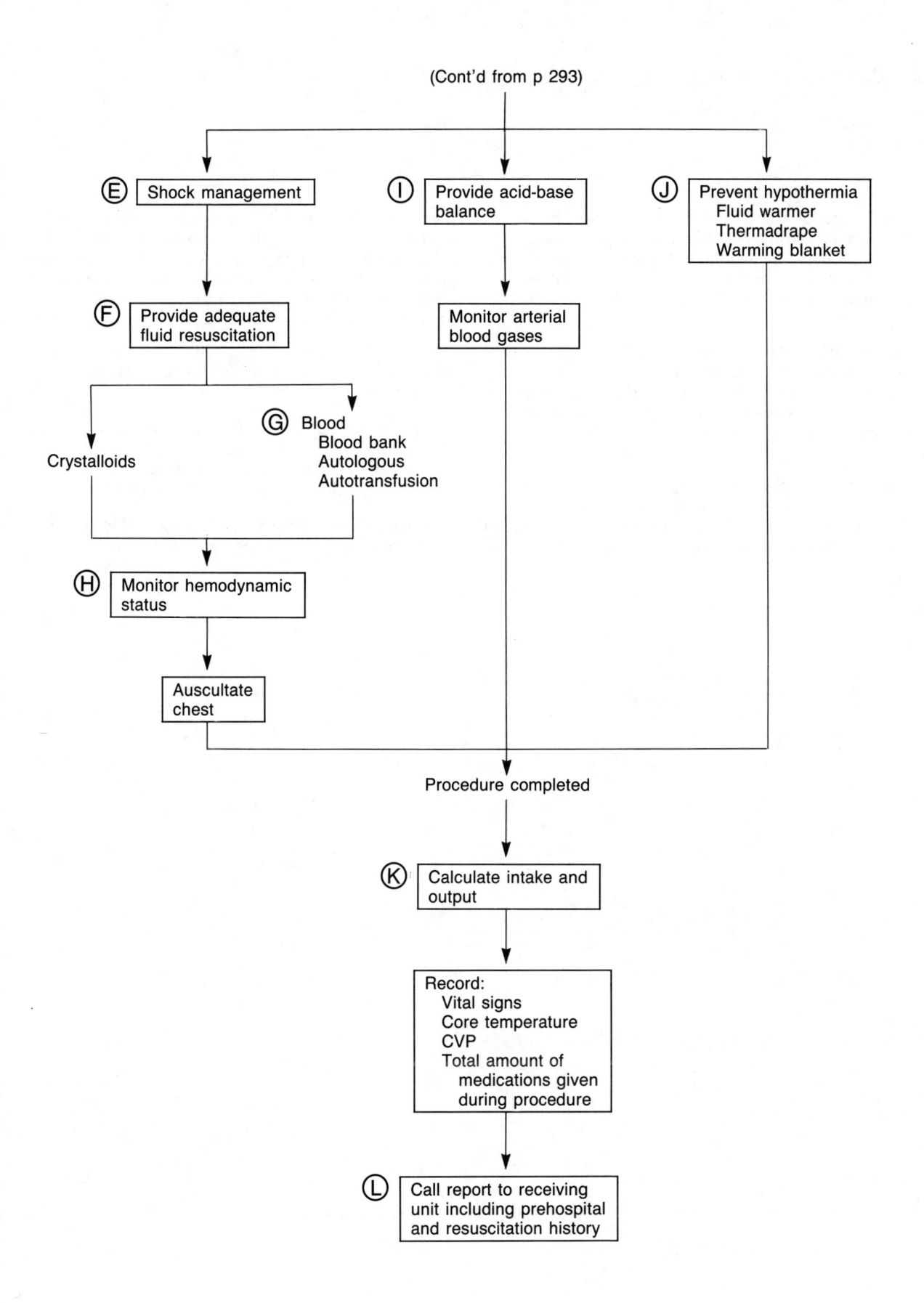

```
                    │
    ┌───────────────┼───────────────┐
    ▼               ▼               ▼
Ⓔ Shock         Ⓘ Provide       Ⓙ Prevent hypothermia
  management      acid-base         Fluid warmer
                  balance           Thermadrape
    │               │               Warming blanket
    ▼               ▼
Ⓕ Provide       Monitor arterial
  adequate        blood gases
  fluid
  resuscitation
    │
    ├───────────────┐
    ▼               ▼
Crystalloids    Ⓖ Blood
                  Blood bank
                  Autologous
                  Autotransfusion
    │
    ▼
Ⓗ Monitor hemodynamic
  status
    │
    ▼
Auscultate
chest
```

Procedure completed

Ⓚ Calculate intake and output

Record:
    Vital signs
    Core temperature
    CVP
    Total amount of medications given during procedure

Ⓛ Call report to receiving unit including prehospital and resuscitation history

MANAGEMENT OF OPEN WOUNDS

Janet Neff

A. Open wounds may result from penetrating or severe blunt trauma. Factors such as the vehicle of injury (razor blade, windshield, bullet, or metal railing), the force exerted, the environmental surroundings, and the location of the wound influence decision making in open wound management.

B. Open wounds are often associated with other injuries. The usual monitoring of airway, breathing, and circulation must be maintained despite rather dramatic tissue trauma. Care of concurrent injuries at the site of the open wound may proceed simultaneously or precede wound management.

C. Substantial oozing may be unrecognized until a pool of blood accumulates below an extremity or a cervical collar. Be sure to check the patient's back to find all open wounds and significant bleeding.

D. Bleeding can be controlled by direct fingertip pressure, a rolled gauze pad with direct pressure, elevation (with splinting if fracture is suspected), ligation or cautery, surgical clips, or tourniquets (last resort). Proper lighting and suction assist physicians to avoid damage to nearby structures during cautery and vascular clamping.

E. An open wound in the epigastrium or an avulsion in the left flank may be associated with significant internal trauma (p 134).

F. Soft tissue trauma, including muscle trauma, is a serious complication of crush injury. Potent toxins that may damage the heart and kidneys are released from compromised muscle. Delayed death is possible.

G. Extremity injuries with open wounds have a high risk for injury to vessels, nerves, tendons, or bone.

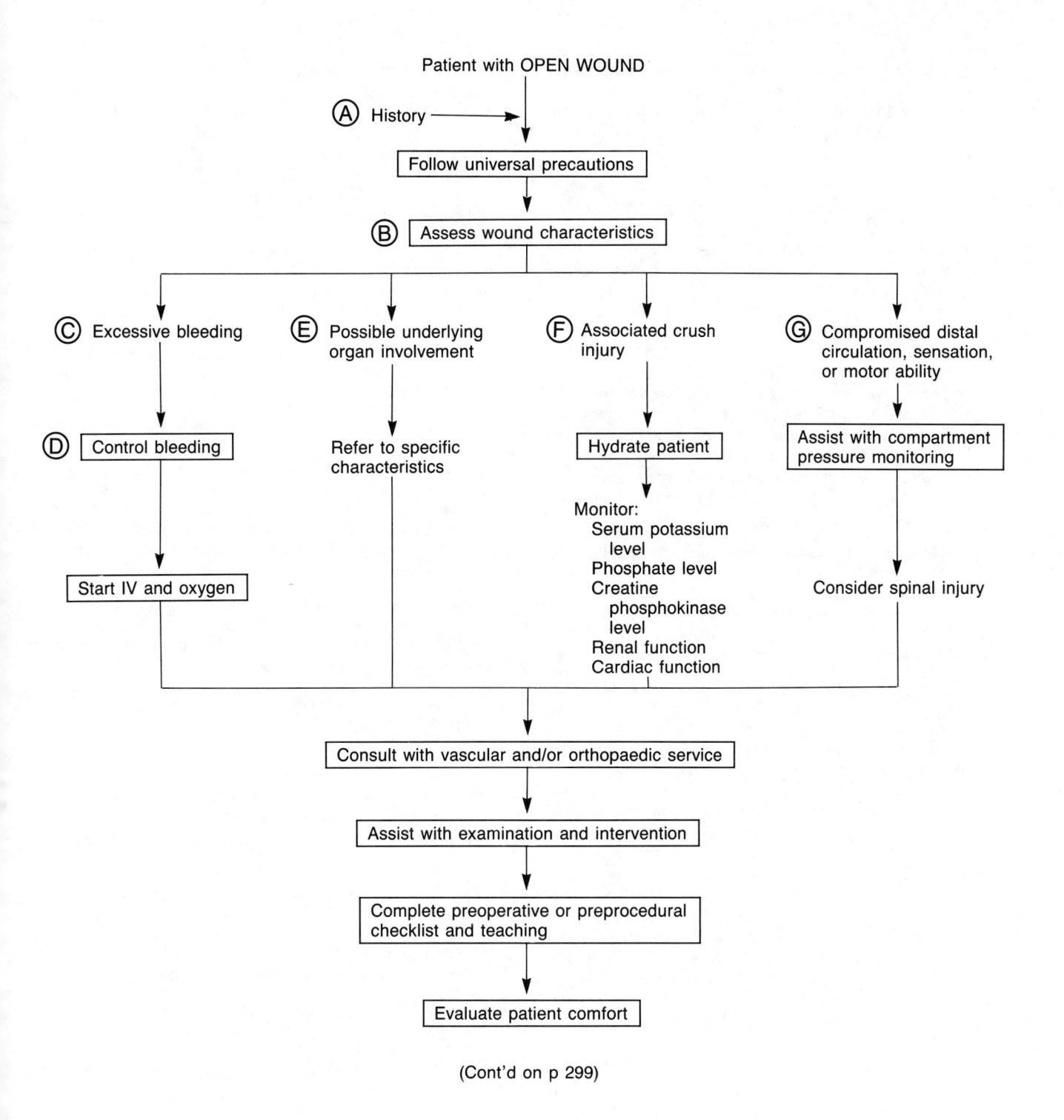

Patient with OPEN WOUND

(A) History ⟶

↓

Follow universal precautions

↓

(B) Assess wound characteristics

↓

- (C) Excessive bleeding
- (E) Possible underlying organ involvement
- (F) Associated crush injury
- (G) Compromised distal circulation, sensation, or motor ability

(C) → (D) Control bleeding → Start IV and oxygen

(E) → Refer to specific characteristics

(F) → Hydrate patient → Monitor:
  Serum potassium level
  Phosphate level
  Creatine phosphokinase level
  Renal function
  Cardiac function

(G) → Assist with compartment pressure monitoring → Consider spinal injury

↓

Consult with vascular and/or orthopaedic service

↓

Assist with examination and intervention

↓

Complete preoperative or preprocedural checklist and teaching

↓

Evaluate patient comfort

(Cont'd on p 299)

H. Culturing wounds during the initial assessment phase is controversial; however, swabbed specimens or tissue biopsies performed by the physician may be obtained. Cultures are often requested in the presence of an open fracture.

I. Prophylactic antibiotics are generally reserved for patients with heavily contaminated wounds or contaminated wounds in the presence of local or systemic factors that impair resistance to infection. These factors include wound ischemia, gross contaminants, delayed wound cleansing, contused tissue, wound hematoma, immune suppression secondary to major trauma, corticosteroid use, malnutrition, obesity, uncontrolled diabetes mellitus, and extremes of age. Prophylactic antibiotics are routinely recommended in open fractures, human bites to the hand, patients at risk for endocarditis, and patients with implanted orthopaedic devices. When it is appropriate to use antibiotics prophylactically, a broad-spectrum antibiotic is chosen and must be present in effective concentration in the wound at time of closure or preoperatively; therefore, intravenous (IV) administration is necessary.

J. Soft tissue anteroposterior, lateral, and oblique films assist in confirming the presence of foreign bodies. These films easily detect metal objects and the vast majority of glass (despite past comment to the contrary). For stubborn cases of glass retention, xerography may be useful. Wood and plastic are more difficult to identify; therefore, local exploration or guided fluoroscopic exploration may be necessary.

K. Topical or injectable agents may be used to induce tissue anesthesia prior to cleansing and suturing. The common topical solution TAC (0.5 percent tetracaine, 1:2000 adrenaline, and 11.8 percent cocaine) provides effective anesthesia and greater compliance during the suturing process in children. The nurse, parent, or patient can hold the sterile saturated gauze pad or cotton ball to the wound for 10 minutes with a gloved hand. Topical lidocaine (Xylocaine) jelly is a useful adjunct prior to cleansing of abrasions; however, large or deeply abraded areas may require systemic analgesia and/or sedation or patient controlled analgesia such as nitrous oxide inhalation. Use of a whirlpool tank may also be beneficial. The onset and duration of action and maximal dose of anesthetic agents must be known for safe and effective use.

L. Irrigation and debridement are the mainstays of wound cleansing. However, overly aggressive irrigation, manual debridement, and use of irritating solutions can damage tissue defenses and increase the risk of infection. Pulsatile irrigation with normal saline through a 35-ml syringe and 19-gauge needle is recommended. If scrubbing is indicated, a surfactant soaked sponge should be used. Surgical debridement may be necessary for devitalized tissue and embedded debris. Shaving of hair is not recommended.

M. Although time since injury has been considered the golden standard in primary closure, it has now been recognized that primary healing of closed, contaminated wounds is a function of the quantitative bacterial load. Immediate closure is usually reserved for wounds caused by shear forces or low energy compressive forces without gross contaminants such as feces, saliva, or specific soil contaminants.

N. Delayed primary closure is intended for contaminated wounds and severely traumatized wounds such as high velocity missile injuries in which tissue viability cannot be immediately ascertained. Repeated sessions of debridement allow maximal salvage of viable tissue and give time for the reparative process and enhance resistance to infection. Closure should commence when fewer than 10^5 organisms per gram of tissue exist.

O. Late tertiary closure is the choice when wounds have remained open well beyond the usual 4- to 7-day period for delayed primary closure or when infected tissue or surrounding cellulitis exists.

P. Skin grafts provide temporary or definitive closure, and flap coverage preserves vital structures exposed in soft tissue losses.

Q. Tetanus prophylaxis should be given within 72 hours of injury. Protocols based on wound type and immunization history should be consulted. The lot number and manufacturer must be documented.

References

Edlich RF, Rodeheaver GT, Morgan RF, Berman DE, Thacker JG. Principles of emergency wound management. Ann Emerg Med 1988; 17(12):20–38.

Immunization Practices Advisory Committee. Recommendations of the immunization practices advisory committee. MMWR 1989; 38(13):205–227.

Stotts N. The most effective method of wound irrigation. Focus Crit Care 1983; 10(5):45–48.

(Cont'd from p 297)

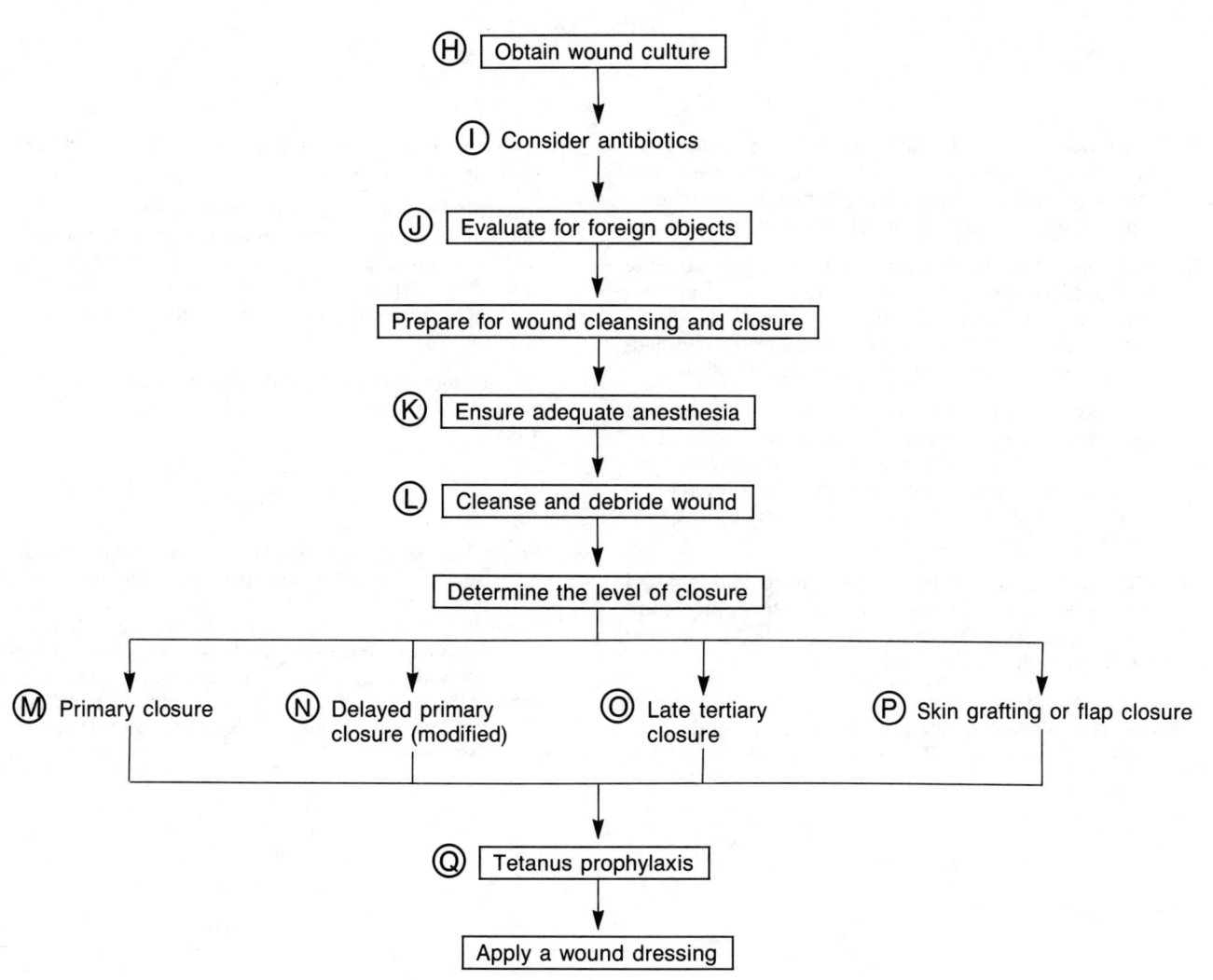

- Ⓗ Obtain wound culture
- Ⓘ Consider antibiotics
- Ⓙ Evaluate for foreign objects
- Prepare for wound cleansing and closure
- Ⓚ Ensure adequate anesthesia
- Ⓛ Cleanse and debride wound
- Determine the level of closure
  - Ⓜ Primary closure
  - Ⓝ Delayed primary closure (modified)
  - Ⓞ Late tertiary closure
  - Ⓟ Skin grafting or flap closure
- Ⓠ Tetanus prophylaxis
- Apply a wound dressing

COAGULATION PROBLEMS

R. Bernard Rochon

A. In the patient with excessive bleeding, the medical history should establish any history of medication use, i.e., aspirin or sodium warfarin (Coumadin). An accurate family history of bleeding tendencies is also useful.

B. The assessment helps to discern whether the bleeding is treatable by surgical intervention, requires replacement of coagulation factors, or both. Vital signs must be carefully monitored and the patient aggressively resuscitated. A chest film rules out or confirms hemothorax.

C. Nonsurgical bleeding occurs in patients with a defect in the coagulation mechanism. These patients manifest diffuse signs of coagulopathy, such as bleeding from intravenous sites and mucous membranes. They require transfusion with specific blood component therapy to correct the defect.

D. Abnormalities of the clotting mechanism are identified by examining platelet count, bleeding time, prothrombin time (PT), activated partial thromboplastin time (aPTT), and fibrinogen level.

E. In trauma patients, the most common abnormality is decreased platelet count secondary to consumption. Patients with prolonged PT and aPTT require transfusion with fresh frozen plasma. Cryoprecipitate is used to restore fibrinogen levels.

F. Surgical bleeding requires an operation for control. Any external signs of bleeding can be treated by tamponade with direct pressure. Stable patients with equivocal findings may require further diagnostic studies, i.e., peritoneal lavage, to rule out the abdomen as a source of blood loss.

G. Resuscitation and monitoring of the patient should continue as the patient is prepared for the operating room (OR).

References

Counts RB, Haisch C, Simon TL, et al. Hemostasis in massively transfused trauma patients. Ann Surg 1979; 190–91.

Sherman LA. DIC in massive transfusion. In: Collins JA, Murawski K, Shafer WA, eds. Massive transfusion in surgery and trauma. New York: Alan R. Liss, 1982.

Sohmer PR, Dawson RB. Transfusion therapy. In: Spittell JA, ed. Clinical medicine. Vol. 5. Hagerstown: Harper & Row, 1984.

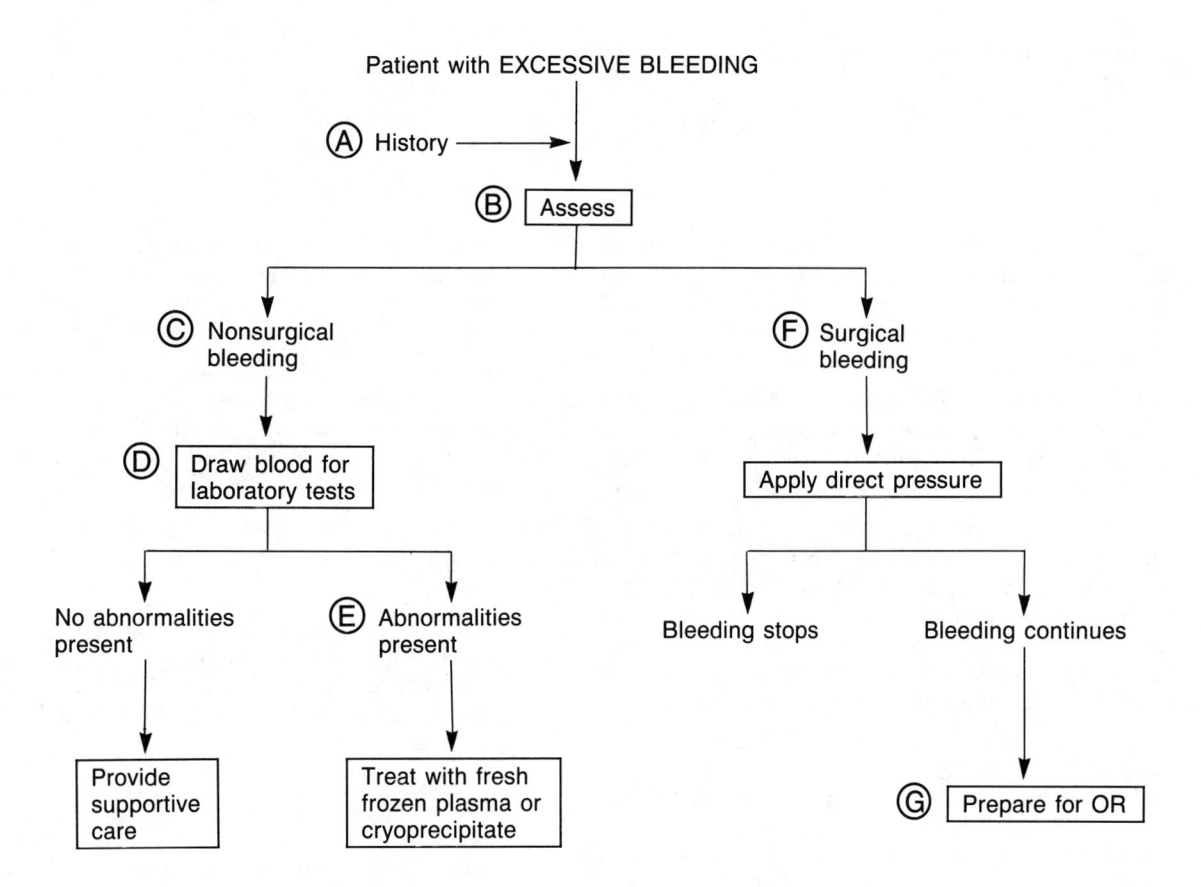

```
Patient with EXCESSIVE BLEEDING
              │
    Ⓐ History ──→
              ▼
         Ⓑ [Assess]
              │
      ┌───────┴───────┐
      ▼               ▼
 Ⓒ Nonsurgical    Ⓕ Surgical
   bleeding         bleeding
      │               │
      ▼               ▼
 Ⓓ [Draw blood for]  [Apply direct pressure]
   [laboratory tests]
      │               │
   ┌──┴──┐        ┌───┴────┐
   ▼     ▼        ▼        ▼
No abnormalities  Ⓔ Abnormalities   Bleeding stops   Bleeding continues
present            present
   ▼               ▼                                  ▼
[Provide         [Treat with fresh              Ⓖ [Prepare for OR]
supportive       frozen plasma or
care]            cryoprecipitate]
```

FEBRILE SYNDROMES

Janet Neff

A. Multiple sources can be responsible for fever in the multiple trauma patient. The mechanism of injury, specific injuries sustained, and current interventions can help to determine the probable cause for a rise in body temperature.

B. Sepsis is a well known complication of trauma, often leading to death. Endotoxins (exogenous pyrogens) act to release endogenous pyrogens such as prostaglandins, which stimulate fever.

C. Injury to the preoptic or rostral hypothalamic region of the brain may result in central hyperthermia. It is believed that prostaglandin (an endogenous pyrogen) is also responsible for fever in cerebral trauma. Injury to brain tissue does alter cellular metabolism, thereby resulting in synthesis and release of prostaglandins. Fever also adversely affects intracranial pressure.

D. Aseptic meningitis is caused by irritation of the meninges without evidence of an infectious source. Surgical intervention and extravasated blood in the cerebrospinal fluid creates an aseptic meningeal irritation. Intraventricular hemorrhage can evoke an intense, almost immediate hyperpyrexia, which is believed to be related to concurrent tissue trauma.

E. Cultures are often obtained in trauma patients when temperatures are elevated to identify and avert sepsis promptly. All possible sources should be cultured, including sites of invasive therapies. Significant hyperthermia within the first 24 hours of trauma is often related to central hyperthermia in the patient with penetrating or closed head injury.

F. Antibiotics are ordered based on culture results or the presumed source of infection. Multiple antibiotic therapy may be instituted. Shivering may result from cooling measures, thereby necessitating drugs such as diazepam or neuromuscular blockers. Chlorpromazine lowers seizure threshold and therefore should be avoided.

G. Diagnostic studies are essential in determination of the source of infection, if present. Chest films to detect infiltrates, effusions, and pneumonia and computed tomography to identify abscesses are both common.

H. Malignant hyperthermia has a familial incidence and is most common in childhood through young adulthood. It is a complication of anesthesia and creates severe acidosis, hyperkalemia, rapid sustained elevation in body temperature, and eventually disseminated intravascular coagulopathy and renal failure. Common triggering agents include halothane and succinylcholine.

I. Heatstroke, although it is rare, may occur in trauma patients when they have been injured and trapped in a hot environment.

J. In malignant hyperthermia, early signs may allow abandonment of anesthesia. In heatstroke, the patient's level of consciousness drops and emesis may occur, thereby jeopardizing airway patency. Hyperventilation is a natural means of eliminating excess heat and may be noticed or induced.

K. Dantrolene sodium may be administered for malignant hyperthermia. No specific medication is indicated for heatstroke.

L. Antipyretics inhibit prostaglandin synthesis and are often administered to control temperature spikes temporarily. It is controversial whether antipyretics are effective in fever associated with cerebral trauma, and they are not indicated in heat related emergencies.

M. Adequate hydration must be maintained in all patients with fever, but it is especially essential in patients with heatstroke and malignant hyperthermia, for which rapid infusion of cool fluids is paramount. Monitor for fluid overload.

N. Effective cooling techniques in the patient with neurogenic hyperthermia often consist of limiting clothing and use of a bedside fan over moistened skin surfaces to allow evaporative cooling. In severe hyperthermia such as heatstroke or malignant hyperthermia, ice packs, ice water immersion, and intragastric, peritoneal, and extracorporeal cooling may be used.

O. During antipyretic therapy, patients periodically sweat as the fever "breaks." Maintain skin integrity by using good techniques for repositioning and monitoring skin temperature and condition when cooling pads are in use p 399).

References

Holdcroft A. Body temperature control. London: Bailliere Tindall, 1980:75–80; 91–105.
Lipton JM. Fever. New York: Raven Press, 1980:131–137; 165–175.
Lomax P, Schonbaum E, eds. Body temperature: regulation, drug effects, and therapeutic implications. New York: Marcel Dekker, 1979.
Mercer JB, ed. Thermal physiology 1989 proceedings. New York, Elsevier, 1989.

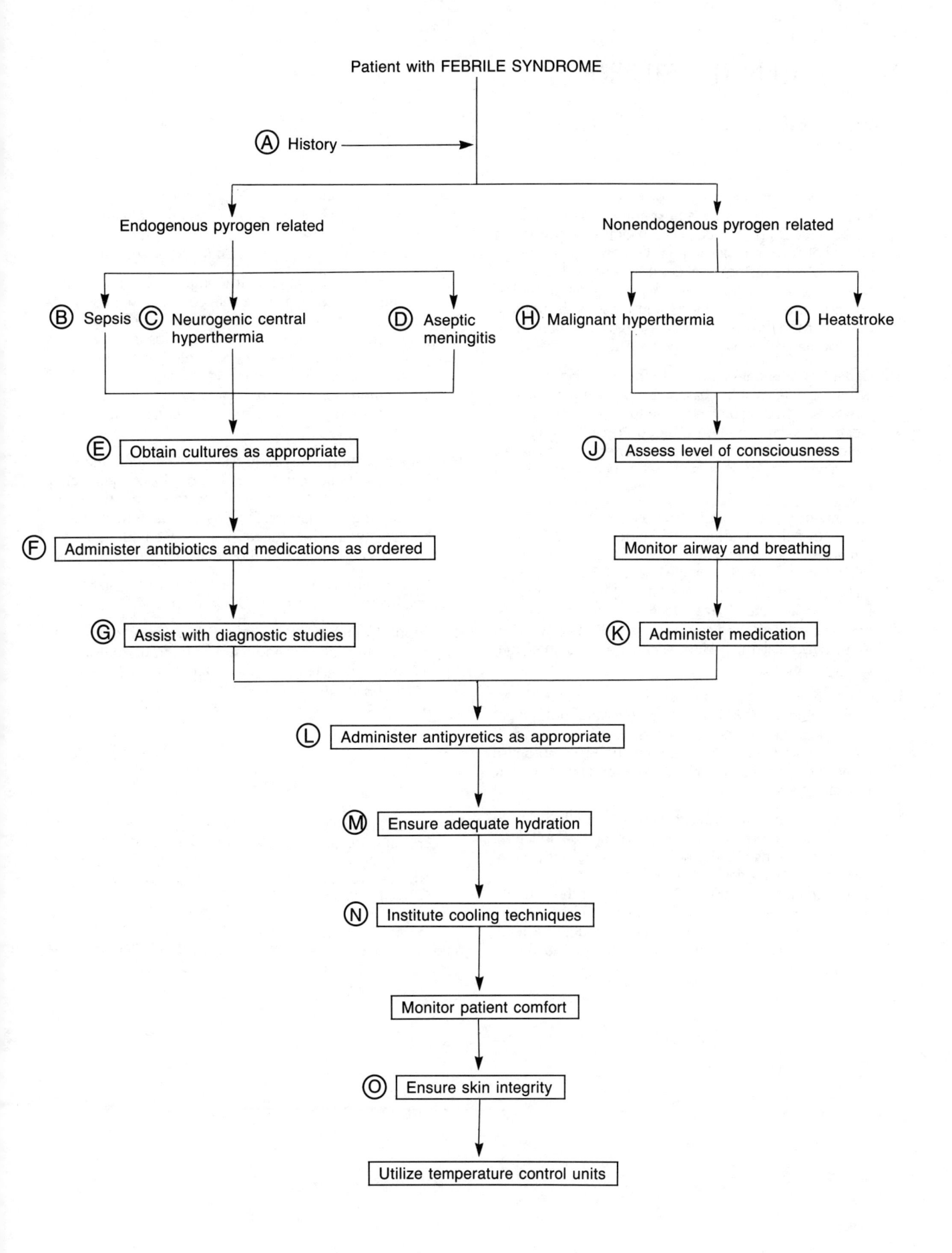

```
                    Patient with FEBRILE SYNDROME
                                │
                    ┌──(A) History ──────────►
                    │                          │
          ┌─────────┴─────────┐     ┌──────────┴──────────┐
    Endogenous pyrogen related     Nonendogenous pyrogen related
          │                                    │
   ┌──────┼──────┐                      ┌──────┴──────┐
(B) Sepsis (C) Neurogenic  (D) Aseptic  (H) Malignant  (I) Heatstroke
           central         meningitis       hyperthermia
           hyperthermia
           │                                    │
  (E) Obtain cultures as appropriate    (J) Assess level of consciousness
           │                                    │
  (F) Administer antibiotics and         Monitor airway and breathing
      medications as ordered                    │
           │                            (K) Administer medication
  (G) Assist with diagnostic studies            │
                         │                      │
                         └──────┬───────────────┘
                                ▼
                  (L) Administer antipyretics as appropriate
                                │
                  (M) Ensure adequate hydration
                                │
                  (N) Institute cooling techniques
                                │
                     Monitor patient comfort
                                │
                  (O) Ensure skin integrity
                                │
                     Utilize temperature control units
```

303

ACUTE RENAL FAILURE

Molly A. Seaman

A. Patients who present with known or suspected acute renal failure (ARF) as a result of trauma have received an ischemic insult. This decrease in kidney perfusion can occur because of hypovolemia, hemorrhage, burns, or surgery. As the history is taken, it is important to identify those patients who are at risk for developing further organ failure (i.e., the elderly and those with multiple trauma). Mortality rates can be as high as 50 percent in the trauma patient who develops ARF.

B. Careful assessment on arrival to the intensive care unit is important to establish baseline data. Complete laboratory tests should be ordered, as follows: serum and urine electrolytes, creatine levels, blood urea nitrogen, complete blood count with differential, arterial blood gases, serum amylase, lipase, and urine for specific gravity and protein.

C. Patients may present in various stages of renal insufficiency or failure. During the oliguric phase, urine output is less than 400 ml per day. The patient exhibits an inability to excrete metabolic waste or fluids and to regulate electrolytes. During the diuretic phase, the patient is able to excrete a great deal of urine. Imbalances, however, still exist and complications must be watched for (i.e., hypokalemia, acidosis, fluid overload, infection, and pericarditis).

D. Carefully evaluate blood pressure, central venous pressure, pulmonary capillary wedge pressure, pulmonary artery pressure, and cardiac output. Elevation may indicate fluid overload and may result in further compromise to the already traumatic patient. Decreased pressures may indicate bleeding.

E. Careful monitoring of intake and output is needed to evaluate improvement or deterioration of renal function. Fluid restrictions may be necessary to prevent pulmonary or cerebral edema. The physician may also order a fluid challenge of 100 to 500 ml to assess the patient's ability to excrete urine. Watch the patient closely for increasing shortness of breath, extra heart sounds, distended neck veins, wheezing, or rales. Weigh and record weight daily.

F. Frequent laboratory tests may be needed to monitor potassium and sodium levels. Elevated potassium levels may result in dangerous arrhythmias; therefore, it is important to keep the patient on a cardiac monitor.

G. Patients who do not exhibit uremic or life threatening conditions can be managed with conservative treatment. Underlying causes for renal failure must of course be managed first (i.e., bleeding and fluid loss secondary to trauma). Hyperkalemia may be controlled through diet restrictions, and by monitoring medication and fluid preparations for excess potassium. Administer medications to bind and remove excess potassium (cation-exchange resins).

H. Patients with progressively rising potassium along with severe metabolic acidosis and fluid overload require rapid intervention. Dialysis is indicated to correct these life threatening imbalances. Dialysis may be done either by hemodialysis or peritoneal dialysis. Hemodialysis is a much more efficient method than peritoneal dialysis.

I. Continue to monitor the patient closely for response to treatment to adjust or modify therapy.

J. Supportive treatment includes (1) promotion of comfort (i.e., controlling pain and nausea); (2) injury prevention (i.e., preventing falls, infection, or drug toxicity); and (3) providing emotional support to the patient and/or family during this period of change and rehabilitation.

References

Johnson BC, Wells SJ, Hoffmeister D, Dungca CU. Standards for critical care. St. Louis: CV Mosby, 1988:399.

Farley HF, Miller DL. Renal failure. In: Phipps WJ, Long B, Woods NF, eds. Med-surg nursing concepts and practice. 3rd ed. St. Louis: CV Mosby, 1987:1655.

Lindenfeld SM. Acute renal failure. In: Don H, ed. Decision making in critical care. St. Louis: CV Mosby, 1985:144.

Toto KH. Acute renal failure. In: Mancini ME, ed. Decision making in emergency nursing. Toronto: BC Decker, 1987:148.

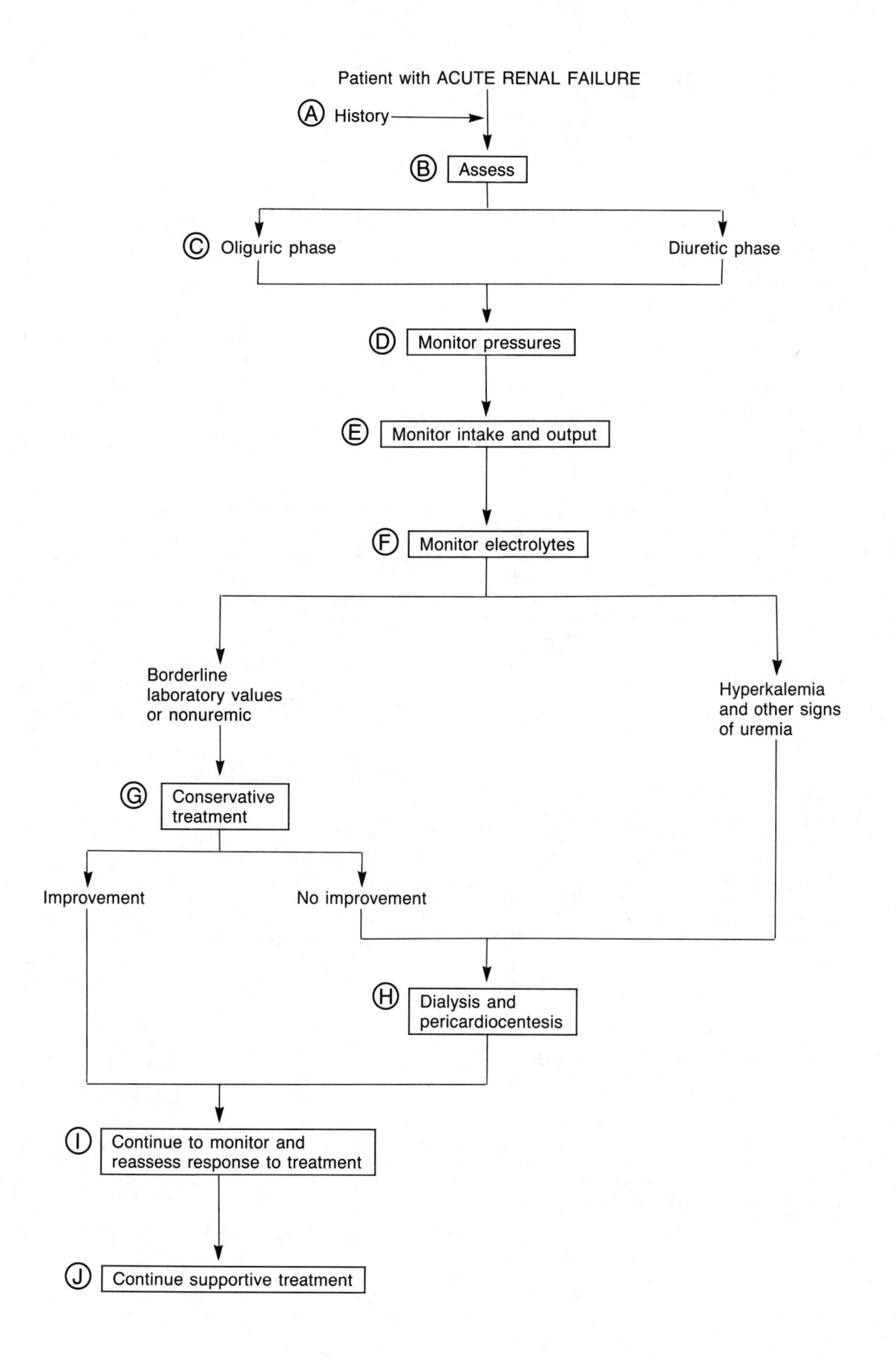

```
Patient with ACUTE RENAL FAILURE
      │
  Ⓐ History ──►
                │
              Ⓑ Assess
         ┌──────┴──────┐
         ▼             ▼
  Ⓒ Oliguric phase   Diuretic phase
         └──────┬──────┘
                ▼
         Ⓓ Monitor pressures
                ▼
         Ⓔ Monitor intake and output
                ▼
         Ⓕ Monitor electrolytes
         ┌──────────────┴──────────────┐
         ▼                             ▼
  Borderline                    Hyperkalemia
  laboratory values             and other signs
  or nonuremic                  of uremia
         ▼
  Ⓖ Conservative
    treatment
   ┌─────┴─────┐
   ▼           ▼
Improvement  No improvement
                   │
                   ▼
         Ⓗ Dialysis and
           pericardiocentesis
   │               │
   └───────┬───────┘
           ▼
  Ⓘ Continue to monitor and
    reassess response to treatment
           ▼
  Ⓙ Continue supportive treatment
```

305

GAS GANGRENE INFECTION

Sheena M. Ferguson

A. Typically, gas gangrene infection occurs from traumatic injury with a deep muscle laceration, from surgical intervention (often involving the bowel), or from vascular insufficiency (as with diabetes). Gas gangrene is the most common type of clostridial infection after an open orthopaedic injury. *Clostridium perfringens* is a large, anaerobic, gram-positive rod that is saprophytic and ubiquitous. The endospore form of the bacterium is in a dormant phase, but when the spore is introduced into optimal growth conditions, it can convert back to a vegetative state cell within minutes. Optimal conditions include a warm, moist, necrotic, and anaerobic environment, such as a deep muscle laceration. The *C. perfringens* bacterium secretes many toxins, specifically the alpha-toxin, or lecithinase, which is hemolytic, destroys platelets and cell membranes, and alters capillary permeability. As the toxin destroys the cells, there is liquefaction of the muscle fibers. The anaerobic processes in the metabolic pathway result in the production of insoluble gases such as hydrogen and nitrogen, which result in gas forming infections. Clinical identification of *Clostridium* infection is often difficult. *Escherichia coli*, *Klebsiella*, *Enterobacter*, and *Pseudomonas* may also lead to gas forming infections. The *Clostridium* species is responsible for 90 percent of gas gangrene infections. Of these infections, 80 percent are caused by the *Clostridium perfringens* organism.

B. Early clinical detection and timely treatment can significantly alter the overwhelming morbidity and mortality associated with gas gangrene infection. Local effects include severe pain and tense swelling and edema, palpable crepitance and frothiness from gases, color with a white and blue marbling effect, cooler temperature than in other areas, thin hemorrhagic exudate with bullae formation, and a sweet putrid odor. Systemic effects include tachycardia and hypertension, agitation and/or delirium, fever and elevated white blood cell count, coma prior to death, and a general toxic presentation.

C. Sterile needle aspiration and Gram stain are helpful in making the diagnosis. In advanced cases, radiographic studies reveal gas trapped in the tissues. Occasionally, the patient has a deep-seated infection with muscle necrosis but with only minimal clinically evident skin changes that are suggestive of a simple cellulitis. Clinical deterioration that is inconsistent with the appearance of the wound requires a high index of suspicion that a deeper infective process is present. Direct visualization of the myonecrosis is considered critical in making a diagnosis of gas gangrene. The presence of the *Clostridium* bacterium in the wound does not necessarily indicate a severe infective process.

D. Parenteral penicillin, 20 million units per day, is usually the drug of choice. In situations in which allergy to penicillin is present, other antibiotics may be used.

E. Surgical debridement of all necrotic tissue is necessary. Tissue may appear pale and edematous, and the muscle does not contract. Deeper muscle appears beefy red and nonviable to a black and gangrenous patchwork.

F. The wound should be left open to allow drainage as well as visualization and further debridement.

G. The use of hyperbaric oxygen treatment remains controversial. The therapy delivers increased oxygen tensions (250 to 300 mm Hg) to the tissues. Although not high enough to kill the Clostridium, the bacteria's ability to secrete alpha-toxin is blocked. Medical centers without a hyperbaric oxygen chamber have acceptable mortality rates. This would indicate that expert medical and surgical management is probably more important than hyperbaric oxygen treatment in treating gas gangrene infections.

H. The reappearance of nonviable muscle requires further surgical debridement. In fact, repeated debridement is usually necessary.

I. The tissues appear viable, and the toxic systemic effects of the infection are resolving.

J. The wound may require extensive reconstructive surgery.

References

Caplan E, Kluge R. Gas gangrene. Arch Int Med 1976; 136:788–791.

Hoyt N. Infections following orthopedic surgery. Orthop Nurs 1986; 5(6):19–24.

Kasper DL. Other clostridial infection. In: Braunwald E, Isselbacher KJ, Petersdorf RG, et al, eds. Harrison's principles of internal medicine. 11th ed. New York: McGraw-Hill, 1988:563–567.

Rush D, Kelly J, Nichols R. Prevention and management of common infections after trauma. In: Mattox K, Moore E, Feliciano D, eds. Trauma. Norwalk, CT: Appleton-Lange, 1988:223–236.

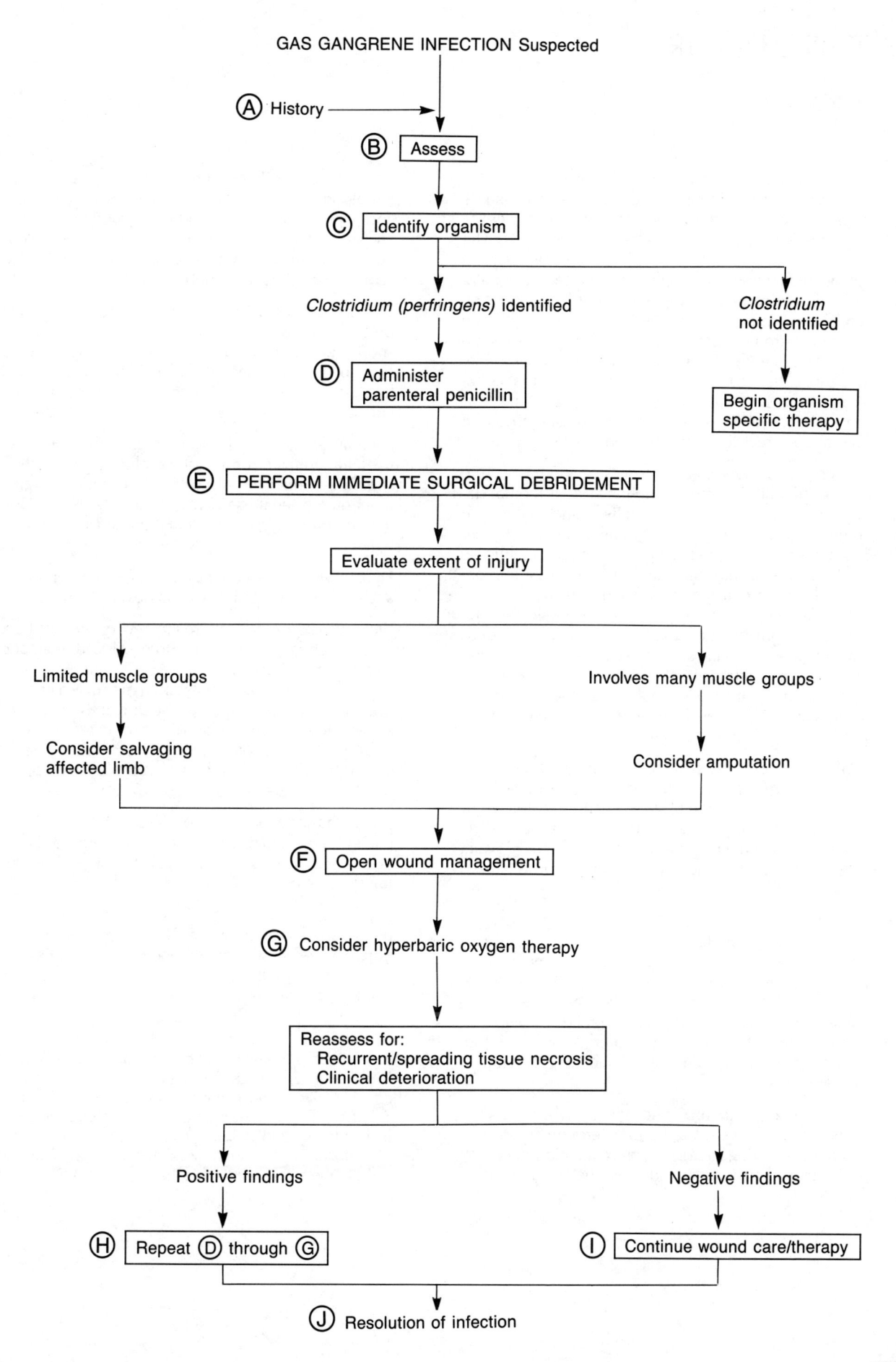

```
                    GAS GANGRENE INFECTION Suspected
                                    │
        Ⓐ History ──────────────────▶│
                                    ▼
                            Ⓑ │ Assess │
                                    │
                                    ▼
                         Ⓒ │ Identify organism │
                                    │
                    ┌───────────────┴───────────────┐
                    │                               │
         Clostridium (perfringens) identified    Clostridium
                    │                            not identified
                    ▼                               │
                Ⓓ │ Administer                     ▼
                    parenteral penicillin │   ┌─────────────────┐
                    │                         │ Begin organism  │
                    ▼                         │ specific therapy│
         Ⓔ │ PERFORM IMMEDIATE SURGICAL DEBRIDEMENT │
                    │
                    ▼
            │ Evaluate extent of injury │
                    │
        ┌───────────┴───────────┐
        │                       │
  Limited muscle groups    Involves many muscle groups
        │                       │
        ▼                       ▼
   Consider salvaging       Consider amputation
   affected limb
        │                       │
        └───────────┬───────────┘
                    ▼
            Ⓕ │ Open wound management │
                    │
                    ▼
        Ⓖ Consider hyperbaric oxygen therapy
                    │
                    ▼
        ┌───────────────────────────┐
        │ Reassess for:             │
        │   Recurrent/spreading tissue necrosis │
        │   Clinical deterioration  │
        └───────────────────────────┘
                    │
        ┌───────────┴───────────┐
   Positive findings         Negative findings
        │                       │
        ▼                       ▼
  Ⓗ │ Repeat Ⓓ through Ⓖ │   Ⓘ │ Continue wound care/therapy │
        │                       │
        └───────────┬───────────┘
                    ▼
            Ⓙ Resolution of infection
```

HEPATIC FAILURE

Nathan Coates

A. Hepatic failure may be of new onset or result from an acute worsening of chronic liver disease. Mortality ranges from 66 percent (in those less than 15 years of age) to 95 percent (in those over the age of 45 years). The pathophysiology of liver failure is attributable more to the loss of function rather than to actual death of hepatocytes. A prediction of the degree of cellular dysfunction cannot be made purely on the basis of the magnitude of liver function test abnormalities. False neurotransmitters such as gamma-aminobutyric acid and the inability to regulate the serum glucose level affect cerebral cellular function. Cerebral swelling increases as coma worsens; whether this swelling is caused by altered blood flow or by direct toxic effects is unknown.

B. Appreciation of the onset and early stages of liver failure may be difficult. The most prominent sign is mental status change. Dramatically elevated liver function tests are common. An elevated prothrombin time with severe hypoglycemia or difficulty controlling the serum glucose level may be an indication of hepatocyte dysfunction. An early indication may be a sudden increase in the levels of drugs metabolized by the liver. Elevated ammonia levels indicate hepatocyte dysfunction, as does marked increased in the blood urea nitrogen. An increase in the serum creatinine level may be a harbinger of renal dysfunction from hepatorenal syndrome. Electroencephalogram wave slowing may be an early indicator of coma, but it is not diagnostic.

C. Well recognized signs of hepatic failure are progressive jaundice, hemorrhagic tendencies from an elevated prothrombin time, and mental status changes. Asterixis, or liver flap, is the most characteristic peripheral neurologic finding, but it is not diagnostic. Fetor hepaticus, a sweet musty odor, is also noted and is thought to be caused by indole or mercaptan production.

D. Mental state alterations are the center of diagnosis and staging, ranging from lethargy to frank coma. Four stages are recognized, as follows: (1) minimal alteration; (2) confusion, disorientation, and drowsiness; (3) light coma; and (4) deep stupor. Sluggish pupillary response may occur as coma and accompanying cerebral edema worsen. Other origins of cerebral dysfunction must be excluded, such as subdural hematoma, diabetic ketoacidosis, or meningitis.

E. Determining the etiology of hepatic failure is not always straightforward. The goals are to determine and to correct the underlying etiology, to prevent the onset of worsening of encephalopathy, and to rest the remaining liver.

F. Nitrogenous overload usually results from gastrointestinal blood losses. Common sources are varices, gastritis and peptic ulceration. Blood is removed with lactulose and sorbitol, either by nasogastric or rectal tube. Neomycin diminishes bacterial breakdown of blood and subsequent protein production.

G. The metabolism of excessive blood products or dietary protein may overwhelm the liver. Sources of ammonia should be diminished or removed. If total parenteral nutrition is being used, consider changing to a form that has lesser amounts of aromatic amino acids and higher concentrations of arginine and branched chains.

H. A common cause of hepatic coma is the use of sedatives, tranquilizers, or narcotic analgesics. Hypnotic use should be limited or discontinued because marginally functioning hepatocytes may be easily overwhelmed, thereby prolonging the circulation and obtunding the patient.

I. Hepatocyte dysfunction may be the result of hypovolemic and/or cardiogenic shock or hypoxia.

J. Other causes of liver failure are new onset viral hepatitis, toxic chemical exposure, drug induced or alcoholic hepatitis, or severe infection. Abnormalities of electrolytes such as sodium or potassium may play a contributing role. Hypoglycemia must be diligently searched for and treated. Because alkalosis encourages ammonium to leave the gastrointestinal tract, ventilator settings should be adjusted accordingly. Coagulation defects may need to be corrected by fresh frozen plasma.

K. The high mortality rate associated with liver failure has encouraged alternative methods of care, such as hemodialysis, exchange transfusion, plasmapheresis, and even transplantation.

L. Signs of potentially fatal outcome are convulsions, progressive elevation of coagulation times, severe reduction in acute phase proteins, and laboratory evidence of liver parenchymal loss.

References

Bernuau J, Reuff B, Benhamou JP. Fulminant and subfulminant liver failure. Semin Liver Dis 1986; 6:97–106.

Maddrey WC. Drug and chemical-induced hepatic injury. In: Schiff L, Schiff E, eds. Diseases of the liver. Philadelphia: JB Lippincott, 1987:2922–2956.

Zieve L. Hepatic encephalopathy. In: Schiff L, Schiff E, eds. Diseases of the liver. Philadelphia: JB Lippincott, 1987:925–948.

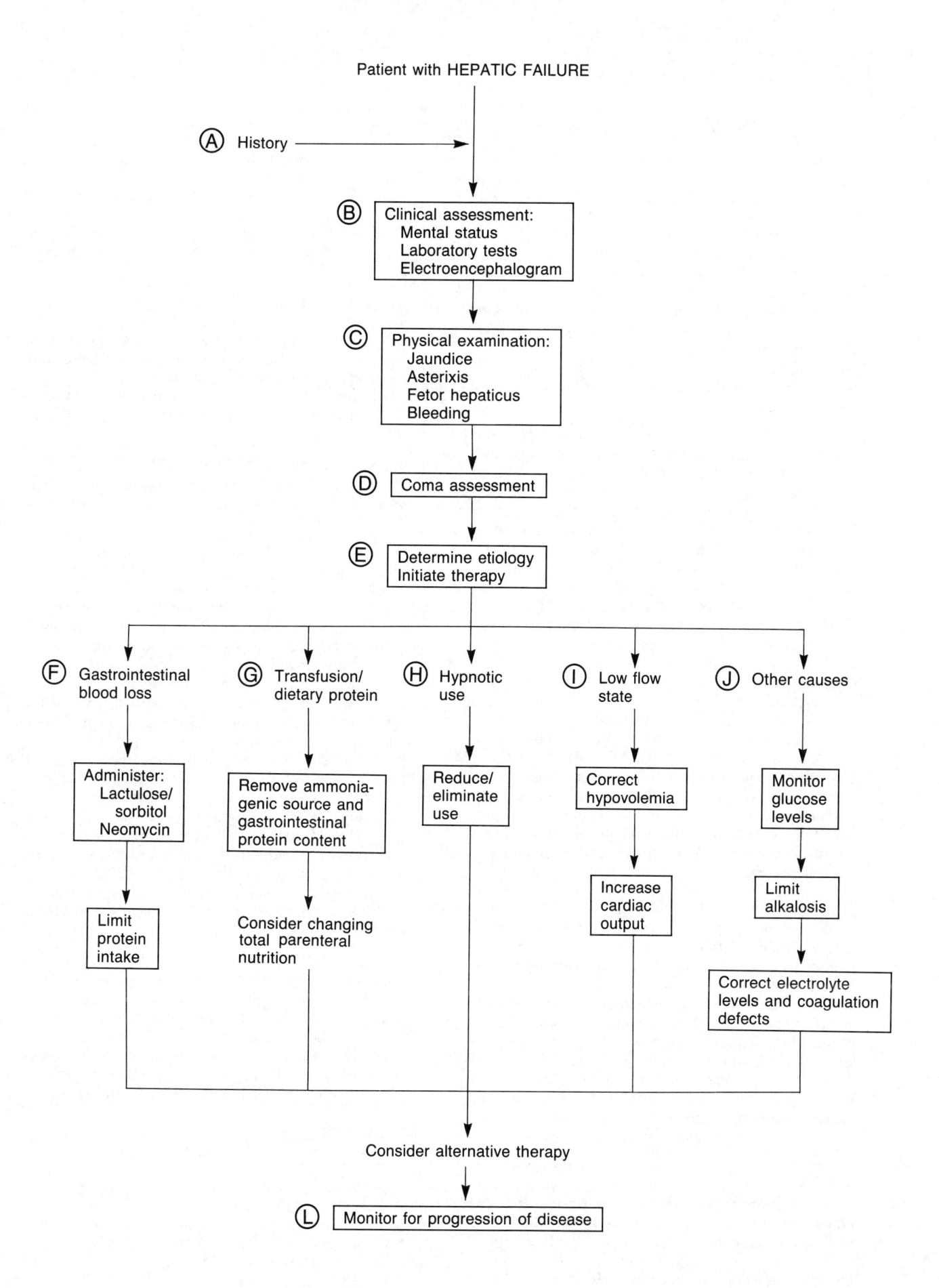

```
Patient with HEPATIC FAILURE
                │
(A) History ───▶│
                ▼
(B) Clinical assessment:
       Mental status
       Laboratory tests
       Electroencephalogram
                │
                ▼
(C) Physical examination:
       Jaundice
       Asterixis
       Fetor hepaticus
       Bleeding
                │
                ▼
(D) Coma assessment
                │
                ▼
(E) Determine etiology
    Initiate therapy
```

- (F) Gastrointestinal blood loss → Administer: Lactulose/sorbitol Neomycin → Limit protein intake
- (G) Transfusion/dietary protein → Remove ammoniagenic source and gastrointestinal protein content → Consider changing total parenteral nutrition
- (H) Hypnotic use → Reduce/eliminate use
- (I) Low flow state → Correct hypovolemia → Increase cardiac output
- (J) Other causes → Monitor glucose levels → Limit alkalosis → Correct electrolyte levels and coagulation defects

Consider alternative therapy

(L) Monitor for progression of disease

309

RESPIRATORY FAILURE

Joseph P. Osterkamp

A. Adult respiratory distress syndrome (ARDS) is a descriptive term applied to many acute, diffuse infiltrating lung lesions of various etiologies that cause severe arterial hypoxemia. Conditions that may lead to ARDS include, but are not limited to, diffuse pulmonary infections, aspiration, inhalation of toxins and irritants, postcardiopulmonary bypass, thoracic trauma with pulmonary contusion, and massive soft tissue and skeletal trauma. The common manifestations of ARDS are pulmonary edema, decreased pulmonary compliance, and progressive hypoxemia without elevated pulmonary capillary hydrostatic pressure.

B. Increased permeability of the alveolar-capillary membranes occurs either via direct insult from acidity or toxins or indirectly through white blood cell produced mediators (prostaglandins, leukotrienes, and thromboxanes). This increase in permeability allows leakage of fluids, fibrinogen, and cellular components into the alveoli, thereby causing alveolar collapse and interference with normal surfactant activity. This, in turn, causes severe ventilation-perfusion imbalance and shunting of blood through collapse and edematous pulmonary beds. The lungs become less compliant and require increased inspiratory pressures for spontaneous ventilation. Acute respiratory failure develops, manifested by hypoxemia, increased respiratory rate, decreased tidal volume, and deterioration in gas exchange. The initial clinical signs of ARDS are often an increased respiratory rate and dyspnea. The lung fields may appear clear on initial chest film or may have only minimal interstitial infiltrations. Arterial blood gas (ABG) measurements demonstrate a decreased PaO_2 and $PaCO_2$. This occurs secondary to the increased respiratory rate, and ventilation and perfusion provide symptomatic relief and alleviate the initial decreased PaO_2. As respiratory failure progresses, the patient experiences increasing dyspnea, tachypnea, and cyanosis. Chest films at this stage reveal diffuse bilateral interstitial and alveolar infiltrates. ABGs demonstrate an increased alveolar-arterial oxygen level secondary to right-to-left shunting of blood through the pulmonary vasculature. This is generally not correctable by administration of oxygen via face mask or nasal prongs. Intubation and administration of positive end-expiratory pressure (PEEP) are needed to correct the increasing hypoxemia. This therapy is designed to increase lung volume by opening previously closed airways and thus improving oxygenation. Large tidal volumes (12 to 15 ml/kg) at a respiratory rate of 12 to 15 breaths per minute with high inflation pressures are often required to achieve adequate arterial oxygenation.

C. If the patient is able to initiate spontaneous respiratory efforts, synchronized intermittent mandatory ventilation (SIMV) delivers periodic mandatory breaths that are timed with the patient's spontaneous inspiration. This permits adequate inspiratory volumes and limits spontaneous expiration during inflation cycle, thereby avoiding high inspiratory pressures and delivery of small tidal volumes. If the spontaneous respiratory rate is so rapid that expiratory efforts occur before the SIMV mode ventilator delivers the mandatory breath, assist control mode is usually required in conjunction with sedation and/or paralysis.

D. If oxygen saturation continues to improve with mechanical ventilation and vigorous pulmonary care, gradual weaning is initiated. Initially, as respiratory status stabilizes, FIO_2 should be decreased to 50 percent or less, followed by gradual decrease in PEEP. Continuous assessment of oxygen saturation, ABGs, respiratory rate, and chest films is needed to monitor resolution of early ARDS.

E. If oxygen saturation continues to decrease to less than 90 percent as ARDS progresses and interstitial fibrosis develops, PEEP and FIO_2 are increased in an attempt to correct hypoxemia.

F. In the patient with ARDS who is critically ill and unstable, a pulmonary artery catheter assists in the management of supportive therapy such as fluid hydration, volume status evaluation, measurement of mixed venous oxygen, and calculation of oxygen consumption. A general guideline is to maintain the pulmonary capillary wedge pressure as low as is compatible with a reasonable cardiac output, mean arterial pressure, urine output, and mixed venous oxygen. Inotropic and vasoactive agents may be of additional benefit to achieve these goals. Dopamine and/or dobutamine are generally the initial agents used to maintain an appropriate cardiac output and mixed venous PO_2. Overhydration can complicate ARDS; however, adequate hydration to maintain perfusion is also essential. Blood volume and electrolyte balance should be maintained with plasma products and crystalloids. Adequate nutritional support is essential to meet the increased metabolic demands. Close monitoring for nosocomial pneumonia is important, and antibiotic therapy should be initiated early if symptoms occur.

G. If ARDS persists for longer than 7 to 10 days, interstitial fibrosis can occur secondary to mononuclear cell infiltration. Areas of infection become evident as a result of impaired bacterial clearance. Progressive multiorgan system failure is a potential complication at this stage. As the disease progresses, the lungs become fibrotic; the process is not easily reversible because of gradual and progressive impairment of gas exchange and ventilation.

References

American College of Surgeons. Early care of the injured patient. Philadelphia: WB Saunders, 1976.
Blaisdell FW, Lewis FR. Respiratory distress syndrome of shock and trauma. Philadelphia: WB Saunders, 1977.
Shires GT. Care of the trauma patient. New York: McGraw-Hill, 1979: 576–591.

Patient with RESPIRATORY FAILURE/ARDS

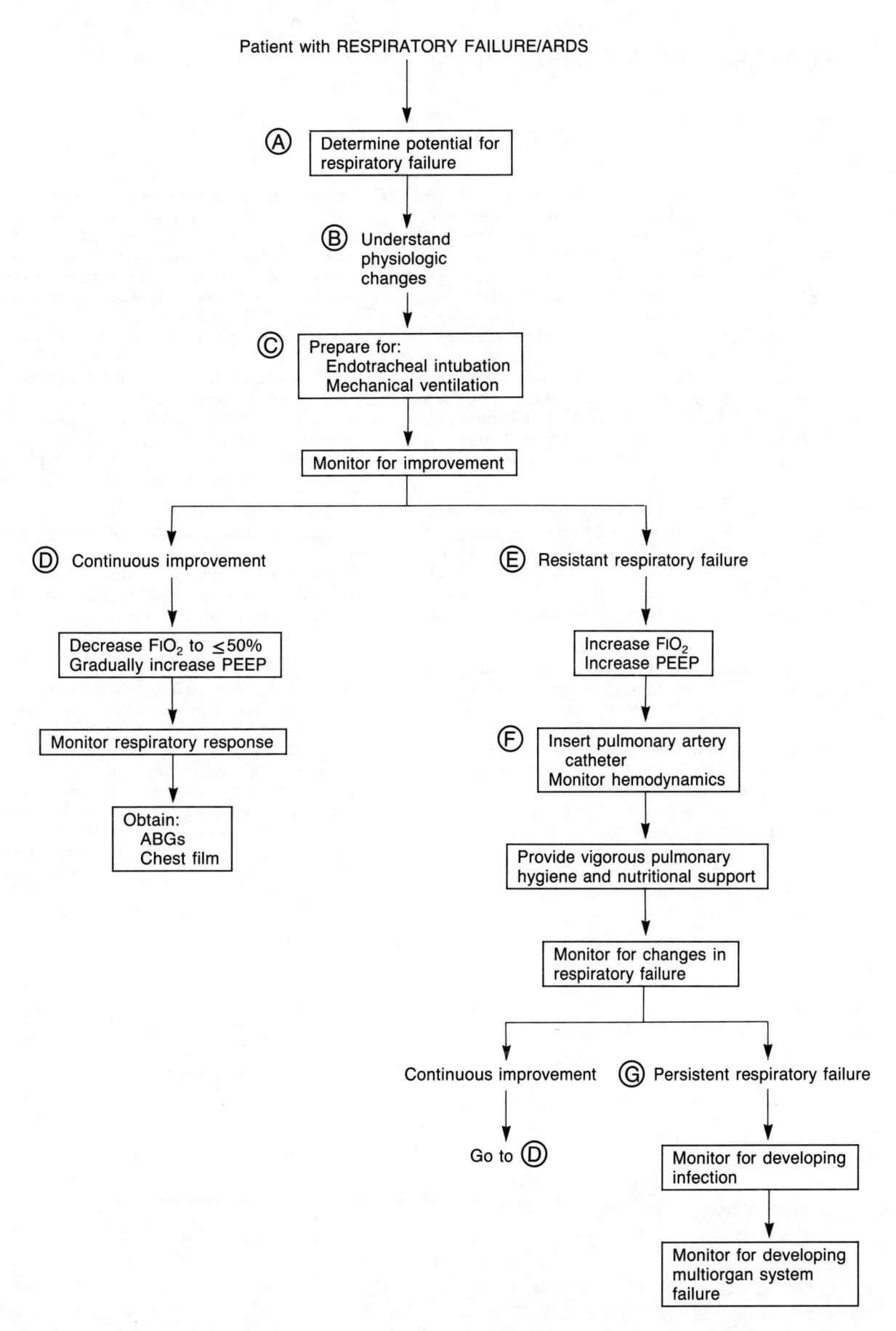

- (A) Determine potential for respiratory failure
- (B) Understand physiologic changes
- (C) Prepare for:
  - Endotracheal intubation
  - Mechanical ventilation

Monitor for improvement

- (D) Continuous improvement
  - Decrease FIO_2 to $\leq 50\%$
  - Gradually increase PEEP
  - Monitor respiratory response
  - Obtain:
    - ABGs
    - Chest film

- (E) Resistant respiratory failure
  - Increase FIO_2
  - Increase PEEP
  - (F) Insert pulmonary artery catheter; Monitor hemodynamics
  - Provide vigorous pulmonary hygiene and nutritional support
  - Monitor for changes in respiratory failure
    - Continuous improvement → Go to (D)
    - (G) Persistent respiratory failure
      - Monitor for developing infection
      - Monitor for developing multiorgan system failure

Shoemaker W, Appel P. Pathophysiology of adult respiratory distress syndrome after sepsis and surgical operations. Crit Care Med 1985; 13:166–172.

Weigelt IA, Mitchele RA, Synder WH. Early positive end expiratory pressure in the adult respiratory distress syndrome. Arch Surg 1979; 114:497–499.

MECHANICAL VENTILATION

Joseph P. Osterkamp

A. Mechanical ventilators allow control of ventilation and oxygenation by regulation of tidal volume, respiratory rate, inspiratory flow, airway pressure, and percentage of oxygen (FIO_2) delivered to the patient. Basic initial ventilator settings include a rate of 10 to 12 breaths per minute at a tidal volume of 10 ml/kg to yield a minute ventilation of 100 ml/kg per minute. The FIO_2 is generally set at 50 percent, and a positive-end expiratory pressure (PEEP) at 5 cm H_2O is used to prevent alveolar atelectasis. Peak inspiratory pressures are generally gauged on the ventilator and are determined by the tidal volume and compliance of the lungs. Inspiratory pressures are elevated with an increase in tidal volume or with a decrease in pulmonary compliance.

B. Once the patient has been placed on mechanical ventilation, a chest film is obtained to assess endotracheal tube placement and lung fields. Arterial blood gas (ABG) measurements are obtained to assess oxygenation and ventilation. Frequent suctioning of the endotracheal tube may be required if copious secretions or blood is present.

C. Various modes of ventilation may be used, along with decreasing PEEP and FIO_2, to facilitate weaning from mechanical ventilation. Intermittent mandatory ventilation is useful for alert of spontaneously breathing patients. This assist mode assures delivery of a set number of breaths at a desired tidal volume while allowing the patient to breathe spontaneously between ventilator inhalations. Continuous positive airway pressure mode is used in patients who have adequate spontaneous respirations and do not require additional breaths. It is generally used only intermittently prior to weaning the patient completely from mechanical ventilation.

D. Weaning parameters are generally measured and analyzed with improving respiratory status. The following are indications for weaning and extubation: (1) spontaneous respiratory rate lower than 25 breaths per minute; (2) tidal volume greater than 5 ml/kg; (3) forced vital capacity of 10 ml/kg; and (4) negative inspiratory force of 20 cm H_2O or greater. The transition to spontaneous respiration should be rapid, with the ventilator changed to the continuous positive airway pressure mode and constant monitoring of the patient's respiratory rate and hemodynamic status. If the patient maintains an adequate respiratory rate and heart rate and fulfills weaning parameters, extubation is indicated. A follow-up assessment of the patient's ability to ventilate and oxygenate spontaneously and effectively should occur.

E. If the PCO_2 is elevated, ventilatory rate may be increased to 15 to 20 breaths per minute, along with an increase in the tidal volume to 15 ml/kg. It should be remembered that the rate is increased prior to increasing tidal volume to avoid inappropriate high peak inspiratory pressures. Under usual circumstances, 300 ml/kg per minute is a maximal value for ventilation to avoid excessive peak inspiratory pressures or ventilatory rate.

F. If the oxygenation is inadequate with the PO_2 less than 60 mm Hg, despite the initial ventilator settings, the first step to improve oxygenation is to increase the FIO_2 to 0.5 to 0.7 and to increase PEEP to 5 to 12 cm H_2O. An increase in PEEP above 5 cm H_2O may compromise systemic oxygen delivery by decreasing cardiac output secondary to a decrease in venous return to the heart. Therefore, adjustments in PEEP may require the placement of a pulmonary artery catheter to allow measurements of mixed venous oxygen saturation and cardiac output.

```
                    Patient on MECHANICAL VENTILATION
                                    │
    History ────────────────────────┤
                                    ▼
                          ⒶAssess current ventilator
                              settings
                                    │
                                    ▼
                          Ⓑ Monitor:
                              Chest films
                              ABGs
        ┌───────────────────────────┼───────────────────────────┐
        ▼                           ▼                           ▼
   Po₂ ≥60 mm Hg              Pco₂ >45 mm Hg              Po₂ <60 mm Hg
   Pco₂ ≤45 mm Hg
        │                           │                           │
        ▼                           ▼                           ▼
   ⒸTrial intermittent        ⒺIncrease:                  ⒻMaintain PEEP at
     mandatory ventilation      Respiratory rate to         5–10 cm H₂O
     or continuous              15–20 breathes/min          Increase FiO₂ to
     positive airway            Tidal volume to 15 ml/kg    0.5–0.7
     pressure                                               Measure mixed
                                                            venous oxygen
                                                            saturation to adjust
                                                            PEEP
        ▼
   Decrease:
     FiO₂ to maintain
     oxygen ≥25%
     PEEP to 0 cm H₂O
        ▼
   ⒹMeasure weaning
     parameters

                                            (Cont'd on p 315)
```

G. If the PCO_2 is still elevated, the patient may require further sedation and paralysis to decrease consumption of oxygen and production of carbon dioxide.

H. If oxygenation still remains inadequate, other variables to maximize oxygen delivery should be optimized. Hemoglobin concentration, cardiac output, and oxygen consumption should be regulated by administration of red blood cells, fluids, and inotropic agents. Early treatment of infections and sedation with paralysis are also indicated.

I. If the PCO_2 remains elevated, the patient may be allowed to equilibrate at a high PCO_2, or extracorporeal circulation may be instituted.

J. The patient may need to be placed on inverse ratio ventilation to improve inadequate oxygenation after optimizing PEEP, FIO_2, and oxygen delivery. FIO_2 greater than 0.6 to 0.7 should be avoided to help prevent oxygen toxicity to the lung. Extracorporeal circulation may also be tried as a last effort.

References

American College of Surgeons. Early care of the injured patient. Philadelphia: WB Saunders, 1976.

Blaisdell FW, Lewis FR. Respiratory distress syndrome of shock and trauma. Philadelphia: WB Saunders, 1977.

Shires GT. Care of the trauma patient. New York: McGraw-Hill, 1979: 576–591.

Weigelt IA, Mitchele RA, Synder WH. Early positive end expiratory pressure in the adult respiratory distress syndrome. Arch Surg 1979; 114:497–499.

(Cont'd from p 313)

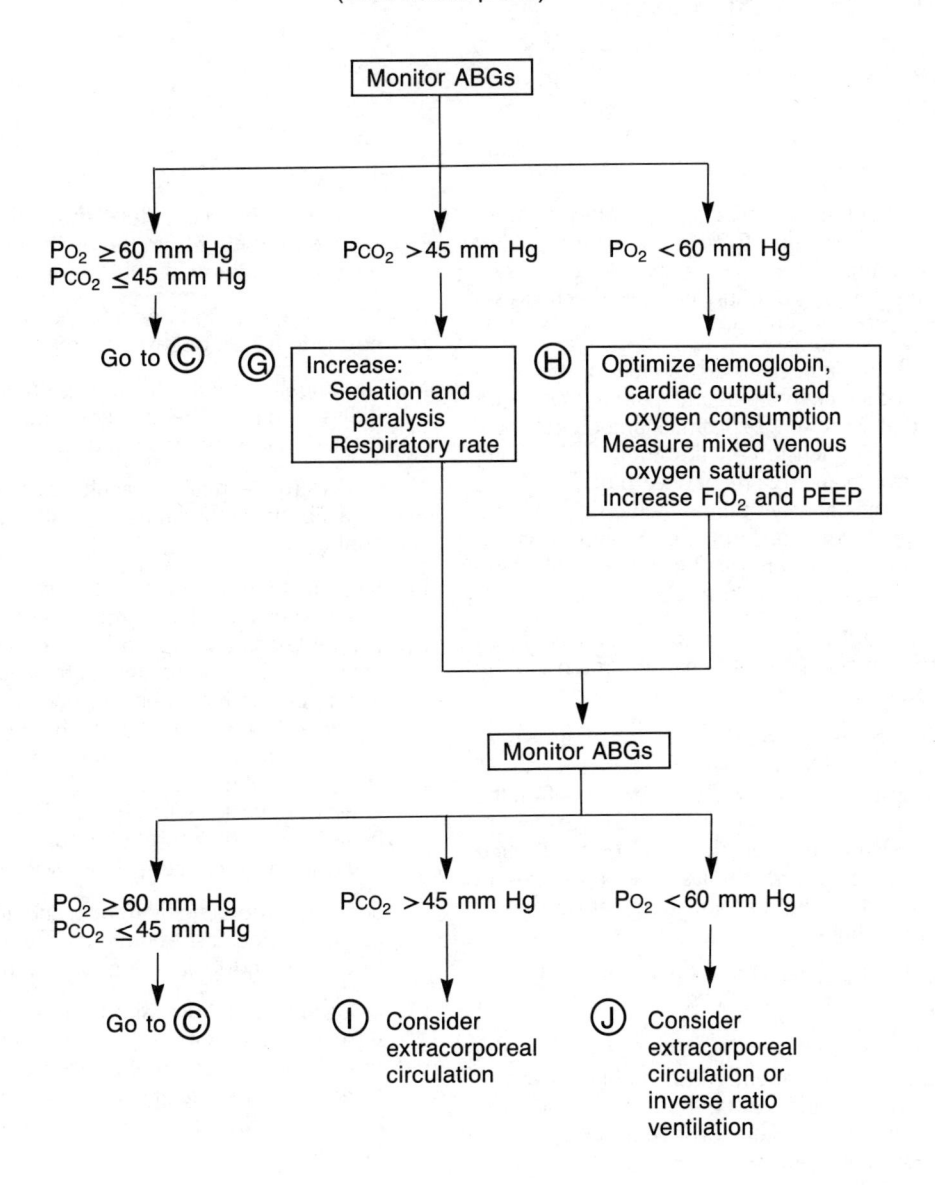

```
                    ┌─────────────┐
                    │ Monitor ABGs│
                    └──────┬──────┘
         ┌─────────────────┼─────────────────┐
         ▼                 ▼                 ▼
   Po₂ ≥60 mm Hg    Pco₂ >45 mm Hg     Po₂ <60 mm Hg
   Pco₂ ≤45 mm Hg
         │                 │                 │
         ▼                 ▼                 ▼
       Go to Ⓒ     Ⓖ ┌──────────┐   Ⓗ ┌──────────────────┐
                     │Increase: │      │Optimize hemoglobin,│
                     │Sedation and│    │cardiac output, and │
                     │paralysis │      │oxygen consumption  │
                     │Respiratory rate│ │Measure mixed venous│
                     └────┬─────┘      │oxygen saturation   │
                          │            │Increase FiO₂ and PEEP│
                          │            └────────┬───────────┘
                          └─────────┬───────────┘
                                    ▼
                            ┌─────────────┐
                            │ Monitor ABGs│
                            └──────┬──────┘
              ┌────────────────────┼────────────────────┐
              ▼                    ▼                    ▼
        Po₂ ≥60 mm Hg       Pco₂ >45 mm Hg        Po₂ <60 mm Hg
        Pco₂ ≤45 mm Hg
              │                    │                    │
              ▼                    ▼                    ▼
           Go to Ⓒ         Ⓘ Consider            Ⓙ Consider
                              extracorporeal         extracorporeal
                              circulation            circulation or
                                                     inverse ratio
                                                     ventilation
```

315

CARDIOGENIC SHOCK

Barbara A. Bielawski
Paula Tanabe

A. The history should include mechanisms of injury, prehospital care, and allergies. Particular attention should be paid to steering wheel damage and the use of seat belts (if the mechanisms of injury is a motor vehicle accident) and past cardiac history.

B. The chest wall should be assessed for areas of ecchymosis. Cardiogenic shock in the trauma patient may result from myocardial contusion, pericardial tamponade, myocardial infarction, or tension pneumothorax. Therefore, rapid identification and treatment of cardiogenic shock are essential. Signs and symptoms include chest pain; decreased level of consciousness; hypotension; bradycardia; rapid shallow respirations; pale, cool, clammy skin; and cardiac dysrhythmias.

C. A patient with stable vital signs and a normal ECG, but with a significant history, should be monitored closely for any potential changes.

D. Serial ECGs provide the opportunity for diagnosis of changes indicative of myocardial infarction, such as ST elevations. Elevated cardiac isoenzyme levels confirm the diagnosis. Cardiac monitoring provides for early identification of arrhythmias. If an abnormal ECG, elevated enzyme levels, cardiac arrhythmias, or deterioration in vital signs occurs, follow the procedure set out below for abnormal findings.

E. Maintaining the airway, breathing, and circulation (ABCs) must always be the first priority.

F. Oxygen therapy should be administered based on the individual status of the patient. If critical, high flow oxygen with a non-rebreather device should be considered. Endotracheal intubation is the most definitive intervention for airway management.

G. Peripheral access should be obtained with two large bore intravenous (IV) catheters. The rate of administration of Ringer's lactate or normal saline is dependent on the patient's condition.

H. A brisk rise in central venous pressure after the administration of fluid, in association with slight or no improvement in cardiac output, is usually indicative of cardiac tamponade or mediastinal compression. Central venous pressure monitoring acts as a guide in determining the rate of fluid administration.

I. A chest film can identify tension pneumothorax as a possible etiology of cardiogenic shock.

J. The confirmation of tension pneumothorax, with or without a chest film, is treated by the insertion of a chest tube.

K. If the patient exhibits Beck's triad (i.e., muffled heart sounds, hypotension, and elevated venous pressure), pericardial tamponade should be suspected, and an immediate pericardiocentesis should be performed. After aspiration of fluid from the pericardial sac, an improvement in condition should be noted.

L. If the patient's condition does not improve, plans should be made for an open thoracotomy or for surgery.

M. Continually monitor for the recurrence of Beck's triad. If these symptoms recur, pericardiocentesis is again performed, and surgery should be considered.

N. Congestive heart failure, acute myocardial infarction, and atrial fibrillation or flutter may result in altered myocardial contractility.

O. Digoxin, dopamine, dobutamine, and the combined ionotropic and chronotropic effects of isoproterenol (Isuprel) decrease the workload of the left ventricle, increase cardiac output, and increase coronary artery perfusion. Dopamine is beneficial because it increases renal artery perfusion. Dobutamine has the advantage of inotropic stimulation without resulting tachycardia. Isoproterenol has been described as the drug of choice when immediate treatment is indicated. Digoxin has also been identified as a mild inotropic drug; its use is indicated for the treatment of atrial fibrillation or flutter.

P. Sodium nitroprusside (Nipride) and nitroglycerine are indicated to decrease ventricular afterload and peripheral resistance and to increase cardiac output.

Q. Lidocaine, bretylium, and procainamide hydrochloride (Pronestyl) are indicated for the treatment of ventricular arrhythmias. Propranolol hydrochloride (Inderal) is indicated for the treatment of resistant sinus tachycardia. Verapamil is indicated for the treatment of resistant atrial tachyarrhythmias.

References

McQuillan K, Wiles C. Initial management of traumatic shock. In: Cardona V, Hurn P, Bastnagel Mason P, Scanlon-Schlipp A, Veise-Berry S, eds. Trauma nursing from resuscitation through rehabilitation. Philadelphia: WB Saunders, 1988:160–181.

Sheehy S, Mavin J, Jimmerson-Le Duc C. Manual of clinical trauma care: the first hour. St. Louis: CV Mosby, 1989: 249–268.

Shires GT III, Fantini G, Shires G. Management of shock. In: Mattox K, Moore E, Feliciano D, eds. Trauma. Norwalk, CT: Appleton & Lange, 1988:139–157.

Thal E, Raess D. Early recognition and treatment of shock. In: Richardson J, Polk H Jr, Flint L, eds. Trauma clinical care and pathophysiology. Chicago: Year Book, 1987:32–40.

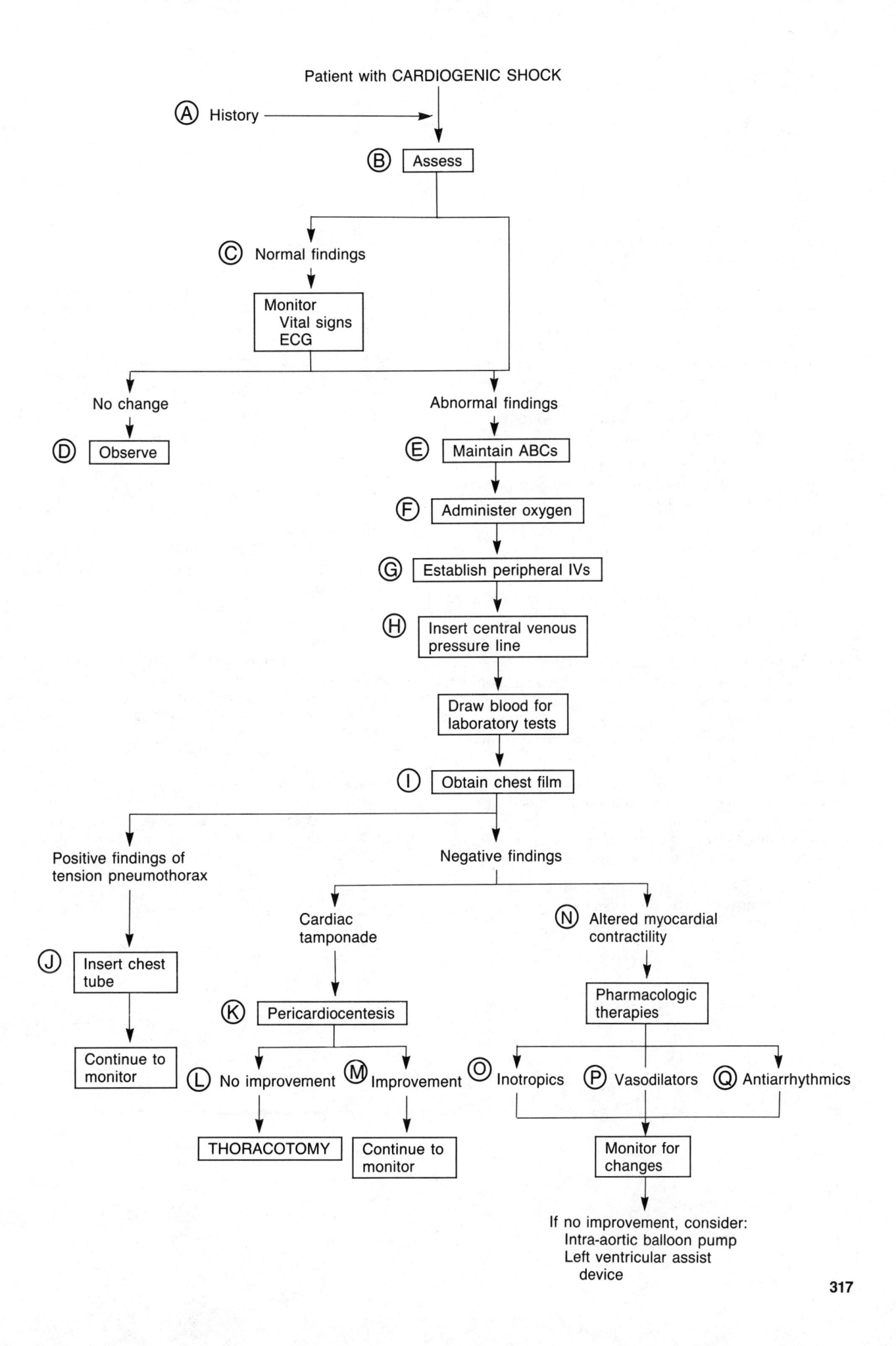

```
                    Patient with CARDIOGENIC SHOCK
    Ⓐ History ─────────────────────▶
                                      ↓
                                Ⓑ  Assess
                                      ↓
                    ┌─────────────────┴─────────────────┐
                    ↓                                   ↓
           Ⓒ Normal findings                      Abnormal findings
                    ↓                                   ↓
              ┌───────────┐                      Ⓔ Maintain ABCs
              │ Monitor   │                             ↓
              │ Vital signs│                     Ⓕ Administer oxygen
              │ ECG       │                             ↓
              └───────────┘                     Ⓖ Establish peripheral IVs
                    ↓                                   ↓
              No change                          Ⓗ Insert central venous
                    ↓                                pressure line
              Ⓓ Observe                                 ↓
                                                  Draw blood for
                                                  laboratory tests
                                                        ↓
                                                Ⓘ Obtain chest film
```

Positive findings of tension pneumothorax → Ⓙ Insert chest tube → Continue to monitor

Negative findings:
- Cardiac tamponade → Ⓚ Pericardiocentesis → Ⓛ No improvement → THORACOTOMY; Ⓜ Improvement → Continue to monitor
- Ⓝ Altered myocardial contractility → Pharmacologic therapies → Ⓞ Inotropics, Ⓟ Vasodilators, Ⓠ Antiarrhythmics → Monitor for changes

If no improvement, consider:
Intra-aortic balloon pump
Left ventricular assist device

NEUROGENIC SHOCK

Barbara A. Bielawski
Paula Tanabe

A. The history should include the mechanism of injury, prehospital care, medications taken, and allergies. Particular attention should be paid to potential spinal cord injury.

B. Neurogenic shock may result from a spinal cord injury above the T6 level or from brain stem injury at the level of the medulla. Causes include loss of sympathetic tone, which results in peripheral vasodilation and hypotension. Signs and symptoms include neurologic deficit; normal or decreased pulse; hypotension; widened pulse pressure; warm, dry, flushed skin; rapid, shallow respirations; or the absence of respiration.

C. A spinal cord or head injured patient with normal vital signs and intact sensorimotor function should be monitored closely for changes.

D. Maintenance of airway, breathing, and circulation (ABC's) should always be the first priority.

E. If a neurologic deficit is present or an abnormality is present on x-ray examination, spinal immobilization should continue until more definitive treatment is provided.

F. A pneumatic antishock garment (PASG) or military antishock trousers are indicated in the early management of neurogenic shock to improve blood pressure temporarily while fluid resuscitation is begun. Contraindications include pulmonary embolus, congestive heart failure, pregnancy, or increased intracranial pressure.

G. In the presence of spinal cord or head injury without other associated trauma, intravenous (IV) fluids must be administered cautiously. Hypotension results from vasodilation following spinal shock. Ringer's lactate should be administered at a rate of 1 mg/kg per hour.

H. Continued monitoring of vital signs for evidence of other injury is imperative. Blood loss must be ruled out as a cause of hypotension. The pulse rate should be slow, unless hypovolemia is present.

I. By placing a central venous pressure line, fluid resuscitation can be monitored more accurately. The goal is to maintain a normal or slightly low central venous pressure reading.

J. Neurogenic shock can be caused by gastric dilation alone. Placement of a nasogastric tube with suction can be an effective treatment. The placement of a Foley catheter allows for accurate assessment of urine output.

K. To support arterial pressure, vasopressors such as phenylephrine can be used with caution; renal ischemia and cardiac arrhythmias are potential complications. The central venous pressure should be maintained at a point at which it rises slightly with rapid administration of fluid, thus assuring adequate fluid volume. The initial dose of phenylephrine is 30 μg per minute. The dose can then be titrated to a desirable blood pressure, with a dosage range of 20 to 200 μg per minute.

References

McQuillan K, Wiles C. Initial management of traumatic shock. In: Cardona V, Hurn P, Bastnagel Mason P, Scanlon-Schlipp A, Veise-Berry S, eds. Trauma nursing from resuscitation through rehabilitation. Philadelphia: WB Saunders, 1988:160–181.

Scott J. Cervical spine injury. In: Mancini M, ed. Decision making in emergency nursing. Toronto: BC Decker, 1987:40.

Sheehy S, Mavin J, Jimmerson-Le Duc C.. Manual of clinical trauma care: the first hour. St. Louis: CV Mosby, 1989:249–268.

Shires GT III, Fantini G, Shires G. Management of shock. In: Mattox K, Moore E, Feliciano D, eds. Trauma. Norwalk, CT: Appleton & Lange, 1988:139–157.

Thal E, Raess D. Early recognition and treatment of shock. In: Richardson J, Polk H Jr, Flint L, eds. Trauma clinical care and pathophysiology. Chicago: Year Book, 1987:32–40.

Patient with NEUROGENIC SHOCK

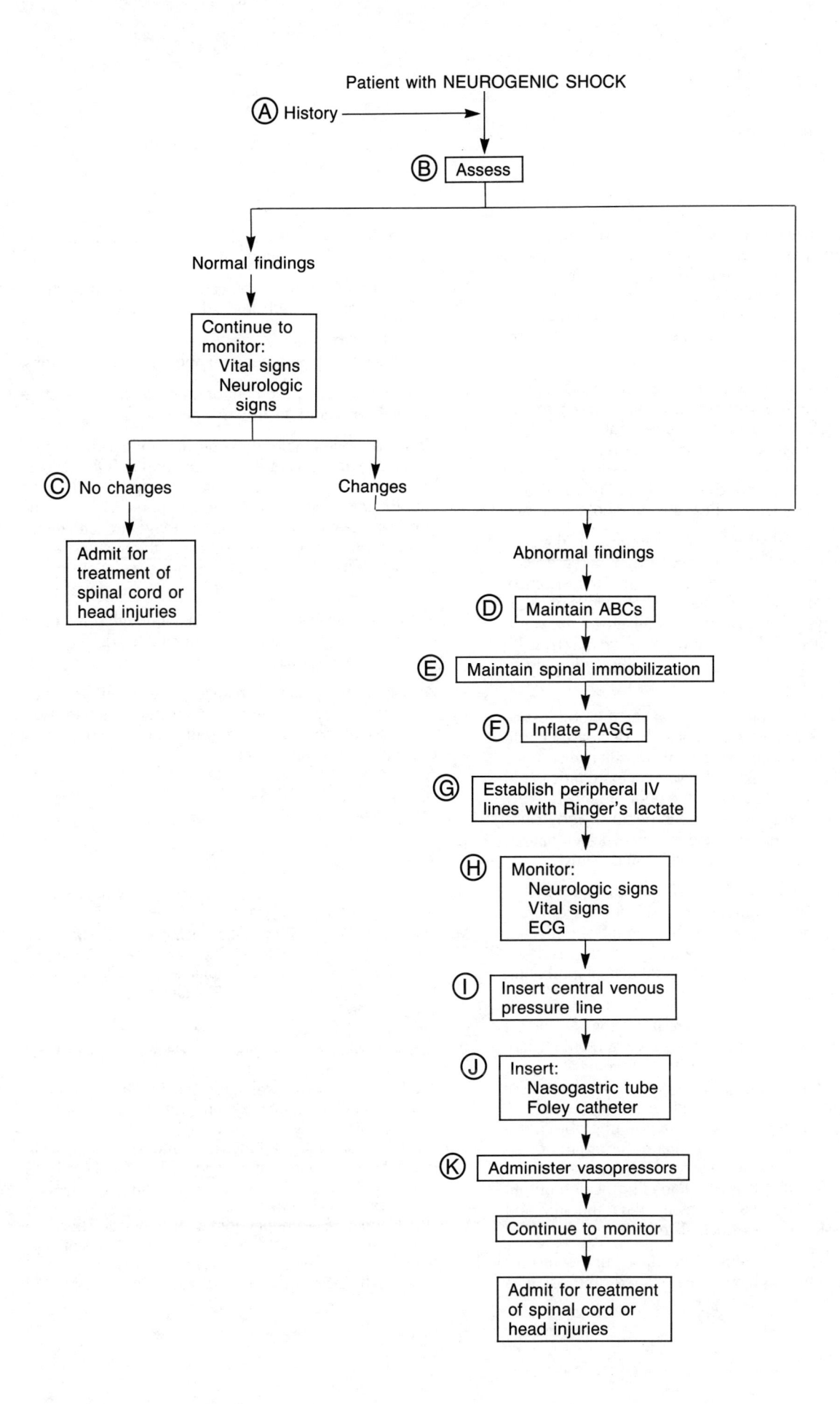

(A) History ⟶

(B) Assess

Normal findings

Continue to monitor:
 Vital signs
 Neurologic signs

(C) No changes

Admit for treatment of spinal cord or head injuries

Changes

Abnormal findings

(D) Maintain ABCs

(E) Maintain spinal immobilization

(F) Inflate PASG

(G) Establish peripheral IV lines with Ringer's lactate

(H) Monitor:
 Neurologic signs
 Vital signs
 ECG

(I) Insert central venous pressure line

(J) Insert:
 Nasogastric tube
 Foley catheter

(K) Administer vasopressors

Continue to monitor

Admit for treatment of spinal cord or head injuries

319

SEPTIC SHOCK

Barbara A. Bielawski
Paula Tanabe

A. History should include the mechanism of injury, prehospital care, past medical history, medications taken, allergies, actual and potential injuries, instrumentation, and invasive procedures. Sepsis is uncommon immediately following a traumatic event, but it becomes suspect if preinjury infective foci exist or a delay in transport occurred.

B. Septic shock is a frequent complication of the multiply traumatized patient. Its mortality rate is 50 percent. Predisposing factors include extremes of age, burns, pre-existing immunosuppression, chronic disease, invasive procedures, surgery, and the stress response. Gram-negative bacilli, gram-positive organisms, and fungi contribute to hemodynamic failure and metabolic changes.

C. The hyperdynamic state is most common in the normovolemic patient. It is evidenced by an increased cardiac output, decreased peripheral vascular resistance, hypotension, normal or elevated central venous pressure (CVP), hyperventilation, respiratory alkalosis, and warm dry extremities. Chills and fever may or may not be present, dependent on the patient's ability to initiate an immune response.

D. The hypodynamic state occurs with acute blood loss or third space losses and is evidenced by decreased cardiac output, increased peripheral vascular resistance hypotension, decreased CVP, cyanotic extremities, and metabolic acidosis. Owing to the poor prognosis, early identification and treatment are imperative. Early signs and symptoms include the triad of mild hyperventilation, respiratory alkalosis, and altered mental status.

E. A chest film should be obtained to rule out a possible source of infection, although by itself it does not provide a definitive diagnosis. Oxygen should be delivered based on initial and serial arterial blood gas results. If respiratory failure is suspected, endotracheal intubation should be instituted.

F. In the hyperdynamic state, fluid resuscitation is achieved with Ringer's lactate, based on the CVP and pulmonary capillary wedge pressure (PCWP) readings. In the hypodynamic state, immediate correction of hypovolemia is essential and is achieved with Ringer's lactate, blood replacement (based on hemoglobin and hematocrit levels), and administration of plasma or albumin. The rate and volume of fluid replacement are dependent on the PCWP and CVP readings. Urine output must be monitored hourly to assess renal function and the progression of the shock state.

G. Antibiotics are not withheld pending culture results. Broad-spectrum antibiotics are started immediately. When the particular site is identified, site specific antibiotics should be administered.

H. The septic shock state can occasionally resolve with antibiotic treatment and fluid administration alone.

I. Lack of improvement within 6 to 12 hours after antibiotic therapy indicates a need for additional interventions.

J. Often surgical debridement or drainage of the infection is required before an improvement occurs.

K. With continued hemodynamic instability, the use of vasoactive agents is indicated. Dopamine is the drug of choice because of its beta 2 stimulatory effect. Dosage should range from 2 to 5 $\mu g/kg$ per minute. Dobutamine and isoproterenol (Isuprel) may increase myocardial oxygen demands. Therefore, if chosen, the smallest effective dose should be used. In the presence of current or pre-existing heart failure, digoxin may be effective.

L. The use of steroids is controversial, although some cases have shown improvement. A recommended dose for therapy is not agreed on.

M. Persistent shock state can lead to renal failure, adult respiratory distress syndrome, and disseminated intravascular coagulation. Early recognition and treatment may prevent irreversible damage.

References

Hardaway R, ed. Shock, the reversible stage of dying. Littleton: PSG Publishing, 1988:178–197.

McQuillan KA, Wiles CE III. Initial management of traumatic shock. In: Cardona V, Hurn P, Bastnagel-Mason P, Scanlon-Schlipp A, Veise-Berry S, eds. Trauma nursing from resuscitation through rehabilitation. Philadelphia: WB Saunders, 1988:160–161.

Shires GT III, Fantini GA, Shires GT. Management of shock. In: Mattox K, Moore E, Feliciano D, eds. Trauma. Norwalk, CT: Appleton & Lange, 1988:139–157.

Thal ER, Raess DH. Early recognition of shock. In: Meyers MH, ed. The multiply injured patient with complex fractures. Philadelphia: Lea & Febiger, 1984:32–40.

Trunkey DD, Carmona R, Tortella B. Shock: cardiovascular pathophysiology and treatment. In: Richardson JD, Polk HC Jr, Flint CM, eds. Trauma clinical care and pathophysiology. Chicago: Year Book, 1987:13–37.

Vary TC, Linberg SE. Pathophysiology of traumatic shock. In: Cardona V, Hurn P, Bastnagel-Mason P, Scanlon-Schlipp A, Veise-Berry S, eds. Trauma nursing from resuscitation through rehabilitation. Philadelphia: WB Saunders, 1988:127–157.

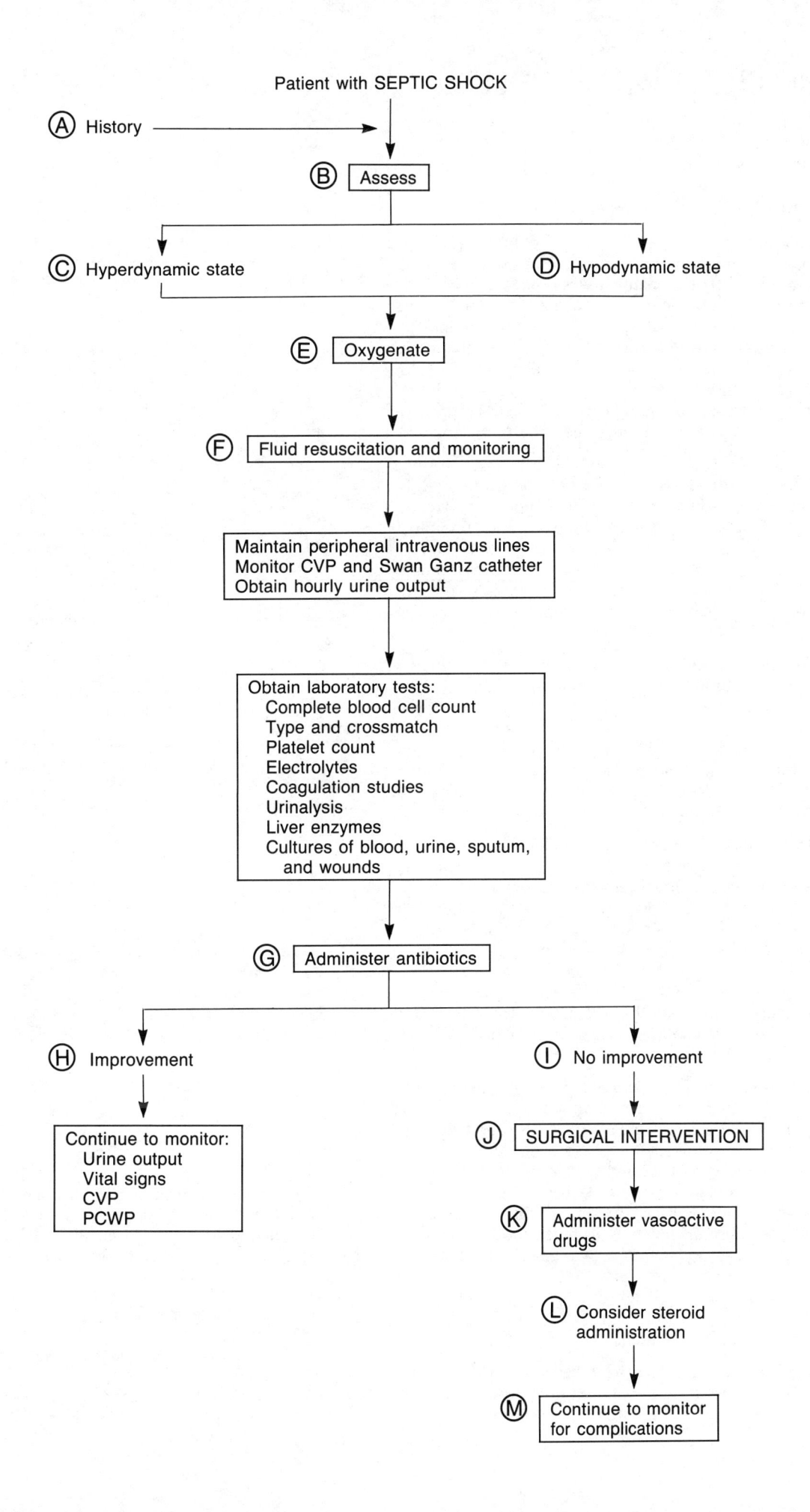

```
                    Patient with SEPTIC SHOCK
    Ⓐ History ─────────────►    │
                                 ▼
                             Ⓑ ┌──────┐
                               │Assess│
                               └──────┘
                        ┌────────┴────────┐
                        ▼                 ▼
               Ⓒ Hyperdynamic state   Ⓓ Hypodynamic state
                        └────────┬────────┘
                                 ▼
                             Ⓔ ┌─────────┐
                               │Oxygenate│
                               └─────────┘
                                 ▼
                             Ⓕ ┌──────────────────────────────┐
                               │Fluid resuscitation and monitoring│
                               └──────────────────────────────┘
                                 ▼
                  ┌─────────────────────────────────────┐
                  │Maintain peripheral intravenous lines│
                  │Monitor CVP and Swan Ganz catheter   │
                  │Obtain hourly urine output           │
                  └─────────────────────────────────────┘
                                 ▼
                  ┌─────────────────────────────────────┐
                  │Obtain laboratory tests:             │
                  │    Complete blood cell count        │
                  │    Type and crossmatch              │
                  │    Platelet count                   │
                  │    Electrolytes                     │
                  │    Coagulation studies              │
                  │    Urinalysis                       │
                  │    Liver enzymes                    │
                  │    Cultures of blood, urine, sputum,│
                  │      and wounds                     │
                  └─────────────────────────────────────┘
                                 ▼
                             Ⓖ ┌────────────────────┐
                               │Administer antibiotics│
                               └────────────────────┘
                        ┌────────┴────────┐
                        ▼                 ▼
                  Ⓗ Improvement      Ⓘ No improvement
                        ▼                 ▼
          ┌──────────────────┐     Ⓙ ┌─────────────────────┐
          │Continue to monitor:│      │SURGICAL INTERVENTION│
          │   Urine output   │       └─────────────────────┘
          │   Vital signs    │                 ▼
          │   CVP            │           Ⓚ ┌──────────────────┐
          │   PCWP           │             │Administer vasoactive│
          └──────────────────┘             │drugs             │
                                           └──────────────────┘
                                                 ▼
                                           Ⓛ ┌──────────────────┐
                                             │Consider steroid  │
                                             │administration    │
                                             └──────────────────┘
                                                 ▼
                                           Ⓜ ┌──────────────────┐
                                             │Continue to monitor│
                                             │for complications │
                                             └──────────────────┘
```

MULTIPLE ORGAN FAILURE

Kathleen C. Solotkin
Mary C. McCarthy

A. Multiple organ failure (MOF) is a clinical syndrome characterized by progressive failure of two or more organ systems. The mortality rate is over 60 percent, and it is the most common cause of death in severely injured patients who survive the initial 48 hours after injury. Inadequate organ perfusion, hypoxia, and infection are contributing factors in the development of MOF. Multiple transfusions, extensive tissue damage, and pre-existing disease have also been implicated. Progressive system injury occurs through the release of cytokinins and other toxic mediators.

B. A detailed initial assessment should be made of every severely injured patient. Particularly important is a complete physical examination; pulmonary and abdominal examinations are critical. Certain mechanisms of injury place the patient at increased risk for the development of MOF. Patients with contaminated wounds, severe pulmonary contusions, and extensive burns are at greatest risk.

C. Baseline laboratory data should be obtained, including complete blood cell count; prothrombin time; partial thromboplastin time; platelet, electrolyte, blood-urea nitrogen, creatinine, glucose, and amylase levels; and liver functions (SGOT, alkaline phosphatase, and bilirubin). Arterial blood gases and a baseline chest film should be obtained. Serial studies should be drawn, with the time interval dependent on the patient's condition.

D. Deterioration in the patient's condition classically occurs after the initial 48 hours post injury. Early MOF (i.e., days 2 to 7) is commonly a prodromal phase that resembles sepsis. By days 7 to 14, multiple organ dysfunction is usually evident. After day 14, a period of late organ failure develops, with the patient becoming hemodynamically unstable. The syndrome progresses to a preterminal phase with cardiovascular failure, reduced oxygen extraction, and severe lactic acidosis. The criteria for MOF are variable; however, the definitions in Table 1 may prove useful.

E. MOF is characterized by a hyperdynamic, hypermetabolic state similar to that seen in sepsis. The most commonly involved organs are the lungs, liver, and kidneys. Assessments should include close observation of all organ systems. Early signs and symptoms of infection and pulmonary deterioration (i.e., tachypnea and increasing oxygen requirements) are most frequently encountered. Increased liver function tests, jaundice, prolonged bleeding, petechiae, and hematuria may be seen. Renal failure may be oliguric or high output. Hemodynamic instability, central nervous system changes (e.g., confusion to obtundation), and gastrointestinal bleeding from stress ulceration may be present.

F. Nursing energies should be directed at closely observing the patient for the evolution of clinical syndromes and at continuously monitoring the patient.

TABLE 1   Criteria for Multiple Organ Failure

Pulmonary	Hypoxia that requires mechanical ventilation for 5 or more days
	FIO_2 greater than 40% ± positive-end expiratory pressure
Renal	Creatinine level greater than 2 mg/dl or doubling of admission creatinine level with less than 500 ml urine output per 24 h
Liver	Bilirubin level greater than 2 mg/dl with SGOT and lactate dehydrogenase twice the normal level
Gastrointestinal	Endoscopically confirmed stress ulcerations
	2 units blood replacement within 24 h for upper gastrointestinal bleeding
	Acalculous cholecystitis
Coagulation	Thrombocytopenia
	Prolonged prothrombin time and partial thromboplastin time
	Hypofibrinogenemia
	Presence of fibrin split products (i.e., disseminated intravascular coagulation)
Cardiac	Hypotension
	Cardiac index less than 2.5 L/m²
	No evidence of infarction
Central nervous system	Response only to painful stimuli

G. Treatment is directed at control and correction of precipitating factors, treatment of infection, hemodynamic support, nutritional support, and prevention of further deterioration. If MOF is unsuccessfully controlled, the end result is a hypodynamic state, cardiovascular collapse, and death.

References

Bessey PQ. Metabolic response to critical illness. In: Wilmore D, ed. Care of the surgical patient. Volume 1 Critical Care. New York, Scientific American, 1989.

Borzotta AP, Polk HC. Multiple system organ failure. Surg Clin North Am 1983; 63(2):315–333.

DeCamp MM, Demling RH. Concepts in emergency and critical care: posttraumatic multisystem organ failure. JAMA 1988; 260:530–534.

Fry DE. Multiple system organ failure. Surg Clin North Am 1983; 66(1):107–122.

Moore EE, Eiseman B, VanWay CW. Critical decisions in trauma. St. Louis: CV Mosby, 1984:414–418.

Patient with SHOCK AND TISSUE TRAUMA

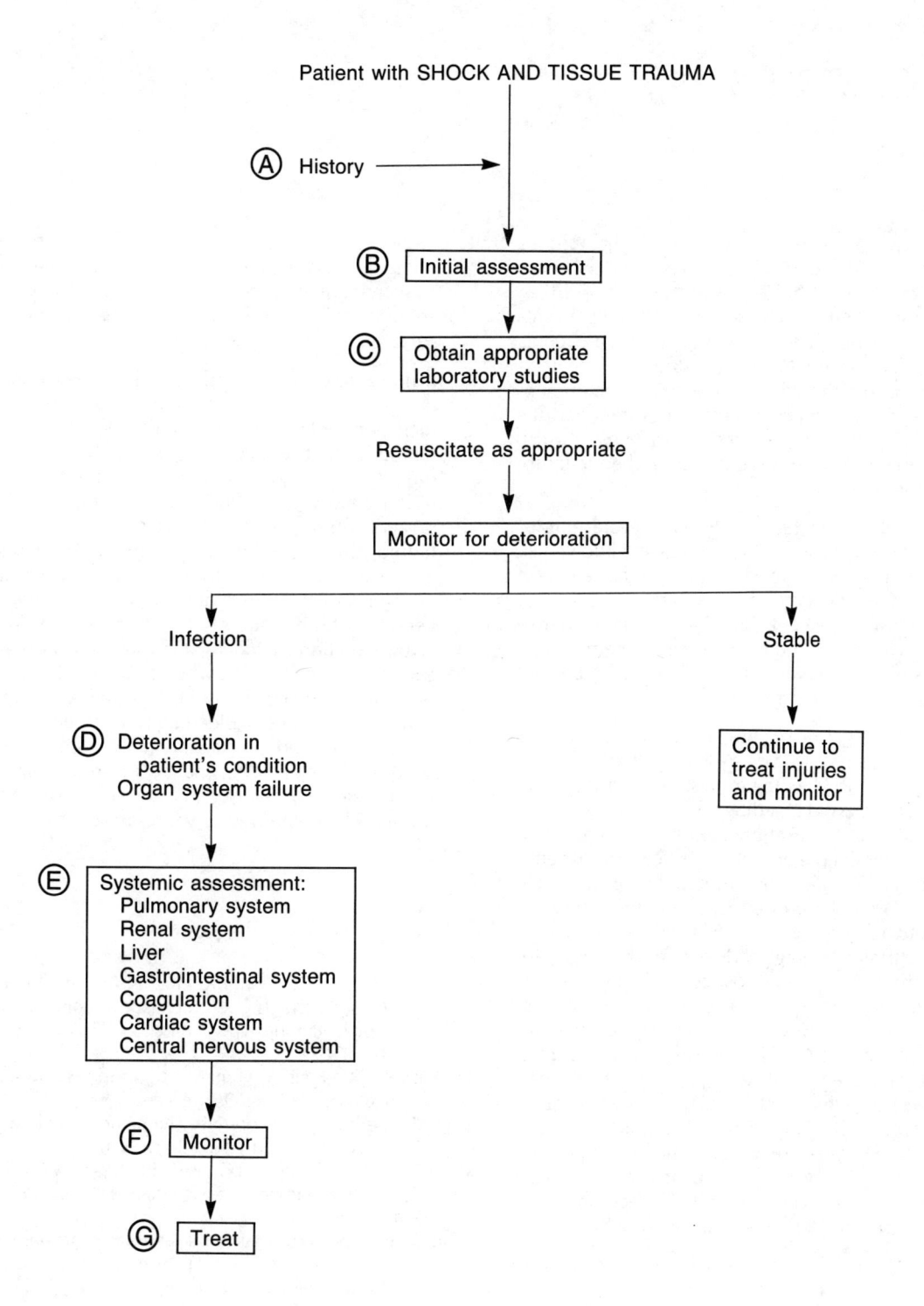

Ⓐ History ⟶

Ⓑ Initial assessment

Ⓒ Obtain appropriate laboratory studies

Resuscitate as appropriate

Monitor for deterioration

- Infection
- Stable

Ⓓ Deterioration in patient's condition
Organ system failure

Ⓔ Systemic assessment:
- Pulmonary system
- Renal system
- Liver
- Gastrointestinal system
- Coagulation
- Cardiac system
- Central nervous system

Ⓕ Monitor

Ⓖ Treat

Continue to treat injuries and monitor

STRESS GASTRITIS

John A. Weigelt

A. Patients at low risk are those who have minimal injuries (i.e., injury severity score of 15 or less) and who are without known risk factors (e.g., shock, sepsis, or organ failure). These patients would be expected to regain gastrointestinal function within 1 to 3 days. These patients are at extremely low risk for stress gastritis, and the need for any type of prophylaxis is unclear. Our recommendations are that they receive no specific stress gastritis prophylaxis. The most important concern with a low-risk patient is rapid resuscitation to prevent ischemic injury to the gastric mucosa.

B. Patients at high risk include those with severe injuries (i.e., injury severity score of 15 or more) and known risk factors including shock, sepsis, and/or organ failure of any type. The incidence of stress gastritis in these patients is at least 25 percent if untreated. The incidence of bleeding is between 5 and 10 percent. The mortality rate from stress gastritis is estimated at 3 to 5 percent of patients who develop the syndrome.

C. Monitoring of the gastric pH level helps to select options for stress gastritis prophylaxis. A gastric pH level of 3.5 is adequate to avoid bleeding from stress gastritis. Other pH levels used to avoid bleeding have been between 4.5 to 6. Recently, gastric alkalinization has been associated with nosocomial pneumonia in critically ill patients. Aggressive alkalinization might increase the incidence of pneumonia. A pH level of 3.5 is a compromise between the two following ideas: first, that alkalinization prevents gastritis bleeding, and second, that excessive alkalinization promotes nosocomial pneumonia. Monitoring of the gastric pH level can be done with standard nitrazine paper. However, the lowest pH level this paper can measure is 4.5. Thus, a patient with a pH level of 4.5, as measured by nitrazine paper, can have a gastric pH level anywhere between 1 and 4.5. Recently, indwelling pH probes have been incorporated into standard nasogastric tubes. These tubes offer the opportunity to monitor the gastric pH level accurately over a wide range of values. This type of monitor is recommended in selecting patients for stress gastritis prophylaxis.

D. A gastric pH level of greater than 3.5 indicates that no further treatment is needed.

E. A gastric pH level of 3.5 or less indicates treatment by antacids every 1 to 2 hours. The goal of this therapy is to keep the gastric pH level above 3.5. Hourly pH monitoring is continued. The average dose is 15 to 30 ml every 2 hours.

F. If the gastric pH level is 3.5 or less for 2 consecutive hours, additional therapy is given. The antacids may be increased, or H2 blockers can be added. Cimetidine and ranitidine are two commonly used H2 blockers. Cimetidine is usually given intravenously at a dose of 300 to 400 mg every 4 to 6 hours, and ranitidine is given at a dose of 150 mg every 12 hours. Continuous infusion of both agents is possible. It is common to include these agents in parenteral nutrition solutions when they are given as constant infusions. Additionally, prophylactic agents include sucralfate and prostaglandin E_2. Cytoprotection is the mechanism of action of these agents. It is unclear yet whether they have any benefit over the use of antacids or H2 blockers. In some studies a higher incidence of bleeding is recorded with the use of sulcrafate and prostaglandin E_2. Neither agent increases gastric pH level, and it is suggested that their use is associated with a lower incidence of nosocomial pneumonia. This benefit is as yet unproven.

References

Driks MR, Craven DE, Celli BR, et al. Nosocomial pneumonia in intubated patients given sucralfate as compared with antacids or histamine type 2 blockers. N Engl J Med 1987; 317:1376–1382.

Durham RM, Weigelt JA. Monitoring gastric pH levels. Surg Gynecol Obstet 1989; 169(1):14–16.

Silen W, Merhav A, Simson JNL. The pathophysiology of stress ulcer disease. World J Surg 1981; 5:165–174.

Weigelt JA, Aurbakken CM, Gewertz BL, Snyder WH III. Cimetidine vs antacid in prophylaxis for stress ulceration. Arch Surg 1981; 116:597–601.

Zinner MJ, Rypins EB, Martin LR, et al. Misoprostal versus antacid titration for preventing stress ulcers in postoperative surgical ICU patients. Ann Surg 1989; 210(5):590–595.

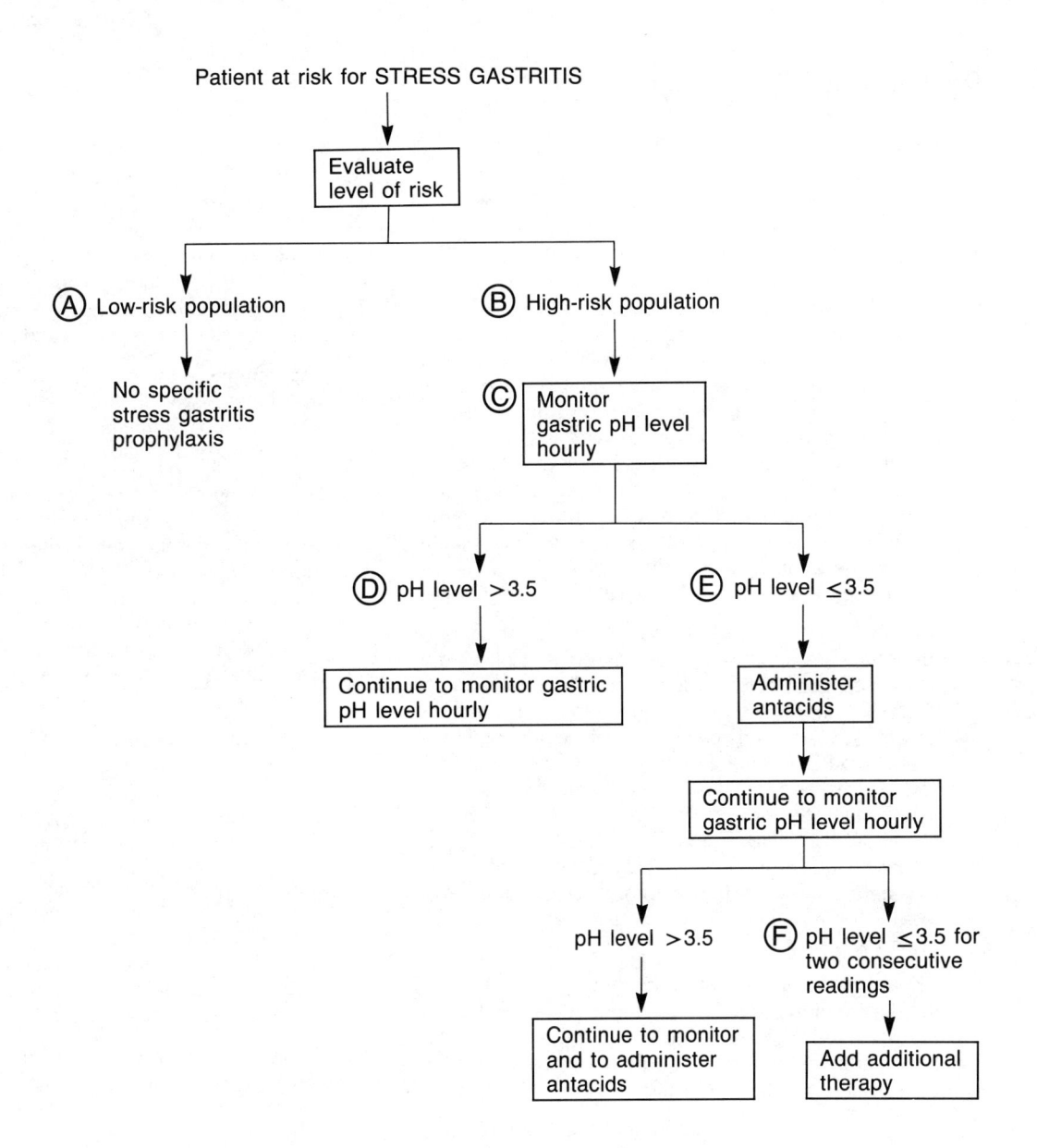

```
Patient at risk for STRESS GASTRITIS
                │
                ▼
        ┌───────────────┐
        │   Evaluate    │
        │ level of risk │
        └───────────────┘
         │             │
         ▼             ▼
(A) Low-risk      (B) High-risk
    population        population
         │             │
         ▼             ▼
  No specific    (C) ┌──────────────┐
  stress gastritis   │   Monitor    │
  prophylaxis        │ gastric pH   │
                     │ level hourly │
                     └──────────────┘
                      │           │
                      ▼           ▼
              (D) pH level    (E) pH level
                  >3.5            ≤3.5
                   │               │
                   ▼               ▼
          ┌──────────────┐   ┌────────────┐
          │ Continue to  │   │ Administer │
          │ monitor      │   │ antacids   │
          │ gastric pH   │   └────────────┘
          │ level hourly │         │
          └──────────────┘         ▼
                          ┌──────────────────┐
                          │ Continue to      │
                          │ monitor gastric  │
                          │ pH level hourly  │
                          └──────────────────┘
                              │         │
                              ▼         ▼
                        pH level   (F) pH level ≤3.5 for
                        >3.5           two consecutive
                         │             readings
                         ▼              │
                ┌──────────────┐        ▼
                │ Continue to  │  ┌────────────┐
                │ monitor and  │  │ Add        │
                │ to administer│  │ additional │
                │ antacids     │  │ therapy    │
                └──────────────┘  └────────────┘
```

PULMONARY EMBOLISM

Jodi Luke

A. Pulmonary embolism (PE) occurs in over five million patients each year, with 100,000 fatalities. Eighty percent of the deaths occur within 2 hours of the onset of symptoms, usually before the diagnosis is made. Any patient who presents with a sudden, unexplained shortness of breath should be evaluated for potential PE. Risk factors include a history of previous deep vein thrombosis or PE, varicose veins, oral contraceptive use, pregnancy, obesity, cardiopulmonary disease, major surgeries, cancer, and long periods of sitting or bed rest. Any injury to the legs, whether caused by surgery or trauma, places the patient at high risk because emboli usually form in the lower extremities and migrate to the lungs. PE is more common in blacks than in whites or orientals.

B. Initially the patient may be asymptomatic or may have pleuritic chest pain, syncope, dyspnea, tachycardia, tachypnea, hemoptysis, pulmonary hypertension, or signs of compromised right ventricular heart function. Shock, cyanosis, and hypotension may be present if there is massive PE. A careful history for these symptoms is essential. Tachycardia is usually present. Blood pressure may be elevated or decreased as in a massive PE with cardiovascular collapse. An elevated temperature may indicate a septic embolism or a pulmonary infection that may be the source of the symptoms. Unexplained restlessness or apprehension may be early signs of hypoxia or shock.

C. Arterial blood gases (ABGs) are crucial in determining the degree of hypoxemia. An arterial PO_2 above 90 mm Hg is a good indication that a large PE is not present. Serum enzymes may be monitored to differentiate acute myocardial infarction from the PE.

D. Oxygen may be administered after the ABGs to maintain the PO_2 above 60 mm Hg. Intubation may be required.

E. An ECG may assist in differentiating between a PE and an acute myocardial infarction. Right ventricular overload may be seen on the ECG following a massive PE.

F. A chest film can assist in determining other causes, such as pneumonia or pleural effusion, for the symptoms but cannot give a conclusive diagnosis of PE.

G. The early institution of an intravenous (IV) access in the patient with impending circulatory collapse is essential. An IV will also be necessary to perform the ventilation-perfusion scan and angiography.

H. A negative ventilation-perfusion scan can completely rule out the diagnosis of PE. A positive scan is not conclusive because other pulmonary conditions may cause abnormal scans. Positive results indicate the need for angiography.

I. Patients in circulatory or impending circulatory collapse with resulting hypotension may require pharmacologic support. Isoproterenol (isuprel) and digitalis may be used to improve myocardial function. Invasive hemodynamic monitoring via pulmonary artery catheter is used to monitor cardiac function. The use of antiembolization stockings promotes venous return and prevents clot formation.

J. Angiography is the only test that can provide a conclusive diagnosis of PE. The test is considered positive if an intraluminal filling defect can be identified or if there is a sharp cutoff of lobar or segmental vessels.

K. The treatment of choice is continuous heparin infusion. The goal is to treat the underlying cause and prevent the formation of further emboli. The partial prothrombin time should be lengthened 1.5 to 2.5 times the control. The initial heparin bolus of 5,000 to 10,000 USP units is to be given at the time the continuous heparin infusion is begun. Run the heparin infusion at 10 to 15 units/kg per hour. Closely monitor clotting times, especially on days 3 through 5 when bleeding is mostly likely.

L. An embolectomy, or removal of the clot, may be performed. This entails major thoracic surgery and is usually reserved for an acute massive PE. Recurrent emboli may require partial interruption of the vena cava through the use of filters, clips, or ligation.

M. Closely monitor for exsanguination. Observe secretions for occult blood. Maintain pressure on venipuncture sites for an extended period of time. Avoid arterial punctures, particularly in areas such as the groin that are difficult to monitor. Teach the patient to avoid insults to the integrity of the mucous membrane and skin.

N. Using antiembolization stockings, avoiding dehydration, elevating lower extremities, performing active and passive range of motion exercises, and controlling signs of congestive heart failure with medications are all ways of preventing venous stasis and resulting emboli. Long-term anticoagulation therapy with warfarin is common following PE.

O. Instruct the patient on use of anticoagulation medication and on early recognition of the signs and symptoms of recurring deep vein thrombosis and PE.

References

Kinney MR, Packa DR, Dunbar SB. AACN'S clinical reference for critical care nursing. New York: McGraw-Hill, 1988: 748–755.

Kirsh MM, Sloan H. Blunt chest trauma, general principles of management. Boston: Little, Brown, 1977:19–43.

Mancini ME, ed. Decision making in emergency nursing. Toronto: BC Decker, 1987:86–87.

Schwartz SI, Shires TG, Spencer FC, Storer EH, eds. Principles of surgery. New York: McGraw-Hill, 1979:985–996.

Shires TG. Principles of trauma care. New York: McGraw-Hill, 1985:541–547.

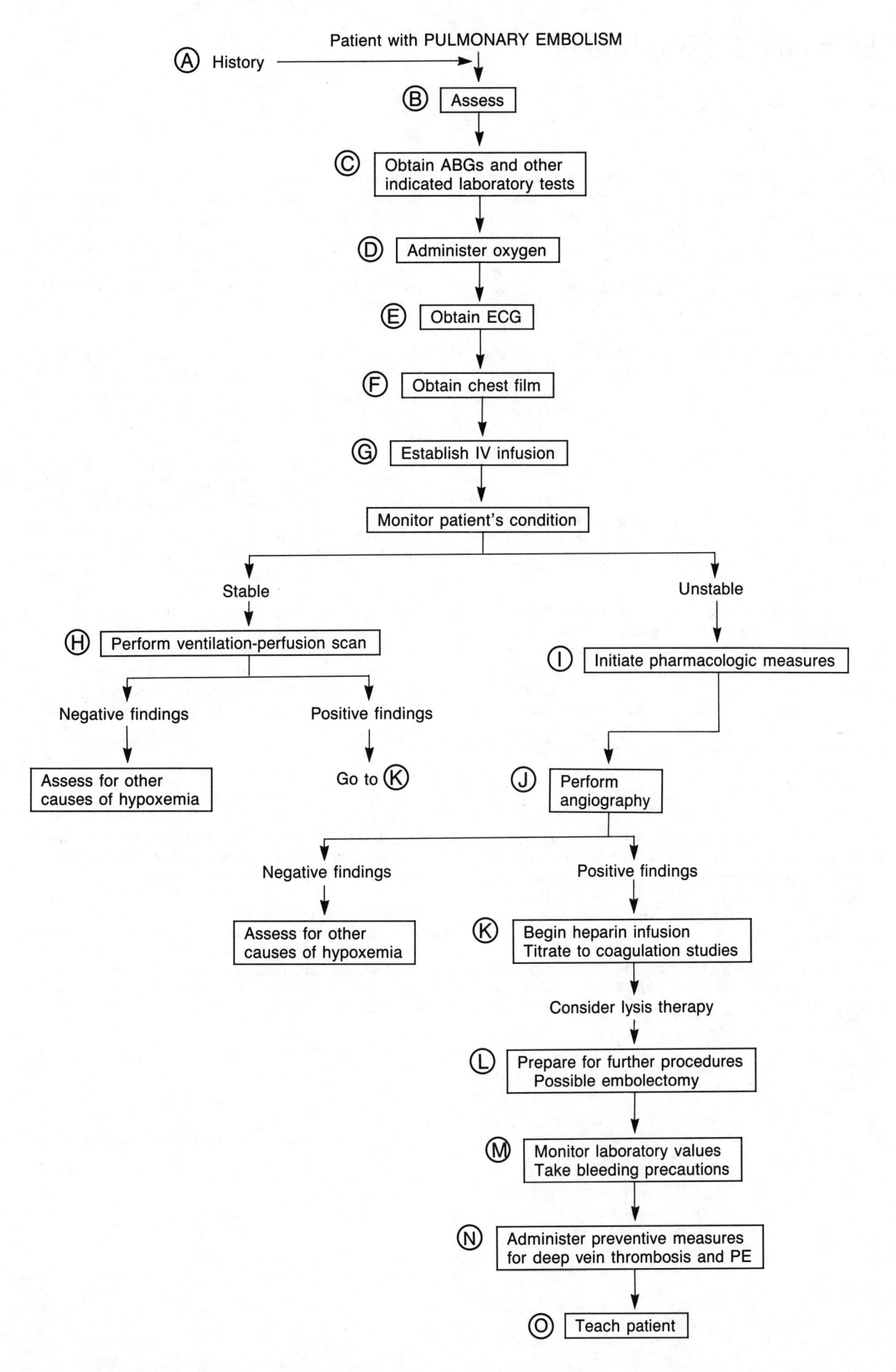

Patient with PULMONARY EMBOLISM

- (A) History
- (B) Assess
- (C) Obtain ABGs and other indicated laboratory tests
- (D) Administer oxygen
- (E) Obtain ECG
- (F) Obtain chest film
- (G) Establish IV infusion

Monitor patient's condition

Stable
- (H) Perform ventilation-perfusion scan
  - Negative findings → Assess for other causes of hypoxemia
  - Positive findings → Go to (K)

Unstable
- (I) Initiate pharmacologic measures
- (J) Perform angiography
  - Negative findings → Assess for other causes of hypoxemia
  - Positive findings → (K) Begin heparin infusion; Titrate to coagulation studies

Consider lysis therapy

- (L) Prepare for further procedures; Possible embolectomy
- (M) Monitor laboratory values; Take bleeding precautions
- (N) Administer preventive measures for deep vein thrombosis and PE
- (O) Teach patient

327

DEEP VEIN THROMBOSIS

Thomas S. Helpenstell

A. The triad of vein wall injury, hypercoagulability, and venous stasis predispose a patient to deep vein thrombosis (DVT). The incidence of DVT in the trauma patient is 20 to 30 percent. Complications of DVT include postphlebitic syndrome, venous insufficiency, and pulmonary embolism (PE). Local thromboses and a secondary consumption coagulopathy, followed by an increased production of platelets and clotting factors, are the physiologic responses to trauma. Thus, for the first few days a trauma patient has a tendency to bleed easily, and after approximately 5 to 7 days the patient will be prone to forming DVT. Hypotension, hypothermia, hypovolemia, and immobilization all stimulate thrombosis. Other risk factors for DVT include an age greater than 60 years, polycythemia, obstructed venous return, pregnancy, cancer, obesity, prior history of DVT, shock, and cardiac disease.

B. Patients with fractures of the pelvis or lower extremities have a higher (over 40 percent) incidence of DVT. Patients with head injuries or spinal cord injuries have a 30 to 40 percent incidence of DVT.

C. Any patient with pelvic or lower extremity fractures, especially elderly patients with hip fractures, should have prophylaxis for at least 7 days—and until ambulatory—unless contraindicated by other problems. Low dose warfarin (Coumadin), dextran, and external pneumatic compression (EPC) hose have all been shown to be effective. Elastic compression stockings (TEDs) are probably effective. Aspirin and subcutaneous heparin have not been shown to be effective. The peak incidence of DVT is 1 to 2 weeks postinjury. Anticoagulation should not be started until all acute bleeding has been controlled.

D. Head injured patients should not be anticoagulated. External pneumatic compression hose or elastic compression stockings are best for head injured or spinal cord injured patients. Low dose heparin is also effective, and rotating beds may be effective, for patients with spinal cord injuries.

E. Signs and symptoms of DVT include leg swelling, pain, erythema, warmth, tenderness, Homans' sign, fever, and tachycardia.

F. Differential diagnoses for DVT include lymphedema, cellulitis, Baker's cyst, contusion, fracture, and cardiac or renal failure.

G. Signs and symptoms of PE include dyspnea, tachypnea, hypoxia, cough, hemoptysis, pleuritic rub, fever, chest pain, tachycardia, right heart failure, atrial fibrillation, depressed S-T segment on ECG, change in mental status, and anxiety.

H. Differential diagnoses for PE include fat emboli syndrome, sepsis, pneumothorax, pulmonary or cardiac contusion, atelectasis, pneumonia, rib fractures, fluid overload, congestive heart failure, angina, myocardial infarction, pleuritis, asthma, and pericarditis.

I. Pulmonary angiography is the most accurate test for PE. Consider ventilation and perfusion scanning only in a stable, cooperative patient with a normal chest film.

J. Treatment for confirmed DVT or PE is as follows: Administer heparin, 100 units/kg via intravenous bolus, then 1000 to 2000 units per hour. Adjust heparin to keep partial thromboplastin time 1.5 to 2 times the normal level. Begin warfarin in 3 to 4 days, 10 mg by mouth daily, for 3 days. Adjust warfarin to keep 2 to 2.5 times the control level. Continue heparin until warfarin is therapeutic. Continue warfarin for a total of 3 months for DVT and 6 months for PE. Consider using a vena cava filter in the patient with a contraindication to anticoagulation.

References

Becker DM, et al. Prevention of deep vein thrombosis in patients with acute spinal cord injuries: use of rotating treatment tables. Neurosurgery 1987; 20(5):675–677.

Knudson MM, Collins JA. Disorders of hemostasis and coagulation in injured patients. Adv Trauma 1989; 4:141–163.

National Institutes of Health Consensus Development Conference Statement. Prevention of venous thrombosis and pulmonary embolism 1986; 6(2).

Way LW. Current surgical diagnosis and treatment. 7th ed. Los Altos, CA: Lange Medical Publications, 1985:716–727.

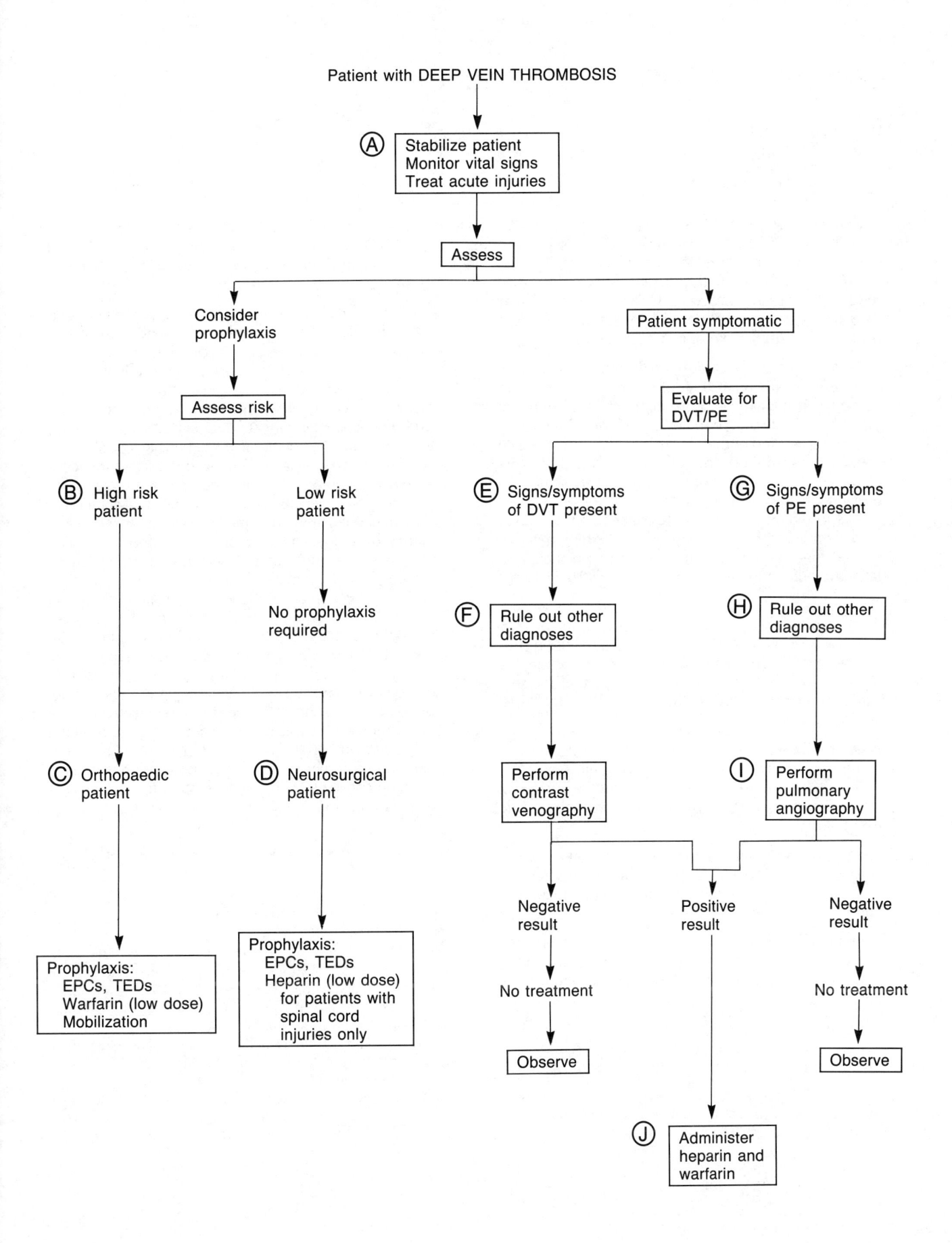

Patient with DEEP VEIN THROMBOSIS

- **A** Stabilize patient / Monitor vital signs / Treat acute injuries
- Assess
  - Consider prophylaxis
    - Assess risk
      - **B** High risk patient
        - **C** Orthopaedic patient
          - Prophylaxis: EPCs, TEDs / Warfarin (low dose) / Mobilization
        - **D** Neurosurgical patient
          - Prophylaxis: EPCs, TEDs / Heparin (low dose) for patients with spinal cord injuries only
      - Low risk patient
        - No prophylaxis required
  - Patient symptomatic
    - Evaluate for DVT/PE
      - **E** Signs/symptoms of DVT present
        - **F** Rule out other diagnoses
          - Perform contrast venography
            - Negative result → No treatment → Observe
            - Positive result → **J** Administer heparin and warfarin
      - **G** Signs/symptoms of PE present
        - **H** Rule out other diagnoses
          - **I** Perform pulmonary angiography
            - Negative result → No treatment → Observe

THERAPY FOR INFECTIOUS PROCESSES

Kathleen C. Solotkin
Mary C. McCarthy

A. Multiply injured patients are vulnerable to infection, especially when the body's defenses are violated by open or contaminated wounds. Host factors, such as diabetes, obesity, steroids, malnutrition, and shock, may also reduce resistance to infection. Delay in treatment may increase the risk of infection, and nosocomial infections may develop during prolonged hospital stays.

B. Patient assessment includes monitoring for infection; common findings are leukocytosis, fever, and hemodynamic changes. Pain, erythema, and purulent drainage indicate skin or soft tissue infection. Pulmonary symptoms include purulent sputum, diminished breath sounds, rales, and rhonchi. Abdominal findings may include tenderness, distention, or ileus. Urinary symptoms depend on upper or lower tract involvement. Sepsis results in decreased vascular resistance and increased cardiac output. These patients initially exhibit a warm, flushed appearance with tachycardia and tachypnea, with late development of decompensation and "cold shock."

C. Cultures of sputum, urine, blood, wound drainage, and other suspected sites should be obtained. Antibiotic therapy may need to be initiated before final culture results are available. Broad-spectrum coverage should be reserved for specific indications. When culture and sensitivity results are available, therapy should be adjusted accordingly.

D. Patients with skin and soft tissue infections may require incision and drainage in addition to systemic antibiotics. Ongoing wound assessment and care and instruction of the patient and family in preparation for discharge are essential.

E. The diagnosis of intra-abdominal infection may require advanced technologies. Critically ill patients require preparation for and monitoring during any procedures and during the perioperative period.

F. Pneumonia is a frequent complication in the trauma patient. Care involves assessing the need for analgesia to reduce splinting, frequent position changes, and pulmonary toilet.

G. Indwelling urinary catheters may predispose the patient to the development of infection. Catheters should be kept in a dependent position to prevent reflux, and the perineum should be kept clean.

H. Systemic infections are critical in an otherwise recovering patient (see p 316).

I. Intravascular catheters may be "seeded" during bacteremia. Access sites should be assessed frequently and changed if infection is suspected. Antibiotics may be required if cellulitis or thrombophlebitis persists.

J. Antibiotics may be life saving but have potentially serious side effects, including the emergence of resistant organisms and the development of superinfection. Antibiotic selection should be based on the following factors: suspected source of infection, the identity of the organism, severity of the infection, patient factors (adequacy of hepatic and renal function and drug allergies), and susceptibilities of the suspected organisms. Skin and soft tissue infections usually involve *Staphylococcus aureus* or streptococci unless complicating factors are present. First-generation cephalosporins or nafcillin is the drug of choice. Intra-abdominal infections are generally caused by a mixed flora, including gram-positive cocci, gram-negative rods, and anaerobes. Broad-spectrum coverage, e.g., imipenem-cilastatin or ampicillin-clindamycin, ampicillin-sulbactam, or cephalosporins in combination with aminoglycosides, may be required. Nosocomial pneumonias are responsive to third generation cephalosporins, with the addition of a second drug in compromised patients. Urinary tract infections, usually caused by colonization with gram-negative rods, may require quinolines or other appropriate drugs depending on culture results. Treatment of bacteremia relies on the suspected primary source. Once infection is resolved, energies should be directed at the prevention of reinfection and constant vigilance for symptoms of a recurrent or new infection.

References

Cardona VD, Hurn PD, Mason PJ, Schlipp AM, Viese-Berry SW. Trauma nursing: from resuscitation through rehabilitation. Philadelphia: WB Saunders, 1988:234–256.

Moore EE, Eiseman B, Van Way CW. Critical decision in trauma. St. Louis: CV Mosby, 1984:414–418.

Norwood SH. The prevalence and importance of nosocomial infections. In: Civetta JM, Taylor RW, Kirby RR, eds. Critical Care. Philadelphia: JB Lippincott, 1988:757–767.

Sabath LD, Simmons RL, Howard RJ. Antimicrobial agents. In: Howard RJ, Simmons RL, eds. Surgical infectious diseases. Norwalk CT: Appleton & Lange, 1988:259–306.

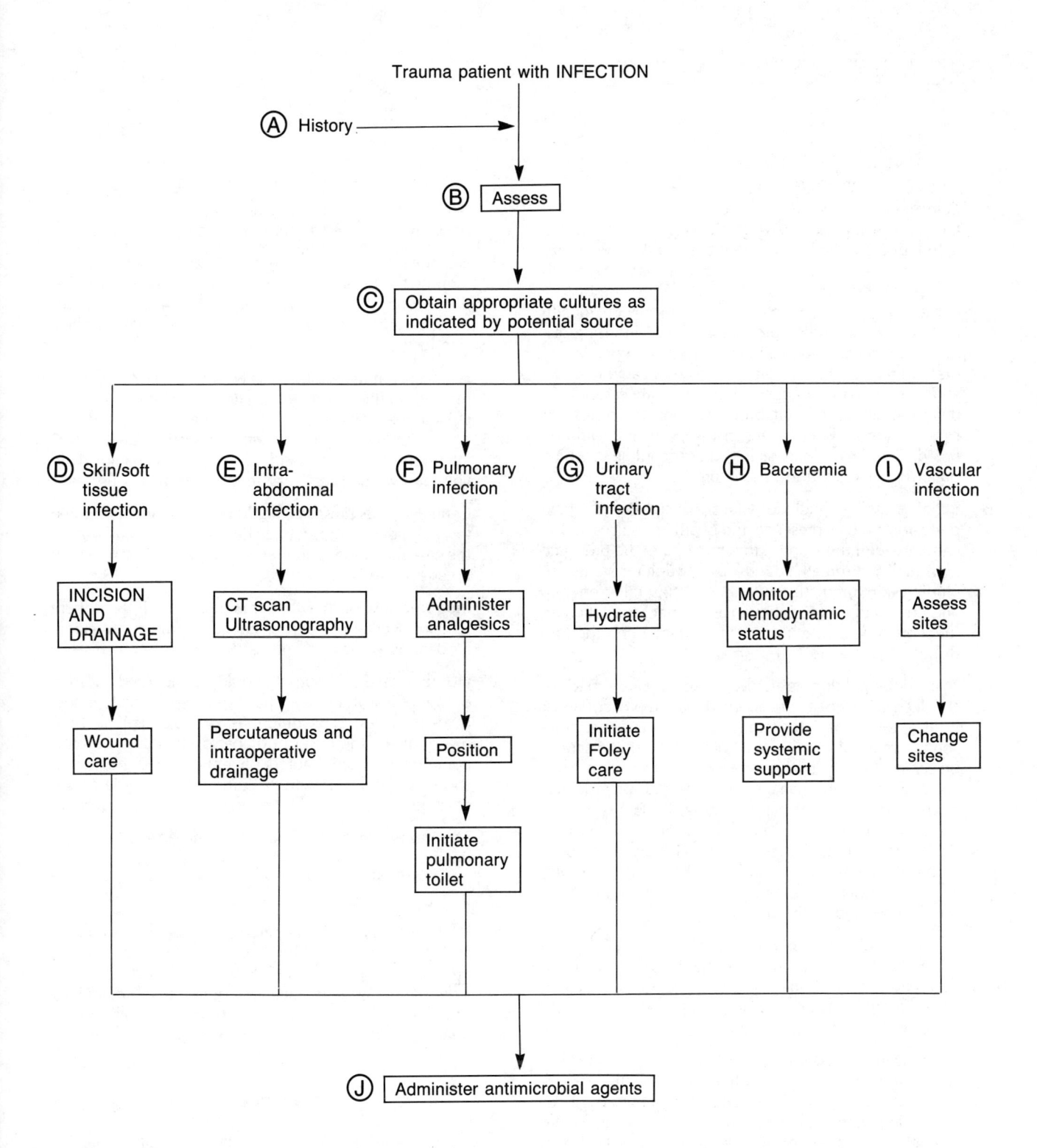

```
Trauma patient with INFECTION
            │
Ⓐ History ──┤
            ▼
         Ⓑ Assess
            │
            ▼
Ⓒ Obtain appropriate cultures as
  indicated by potential source
            │
  ┌─────┬─────┬─────┬─────┬─────┬─────┐
  ▼     ▼     ▼     ▼     ▼     ▼
Ⓓ Skin/ Ⓔ Intra- Ⓕ Pulmonary Ⓖ Urinary Ⓗ Bacteremia Ⓘ Vascular
  soft   abdominal  infection   tract                  infection
  tissue infection              infection
  infection
```

- Ⓓ → INCISION AND DRAINAGE → Wound care
- Ⓔ → CT scan Ultrasonography → Percutaneous and intraoperative drainage
- Ⓕ → Administer analgesics → Position → Initiate pulmonary toilet
- Ⓖ → Hydrate → Initiate Foley care
- Ⓗ → Monitor hemodynamic status → Provide systemic support
- Ⓘ → Assess sites → Change sites

Ⓙ Administer antimicrobial agents

ORGAN PROCUREMENT

Jodi Luke

A. In recent years medical advances have greatly increased the survival rate of organ recipients. However, the demand for organs still far exceeds the supply. The importance of identifying potential donors is the key to increasing the number of organs available. The history of the traumatic event and the patient's previous health and lifestyle, including pre-existing heart and lung disease, infections, diabetes, malignancies (except primary brain tumors and skin cancer), communicable disease, and history of intravenous (IV) drug use, are essential in determining donor suitability. Periods of prolonged hypotension and high doses of vasopressors should be noted. Criteria for donor status differ according to which organ or organs are to be procured.

B. Initial assessment includes vital signs; signs of adequate perfusion such as presence and quality of pulses, color, capillary refill time, and skin temperature; the presence and quality of breath sounds; and hydration status, including skin turgor, distended neck veins, rales, edema, and urinary output. Continued assessment of vital organ function is necessary to prevent ischemia and the loss of potential organs for transplant.

C. Many potential donors are overlooked because medical staff lack knowledge concerning donation procedures or hesitate to approach the family. Organ procurement personnel are usually available 24 hours per day and should be contacted early in any suspected donor situation. They can assist in donor management as well as provide personnel experienced in approaching the family. Organ procurement personnel must be informed of the diagnosis, date of admission, past medical history, blood pressure (BP), central venous pressure (CVP), urine output, serum creatinine level, urinalysis, current medications, blood type, and body weight.

D. The irreversibility of brain death should be clearly explained to the family. There should be no confusion on their part as to the patient's survival. Although the heart continues to beat and breathing continues on the ventilator, brain death is permanent.

E. Brain death criteria vary according to state and institution, but the following guidelines are generally accepted measures of brain death. The neurologist or neurosurgeon must establish unreceptivity and unresponsiveness. The patient must have no reflexes and be in an irreversible coma; central nervous system activity, movement, and spontaneous respirations must be absent. There should be very little or no electrical activity on the electroencephalogram.

F. Legal consent must be obtained even if the donor has signed an organ donation card. A knowledgeable person should be available to answer questions and to explain the organ donation procedure to the family.

G. Numerous laboratory tests as well as tissue typing and serology are necessary to determine organ function.

H. Electrocardiography and chest films are performed to determine the presence of underlying disease or injury. A high quality chest film is essential in the heart-lung transplant because it is used to determine the necessary chest size in the recipient.

I. Hypotension may result from hemorrhage or damage to the central nervous system, with a resultant loss of vascular tone. Replacement of volume can be achieved with normal saline, Ringer's lactate, or blood products. Strict attention should be paid to volume status to avoid volume overload that may render the organs useless.

J. Central venous pressure should be frequently monitored to evaluate the fluid status. The transplant team will set the maintenance parameters, depending on which organs are to be harvested.

K. Inotropic support may become necessary if the patient remains hypotensive despite adequate fluid resuscitation. Dopamine or dobutamine is the drug of choice.

L. Hourly intake and output should be recorded. A urine output of less than 50 ml per hour may indicate inadequate perfusion. Large outputs of 200 to 300 ml per hour may indicate the onset of diabetes insipidus, which is common in head injured patients. The urine output should be replaced with IV fluids; however, if large urinary output persists, a Pitressin drip may be indicated.

M. Thermoregulation may be lost in the head injured patient, thereby decreasing perfusion and increasing ischemia. Maintaining the core body temperature close to 37° C is essential.

N. Ventilator support is maintained until the organs are harvested. Oxygenation should be frequently evaluated with arterial blood gases (ABGs). Strict aseptic technique and stringent pulmonary toilet are required to maintain lung function and to avoid complications, especially in the heart-lung donor.

References

Cardona VD, Hurn PD, Mason PJ, Schlipp AM, Veise-Berry SW. Trauma nursing from resuscitation through rehabilitation. Philadelphia: WB Saunders, 1988:785–798.

Kinney MR, Packa DR, Dunbar SB. AACN's clinical reference for critical-care nursing. New York: McGraw-Hill, 1988:1566–1573.

Schwartz SI, Shires TG, Spencer FC, Storer EH, eds. Principles of surgery. New York: McGraw-Hill, 1979:447–449.

Toto K. Organ Procurement. In: Mancini ME, ed. Decision making in emergency nursing. Toronto: BC Decker, 1987:160–161.

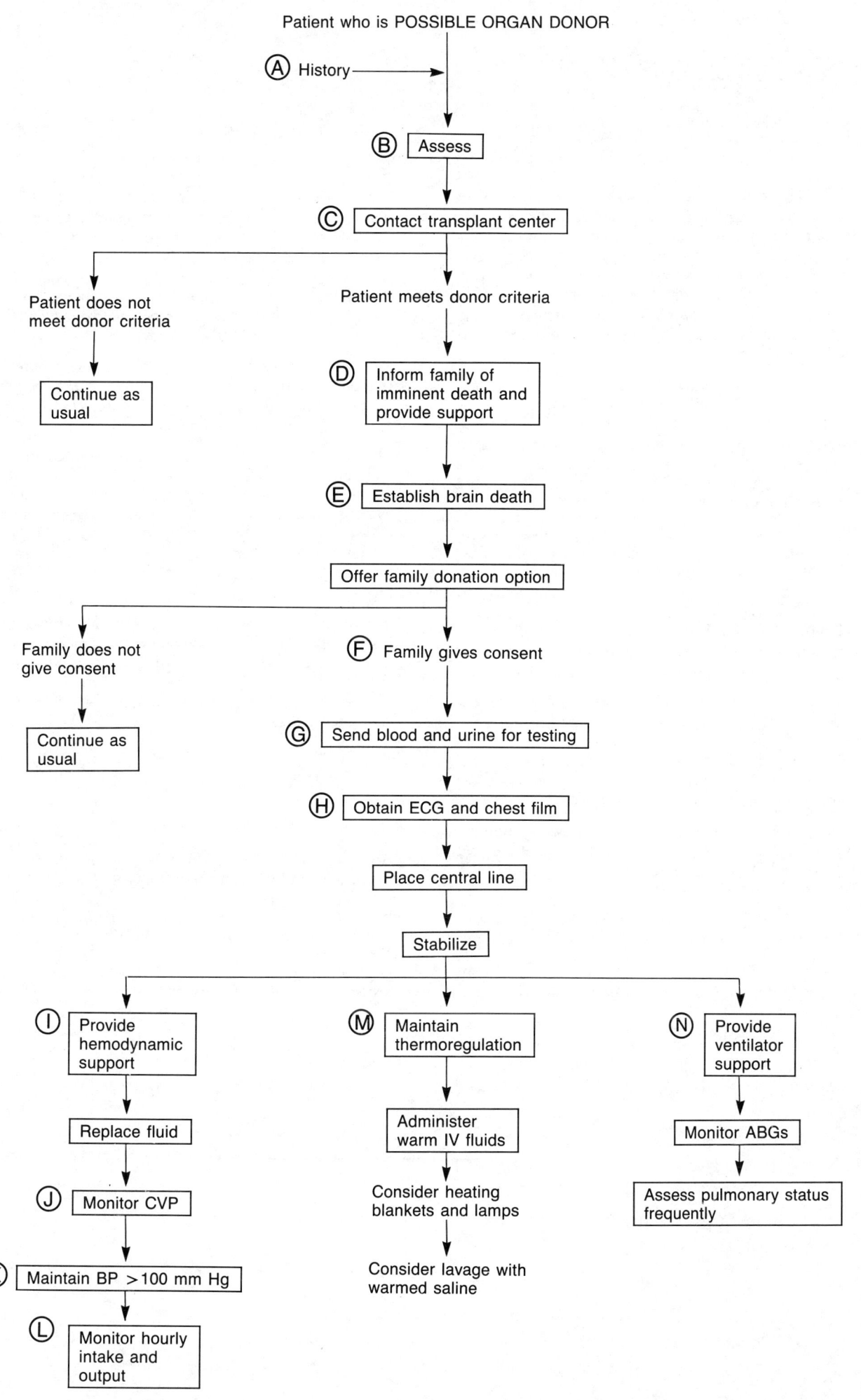

```
Patient who is POSSIBLE ORGAN DONOR
                │
        (A) History ──────►
                │
                ▼
            (B) Assess
                │
                ▼
        (C) Contact transplant center
         │                    │
Patient does not         Patient meets donor criteria
meet donor criteria              │
         │                       ▼
         ▼               (D) Inform family of
    Continue as              imminent death and
    usual                    provide support
                                 │
                                 ▼
                         (E) Establish brain death
                                 │
                                 ▼
                         Offer family donation option
              │                  │
    Family does not        (F) Family gives consent
    give consent                 │
         │                       ▼
         ▼               (G) Send blood and urine for testing
    Continue as                  │
    usual                        ▼
                         (H) Obtain ECG and chest film
                                 │
                                 ▼
                         Place central line
                                 │
                                 ▼
                             Stabilize
              ┌──────────────────┼──────────────────┐
              ▼                  ▼                  ▼
       (I) Provide        (M) Maintain         (N) Provide
       hemodynamic        thermoregulation     ventilator
       support                  │              support
              │                 ▼                  │
              ▼          Administer                ▼
       Replace fluid     warm IV fluids       Monitor ABGs
              │                 │                  │
              ▼                 ▼                  ▼
       (J) Monitor CVP   Consider heating    Assess pulmonary status
              │          blankets and lamps   frequently
              ▼                 │
       (K) Maintain BP >100 mm Hg
              │                 ▼
              ▼          Consider lavage with
       (L) Monitor hourly warmed saline
       intake and
       output
```

333

CRISIS INTERVENTION

Melanie Daetweiler Boone

A. Crisis may be holistically defined as any injurious event that causes disruption in some aspect of lifestyle. This includes the psychosocial responses of all those connected to the event. Whatever the range of those responses, they are based on the individual perception of each person involved. The main goal of crisis intervention is to support the patient and/or family and to achieve a state of equilibrium that is self-sustaining and powered by usual coping resources.

B. Psychosocial assessment focuses on the psychological aspects of the traumatic injury and the concrete stresses on the social situation of both patient and family. The assessment should help determine premorbid personalities, pre-existing family dynamics, the need for housing that is accessible to the hospital, loss of income, transportation difficulties, and child care.

C. The treatment team should develop a positive working relationship with the patient and family as soon as possible. This relationship should be based on clear and concise information that includes giving information to welcome and orient the patient and family to the hospital system and explaining hospital policies and care procedures. Active listening to the patient's and family's needs and concerns is appropriate at this time.

D. A communication program should be established to provide for the flow of health information between the patient, staff, and family. If the patient is nonvocal, the treatment professional should set up nonverbal communication as soon as possible via blinking and/or a communication board.

E. In the early stages of acute care, one way communication emanates primarily from staff to the patient and family, while the family interacts with the patient from outside the system.

F. Development of trust and treatment alliances allows strong two way communication among all concerned.

G. Providing information that is accurate, clear, and concise allays anxiety and the feeling of helplessness that accompanies trauma. Information should be delivered in a simple, uncomplicated style. Technical and complex explanations should be avoided. A calm, reassuring manner of delivering information is vital. Treatment professionals should resist pressures to speculate on questions they cannot answer accurately. More damage can be done by giving inaccurate or misleading information than by honestly stating, "I don't know."

H. Reinforcing independence helps to improve treatment outcomes and long-term adjustment to disability. Whenever possible, the patient's helplessness and dependence should be minimized.

I. The family should be informed of the care plan and invited and encouraged to participate in some way, e.g., via assisting with feeding, positioning, or personal hygiene. Realistic time and adequate space should be allowed for visiting. Minimize interruption during visits. All appropriate support within the hospital system should be offered to families.

J. It is not helpful to provide truthful, however conservative, predictions about prognosis, especially during the first 2 weeks of the acute care phase. Remember: People need to hear about their injuries; however, this need should be gauged by assessing the patient's readiness to accept the truth. It is possible to tell the truth without taking away hope.

References

Auvenshine CD, Noffsinger RL. Counseling: an introduction for the health and human services. Chicago: University Park Press, 1984:78–79.

Combs AW, Avilla DL. Helping relationships: basic concepts for the helping professions. 3rd ed. Allyn and Bacon, 1985:34–38.

Krueger DW, ed. Rehabilitation psychology: a comprehensive textbook. Rockville, MD: Aspen, 1984:25–35.

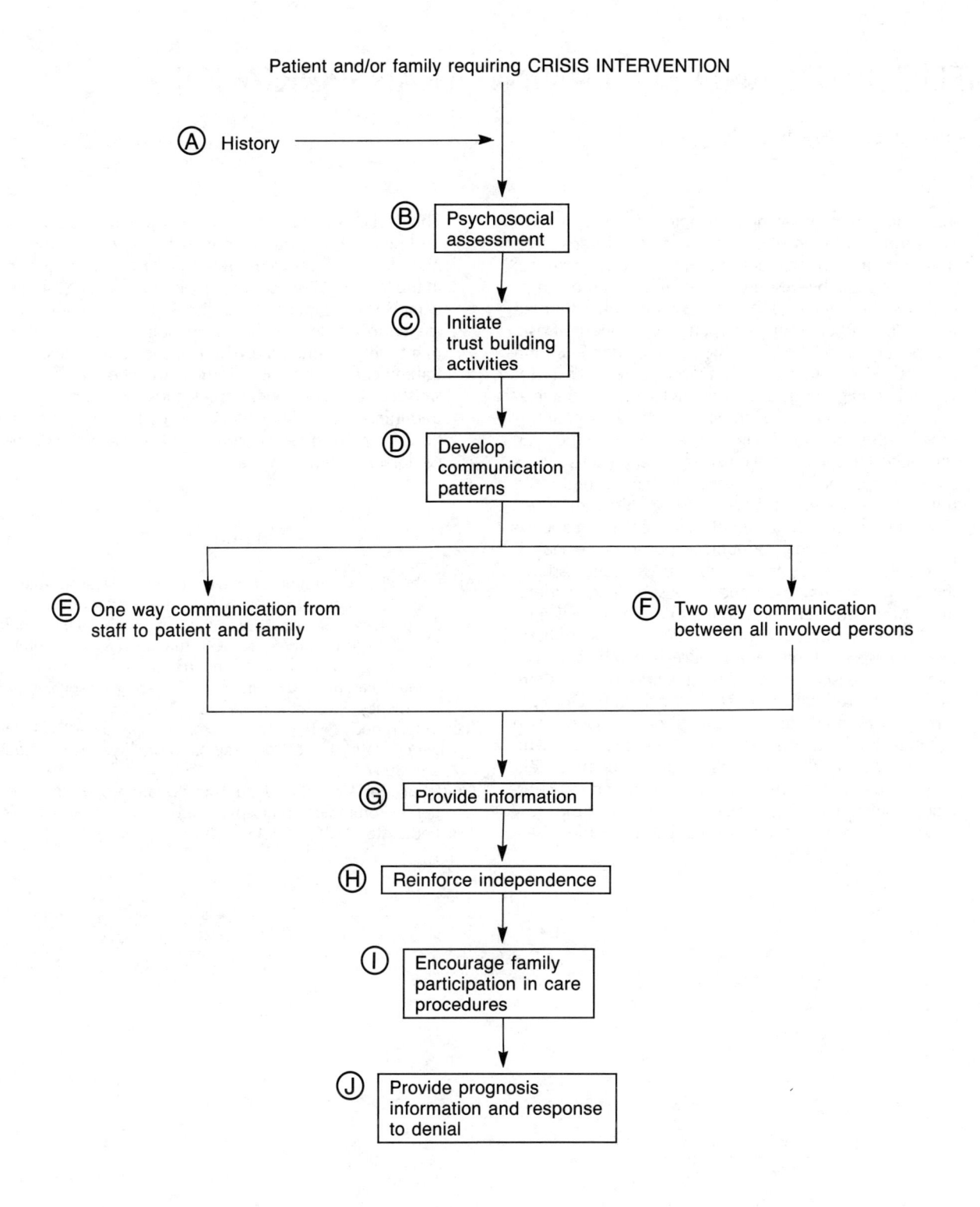

Patient and/or family requiring CRISIS INTERVENTION

- **A** History
- **B** Psychosocial assessment
- **C** Initiate trust building activities
- **D** Develop communication patterns
- **E** One way communication from staff to patient and family
- **F** Two way communication between all involved persons
- **G** Provide information
- **H** Reinforce independence
- **I** Encourage family participation in care procedures
- **J** Provide prognosis information and response to denial

HELICOPTER AND FIXED-WING TRANSPORTATION

Robert J. O'Malley

A. Incorporation of rotor-wing (helicopter) air medical transportation into the local emergency medical transportation system is dependent on several considerations, including available resources. This incorporation must comprise an organized response system rather than an incidental and convenient response to a patient at risk. The general factors to be considered include the terrain and the existing transportation infrastructures that provide for rapid ground transportation. Determine the relative transportation time of ground vehicles during various times of the day and during various seasons of the year. Virtually all hospital based emergency helicopter services are staffed by at least one specially trained registered nurse; many are staffed by physicians. This level of service must be compared with the relative training and experience of customary ground response personnel. If helicopter resources are available for scene transports, the use of the service depends on a specific consideration of the above criteria applied to the particular incident. Are there physiologic indicators such as difficult airway, suspected spinal cord injury, hypotension, dyspnea, or decreased neurologic status present? Are there multiple injured patients needing evacuation? Does the terrain or road conditions make ground transportation difficult? Is a helicopter needed to find the patient who is injured? Will helicopter transportation save the patient at least 10 minutes over conventional ground transportation? Will the training and experience level of the crew make a difference in the treatment of the patient?

B. The decision to transport via helicopter from a community hospital to a trauma center requires assessing the need for rapid transportation and for a team of experts in the transportation of critically injured patients. Trauma centers should identify facilities that are in an appropriate territory so that the helicopter automatically responds in a timely manner. If a patient needs the services of a trauma center and the administrative requirements are satisfied, the use of helicopter transport is appropriate to minimize out-of-hospital time and to reduce the time between request for transfer and the arrival at the trauma center for a definitive care.

References

Air Ambulance Guidelines, US Department of Transportation, National Highway Traffic Safety Administration.

Air Ambulance Operations, Committee on Trauma of the American College of Surgeons, ACS Bulletin, October 1984.

Air Medical Crew National Standard Curriculum, Instructor Manual. Pasadena, CA: American Society of Hospital Based Emergency Air Medical Services, 1988.

Baxt WG, Moody P. The impact of rotorcraft aeromedical emergency care service on trauma mortality. JAMA 1983; 249:3047–3051.

Guidelines for Air and Ground Transportation of Pediatric Patients, Committee on Hospital Care, American Academy of Pediatrics. 1986; 78:943–950.

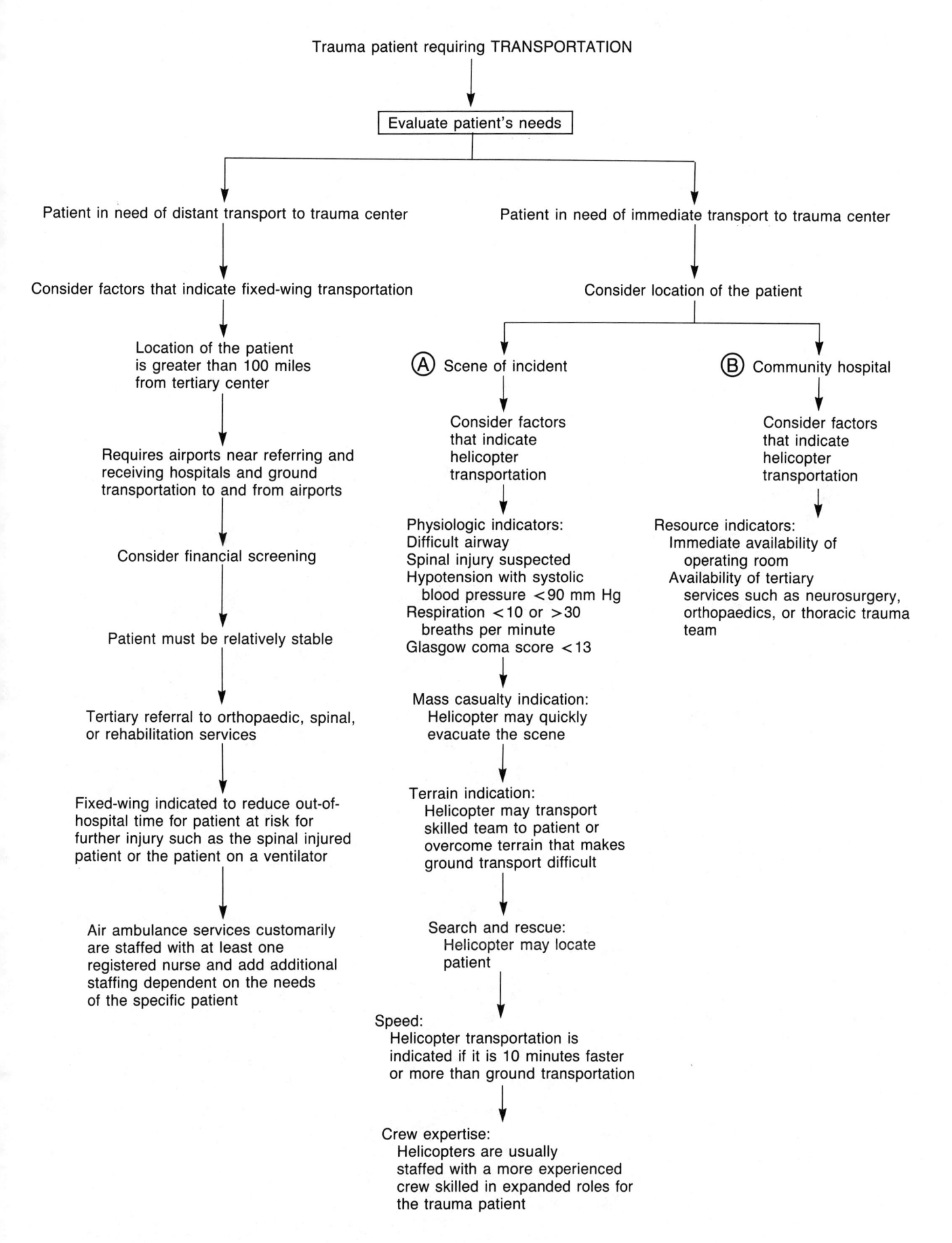

```
                          Trauma patient requiring TRANSPORTATION
                                            │
                                            ▼
                                 ┌──────────────────────┐
                                 │ Evaluate patient's needs │
                                 └──────────────────────┘
                    ┌───────────────────────┴────────────────────────┐
                    ▼                                                ▼
Patient in need of distant transport to trauma center    Patient in need of immediate transport to trauma center
                    │                                                │
                    ▼                                                ▼
Consider factors that indicate fixed-wing transportation    Consider location of the patient
                    │                                    ┌───────────┴───────────┐
                    ▼                                    ▼                       ▼
         Location of the patient               Ⓐ Scene of incident        Ⓑ Community hospital
         is greater than 100 miles                      │                       │
         from tertiary center                           ▼                       ▼
                    │                           Consider factors        Consider factors
                    ▼                           that indicate           that indicate
         Requires airports near referring and   helicopter              helicopter
         receiving hospitals and ground         transportation          transportation
         transportation to and from airports           │                       │
                    │                                  ▼                       ▼
                    ▼                           Physiologic indicators:  Resource indicators:
         Consider financial screening              Difficult airway         Immediate availability of
                    │                              Spinal injury suspected     operating room
                    ▼                              Hypotension with systolic Availability of tertiary
         Patient must be relatively stable          blood pressure <90 mm Hg   services such as neurosurgery,
                    │                              Respiration <10 or >30     orthopaedics, or thoracic trauma
                    ▼                               breaths per minute        team
         Tertiary referral to orthopaedic, spinal,  Glasgow coma score <13
         or rehabilitation services                        │
                    │                                      ▼
                    ▼                           Mass casualty indication:
         Fixed-wing indicated to reduce out-of-    Helicopter may quickly
         hospital time for patient at risk for     evacuate the scene
         further injury such as the spinal injured         │
         patient or the patient on a ventilator            ▼
                    │                           Terrain indication:
                    ▼                              Helicopter may transport
         Air ambulance services customarily        skilled team to patient or
         are staffed with at least one             overcome terrain that makes
         registered nurse and add additional       ground transport difficult
         staffing dependent on the needs                   │
         of the specific patient                           ▼
                                                Search and rescue:
                                                   Helicopter may locate
                                                   patient
                                                          │
                                                          ▼
                                                Speed:
                                                   Helicopter transportation is
                                                   indicated if it is 10 minutes faster
                                                   or more than ground transportation
                                                          │
                                                          ▼
                                                Crew expertise:
                                                   Helicopters are usually
                                                   staffed with a more experienced
                                                   crew skilled in expanded roles for
                                                   the trauma patient
```

REHABILITATION

Rehabilitation of the Head-Injury Patient
Rehabilitation of the Spinal Cord–Injured Patient
Rehabilitation After Upper Extremity Amputation
Rehabilitation After Lower Extremity Amputation
Rehabilitation of the Burn-Injured Patient

REHABILITATION OF THE HEAD-INJURED PATIENT

Sharon V. Morel

A. The history and physical examination address the etiology of the injury, site of impact, classification, and direct and secondary effects of head trauma. They include preexisting and concurrent medical problems or complications; level of consciousness; results of previous diagnostic tests, e.g., EEG, computed tomography scan, and magnetic resonance imaging, and assessment of cranial nerves and reflexes. The history and physical examination are used as a guide for the interdisciplinary team to assess the extent of the patient's loss in physical mobility, communication, behavior, social adaptive ability, and actual brain deficits. The patient's and family's expectations about rehabilitation and their knowledge and understanding of the injury are assessed.

B. Rehabilitation involves an intensely structured program that provides specialized services. Each member of the interdisciplinary team evaluates and implements a patient specific treatment plan. One method of pinpointing the patient's level of dysfunction is through the use of the Rancho Los Amigos scale, which defines eight levels in the recovery process (Table 1). These levels are grouped for use as three phases of cognitive rehabilitation, as follows: the stimulation phase, the structured oriented phase, and the reintegration phase (Table 2). The behavioral and cognitive capacities during the various phases of recovery dictate the intervention methods that will be appropriate and successful; concepts and tasks progress from simple to more complex. This method allows development and implementation of a care plan that addresses mobility, sensory and perceptual deficits, activities of daily living (ADL), diet and feeding, bowel and bladder function, communication, psychosocial adaptation, prevention of complications, and patient and family teaching.

C. Depending on the severity of injury, the following posture disorders may be seen: decerebrate and decorticate posture, spasticity, bradykinesia, ataxia, apraxia, paresis, plegia, dyskinesia, and tremors.

D. Abnormal posturing and spasticity can lead to muscle contractures. The physical therapist designs a program to decrease the patient's abnormal responses and to encourage appropriate motor responses. The nurse follows through by ensuring proper positioning of the patient.

E. Bed activities include turning and positioning every 2 hours initially and passive range of motion exercises twice a day with stretching of the spastic muscles. To prevent deep vein thrombosis, antiembolic stockings may be worn. High top sneakers may be used to prevent foot drop. Bed mobility and the elevation process begin as soon as the patient is medically stable. Depending on the extent of mobility disorders, splints, casts, braces, and muscle straightening exercises may be required.

TABLE 1 Ranchos Los Amigos Scale*: Cognitive Levels Associated with Traumatic Brain Injury

Level	Descriptive Characteristics
I No response	No response to any stimuli
II Generalized response	Responses are nonpurposeful and inconsistent; posturing and reflex responses may be evident
III Localized response	Localized and purposeful responses; follows commands inconsistently; responses often related to discomfort, e.g., pulls tubes
IV Confused, agitated, inappropriate	Severely impaired information processing; responding to internal confusion; attention span very limited; behavior often bizarre; short-term memory impaired; dependent in all aspects of care; safety of major concern
V Confused, nonagitated, inappropriate	Remains distractable; with direction and assistance, can perform previously learned tasks; performance deteriorates when structure decreases or complexity increases
VI Confused, appropriate	Less concrete; memory problems persist, but more aware of not knowing correct answer; completes previously learned tasks with supervision
VII Automatic or appropriate	Oriented consistently; initiates tasks and carries out routines; more awareness of self and others, but lacks insight and judgment and problem solving ability
VIII Purposeful, appropriate	Demonstrates more responsibility for self; able to learn new tasks; new situations, variations in routines can be stressful; more aware of deficits

*Developed by Hagen C, Malkmus D, Durham P. Revised, 1974, by Malkmus D, Stenderup K.
From Hagen C, Malkmus D, Durham P. Levels of cognitive functioning. In: Rehabilitation of the head injured adult: comprehensive physical management. Downey, CA: Professional Staff Association of Rancho Los Amigos Hospital, Inc, 1979:87–88.

TABLE 2 Phases of Cognitive Rehabilitation

Phase	Behavioral Level
Stimulation phase	Behavioral level I, II, III
Structured oriented phase	Behavioral level IV, V, VI
Reintegration phase	Behavioral level VII, VIII

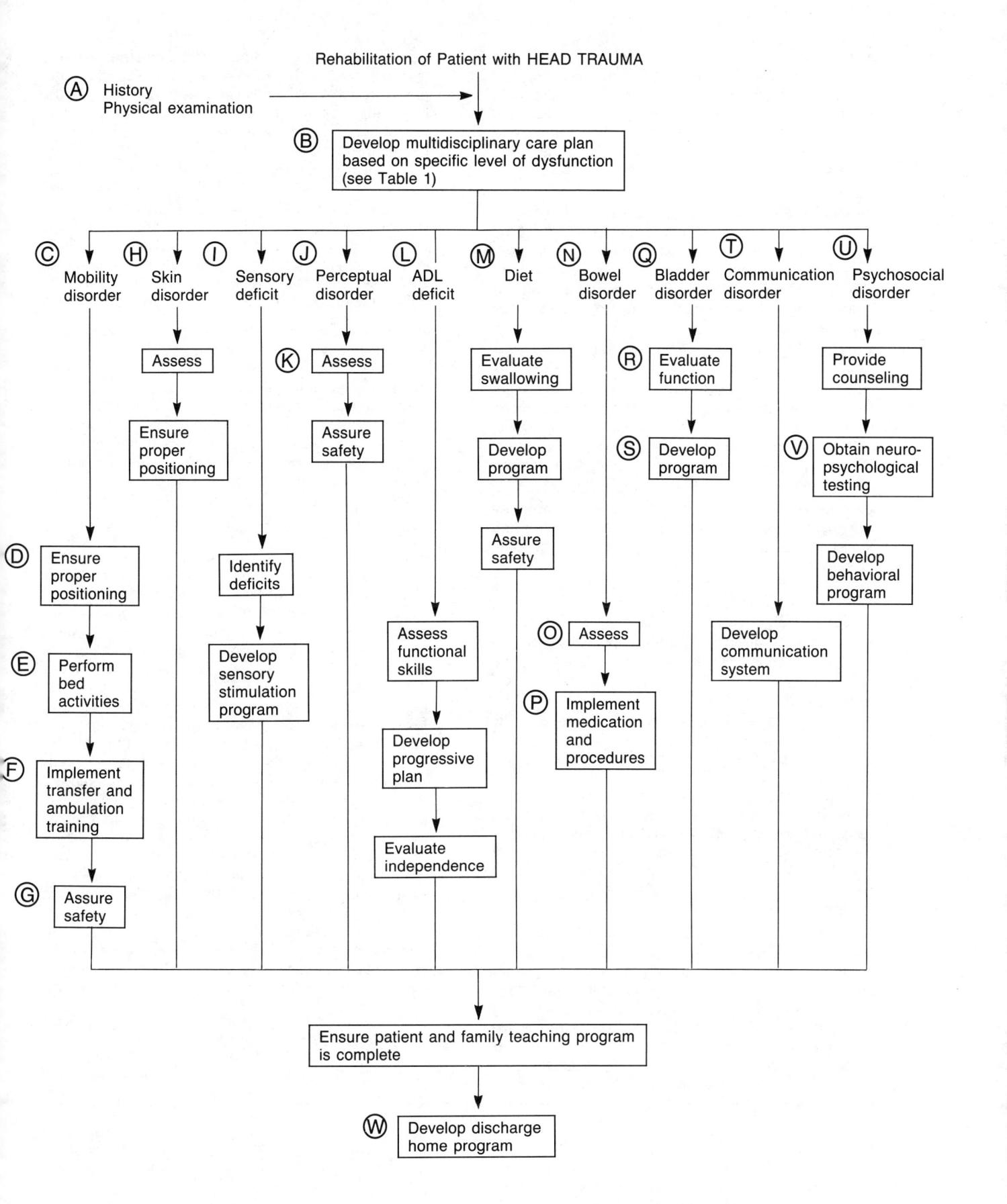

Rehabilitation of Patient with HEAD TRAUMA

(A) History / Physical examination →

(B) Develop multidisciplinary care plan based on specific level of dysfunction (see Table 1)

- **(C)** Mobility disorder
  - **(D)** Ensure proper positioning
  - **(E)** Perform bed activities
  - **(F)** Implement transfer and ambulation training
  - **(G)** Assure safety
- **(H)** Skin disorder
  - Assess
  - Ensure proper positioning
- **(I)** Sensory deficit
  - **(K)** Identify deficits
  - Develop sensory stimulation program
- **(J)** Perceptual disorder
  - Assess
  - Assure safety
- **(L)** ADL deficit
  - Assess functional skills
  - Develop progressive plan
  - Evaluate independence
- **(M)** Diet
  - Evaluate swallowing
  - Develop program
  - Assure safety
- **(N)** Bowel disorder
  - **(O)** Assess
  - **(P)** Implement medication and procedures
- **(Q)** Bladder disorder
  - **(R)** Evaluate function
  - **(S)** Develop program
- **(T)** Communication disorder
  - Develop communication system
- **(U)** Psychosocial disorder
  - Provide counseling
  - **(V)** Obtain neuro-psychological testing
  - Develop behavioral program

Ensure patient and family teaching program is complete

(W) Develop discharge home program

F. As balance and tolerance to sitting develop, transfer to a wheelchair with high extension (and neck brace, if needed) can begin. As endurance, balance, and strength continue to develop, wheelchair activity is advanced. Next, transfer training, wheelchair safety, standing, and ambulation training are implemented. Carefully monitor the effects of each activity on mobility and on skin integrity.

G. Mobility progression must be monitored closely and safety measures must be implemented because of the cognitive deficits associated with head trauma. Monitoring devices with an egress monitoring system, such as a door alarm, are attached to the patient's wheelchair or arm to prevent elopement or wandering into areas of potential harm.

H. The patient is at risk for complications and infections because of decreased body defenses and drug therapy side effects. Spasticity and alteration in the temperature regulation process also enhance the risk for skin impairment. Interventions include correct body positioning; gradually increasing time spent in one position; daily inspection of skin color, elasticity, moisture, edema, cleanliness, lesions, and scars; good nutrition; and skin care.

I. Evaluate the patient's response to all types of sensory input, including smell, taste, hearing, and cutaneous and kinesthetic response. Implement a program to stimulate all sensory systems. Family members can contribute information about the patient's likes and interests to enhance auditory input. Pictures from home may be used for visual stimuli. The occupational therapist offers a variety of more sophisticated sensory input modalities. As the patient approaches level III, all disciplines are involved in activities that solicit the patient's responses and develop prefunctional skills.

J. Assess for perceptual deficits that interfere with the ability to know the body's capacity for movement, to move in space, to manipulate objects appropriately, and to accommodate to time and space. Assess for deficits in the perception of self, illness, and spatial relationships; agnosia (inability to recognize familiar environmental objects); and apraxia (inability to carry out learned voluntary movement without the presence of paralysis). Assess for anosognosia, which is a denial of disability or a lack of awareness of paralysis or paresis of the involved side or extremity.

K. Interventions include constant monitoring for safety and teaching the patient to use intact senses to identify environmental stimuli. Use the drill method of teaching to assist in relearning stimuli. Reteach forgotten skills, and correct any misuse of equipment or incorrect actions. Assess for visual deficits, which include decreased acuity, hemianopsia, and diplopia. (Treatment for diplopia comprises an eye patch over the affected eye.) Teach the patient to use other senses to gather information and to compensate for decreased visual fields by turning the head and scanning the area.

L. Helping the patient to relearn ADL begins with assessment of intact functional skills, of those that are lost, and of those that cannot be accomplished without some help. The occupational therapist performs a functional evaluation and sets up a program for practice of ADLs, such as bathing, dressing, feeding, hair and oral hygiene, and home care skills. The nurse reinforces the program and provides opportunity for practice. The program starts with beginning a routine of self care with assistance, supervision, or cuing from the therapist or nurse. Simple step-by-step instruction is given in an established daily routine. Assistive and orthotic devices are provided as needed for self care. As the patient progresses through the cognitive levels in the recovery progress, self care responsibilities are increased. These responsibilities include conducting all aspects of hygiene, arriving at therapies on time, and coming to the nurses' station at designated times for medication. Memory cues such as cards with daily schedules of activities and times assist the patient.

M. A major complication of head trauma is impaired swallowing. Initially nutrition may be given by tube feeding. The dietician assesses the tube feedings to ensure adequate calories, water, and other electrolytes are maintaining adequate nutrition. Calorie counts and weight are monitored closely. A comprehensive treatment program for the swallowing disorder is initiated by the speech therapist and the occupational therapist in collaboration with other team members. As the patient progresses through the recovery phases, becomes more responsive to stimuli, and can follow one or two step commands, a videofluoroscopic swallow study is done to confirm the safety of oral feeding with specific consistency or to rule out the use of oral feedings due to observed aspiration of barium in the lungs. Problems such as decreased sensation, pooling, or incomplete protection of the airway can be observed on film. Techniques to compensate for these or other difficulties can be implemented. The speech and occupational therapists select appropriate food to enhance swallowing retraining and oral feeding therapy. Families are instructed on how to give verbal cues, how to support the chin to maintain the head in erect position, and how to stimulate the swallowing reflex. When the patient is able to take in sufficient calories by mouth, the feeding tube is removed. As the patient progresses to the confused or agitated level, dietary intake should be closely monitored; this is a time when excessive eating, refusal to eat, and eating of only certain foods may be evident. Placing only two items from a meal tray in front of the patient produces better results than serving the entire tray at one time. The goal of the feeding program is safe, adequate, independent eating. The need for adaptive eating utensils, compensatory techniques in swallowing, restriction of specific food consistencies, and nutritional supplements may be long-term. Continued supervision and assistance may be needed even after discharge.

N. Cerebral damage disrupts inhibitory and facilitory mechanisms in the brain for defecation. The reflex arcs to and from the bowel are intact, and elimination occurs by reflex actions; the major problem is incontinence. Diarrhea is another common problem because of the patient's intolerance of particular tube feedings or of the use of drugs that affect the flora of the gastrointestinal tract. The goals of a bowel program are to establish a pattern of bowel evacuation on a regular time schedule that meets the individual's needs and to prevent incontinence, constipation, or impaction.

O. Bowel assessment includes premorbid habits, diet, fluid intake, and activity level (e.g., ability to sit on a toilet or commode with assistance). The time of day, as based on the patient's previous pattern, should be established for the bowel program.

P. Suppositories (glycerin or dulcolax) given 15 to 30 minutes after meals capitalize on the gastrocolic reflex action. Assist the patient to the toilet or commode if possible. Implement the bowel program every other day until evacuation occurs routinely during a specific time frame. If diet allows, increase fruit and juices along with fiber and bran to facilitate bowel function. As the patient's mobility and cognition improve, bowel function will improve.

Q. As soon as possible, the Foley catheter is removed, and an intermittent catheterization program is implemented to maintain muscle tone and to prevent overdistention and infection by completely emptying the bladder at timely intervals.

R. A complete urologic profile and assessment are performed. These may include urine culture and sensitivity; intravenous pyelography; cystourethrography; cystometrics with urethral profile pressures; kidney, ureter, and bladder assessment; electromyography, renal scan; and renal ultrasonography. The bladder program that is initiated is based on the results of the assessment and the type of bladder dysfunction.

S. Uninhibited neurogenic bladder (i.e., mixed motor neuron) usually results from head injury. Symptoms are urgency, frequency, nocturia, and incontinence. Because sensation and control are diminished rather than lost, bladder training is more easily achieved. Timing is critical to the success of the program. The patient must be conscious, alert, and oriented. A time voiding program is implemented after the patient is checked every 2 hours for 2 to 3 days to establish voiding patterns. Postvoid residual urine is checked to ensure that it is within acceptable limits (i.e., 50 to 100 ml). The intake record should be correlated with voiding patterns. Establish the voiding schedule at periodic intervals (every 2 hours) on a bedside commode or toilet and readjust as incontinence diminishes.

T. Alteration in communication may involve impairment of comprehension of spoken language, speech, reading, writing, and listening. A comprehensive evaluation and treatment program are implemented by the speech therapist. The patient may hear and process incoming information despite being unable to talk. Work out a yes-no communication system with eye blinks, head nods, finger movements, or yes-no cards. Give positive sensory input in as many modalities as possible, such as radio, television, touch, smell, and conversation. As the patient progresses through the recovery levels and aphasia is reduced in severity, the speech therapist will provide an altered communication system or device that acts as a means of expression; this can comprise a picture board, alphabet board, electronic device, and/or simple demonstrations and gestures. When the patient begins to speak, he or she may swear and use language inappropriately. Encourage the use of appropriate language and continue to support and encourage speech efforts. Speak slowly and give the patient time to comprehend and respond. Help the patient to follow simple commands and to identify familiar objects. Give the patient every possible opportunity to succeed in speech efforts.

U. Behavioral and/or cognitive deficits can be overwhelming for family members. Support and ongoing counseling for the patient and the family are important while the patient progresses through the stages of recovery. During the course of recovery, severe psychological and emotional responses occur. The patient may respond from coma to a process of awakening over several weeks. Rapid fluctuations in orientation may occur at any time, but usually the patient becomes more disoriented toward the end of the day. The patient is easily distracted because of difficulty focusing on, and attending to, external and internal stimuli. Illusions may occur because the sleep-wake cycle is disturbed. Restlessness and agitation are often exhibited when the patient first becomes aware of the surroundings. Bizarre behavior, such as outbursts, aggression, disinhibition, hallucinations, delirium, and incoherent verbalization, may be evident.

V. Consultation with the neuropsychology staff is key to successful management. The neuropsychologist evaluates and develops strategies for all the disciplines to improve the patient's behavior and information processing. The goals during this period are providing a safe environment, fostering basic input, and preventing inappropriate response patterning. A calm, quiet, safe environment with consistent caretakers is important. The judicious use of restraining devices may be necessary to avoid falls and injuries. Choice and the amount of stimulation given to the patient need to be restricted. The patient's participation in relearning skills is limited during this phase. Medications are only used as a last resort. Serial neuropsychological testing is valuable in assessing progress and program planning; this is done by the neuropsychologist.

W. The focus of a home program is to facilitate the reintegration phase of levels VII and VIII. The reintegration phase integrates three parts of cognitive growth, as follows: activities related to self, to the home, and to the community. Day passes and therapeutic overnight passes during hospitalization help to prepare the patient and the family for discharge and for the reintegration phase. Referrals to community settings or to day treatment programs are provided as needed. Neuromedical and neuropsychological follow-up appointments are given on discharge. Self help groups, vocational rehabilitation, and the National Head Injury Foundation are all resources for the patient and the family.

References

Baggerly J. Rehabilitation of the adult with head trauma. Nurs Clin North Am 1986; 21(4):577–586.

Bottcher S. Cognitive retraining: a nursing approach to rehabilitation of the brain injured. Nurs Clin North Am 1989; 24(1):193–207.

Hickey J. The clinical practice of neurological and neurosurgical nursing. 2nd ed. Philadelphia: JB Lippincott, 1986.

Sayles S, ed. Rehabilitation nursing: concepts and practice. Evanston, IL: Rehabilitation Nursing Institute, 1981.

Vogt G, Miller E. Mosby's manual of neurological care. St. Louis: CV Mosby, 1985.

REHABILITATION OF THE SPINAL CORD–INJURED PATIENT

Sharon V. Morel

A. The history and physical examination assist in determining functional goals and potential for rehabilitation. The medical history should emphasize the segmental level of the injury, completeness of the injury, evaluation of determatomes, evaluation of motor level, reflex activity, and pre-existing and concurrent medical problems or complications. The patient's expectations of rehabilitation and his or her knowledge and understanding of the injury should be addressed.

B. The biopsychosocial alterations after spinal cord injury (SCI) demand an integrated and collaborative multidisciplinary approach. Focus is on developing comprehensive patient and family care plans related to mobility; skin; activities of dally living (ADL), bowel and bladder function, respiration; psychosocial adaptation; and patient and family teaching.

C. Mobility assessment by the physical therapist includes evaluation of all extremities, mental status, range of motion, endurance, muscles, and spinal stability. If spinal stability is established through surgical intervention and/or an orthotic device, bed mobility and the elevation process can begin. To avoid cardiovascular insult, the process of mobilization must be gradual. The physical therapist will implement a program for mobility training.

D. Bed activities include turning and positioning every 2 hours, which is advanced as tolerated. Passive or assisted passive range of motion exercises must be done at least twice a day, with passive stretching of spastic muscles. Use the prone position as soon as cardiovascular status and spinal stability permit.

E. In preparation for transfer out of bed, the head of the bed can be gradually elevated by 10 increments; vital signs should be monitored during this time. To prevent orthostatic hypotension, use abdominal binders with elastic stockings. When tolerance to sitting develops, a two person transfer to a wheelchair, with the back of the wheelchair in a recline position of 30 degrees and legs elevated, can occur. Gradually raise the back of the wheelchair while lowering the legs to a position the patient can tolerate. Increase wheelchair tolerance by increasing sitting time. For balance activity, help the patient to sit on the side of the bed, As endurance, balance, and muscle strengthening increase, advanced wheelchair activities, mobility, and transfer training are implemented. Because of sensorimotor deficits, pressure relief and weight shift techniques are implemented every 15 to 30 minutes while the patient is in the wheelchair. Therapy should progress to lateral weight shifts, push ups, and weight relief via forward learning. Provide constant teaching and reinforcement until pressure relief techniques are automatic behaviors.

F. The patient with SCI is at risk for skin integrity impairment because of decreased sensation, paralysis, paresis, musculoskeletal problems, and altered health status. Assess skin color, elasticity, moisture, edema, cleanliness, hyperemia, lesions, and scars.

G. Interventions include ensuring correct body positioning in bed and in the wheelchair; all bony prominences should be supported in a manner that relieves pressure over small surfaces and distributes pressure evenly over larger surface areas. Gradually increase the time spent in one position. Use of pressure relief wheelchair pads and mattresses are beneficial. Good nutrition, skin care, skin protection, weight and pressure relief, and proper transfer techniques are vital for skin integrity maintenance.

H. A complete head-to-toe skin inspection twice a day (before dressing and at bedtime) and before and after application of braces and orthotic devices is important. Assess and massage areas above bony prominences such as the sacrum, trochanter, ischial tuberosities, elbows, and heels. Teach the patient to use a mirror to observe the posterior surface of the body.

I. SCI often causes devastating self care deficits. Assessment of neurologic level, motor ability, and functional capabilities assists in determining self care retraining goals. Functional evaluation includes bathing, dressing, feeding, elimination, hygiene, and home care skills. Retraining usually begins with activities that encourage gross function and progresses to activities that require fine motor coordination, such as buttoning. The occupational therapist evaluates and sets up a program for practice of ADL and provides necessary equipment that enhances the patient's functioning. The nurse reinforces the program and provides opportunity for practice. Equipment needs for a high level quadriplegic (C5 and above) may include a universal cuff with built-up self care devices, an overhead sling, a wheelchair with quad knobs or a motorized environmental control unit, and major home renovation. The lower level SCI patient (C6 and below) needs few assistive devices because of independent hand control.

J. The patient with SCI has lost the ability to initiate or inhibit emptying of the rectum, but the bowel can be regulated through reflex activity. With an upper motor neuron lesion, there is an intact reflex arch (S2 to S4); with a lower motor neuron lesion, there is a reduction in involuntary reflex regulation. The patient with SCI risks paralytic ileus (commonly caused by the hypoactivity of peristalsis), stress ulcers, constipation, hemorrhoids, diarrhea, and impaction. The goal is to prevent complications and to achieve bowel function and continence through a comprehensive bowel program. Bowel assessment includes premorbid habits, diet, fluid intake, activity level (i.e., ability to sit at a 90 degree angle), level of injury, and time since injury.

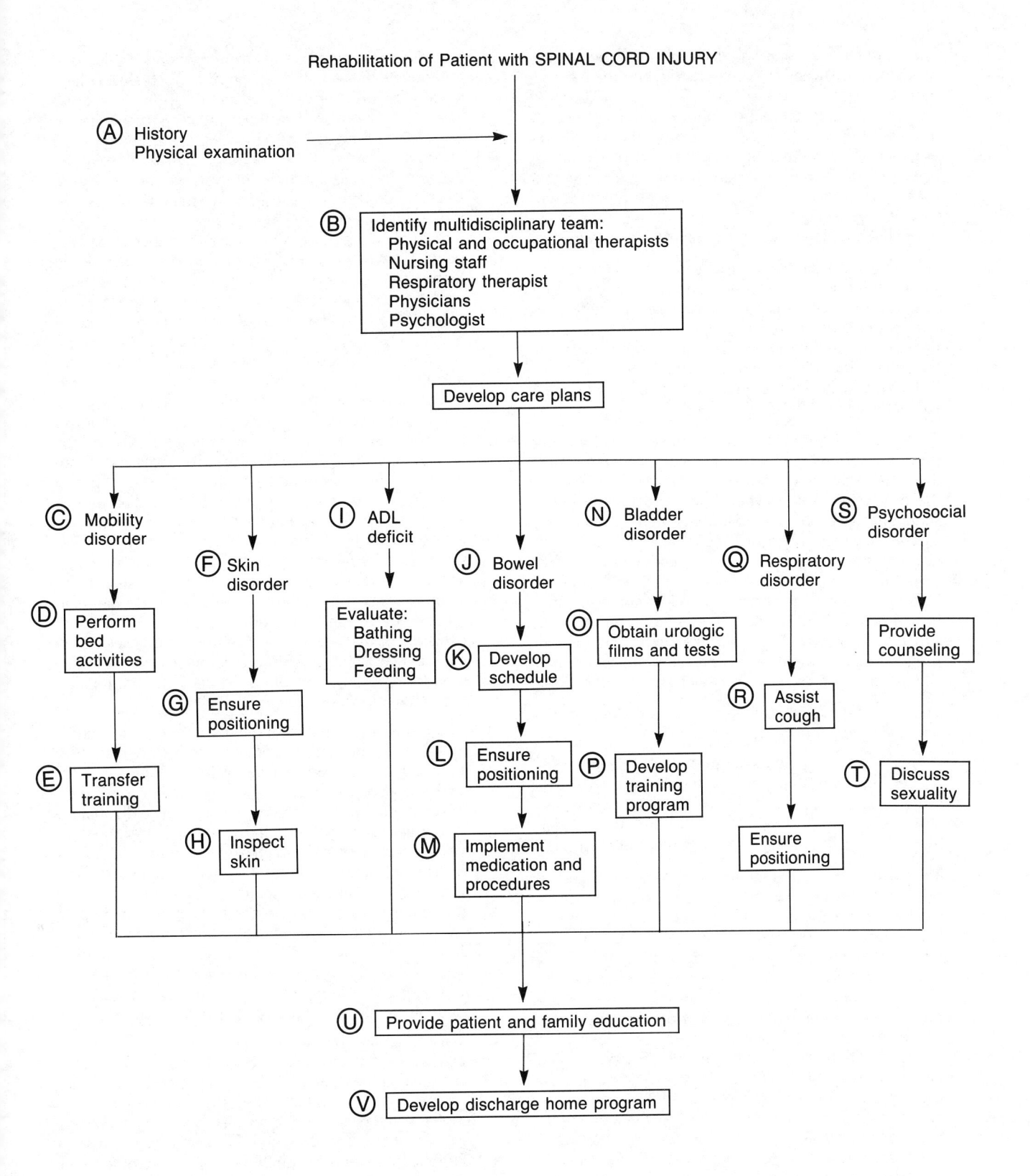

Rehabilitation of Patient with SPINAL CORD INJURY

- (A) History / Physical examination
- (B) Identify multidisciplinary team:
  - Physical and occupational therapists
  - Nursing staff
  - Respiratory therapist
  - Physicians
  - Psychologist
- Develop care plans
- (C) Mobility disorder
  - (D) Perform bed activities
  - (E) Transfer training
- (F) Skin disorder
  - (G) Ensure positioning
  - (H) Inspect skin
- (I) ADL deficit
  - Evaluate: Bathing, Dressing, Feeding
- (J) Bowel disorder
  - (K) Develop schedule
  - (L) Ensure positioning
  - (M) Implement medication and procedures
- (N) Bladder disorder
  - (O) Obtain urologic films and tests
  - (P) Develop training program
- (Q) Respiratory disorder
  - (R) Assist cough
  - Ensure positioning
- (S) Psychosocial disorder
  - Provide counseling
  - (T) Discuss sexuality
- (U) Provide patient and family education
- (V) Develop discharge home program

K. The schedule for the bowel program must provide adequate time for successful emptying and meet the patient's individual needs. The gastrocolic reflex should be used via insertion of rectal suppositories or a mini-enema 30 minutes after meals to facilitate stronger peristalsis and evacuation. Implement the program every other day until evacuation occurs routinely. Some patients may require implementation every day to every third day. Establishing a fixed, routine schedule is important to achieving bowel function and to maintaining continence.

L. Following insertion of the suppository, assist the patient onto a toilet with an elevated padded seat or onto a shower commode chair to take advantage of gravity. Positioning depends on spinal stability and tolerance. If the patient must remain in bed, left side placement assists the descending colon to empty toward the left side. Many SCI individuals need digital stimulation of the anal sphincter or digital removal of stool.

M. There are many products used in a bowel program. Suppositories are inserted above the anal sphincter against the rectal wall and used to set off the reflex and to start the movement of the lower colon and rectum. Stool softeners may be used. Bulk formers such as Metamucil can be used to absorb water and increase mass, thereby causing distention and peristalsis. High fluid intake, high fiber, bran products, and fruit facilitate bowel function. Increased mobility and exercise also increase bowel motility and function. The patient and family must be instructed in bowel anatomy, alteration in function, program management, signs and symptoms of complications, and use of assistive devices and medication.

N. The Foley catheter should be removed and an intermittent catheterization program implemented.

O. A complete urologic assessment should include a urine culture and sensitivity; intravenous pyelography cystourethrography; cystometrics with urethral profile pressures; kidney, ureter, and bladder assessment; electromyography; renal scan; and renal ultrasound.

P. The bladder program is based on the test results and on bladder dysfunction. Hypertonic (i.e., reflex, upper motor neuron) or hypotonic (i.e., areflexic, lower motor neuron) bladder dysfunction usually results from SCI. With an upper motor neuron type of bladder, the long-term goal of bladder management is a reflexive emptying of the bladder with minimal postvoid residual. This is accomplished by intermittent catheterization combined with limited regulated fluid intake; limited fluid intake helps to prevent overdistention of the bladder. The patient and family are taught to stimulate the bladder to empty by tapping on the suprapubic area, by stroking the thighs, and by pulling the pubic hair prior to catheterization. Credé's maneuver and manual pressure over the suprapubic area should be used only with a patient with a hypotonic bladder with flaccid sphincter. As the bladder begins to empty on its own or when stimulated at appropriate intervals, the catheterization schedule (which usually begins every 4 hours) can begin to be tapered. The level of postvoid residual indicates the need for decreasing or increasing frequencies. Consistent postvoid residuals of 50 to 100 ml or 10 percent of the bladder capacity indicate that time intervals can be increased. Regulate fluids or, if necessary, increase frequencies to avoid volumes over 400 ml and overdistention. Use external collecting devices to collect spontaneous voiding between catheterizations. Instruction in catheterization technique (i.e., sterile in the hospital, clean at home) is vital. Even if functionally unable to perform the task, the patient must be able to direct the procedure and be taught the signs and symptoms of urinary tract infection, voiding techniques, care of urinary collection devices and equipment, fluid restriction, and recognition and treatment of autonomic dysreflexia. Autonomic dysreflexia is an emergency situation; it is a vasomotor response to noxious stimuli below the level of injury that occurs in patients with SCI at T6 or above. The signs and symptoms are onset of pounding headache, elevated blood pressure, bradycardia, stuffy nose, flushing, diaphoresis, and goosebumps above the level of the injury. Etiology includes overdistention of bladder or rectum, skin lesions, bladder infections, abdominal pressure, blocked catheters, perineal surgical procedures, and sexual stimulation. In 85 percent of the cases, etiology is bladder related (e.g., overdistention, blocked catheter, urinary tract infection, or bladder stones). Treatment comprises elevating the head of the bed, removing the noxious stimulus, monitoring blood pressure and pulse, and administering medications as ordered.

Q. As a result of neuromuscular impairment, poor mobilization of respiratory secretion, impaired cough response, and reduced vital capacity, the patient is at great risk for respiratory complications. Patients with high cervical involvement (C1 to C5) have the function of the diaphragm and upper accessory muscles directly affected. Ventilatory support or phrenic pacemaker support may be needed. The SCI patient's (T1 to T12) intercostal muscles and abdominal muscles are impaired, thereby limiting lateral costal expansion and forceful exhalation. The goal is to attain the highest level of independent respiratory function that is possible and to maintain adequate ventilation. Intervention includes chest physiotherapy every 4 hours, or more frequently in the initial periods, with gradually increasing intervals between treatments.

R. Assisted cough, by the application of manual force to the abdomen with pressure in an upward direction, assists the diaphragm in mobilizing secretions. Sterile suctioning is done if necessary. Respiratory exercises are implemented by the respiratory therapist. The patient and family are taught self care skills to prevent respiratory complications and to identify signs and symptoms of early respiratory complications.

S. SCI alters the person's body image, self esteem, and role performance. Family lifestyles are simultaneously altered, with family members suffering their own losses. The physical changes of SCI cannot be handled effectively without addressing psychological adaptation. The psychologist or social worker is a valuable resource. Every member of the team should create an environment that is supportive of the multifaceted psychological needs of the patient and the family. The patient and family must be allowed to express behaviors of denial, depression, and anger and hostility. Time must be provided to ventilate and express feelings. The core psychological problem is depression related to multiple and simultaneous losses. The loss of mobility, control, and independence demands immediate changes in lifestyle that threaten psychological security.

T. Sexuality usually surfaces as one of the first concerns of the SCI patient, and it is the last and most difficult concern to resolve. The team must create an environment in which sexuality and sexual function are open for discussion. Sex counseling by a prepared professional includes training in birth control measures, body positioning, and bowel and bladder related issues during intimacy.

U. The patient's ability to perform ADL is one of the most important aspects of the rehabilitation process. Before discharge, the patient and family must be able to demonstrate self care skills, procedures and techniques of medication administration, bowel and bladder program, postural drainage, assisted cough, pulmonary toilet, proper positioning, range of motion, breathing exercises, transfers, pressure relief techniques, and skin care.

V. The focus of a home program is to facilitate continued care of the SCI individual and reintegration into society. Referral to self help groups, vocational rehabilitation, and community resources should be provided.

References

Brenda S. Spinal cord injury nursing education: suggested content. Chicago: American Spinal Injury Foundation, 1983.

Campbell MK. Spinal cord injuries. Top Acute Care Trauma Rehab 1987; 1:62–93.

Hargrove-Drayton S, Reddy AM. Rehabilitation and long term management of spinal cord injured adult. Nurs Clin North Am 1986; 21:599–610.

Kirby N. The individual with high quadraplegia. Nurs Clin North Am 1989; 24:179–190.

Saylee SM. Rehabilitation nursing: concepts and practice. Evanston, IL: Rehabilitation Nursing Institute, 1981.

REHABILITATION AFTER UPPER EXTREMITY AMPUTATION

Anita L. Grudda

A. The history should include the mechanism of injury, level of amputation, pre-existing or concurrent medical complications, previous level of activity, family and home environment, and vocational status. Consider referrals to psychologist, social worker, and vocational rehabilitation counselor.

B. A plaster cast fit with a terminal device may be applied in the operating room; this provides a rigid dressing with uniform contact to the new wound that facilitates edema control and promotes wound healing and early functional use of the extremity.

C. Adequate range of motion in all joints of the involved upper extremity must be achieved and maintained. Active and active-assisted joint range of motion can begin as early as the second postoperative day. Upper extremity muscle strengthening is vital to eventual success in prosthetic training. The strengthening program may include active resistance applied manually by the therapist, cuff weights attached to the residual limb, or weighted pulleys.

D. Proper wound healing requires frequent dressing changes, hydrotherapy, wound care and debridement, and patient education.

E. Shrinking and shaping of the residual limb are imperative to form a firm and tapered stump for proper contact in the prosthetic socket. These are accomplished through the use of compression, such as an elastic ace bandage in a figure-of-eight wrap, with pressure applied distal to proximal; through the use of an intermittent positive pressure compression pump; or with a tubular elastic bandage.

F. Phantom limb sensation is the perception that the nonexistent limb is still present; it is usually stronger and longer lasting in the upper extremity amputee than in the lower extremity amputee. Phantom limb pain is the perception of pain in the nonexistent limb and may be alleviated with transcutaneous electrical nerve stimulation, massage, biofeedback, isometric exercise, or medication. If phantom pain persists, the presence of a neuroma should be explored. Regardless of the presence of phantom limb sensation, a desensitization program of the residual limb that includes massage, tapping, and vibration will improve the patient's tolerance to the eventual pressure in the prosthetic socket.

G. Depending on the level of amputation and on previous hand dominance, the patient may require training in the transfer of dominance as well as training in adaptive equipment to maximize independence in activities of daily living (ADL).

H. Assessment of the patient's readiness for a prosthesis includes evaluation of the shape and skin integrity of the residual limb, mobility and strength in bilateral upper extremities, vocational needs, patients's attitude and motivation as well as desires for function and cosmesis, patient's ability to learn new information, and availability of funding for the prosthesis.

I. Thorough evaluation for fit and function of the prosthesis should include comfort, length, color (if cosmetic), and the efficiency of the control system.

J. Controls training teaches proficient mechanical operation of the prosthesis as the patient gains an awareness of the body motions necessary to control the prosthesis. It is important that the patient not use exaggerated movement for control. Practice in muscular contraction, holding, and relaxing for movement and stability is emphasized.

K. Use training utilizes the skills mastered during controls training for application to specific functional activities, including activities of daily living, vocational activities, and recreational activities.

L. Referrals to vocational rehabilitation, support groups, and social work services may be needed at the time of discharge from therapy. Continual follow-up with the physician and prosthetist should be emphasized at discharge as well as a thorough review of the home program for residual limb skin inspection and hygiene.

References

Atkins DJ, Meier RH, ed. Comprehensive management of the upper-limb amputee. New York: Springer-Verlag, 1989.

Banerjee SN, ed. Rehabilitation management of amputees. Baltimore: Williams & Wilkins, 1982.

Kostuik J, ed. Amputation surgery and rehabilitation. New York: Churchill Livingstone, 1981.

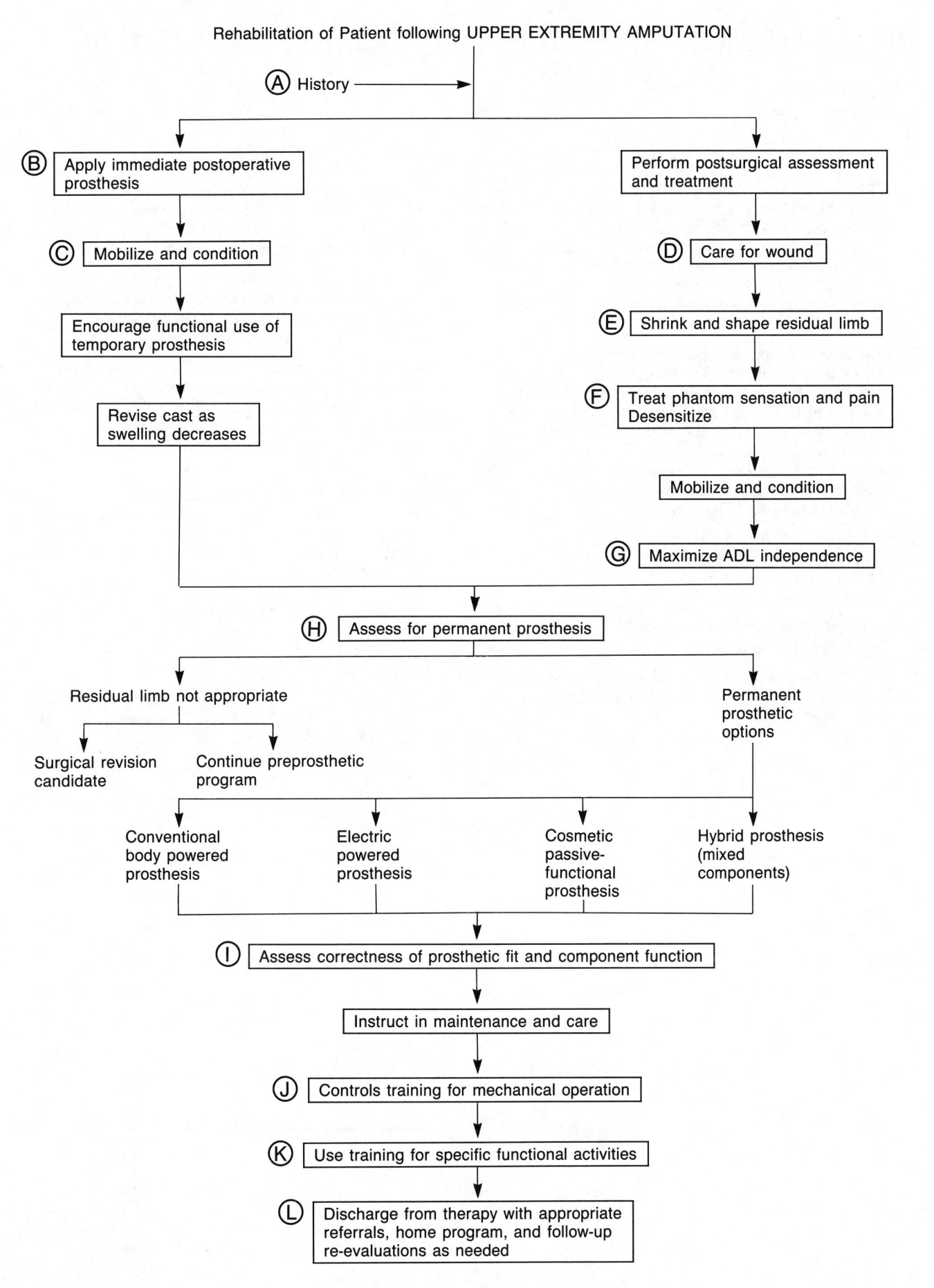

Rehabilitation of Patient following UPPER EXTREMITY AMPUTATION

- **A** History
  - **B** Apply immediate postoperative prosthesis
    - **C** Mobilize and condition
      - Encourage functional use of temporary prosthesis
        - Revise cast as swelling decreases
  - Perform postsurgical assessment and treatment
    - **D** Care for wound
      - **E** Shrink and shape residual limb
        - **F** Treat phantom sensation and pain Desensitize
          - Mobilize and condition
            - **G** Maximize ADL independence

- **H** Assess for permanent prosthesis
  - Residual limb not appropriate
    - Surgical revision candidate
    - Continue preprosthetic program
  - Permanent prosthetic options
    - Conventional body powered prosthesis
    - Electric powered prosthesis
    - Cosmetic passive-functional prosthesis
    - Hybrid prosthesis (mixed components)

- **I** Assess correctness of prosthetic fit and component function
  - Instruct in maintenance and care
    - **J** Controls training for mechanical operation
      - **K** Use training for specific functional activities
        - **L** Discharge from therapy with appropriate referrals, home program, and follow-up re-evaluations as needed

REHABILITATION AFTER LOWER EXTREMITY AMPUTATION

Marina G. Hall
Rebecca P. Jones

A. The history should include the mechanism of injury that resulted in the amputation. The level of amputation and pre-existing or concurrent medical problems such as cardiac problems need to be included. At this time, the patient should be questioned about previous mobility skills, family and home environment, and vocational status. If necessary, consider vocational rehabilitation referrals.

B. The assessment process should include evaluation of all extremities, trunk, mental status, range of motion, strength, coordination, sensation, balance, mobility skills, and potential home environment. A detailed assessment of the residual limb should include the following: range of motion, strength, skin integrity, limb length, shape, circumference, and scar location. Before discharge, the patient's home environment must be assessed. A home health referral should be considered.

C. Range of motion of the residual limb is important in preventing contractures and in assessing the prosthetic fit. It is also a primary consideration for a functional gait pattern.

D. Strength of the extremities is vital in the independent mobility of the amputee.

E. Bed mobility is essential in prevention of decubitus. Achievement of bed mobility is the initial step toward independence.

F. Delayed closure of the wound inhibits prosthetic fit. Appropriate wound care procedures such as hydrotherapy, debridement, dressing changes, and patient and family home program should be implemented.

G. Phantom sensation is common and should not automatically be interpreted as abnormal. If phantom pain persists, a neuroma could exist. A referral to psychiatry or a pain clinic may be necessary.

H. A patient who has a residual limb with paresthesia or hypersensitivity should be instructed in desensitization activities. The patient with a hyposensitive residual limb needs to be instructed in skin precautions and inspection. If hyposensitivity persists, poor prosthetic candidacy may be indicated.

I. Proper bandaging can prevent problems such as dog ears, edema, and a poorly shaped stump. Proper bandaging consists of a figure-of-eight wrap with pressure distal to proximal and medial and lateral on stump ends. If an ace wrap is being used, it should be rewrapped every 4 hours or whenever the wrap slips or loosens. Bandages should be worn at all times except for hygiene and skin inspection.

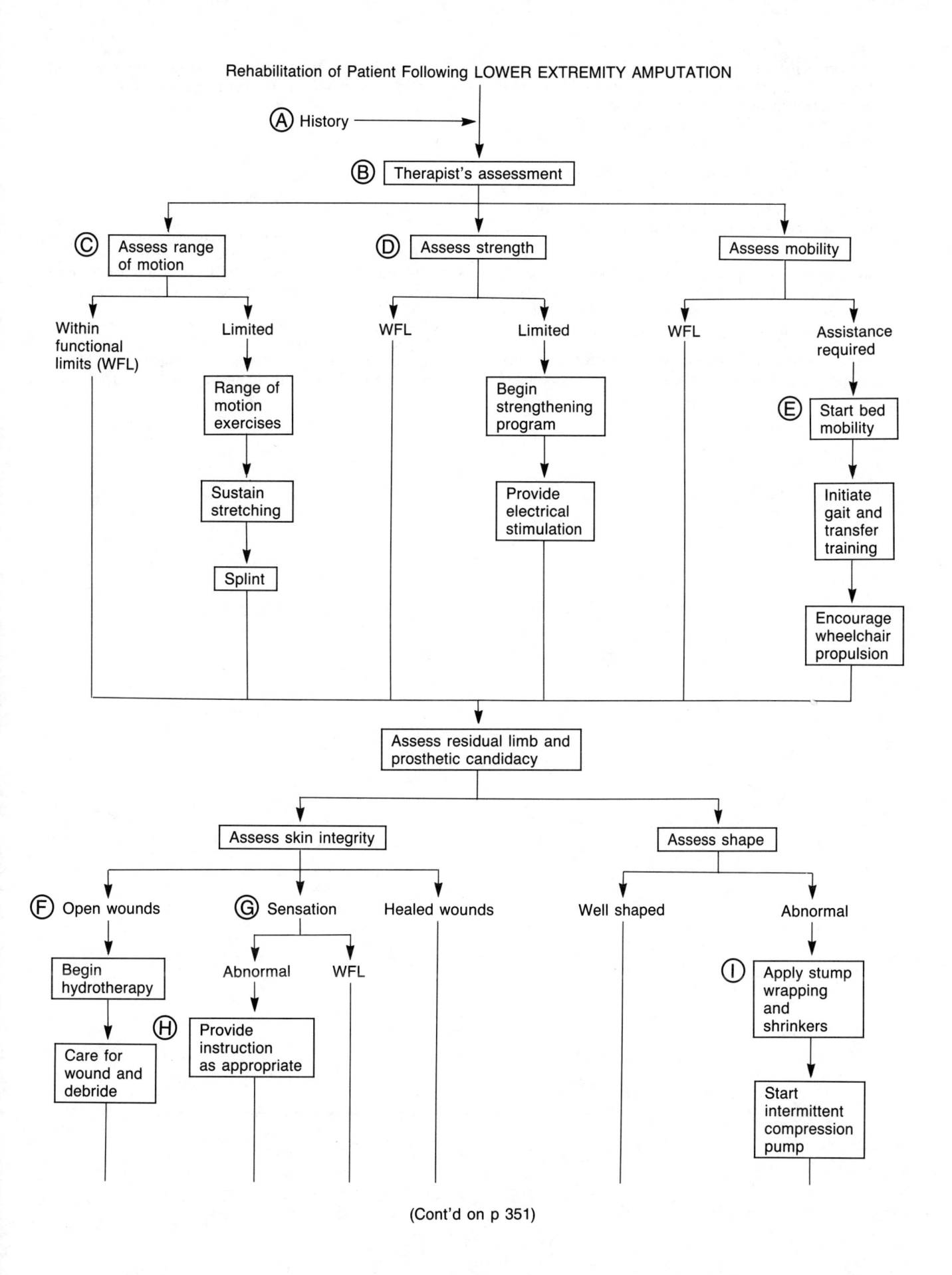

Rehabilitation of Patient Following LOWER EXTREMITY AMPUTATION

- (A) History →
  - (B) Therapist's assessment
    - (C) Assess range of motion
      - Within functional limits (WFL)
      - Limited
        - Range of motion exercises
        - Sustain stretching
        - Splint
    - (D) Assess strength
      - WFL
      - Limited
        - Begin strengthening program
        - Provide electrical stimulation
    - Assess mobility
      - WFL
      - Assistance required
        - (E) Start bed mobility
        - Initiate gait and transfer training
        - Encourage wheelchair propulsion

- Assess residual limb and prosthetic candidacy
  - Assess skin integrity
    - (F) Open wounds
      - Begin hydrotherapy
      - Care for wound and debride
    - (G) Sensation
      - Abnormal
        - (H) Provide instruction as appropriate
      - WFL
    - Healed wounds
  - Assess shape
    - Well shaped
    - Abnormal
      - (I) Apply stump wrapping and shrinkers
      - Start intermittent compression pump

(Cont'd on p 351)

349

J. Early prosthetic fitting with a temporary or preparatory prosthesis is preferred. This prevents problems with deconditioning and contractures and assists with shrinkage of the residual limb. Early prosthetic fitting could be done within 2 to 4 weeks after the incision is healed.

K. Once the patient receives the prosthesis, gait and transfers need to be reassessed. Gait is not a consideration if the prosthesis was made for cosmetic reasons only. Independence, skin inspection, and transfers are the primary goals.

L. Initially, the patient should be instructed to inspect the residual limb after each attempt at wearing. Once shape, size, and pressure areas of the residual limb stabilize, skin inspections are only periodically necessary.

M. Consider referrals to vocational rehabilitation, amputee support groups, social work services, and rehabilitation counseling. It is important to emphasize continued follow-up with the physician and prosthetist.

References

Banerjee SN, ed. Rehabilitation management of amputees. Baltimore: Williams & Wilkins, 1982:359–363.

O'Sullivan SB, Cullen KE, Schmitz TJ. Physical rehabilitation: evaluation and treatment procedures. Philadelphia: FA Davis, 1981:191–220.

Sanders GT. Lower limb amputation: a guide to rehabilitation. Philadelphia: FA Davis, 1986:369–379.

Turek SL. Orthopaedics principles and their applications. 4th ed. Vol. 2. Philadelphia: JB Lippincott, 1984:1678–1739.

(Cont'd from p 349)

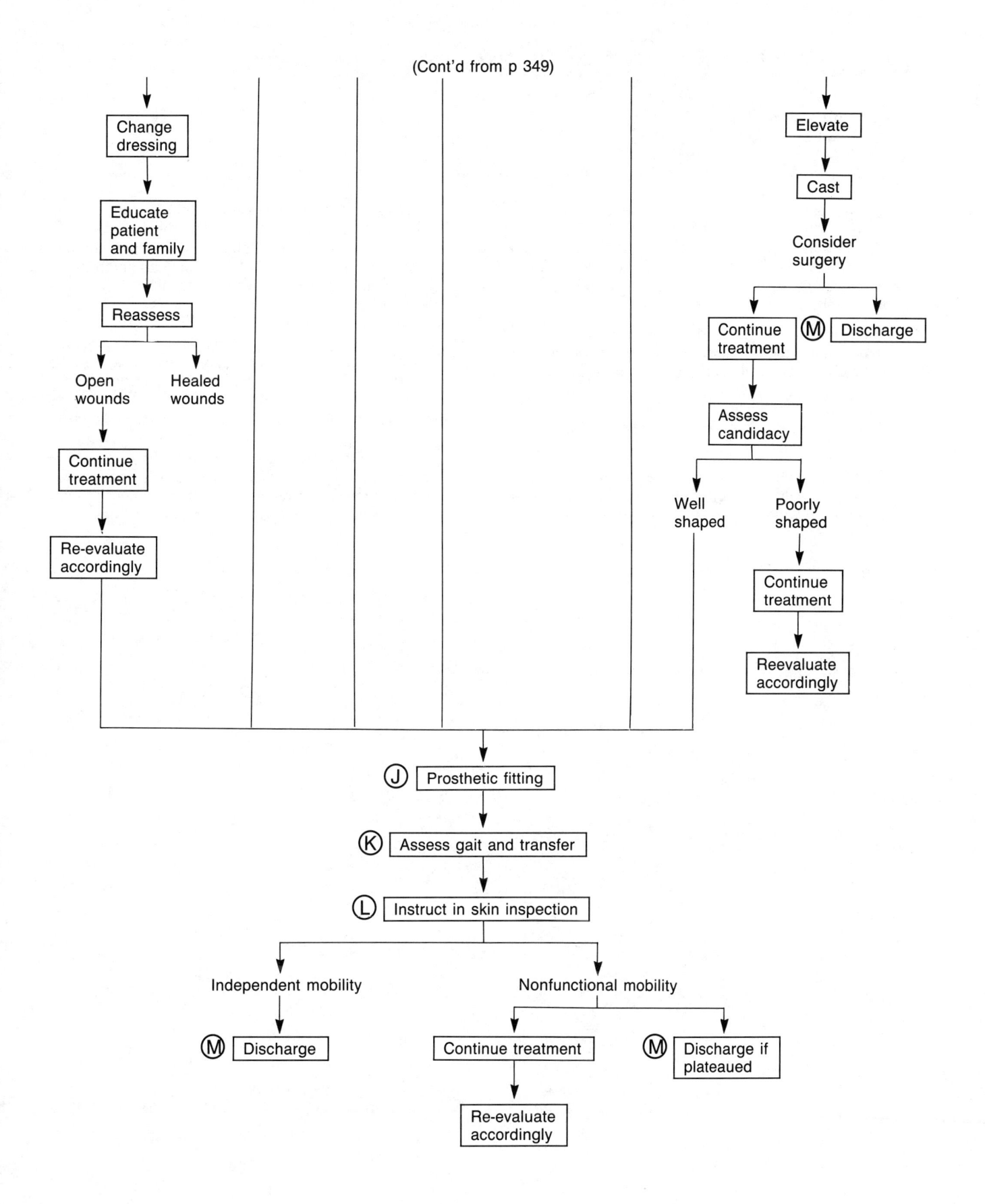

```
      ↓                                              ↓
┌──────────┐                                   ┌──────────┐
│ Change   │                                   │ Elevate  │
│ dressing │                                   └──────────┘
└──────────┘                                         ↓
      ↓                                        ┌──────────┐
┌──────────┐                                   │   Cast   │
│ Educate  │                                   └──────────┘
│ patient  │                                         ↓
│ and family│                                  Consider
└──────────┘                                   surgery
      ↓                                       ┌────┴────┐
┌──────────┐                                  ↓         ↓
│ Reassess │                          ┌──────────┐ Ⓜ ┌──────────┐
└──────────┘                          │ Continue │    │Discharge │
    ┌──┴──┐                           │treatment │    └──────────┘
    ↓     ↓                           └──────────┘
  Open   Healed                             ↓
 wounds  wounds                       ┌──────────┐
    ↓                                 │  Assess  │
┌──────────┐                          │candidacy │
│ Continue │                          └──────────┘
│treatment │                             ┌──┴──┐
└──────────┘                             ↓     ↓
    ↓                                  Well   Poorly
┌──────────┐                          shaped  shaped
│Re-evaluate│                                   ↓
│accordingly│                             ┌──────────┐
└──────────┘                              │ Continue │
                                          │treatment │
                                          └──────────┘
                                                ↓
                                          ┌──────────┐
                                          │Reevaluate│
                                          │accordingly│
                                          └──────────┘

                    Ⓙ ┌─────────────────┐
                      │Prosthetic fitting│
                      └─────────────────┘
                              ↓
                    Ⓚ ┌─────────────────────┐
                      │Assess gait and transfer│
                      └─────────────────────┘
                              ↓
                    Ⓛ ┌─────────────────────┐
                      │Instruct in skin inspection│
                      └─────────────────────┘
                      ┌───────┴────────┐
              Independent mobility  Nonfunctional mobility
                      ↓              ┌────┴────┐
              Ⓜ ┌─────────┐           ↓         ↓
                │Discharge│  ┌──────────────┐ Ⓜ ┌──────────┐
                └─────────┘  │Continue treatment│ │Discharge if│
                             └──────────────┘    │ plateaued │
                                    ↓            └──────────┘
                             ┌────────────┐
                             │Re-evaluate │
                             │accordingly │
                             └────────────┘
```

REHABILITATION OF THE BURN–INJURED PATIENT

Donna Kay Causby
Constance D. Parry

A. A complete history should be obtained, including percentage of body surface area burned, location, depth, type of burn, and date of burn. Complete questioning of the patient should include notation of any associated trauma or pre-existing conditions that may limit functional capacity.

B. The extent of the evaluation depends on the location, depth, percentage of the body surface area burned, and the patient's medical condition. A complete evaluation may take more than one treatment session because of pain and endurance limitations. Precautions and limitations may also be necessary with patients who have undergone recent surgical procedures.

C. Patients with open wounds require a minimum of twice daily treatments for thorough cleansing and debridement of the burn wound. Care must be taken to debride as much as possible while working within the patient's pain tolerance. Once the burn wound has healed, skin must be kept lubricated and mobile. Gradient pressure garments are necessary for hypertrophic scars and must be worn until scar maturity, which is usually 1.5 to 2 years postinjury.

D. In addition to pharmaceutical management of pain, therapists instruct patients in relaxation techniques and the use of modalities such as, and primarily, transcutaneous electrical nerve stimulation (TENS). Desensitization techniques are employed for patients with hypersensitive skin.

E. Because of increased capillary permeability after a burn injury, edema can become a difficult problem to manage. Reduction of edema decreases a patient's risk of contracture development and of possible nerve palsies.

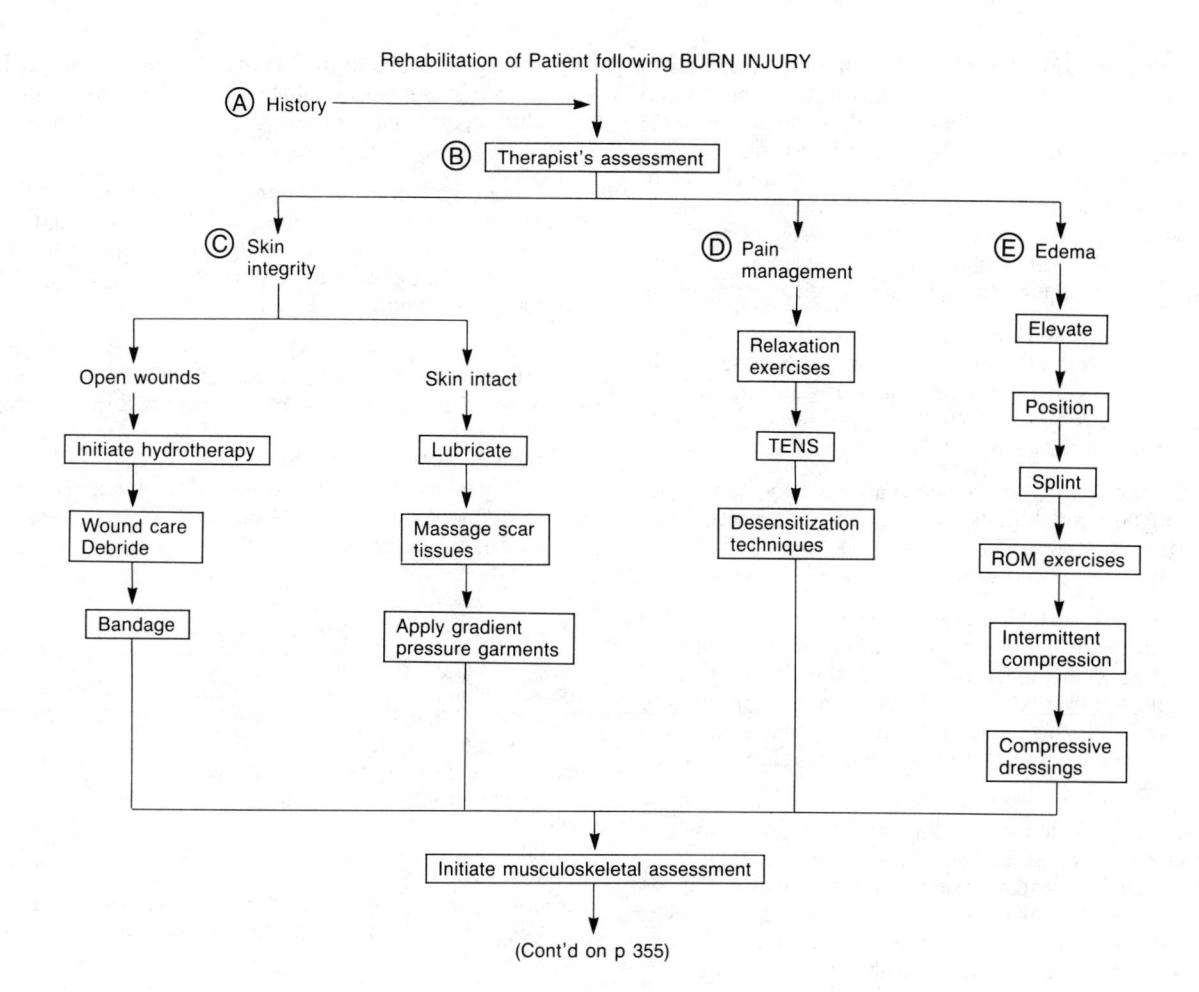

Rehabilitation of Patient following BURN INJURY

- **(A) History** →
- **(B) Therapist's assessment**
  - **(C) Skin integrity**
    - Open wounds
      - Initiate hydrotherapy
      - Wound care / Debride
      - Bandage
    - Skin intact
      - Lubricate
      - Massage scar tissues
      - Apply gradient pressure garments
  - **(D) Pain management**
    - Relaxation exercises
    - TENS
    - Desensitization techniques
  - **(E) Edema**
    - Elevate
    - Position
    - Splint
    - ROM exercises
    - Intermittent compression
    - Compressive dressings

→ Initiate musculoskeletal assessment

(Cont'd on p 355)

F. Range of motion (ROM) evaluation should include joints involved and joints distal and proximal to the burned area. Isolated joint motion as well as functional ROM should be evaluated. To evaluate functional ROM, the entire burned area must be put on a maximal stretch. Evaluation of ROM is restricted after surgical procedures or with an exposed tendon. ROM exercises and positioning should begin within 24 hours of admission and should be held for 3 to 5 days after surgical autografting.

G. The golden rule of burn care dictates that the position of comfort is the position of contracture. Patients should be positioned with the burned area on a stretch. Circumferential burns require alternating positioning programs to maintain ROM in all planes of movement.

H. Splinting must be initiated acutely and continues throughout rehabilitation by a qualified therapist. Serial casting to increase ROM is reserved for patients in whom the majority of the wound has healed.

I. Paraffin and sustained stretch are techniques used once the skin is no longer fragile and the wound is at least 90 percent healed. The temperature of the paraffin should not exceed 118° F and then must be cooled to a semisolid state. Joints must be positioned on a sustained stretch for 20 minutes once paraffin has been applied.

J. Continuous evaluation of the patient's muscle tone and reflexes is necessary, especially in the presence of an electrical burn and after surgical procedures. Central nervous system involvement is commonly seen with electrical injuries up to 2 years postinjury. Peripheral neuropathies are managed with orthotics, muscle reeducation, and modalities that include biofeedback and electrical stimulation.

K. Therapists evaluate the activities of daily living (ADL) skills of patients and initiate retraining of basic skills, including dressing, bathing, and feeding. Adaptive equipment is issued as appropriate.

L. Patients with burns or donor sites located on the extremities often experience limited mobility. Treatment may include retraining for bed mobility, transfers, and gait. Gait should be held for 6 to 10 days after autografting to the lower extremities.

M. A burn injury is devastating to the entire psychological, musculoskeletal, and systemic systems of an individual. All these areas must be incorporated into the treatment program with the ultimate goal of returning the individual to maximal functional capacity. Patient and family education must begin on admission and continue throughout the entire rehabilitation phase to ensure a successful outcome.

References

Fisher S, Helm P. Comprehensive rehabilitation of burns. Baltimore: William & Wilkins, 1984:16–26; 127–135; 188–189; 255–256; 264; 320–326.

Johnson C, O'Shaughnessy E, Ostergren G. Burn management. New York: Raven Press, 1981:5–15; 133–144.

Malick M, Carr J. Manual on management of the burned patient. Pittsburgh: Hamarville Rehabilitation Center, 1982:24–30; 130–138.

Trotter M, Johnson C. The treatment of burn patients. Washington: Health Sciences Learning Resources Center, 1979; 26;37–40.

(Cont'd from p 353)

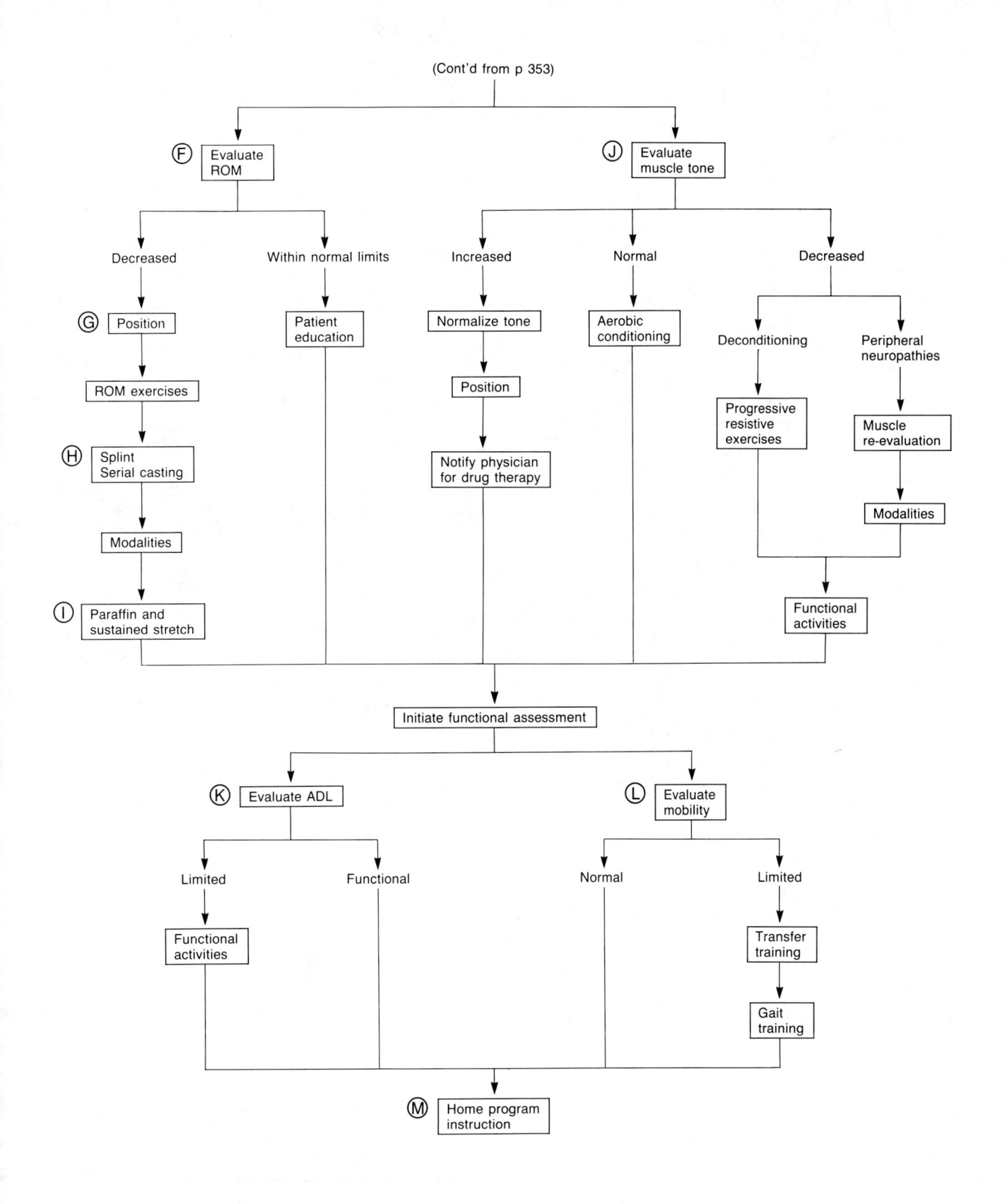

```
                    ┌──────────────┐                          ┌──────────────┐
                    │ Ⓕ Evaluate   │                          │ Ⓙ Evaluate   │
                    │    ROM       │                          │  muscle tone │
                    └──────────────┘                          └──────────────┘
                   Decreased    Within normal limits    Increased      Normal        Decreased
                       │               │                   │             │              │
                ┌──────────┐     ┌──────────┐      ┌──────────────┐  ┌──────────┐   Deconditioning   Peripheral
                │Ⓖ Position│     │ Patient  │      │Normalize tone│  │ Aerobic  │                    neuropathies
                └──────────┘     │education │      └──────────────┘  │conditioning│       │              │
                     │           └──────────┘             │          └──────────┘  ┌──────────────┐ ┌──────────────┐
                ┌──────────────┐                     ┌──────────┐                  │ Progressive  │ │   Muscle     │
                │ROM exercises │                     │ Position │                  │  resistive   │ │re-evaluation │
                └──────────────┘                     └──────────┘                  │  exercises   │ └──────────────┘
                     │                                    │                        └──────────────┘        │
                ┌──────────────┐                     ┌──────────────┐                                ┌──────────┐
                │Ⓗ Splint      │                     │Notify physician│                              │Modalities│
                │ Serial casting│                    │for drug therapy│                              └──────────┘
                └──────────────┘                     └──────────────┘
                     │                                                                    ┌──────────────┐
                ┌──────────┐                                                               │  Functional  │
                │Modalities│                                                               │  activities  │
                └──────────┘                                                               └──────────────┘
                     │
                ┌──────────────┐
                │Ⓘ Paraffin and│
                │sustained stretch│
                └──────────────┘

                          ┌────────────────────────────┐
                          │Initiate functional assessment│
                          └────────────────────────────┘
                          ┌────────────┐         ┌────────────┐
                          │Ⓚ Evaluate  │         │Ⓛ Evaluate  │
                          │   ADL      │         │  mobility  │
                          └────────────┘         └────────────┘
                        Limited    Functional   Normal    Limited
                           │                                 │
                     ┌──────────┐                      ┌──────────┐
                     │Functional│                      │ Transfer │
                     │activities│                      │ training │
                     └──────────┘                      └──────────┘
                                                             │
                                                       ┌──────────┐
                                                       │   Gait   │
                                                       │ training │
                                                       └──────────┘

                                    ┌──────────────┐
                                    │Ⓜ Home program│
                                    │ instruction  │
                                    └──────────────┘
```

355

PROCEDURES: AIRWAY/ VENTILATION MANAGEMENT

Intubation
Cricothyroidotomy
Tracheostomy
Thoracentesis
Tube Thoracostomy
Arterial Blood Gases

INTUBATION

Kevin W. Klein

PURPOSE

To intubate the trachea and protect patient from aspiration.

INDICATIONS

Hypoventilation
Need for hyperventilation
Protection from aspiration of gastric contents or blood
Thermal injury of the larynx
General anesthesia

CONTRAINDICATIONS (RELATIVE)

Cervical spine injury
Severe facial or laryngeal trauma

POTENTIAL COMPLICATIONS

Hypoxemia, hypercarbia, death
Aspiration
Pneumonitis
Laceration
Dental injury
Laryngeal trauma
Increased intraocular pressure
Increased intracranial pressure
Bronchospasm
Arrhythmia
Right bronchial intubation
Esophageal intubation
Cervical cord injury
Mandibular dislocation
Atlanto-occipital dislocation
True vocal cord paralysis

PROCEDURE

1. Assess patient and urgency of intubation
2. Examine airway and decide on oral or nasal intubation and whether the patient should be intubated when asleep or awake
3. Equipment
   a. Oral and nasal airways of appropriate size.
   b. Laryngoscope blades and handles
   c. Tongue blade
   d. Stylet
   e. Appropriately sized endotracheal tubes
   f. Suction, tonsil sucker
   g. Oxygen, face mask, bag
   h. Oxymetazoline spray
   i. Lidocaine ointment, 5%
   j. Lidocaine topical solution, 4%
   k. Gloves, 4 x 4 gauze, tape
   l. ECG monitor, pulse oximeter
   m. Cardiac arrest cart
   n. Intubation pillow
   o. Magill forceps
4. Notify respiratory therapist
5. Explain the procedure to patient, if possible
6. Monitor vital signs throughout
7. Place intravenous catheter
8. Give 30 ml Bicitra either by mouth or by nasogastric tube
9. Position patient on intubation pillow with the plane of the face at the level of the intubator's xyphoid
10. Preoxygenate
11. Oral intubation
    a. Apply cricoid pressure to occlude the esophagus
    b. Sedate and paralyze as needed
    c. Open mouth slightly with right hand; with left hand place the laryngoscope blade to the right of the tongue and move the tongue to the left to expose the epiglottis and larynx. By lifting gently with careful attention to the teeth, the blade will lift the epiglottis to expose the vocal cords. Place the endotracheal tube cuff 1–2 cm past the vocal cords, and gently inflate the cuff with just enough air to prevent leaking with positive pressure ventilation.
12. Nasal intubation
    Prepare the nose with a vasoconstrictor and 4% lidocaine spray. A soft nasal airway lubricated with 5% lidocaine ointment may be used to dilate the nose. The nasal airway should be slightly larger than the endotracheal tube chosen. A transtracheal block may be performed in the patient who is awake by injecting 4 ml of 4% topical lidocaine through the cricoid cartilage using a 1-inch 23-gauge needle. Place the tube gently through the prepared nose to avoid epistaxis. The tube may then be advanced blindly into the larynx or under direct laryngoscopy. Magill forceps may assist with placement.
13. To verify placement, one may auscultate first over the stomach, then the lungs, and measure end-tidal CO
14. Start ventilation
15. Secure the tube

FOLLOW-UP

1. Assess oxygenation and ventilation
2. Check vital signs
3. Consider arterial blood gas sampling or chest films

DOCUMENTATION

Type and size of tube
Route of intubation
Length from tip of tube to teeth
Evidence of ventilation
Complications

References

Barie PS, Shires GT. Initial trauma management of multiple injuries. In: Parrillo JE, ed. Current therapy in critical care medicine. Toronto: BC Decker, 1987:306–314.

Donnan GB, Giesecke AH. Principles of trauma care. New York: McGraw-Hill, 1985:62–84.

CRICOTHYROIDOTOMY

Jorie Klein
Teri Gale

PURPOSE

To provide safe, fast, emergency surgical airway management.

INDICATIONS

When an emergency airway is needed and nasotracheal or endotracheal intubation is either technically impossible or contraindicated
Questionable unstable neck injury, facial trauma
Medical emergencies that occlude the airway
  Epiglottitis
  Acute peritonsillar abscess
  Postsurgical complications

CONTRAINDICATIONS

Pediatric patients under 12 years of age (note: there is a 40–50% incidence of pneumothorax developing after a surgical airway procedure)
Laryngeal trauma when landmarks are not easily identified
Airway obstruction following endotracheal intubation
Primary laryngeal disease

POTENTIAL COMPLICATIONS

Tracheal stenosis
Bleeding that may be difficult to control
Asphyxia
Aspiration
Cellulitis
Esophageal perforation
Exsanguinating hematoma
Tracheal posterior wall perforation
Thyroid perforation
Inadequate ventilation leading to hypoxia or death
Laryngeal stenosis
Laceration of the esophagus
Vocal cord paralysis
Hoarseness

EQUIPMENT

Povidone-iodine (Betadine)
4 × 4 gauze sponges
Gauze packing
12- to 14-gauge over-the-needle catheter
Jet insufflation equipment
  Y-connector and oxygen tubing
Wall mounted oxygen or oxygen tank with flow meter
Syringes, 10 ml
Hemostats
Tracheostomy tube #4, #5
3-mm endotracheal tube
Lidocaine (without epinephrine), 10 ml
Twill tape
Retractors, tracheal hook, tracheal spreader
Mask, gloves, gown, goggles
Electrocautery
Light source
Determine whether needle cricothyroidotomy or surgical cricothyroidotomy is to be attempted first

PROCEDURE

Needle Cricothyroidotomy

1. Assess patient's airway, breathing, and circulation (ABCs) and initiate management of life threatening injuries
2. Communicate potential airway compromise to team
3. Assemble equipment, plug in electrocautery
4. Administer sedation if appropriate
5. Place a rolled sheet between the shoulders to help identify the landmarks, if appropriate (cervical spine cleared)
6. Prepare the overlying cricothyroid area with 10% povidone-iodine solution
7. Direct light source to area
8. Adhere to universal precautions and sterile technique
9. An over-the-needle catheter is opened onto sterile field
10. A #4 tracheostomy tube and a 3-mm pediatric endotracheal tube are opened onto the sterile field
11. The Y-connector is connected to oxygen tubing and flow meter at 15 L per minute (50 psi)
12. Respiratory therapist will set up ventilator and supplemental oxygen with adaptors as indicated
13. Identify the cricothyroid membrane by palpating the inferior border of the thyroid cartilage of the larynx and the superior border of the cricoid cartilage
14. Insert the needle at a 45-degree angle into the lower half of the cricothyroid membrane (Fig. 1)
15. Observe for aspiration of air
16. Assess lung expansion
17. Control bleeding as indicated
18. Secure apparatus
19. Reassess patient

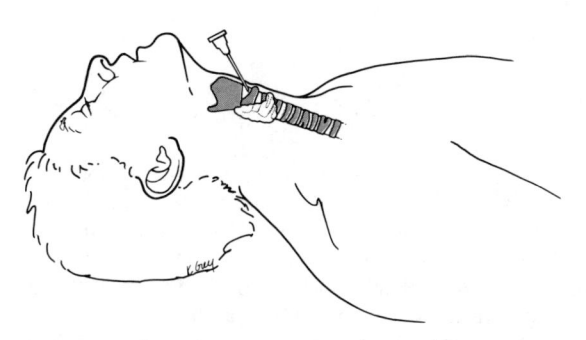

Figure 1 Anatomic landmarks for needle cricothyroidotomy. (Reprinted with permission from Scott J. Cricothyroidotomy. In: Mancini ME, ed. Pocket manual of emergency nursing procedures. Toronto: BC Decker, 1988:2.)

Surgical Cricothyroidotomy

1. Steps 1 through 13 are the same as those for the needle cricothyroidotomy procedure
14. Grasp the thyroid cartilage between the thumb and index finger; make a 2–3-cm incision through the skin over the cricothyroid space
15. Extend the incision through the subcutaneous tissue and down to the cricothyroid membrane
16. Use hemostats to control bleeding in the subcutaneous area
17. Insert #11 blade through the cricothyroid membrane with care to avoid injury to the cricoid cartilage, the thyroid cartilage, and posterior wall of the larynx
18. Extend the incision horizontally to the lateral borders of the cricothyroid membrane
19. Insert a clamp or trousseau dilator through the incision of the cricothyroid membrane and spread
20. Retract the inferior border superiorly with a tracheal hood and insert the appropriately sized tracheostomy tube
21. Secure the tracheal tube placement with umbilical tape
22. Assess lung expansion, ventilate patient
23. Control bleeding as indicated
24. Reassess patient
25. Obtain postprocedure radiograph

FOLLOW-UP

1. Reassess patient's ABCs
2. Obtain repeat arterial blood gas sampling
3. Continue to monitor and document vital signs and level of consciousness every 15 minutes as indicated
4. Continue with ongoing assessment and intervention
5. Notify operating room that patient will need further surgical intervention

DOCUMENTATION

Reassessment of patient
Indication for procedure
Size of tracheal tube placed
Ongoing assessment

References

American College of Surgeons. Advanced trauma life support course. Chicago: American College of Surgeons, 1988:33–56.

Boyd AD. A clinical evaluation of cricothyroidotomy. Surg Gynecol Obstet 1979; 149:365.

Eckstein K. Nursing process in multiple trauma. In: Holloway NM, ed. Emergency department nurses association core curriculum. Philadelphia: WB Saunders, 1985:239.

Scott J. Cricothyroidotomy. In: Mancini ME, ed. Pocket manual of emergency nursing procedures. Toronto: BC Decker, 1988:2–6.

TRACHEOSTOMY

Teri Gale

PURPOSE

To establish a patent airway.

INDICATIONS

Extensive head, facial, oral, or neck injuries present, and need to provide an airway to prevent aspiration
Laryngeal fracture
Intubation to exceed 72–96 hours or longer
Access for suctioning of secretions not otherwise manageable
Necessity to decrease airway dead space volume

CONTRAINDICATIONS

Orotracheal or nasotracheal intubation possible
Tracheobronchitis
Infants under 6 months of age (relative)

POTENTIAL COMPLICATIONS

Infection
Ulceration of tracheal mucosa
Tracheal stenosis
Tracheal malacia
Tracheoesophageal fistula
Hemorrhage
Pneumothorax
Damage to laryngeal nerve
Airway obstruction (i.e., crusting of secretions, herniation of cuff, kinking of tube)

EQUIPMENT

Tracheostomy tray
Lidocaine, 10 ml
Povidone-iodine (Betadine) solution
Three 10-sponge packs of 4 × 4 gauze sponges, gauze packing
Tracheostomy tubes, appropriate sizes
Suction apparatus
Sterile suction catheter kit
Sterile tonsil suction
Oxygen set-up or ventilator as indicated
Electrocautery
Sterile gloves, gown
Mask, goggles, plastic apron
Light source

PROCEDURE

1. Explain procedure to patient, when appropriate
2. Assess patient's airway, breathing, and circulation and initiate management of life threatening injuries
3. Obtain arterial blood gas sampling
4. Communicate the need for procedure to the team
5. Administer sedation if appropriate
6. Place a rolled sheet between the shoulders to help identify the landmarks, if appropriate (cervical spine cleared)
7. Secure the head in a vertical position to prevent movement of patient
8. Prepare the overlying cricothyroid area with 10% povidone-iodine solution
9. Direct light source to area
10. Adhere to universal precautions and sterile technique
11. Open the appropriate size tracheostomy tube onto the sterile field, check balloon for symmetric expansion and leaks
12. Respiratory therapist will set up ventilator with adaptors as indicated
13. Anesthetize the local area by intradermal and subcutaneous injections of 1% lidocaine
14. Initiate a transverse incision, 5 cm in length, approximately 2.5 cm above the suprasternal notch. Carry the incision through the platysma muscle with sharp dissection
15. Separate the anterior cervical musculature in the middle using blunt dissectione, open the pretracheal fascia, and enter the visceral compartment
16. Bluntly dissect the adipose mediastinal tissue from the anterior tracheal wall until the trachea can be clearly identified
17. Grasp the trachea with a tracheal hook or tenaculum and elevate
18. Place a second hook in the same position on the opposite side, further elevating it into the wound
19. Direct the hooks inferiorly to superiorly
20. Make a vertical incision in the second or third tracheal ring with a #15 blade
21. Palpate the innominate artery prior to tracheal incision
22. Introduce the tracheal spreader through the incision and open widely
23. Insert tracheostomy tube and remove obturator
24. Connect patient to ventilator
25. Inflate tracheal balloon slowly, until there is minimal air leak
26. Secure the tracheostomy tube, suction
27. Assess lung expansion, breath sounds
28. Control bleeding as indicated
29. Reassess patient
30. Obtain a postprocedure radiograph

FOLLOW-UP

1. Ventilate patient as indicated
2. Apply sterile dressing around insertion site
3. Do not use cotton filled flats and do not cut 4 × 4 gauze sponge. This may result in bits of fiber being aspirated.
4. Observe patient for pneumothorax
5. Place identical size and tape of tracheostomy tube at head of bed

DOCUMENTATION

Indication for procedure
Procedure, surgeon, and assistant
Size and type of tracheostomy tube
Amount of air needed to establish minimal occlusive volume
Ventilator setting
Radiology report of tube placement
Patient's tolerance and outcome of procedure

References

Hood M. Techniques in general thoracic surgery. Philadelphia: WB Saunders, 1985:39–44

Mims BC. Tracheostomy. In: Mancini ME, ed. Pocket manual of emergency nursing procedures. Toronto: BC Decker, 1988:25–28.

Persons CB. Critical care procedures and protocols: a nursing process approach. Philadelphia: JB Lippincott, 1987:255.

THORACENTESIS

Lisa B. Jones

PURPOSE

To remove pleural fluid and/or possibly air by means of a needle puncture through the chest wall into the pleural space. A needle thoracentesis may also be done to detect the presence of blood in the pleural space following chest trauma.

INDICATIONS

Hemothorax
Pneumothorax
Pleural effusion
Empyema
Hydrothorax

CONTRAINDICATIONS

None

POTENTIAL COMPLICATIONS

Lung damage or reaccumulation of fluid. (Symptoms may include blood-tinged sputum, persistent cough, respiratory distress, or subcutaneous emphysema.)
Mediastinal shift, if large amounts of fluid are removed. (Symptoms may include those of pulmonary edema or cardiac distress caused by a sudden shift in mediastinal contents to the side on which the thoracentesis was performed.)
Infection caused by contamination

EQUIPMENT

Small syringe and needle for local anesthesia
Local anesthetic drug
Syringe, 50 ml
Large bore aspirating needle
Three-way stopcock
Sterile tubing
Sterile specimen container
Sterile drapes
Materials for skin preparation
Small sterile dressing
Sterile gloves

PROCEDURE

1. Inform patient about procedure and indicate to patient the importance of remaining immobile
2. Position patient sitting upright with neck and dorsal spine flexed and arms and shoulders raised. This may be done by having patient sit on edge of bed and lean over a bedside table with arms folded under his head. If patient is unable to sit, place on the unaffected side with arm over head.
3. Expose entire chest and perform aseptic skin preparation. Drape.
4. Inject local anesthetic into intercostal space with a small gauge needle and syringe. (If fluid is present, the thoracentesis site is usually in the seventh or eighth intercostal space at the posterior axillary line. If air is in the pleural cavity, the site is usually in the second or third intercostal space at the midclavicular line.)
5. Advance the thoracentesis needle, attached to a 50-ml syringe and a three-way stopcock, and maintain constant suction on the syringe so it is apparent when the fluid pocket is reached
6. Attach sterile tubing to the other end of stopcock and connect tubing to a receptacle
7. When fluid is obtained, turn stopcock adapter open to receptacle for collection of fluid being aspirated. To reduce dangers of circulatory collapse or acute pulmonary edema, more than 1,200 ml should not be removed at one time.
8. During procedure, observe patient for difficulty in breathing, tightness in chest, tachypnea, tachycardia, vertigo, hypotension, cyanosis, and diaphoresis
9. After needle is withdrawn, apply pressure over puncture site and then apply a small sterile dressing
10. A needle thoracentesis may also be performed with only a needle and syringe to detect the presence of blood following trauma to chest

FOLLOW-UP

1. Place patient on unaffected side for 1 hour
2. Observe patient for tightness in chest, signs of shock (e.g., faintness, falling blood pressure, and weak rapid pulse), and indications of leakage at puncture site. Also observe patient for signs of lung damage or possible reaccumulation of fluid (blood-tinged sputum, cough, respiratory distress, and subcutaneous emphysema). Watch for indications of mediastinal shift toward the affected side and of pyogenic infection.
3. Frequently serum electrolyte blood studies are ordered
4. A chest film may also be ordered to determine effects of procedure

DOCUMENTATION

Respiratory status and vital signs prior to procedure
Patient and family teaching
Type of skin preparation
Times procedure initiated and completed
Type of anesthetic used and any allergic reactions
Total amount, color, and character of fluid removed
Any complications during procedure
Respiratory status (breath sounds) and vital signs following procedures
Any complications following procedures
Sterile dressing applied to site

References

Brunner L, Suddarth D. The Lippincott manual of nursing practice. Philadelphia: JB Lippincott, 1974:122

Jones L. Thoracentesis. In: Mancini ME, ed. Pocket manual of emergency nursing procedures. Toronto: BC Decker, 1988:21–24.

Luckman J, Sorenson K. Diagnosis and evaluation of the patient with a respiratory disorder. In: Luckman J, Sorenson K, eds. Medical-surgical nursing. 1st ed. Philadelphia: WB Saunders, 1974:865.

Tucker S. Patient care standards. St. Louis: CV Mosby, 1975:76.

TUBE THORACOSTOMY

Jorie Klein

PURPOSE

To re-establish negative pressure in chest; to reinflate lung; to evacuate fluid accumulation in chest.

INDICATIONS

Hemothorax
Pneumothorax
Pulmonary restrictions
Prophylaxis, in selected cases of suspected severe lung injury
Diagnostic and therapeutic approach to chest trauma is the same for children and adults. However, a child's chest wall is extremely compliant and allows energy to transfer to the intrathoracic structures, frequently without any evidence of injury on the internal chest wall. Tension pneumothorax or hemopneumothorax is not well tolerated by the child because of mobility of the mediastinal structures. This mobility also makes the child especially sensitive to flail segments.

CONTRAINDICATIONS

None

POTENTIAL COMPLICATIONS

Internal bleeding
Empyema (1–16% of cases develop empyema)
Damage to intercostal nerve, vein, or artery
Damage to mammaryn vessels
Mediastinal emphysema
Reoccurrence of pneumothorax

EQUIPMENT

Povidone-iodine (Betadine)
4 × 4 gauze sponges
Light source
Sedation if indicated
Lidocaine 1% without epinephrine, 20 ml
Syringe, 10 ml, 18- and 23-gauge needle
Chest tube, appropriate size
Chest drainage system, suction
Supplemental oxygen
Thoracostomy tray
Tape
Suture
    2–0, 30 silk cutting needle
    2–0, 30 silk with taper needle
    4–0, monofilament with noncutting needle
Gown, mask, gloves, goggles

PROCEDURE

1. Assess patient's airway, breathing, and circulation
2. Initiate management of life threatening injuries
3. Administer supplemental oxygen as needed
4. Establish intravenous access and ensure adequate fluid resuscitation
5. Obtain baseline arterial blood gas sampling
6. Identify need for thoracostomy
7. Assemble equipment
8. Test suction device
9. Have chest drainage system assembled
10. Identify patient's allergies
11. Explain procedure to patient
12. Place patient on cardiac monitor
13. Place patient in supine position with a sheet roll under affected side at shoulder
14. Place arm over head and restrain as indicated
15. Administer sedation, if indicated
16. Prepare the entire hemithorax with 10% povidone-iodine solution and sterile drape
17. Adhere to universal precautions
18. Maintain sterile environment, sterile field
19. Open chest tube onto sterile field
20. Open suture onto sterile field
21. Anesthetize the skin, subcutaneous tissue, periosteum, around the rib, and the pleura itself with 1% lidocaine
22. Make a 2-cm incision parallel to the inferior border of the rib
23. Carry the incision down through the subcutaneous tissue to the superficial fascia
24. Dissect a subcutaneous tunnel posteriorly and slightly superiorly toward the point of pleural penetration
25. Place the tube on the superior surface of the selected rib
26. Avoid the neurovascular bundle lying below the rib above
27. Enter the pleural space just over the superior margin of the lower rib
28. Use a Kelly clamp to enter the pleural space
29. Place the clamp on the superior margin of the rib and advance through the pleura
30. Spread the pleura open with the clamp, 1–2 cm
31. Confirm thoracic cavity penetration by digitally palpating the lung medially, the diaphragm inferiorly, and the empty space superiorly
32. Bluntly dissect adhesions
33. Grasp the tip of the thoracostomy tube with a Kelly clamp and direct into the pleural space
34. Ensure the tube is not introduced along the subcutaneous tissue
35. Advance the tube posteriorly to lie in the posterior thoracic sulcus
36. Place the tube deeply enough so that the proximal point of the catheter is well inside the pleural space
37. Connect the tube to a chest drainage system and begin suctioning at 20 cm

38. Suture the tube to the skin using a large nonabsorbable suture
39. Place a dry dressing around the tube site
40. Monitor and document the initial chest output
41. Obtain a postprocedure radiograph

FOLLOW-UP

1. Assess respiratory adequacy by observing for changes in respiratory rate or rhythm, symmetry of chest, use of accessory or intercostal muscles, or retractions
2. Auscultate for bilateral breath sounds and hyperresonance
3. Observe for onset of an increase in the presence of subcutaneous emphysema; this may indicate an air leak
4. Note any changes in level of consciousness or skin color
5. Monitor vital signs and chest drainage output every 15 minutes for the first hour, every 30 minutes for the second hour, then every hour until stable
6. Continue to monitor chest drainage every hour and document
7. Continue to reassess patient and intervene as indicated
8. Obtain postprocedure radiograph results

DOCUMENTATION

Initial assessment of patient
Indication for chest tube
Procedure and size of chest tube placed
Outcome of procedure and patient's response
Initial chest output
Ongoing respiratory assessment

References

American College of Surgeons. Advanced trauma life support. Chicago: American College of Surgeons, 1985:73

Graham JM, Mattox KL, Deal AC Jr. Penetrating trauma of the lung. J Trauma 1979; 19:665

Scott J. Tube thoracostomy. In: Mancini ME, ed. Pocket manual of emergency nursing procedures. Toronto: BC Decker, 1988:29–34.

ARTERIAL BLOOD SAMPLING

Janet Neff

PURPOSE

To provide database regarding status of whole body oxygenation, ventilation, and acid-base balance via arterial blood sampling.

INDICATIONS

Change in ventilatory effort or pattern
Change in ventilator settings
Altered tissue perfusion
Signs and symptoms of hypoxia
Periodic monitoring of effective hyperventilation in traumatic head injury
Desire to calculate alveolar-arterial oxygen gradient or oxygen consumption in patient with a pulmonary artery catheter
Validation of pulse oximetry oxygen saturation and corresponding PO_2

CONTRAINDICATIONS

Severe neurovascular deficit in extremity to be punctured for specimen

POTENTIAL COMPLICATIONS

Pain
Peripheral nerve injury
Hematoma
Pseudoaneurysm
Vascular compromise, distal tissue ischemia, and/or necrosis

EQUIPMENT

2 × 2 gauze sponges
Container of crushed ice (cooling prevents reduction in oxygen content related to leukocyte metabolism)
Patient identification label
Laboratory test slip (may be chemistry department or pulmonary function laboratory)
Towel or washcloth roll
Tape elasticized self-adhering bandage (Coban)
Lidocaine (Xylocaine) solution, 1%
25-gauge infiltrating needle
Tuberculin syringe
21- or 23-gauge 1–1.5 inch needle (smaller needles make it more difficult to visualize blood pulsation)
Sodium heparin injection (1000 units per milliliter) for use with glass syringe 5- to 10-ml glass syringe (glass syringes do not allow alteration of gases other than within the blood medium)
3-ml plastic syringe with lyophilized heparin, a dry coating of freeze dried heparin in syringe hub, barrel, and occasionally attached needle. (Plastic syringes have been shown over time to allow exchange of gases from within the plastic matrix of the barrel. As blood is cooled in the ice, its solubility coefficient changes, making the blood more accepting of oxygen molecules from the plastic matrix. Some facilities use plastic syringes to eliminate infection control concerns and in pediatric populations from which smaller volumes are drawn. Liquid heparin can change the pH level unless it is diluted with a sufficiently large volume of blood.)
Rubber plug for end of syringe
Iodophor and alcohol swabs
Gloves

PROCEDURE

1. Explain procedure to patient
2. Wash hands
3. Select the puncture site. The radial artery is generally preferred because of the usual presence of good collateral circulation through the ulnar artery. The brachial artery is easily accessible and larger. The femoral artery is used in the presence of shock, when the peripheral pulsations are too weak to find and successfully puncture the brachial or radial arteries.
4. When the radial artery is selected, Allen's test should be done except in the most emergent situations. This test verifies collateral circulation by the ulnar artery in the event that a thrombus develops in the radial artery after puncture. Compress the radial and ulnar arteries of the selected wrist. Ask the alert patient to make a fist and release it a few times to blanch the hand. (If patient is uncooperative or unconscious, a similar effect can be obtained by elevating the arm.) Release pressure from the ulnar artery only and check for redness in the thenar region of the hand, which indicates perfusion via the ulnar artery. If the hand remains blanched after ulnar artery release, that wrist should not be used for arterial puncture.
5. Prepare the site by cleansing with an iodophor and/or isopropyl alcohol swab. The femoral area needs special attention.
6. Hyperextend the wrist on a rolled towel or washcloth. For brachial artery puncture, the arm should be extended and the hand pronated.
7. Verify lack of allergy to anesthetic, and then draw 0.5 ml of 1% lidocaine without epinephrine into tuberculin syringe with 25-gauge needle. Explain to patient that a slight stick and sting will be experienced, but that it will numb the area for procedure. The lidocaine serves two purposes: first, to reduce pain and thereby avoid changes in ventilation during the procedure, and second, to reduce the incidence of arterial spasm.
8. Palpate puncture site for arterial pulsation and insert the 25-gauge needle subcutaneously but superficial to the artery, injecting 0.1 ml. Then slowly infiltrate more lidocaine into site, aspirating prior to injection to avoid intraarterial injection.

9. Prepare syringe with liquid heparin (not required if using plastic syringes with lyophilized heparin). Draw approximately 1 ml of heparin into syringe. Coat the syringe by pulling the plunger back and forth slowly. Then eject excess heparin, retaining only the heparin that fills the dead space of needle and needle hub.
10. Palpate the artery with index and middle finger and enter at a 45-degree angle with the needle bevel aimed up. Upon entering the artery, a spurt of blood should appear, and the blood should continue to pulsate into the syringe on its own. If the blood does not pulsate, you may have punctured a vein. If a flash of blood is not obtained, insert the needle further. If blood is still not obtained, pull the needle out slowly but remain in the subdermal space. (Sometimes both walls of the artery are punctured and, upon withdrawal, the blood will enter the syringe.) Redirect the needle angle when needle is almost withdrawn. Sometimes the needle will clot or get plugged during attempts at redirection. If arterial blood is still not obtained, withdraw the needle fully and apply pressure. Another site can be attempted.
11. When arterial blood is obtained, fill the syringe to laboratory specifications and smoothly withdraw the needle. Immediately apply firm pressure to the site with gauze. (An assistant is helpful.)
12. Visualize the syringe to check for air bubbles. If present, eject air and blood into gauze with syringe upright until the air is gone. Carefully remove the needle and cap the syringe with rubber plug. (With glass syringes, be careful not to let plunger drop out of barrel.) Rotate the syringe to mix the specimen well with the heparin to prevent clotting.
13. Label the syringe, immediately place in ice.
14. Maintain pressure to puncture site for 5–10 minutes or longer if the patient has a coagulation defect. Coban dressing may be applied snugly over a double folded 2 × 2 gauze but must be removed within a short time to avoid vascular compromise.
15. Complete the laboratory request slip indicating patient temperature, ventilator settings or respiratory rate and FIO_2 in spontaneously breathing patient, and time obtained. The maximal changes in blood gas parameters (per °C) are PO_2 (8%), PCO_2 (3%), and pH (0.014 units). Some authorities advocate reporting blood gas results without correction for body temperature, but most laboratories report the corrected value; therefore an accurate temperature is important. Temperature is one factor that shifts the oxyhemoglobin dissociation curve.
16. If there is uncertainty whether the sample is arterial, either redraw at a new site or draw a venous sample and have both samples analyzed.
17. Evaluate distal perfusion. Report abnormalities immediately.
18. Specimens drawn from arterial lines require withdrawal of "waste" blood to clear the line of fluid from the pressure bag that would dilute the sample and lead to erroneous readings. Volumes required are dependent on the type of equipment set-up.

FOLLOW-UP

1. Assess the site for hemorrhage or hematoma formation
2. Discontinue manual pressure once bleeding is controlled and monitor length of application of pressure bandages
3. Evaluate results of arterial blood gas sampling and report to physician. Institute changes necessary to improve oxygenation or ventilation.
4. Repeat arterial blood gas sampling may be indicated. Changes in arterial oxygen saturation and partial pressure following changes in FIO_2 are dependent on many variables, such as the initial PO_2 value, the degree of parenchymal disease, the tidal volume, functional residual volume, and diffusion. Wash-out (decrease of FIO_2) of oxygen takes longer than wash-in (increase of FIO_2).

DOCUMENTATION

Patient's tolerance of procedure
Dose of lidocaine administered
Time and site of arterial blood gas puncture
Ventilatory status at time of puncture
Neurovascular status of distal tissue pre and post procedure
Laboratory results of obtained specimen

References

Broughton JO. Assessment: respiratory system. In: Hudak CM, Gallo BM, Lohr T, eds. Critical care nursing. Philadelphia: JB Lippincott, 1986:261–282.

Luce JM, Tyler ML, Pierson DJ. Intensive respiratory care. Philadelphia: WB Saunders, 1984; 79–80.

Moran RF, Van Kessel A. Blood gas quality assurance. NSCPT Analyzer 1981; 11(1):18–26.

PROCEDURES: VENOUS/CIRCULATORY ACCESS

Military Anti-Shock Trousers
Peripheral Intravenous Access Exchange
Intraosseous Line

MILITARY ANTI–SHOCK TROUSERS

Erwin R. Thal
Jorie Klein

PURPOSE

To increase blood pressure and tissue perfusion by the application of external counter pressure; to tamponade further bleeding and stabilize fractures of the pelvis. Increased pressure is accomplished by increasing systemic resistance and afterload.

GARMENT

Consists of three compartments, one abdominal and two lower extremity compartments, each of which can be inflated or deflated independently.

INDICATIONS

Cardiac arrest secondary to hypovolemia
Hypotension (blood pressure < 80 mm Hg in adults, < 70 mm Hg in children)
Stabilization of pelvic fractures
Continued hemorrhage secondary to pelvic fracture
Hypotension secondary to spinal cord injury (neurogenic shock)

CONTRAINDICATIONS

Absolute

Congestive heart failure
Pulmonary edema
Cardiogenic shock (myocardial infarction or cardiac tamponade)
Cardiac injury
Suspected diaphragmatic injury

Relative

Impaired pulmonary function, such as pneumothorax and flail chest
Abdominal evisceration
Pregnancy

POTENTIAL COMPLICATIONS

Ischemia
Compartment syndrome
Increased bleeding attributable to elevation of blood pressure

EQUIPMENT

Military anti-shock trousers (MAST)
Blood pressure monitoring equipment

PROCEDURE

Prehospital Inflation

1. Ensure airway, breathing, and circulation are maintained
2. Obtain the patient's vital signs
3. Place the open MAST on the long backboard
4. Transfer the patient to the long board
5. Attach both leg and abdominal Velcro fasteners snugly, attach the tubing of all three compartments to the foot pump, and open the valves to the two extremities. Make certain the abdominal valve is closed.
6. Secure the patient on the long board
7. Reassess vital signs and obtain a physician's order for inflation, if necessary
8. Inflate the leg compartments of the MAST first. Inflate only enough to effect an increase in blood pressure to 100–110 mm Hg. If blood pressure does not respond, close valves to extremity and open abdominal valve. Inflate abdominal compartment unless contraindicated by chest injury.
9. Secure all valves in the closed position
10. Reassess blood pressure
11. Attempts to establish large bore intravenous lines for rapid fluid replacement should be made enroute to the hospital; transport should *not* be delayed

Hospital Inflation

1. Maintain patient's airway, breathing, and circulation
2. Ensure two large bore intravenous lines have been established
3. Identify indication for MAST
4. Place a nasogastric tube and Foley catheter prior to inflating the MAST suit. (A nasogastric tube should be placed in all pediatric trauma patients to decrease the risk of reflux emesis from the MAST suit.)
5. Place MAST under patient by log rolling patient
6. Inflate both legs of MAST suit and reassess blood pressure; if systolic BP is <100 mm Hg, inflate the abdominal compartment, unless contraindicated, and reassess blood pressure
7. Continue to monitor cardiac status and vital signs
8. Garment may be inflated to tamponade bleeding or to stabilize pelvic fractures

9. Obtain x-ray films through the MAST suit if the patient remains unstable
10. Continue to reassess the patient for injury and hemodynamic stability; intervene as indicated
11. Note and record the length of time the garment is inflated

Deflation

1. Assess airway, breathing, and circulation; intervene as indicated; obtain complete vital signs
2. Ensure two large bore intravenous lines have been established
3. Ensure blood is readily available for transfusion
4. Begin deflation with the abdominal compartment and closely monitor the patient's blood pressure. This should be done in small increments. Do *not* let all of the air out at one time. Do not cut the MAST suit
5. Reinflate the compartment if the systolic blood pressure drops below 20 mm Hg
6. After deflating the abdominal compartment, deflate each leg individually using the same technique as for the abdomen
7. Closely monitor the cardiac status and vital signs after deflation
8. Reassess patient
9. Evaluate for potential missed injuries to abdomen, pelvis, lower extremities, and back
10. Continue to monitor and reassess patient

FOLLOW-UP

Place MAST in appropriate place (i.e., Emergency Medical Services room for prehospital use)

DOCUMENTATION

Time and place of inflation (prehospital or at hospital)
Assessment and intervention
Time of deflation and total duration of inflation
Reassessment and vital signs during deflation
Where MAST was placed after removal
Continued assessment and intervention

References

American College of Surgeons. Advanced trauma life support. Chicago: American College of Surgeons, 1988.

Aphahamian C, Gessert G. MAST–associated compartment syndrome (MACS): a review. J Trauma 1989; 29(5).

Markouchick VJ. MAST suit. Moore E, Eiseman B, Van Way III C, eds. Critical decisions in trauma. St. Louis: CV Mosby, 1984:558–563.

Mattox K, Bickell W. Prospective MAST study in 911 patients. J Trauma 1989; 29(8):1104–1112.

McSwain N Jr. Pneumatic anti-shock garment: state of the art. Ann Emerg Med 1988; 17(5):506–519.

PERIPHERAL INTRAVENOUS ACCESS EXCHANGE

Jorie Klein

PURPOSE

To exchange a 20-gauge or larger peripheral intravenous catheter to a large bore (7 F or 8 F) sheath for rapid volume infusion.

INDICATIONS

Rapid volume infusion

CONTRAINDICATIONS

None (when used in patients who require rapid volume fluid infusion)

POTENTIAL COMPLICATIONS

Vessel wall perforation
Infiltration
Catheter embolism
Infection
Inadvertent arterial puncture
Nerve damage
Hematoma
Intravascular clotting and hemorrhage
Fluid overload
Foreign body (loss of the guidewire)
Vessel rupture

EQUIPMENT

Rapid infusion exchange set
Povidone-iodine solution
4 × 4 gauze (10-count package)
Suture
Large bore intravenous administration tubing
Warmed fluid

PROCEDURE

1. Prepare puncture site, indwelling intravenous catheter, and current intravenous administration tube connector with povidone-iodine solution
2. Place tourniquet approximately 12.5 cm above the current intravenous catheter
3. Disconnect the administration tubing from the current intravenous catheter
4. Insert the spring guidewire through the lumen of the catheter into the vein, maintaining a firm grip on the wire at all times
5. If resistance is encountered, hold the catheter in place and carefully withdraw the guidewire; attempt reinsertion
6. Remove the current intravenous catheter once the guidewire is inserted through the catheter into the vein
7. Thread the tapered tip of the dilator over the guidewire and advance to cutaneous puncture site
8. Enlarge the cutaneous puncture site with scalpel, if indicated

9. Grasp the skin and advance the dilator into the vessel with a twisting motion
10. Advance sheath over dilator into vessel using twisting motion
11. Remove the guidewire and dilator, holding the sheath in place (free blood flow indicates proper placement)
12. Attach Luer-Lok administration tubing to sheath hub
13. Use large bore tubing for rapid volume infusion
14. Release tourniquet
15. Secure wing of catheter hub with sutures
16. Apply povidone-iodine ointment to puncture site with small dressing
17. Administer warmed fluid to prevent hypothermia

FOLLOW-UP

1. Periodically assess site for infiltration or hematoma
2. Closely monitor intravenous fluid rate and urinary output
3. Assess temperature
4. Reassess patient

DOCUMENTATION

Size of exchange catheter and procedure
Rate of fluid administration
Type of fluid administered
Vital signs, intake, and output

INTRAOSSEOUS LINE

Patti Sutton-Dietrich

PURPOSE

To place a rigid needle through the bone cortex into the medullary cavity to establish a rapid vascular access in a child when an intravenous (IV) access is difficult or impossible in an emergency situation; to resuscitate a critically ill child with fluids and medications in a safe and effective manner.

INDICATIONS

Children in emergency situations in whom IV access cannot be established within 5 minutes (e.g., hypovolemic states, multiple trauma, burns, near drowning, seizures)

Children in extremis who do not have adequate vascular access and who need resuscitative measures

CONTRAINDICATIONS

Fracture of tibia
Burn at site
Infective process at site
Bone disorders

POTENTIAL COMPLICATIONS

Osteomyelitis
Obstructed needle
Improper placement of needle

EQUIPMENT

16- or 18-gauge hypodermic needle, spinal needle with stylet, or bone marrow needle
Povidone-iodine (Betadine/alcohol swabs)
10-ml syringe prefilled with normal saline
50-ml bag, normal saline
Buretrol
IV fluids as ordered
Central venous pressure dressing kit
1% lidocaine

Procedure

1. Wash hands using aseptic technique
2. Prepare site (anterior medial surface of the tibia below the epiphyseal plate)
3. Localize site if indicated
4. Restrain/immobilize extremity
5. Penetrate skin with needle, directing needle at a 15- to 30-degree angle toward the foot and away from the epiphyseal plate. Use a twisting downward pressure. When a pop is felt, the medullary cavity has been entered. The needle should stand upright without any support.
6. Remove stylet
7. Attach prefilled saline syringe and aspirate for bone marrow
8. Connect IV tubing and administer IV fluids and medications as needed. Fluid should be free flowing without signs of subcutaneous infiltration.
9. Secure needle and place a sterile dressing on site

FOLLOW-UP

1. Assess effectiveness of fluid/medication administration
2. Assess involved extremity for infiltration, infection, and circulatory complications
3. Initiate attempts for a more permanent venous access
4. Assess patient for signs/symptoms of infection after discontinuation of intraosseous line

DOCUMENTATION

Initial assessment of patient
Reason for procedure, including number of IV access attempts prior to intraosseous line
Size and type of needle used
Site used and assessment after initiation of intraosseous line
Type of fluids and medications infused
Response to treatment
Time and date of insertion and discontinuation of line

References

Brieg R. Emergency infusion of catecholamines into bone marrow. Am J Dis Child 1984; 138:810–811.

Kanter RK, Zimmerman JJ, Strauss RH, et al. Pediatric emergency intravenous access. Am J Dis Child 1986; 140:132–134.

Manley L, Haley K, Dick M. Intraosseous infusion: a rapid access for critically ill or injured infants and children. J Emerg Nurs 1988; 14:63–69.

Rosetti V, Thompson BM, Aprahamian C, et al. Difficulty and delay in intravascular access in pediatric arrests: abstract. Ann Emerg Med 1984; 13:406.

Rosetti VA, Thompson BM, Miller J, et al. Intraosseous infusions: an alternative route of pediatric intravascular access. Ann Emerg Med 1985; 14:885.

DIAGNOSTIC PROCEDURES

Arteriogram/Aortogram
Computed Tomography Scan
Diagnostic Peritoneal Lavage
Local Exploration
Magnetic Resonance Imaging
Pericardiocentesis
Paracentesis

ARTERIOGRAM/AORTOGRAM

Lisa B. Jones

PURPOSE

To detect vascular injury; to indicate abnormalities of blood flow attributable to arterial obstruction or narrowing.

INDICATIONS

Suspected arterial injuries caused by trauma
Suspected vascular insufficiency
Suspected intracranial arteriovenous malformation or aneurysm

CONTRAINDICATIONS

Allergy to dye used
Renal insufficiency
Recent cerebral vascular accident

POTENTIAL COMPLICATIONS

Allergic reaction to dye
Arterial injury during procedure
Bleeding
Renal failure

EQUIPMENT

Intravenous catheter and fluid monitoring equipment

PROCEDURE

1. Explain procedure to patient
2. Initiate intravenous fluids
3. Obtain consent and make arrangements with radiologist
4. Transport patient to radiology department for procedure

FOLLOW-UP

1. On return of patient, monitor vital signs every 15 minutes × 4, every 30 minutes × 4, every hour × 4, then every 4 hours.
2. Assess distal pulses for presence and equality with vital signs.
3. Observe site for bleeding and/or hematoma
4. Maintain intravenous fluids
5. Monitor intake and output
6. Instruct patient to remain in low Fowler's position for 6–8 hours after the procedure
7. Prepare patient for surgery if necessary

DOCUMENTATION

Patient teaching and consent
Time to and from radiology department
Vital signs as per follow-up
Pulses (before and after arteriogram)
Presence or absence of bleeding or hematoma from injection site

References

Brunner L, Suddarth D, eds. The Lippincott manual of nursing practice. Philadelphia: JB Lippincott, 1974:318.

Jones L. Arteriogram. In: Mancini ME, ed. Pocket manual of emergency nursing procedures. Toronto: BC Decker, 1988:178–179.

Martin-Paredro V. Risk of renal failure after major arteriography. Arch Surg 1983; 118:1417–1420.

Tucker S, ed. Patient care standards. St. Louis: CV Mosby, 1975:112.

COMPUTED TOMOGRAPHY SCAN

Molly A. Seaman

PURPOSE

To provide a mechanism for identifying occult injuries not seen clearly on examination or on routine radiographs.

INDICATIONS

Closed head injuries
Suspected cervical or thoracic injuries
Blunt abdominal trauma
Bony injuries

CONTRAINDICATIONS

Hemodynamic instability
Penetrating abdominal injuries

POTENTIAL COMPLICATIONS

Allergic reactions to contrast medium
Patient's condition may deteriorate because of delay in performing scan
Resuscitation efforts may be difficult because of space and patient's condition

EQUIPMENT

Scanner
Contrast
Emergency resuscitation equipment (i.e., intubation tubes, monitor/defibrillator, suction, neuroventriculostomy tray)

PROCEDURE

1. Ensure integrity of airway, breathing, and circulation (ABCs) prior to start of procedure
2. Remove metal objects (i.e., jewelry or electrode leads) that would interfere with visualization of suspected injury
3. Maintain intravenous access and monitor patient during procedure
4. If patient is conscious, attempt to explain the procedure quickly and simply. In addition, include family in discussions when possible.
5. Assist radiology technician in moving patient to table
6. Ensure patient is intubated during procedure
7. Patient with worsening neurologic status must be monitored closely during procedure to detect subtle or life threatening changes
8. After the procedure is completed, transport patient back to emergency department operating room as results indicate
9. Patients with contrast studies should receive fluids to facilitate excretion of medium (note: fluids should be given cautiously to the head injured patient)

FOLLOW-UP

1. Neurologic status of head injured patients must be monitored closely
2. Maintain ABCs and continue to monitor until definitive treatment is given
3. Monitor intake and output
4. Prepare patient for operating room and/or admission to appropriate area
5. Remember to keep family informed and updated on patient's condition

DOCUMENTATION

Assessment of patient before, during, and after procedure
Complications encountered or emergency treatment required
Patient's responses to treatment
Radiologist should document findings in patient's medical record

References

Bresler MJ. Computed tomography vs peritoneal lavage in blunt abdominal trauma. Top Emerg Med 1988; 10:59–73.
Mace SE. Emergency evaluation of cervical spine injuries: CT versus plain radiographs. Ann Emerg Med 1985.
Trunkey DD, Federle MP. Special diagnostic testing. In: Trunkey DD, Lewis FR, eds. Current therapy of trauma–2. Toronto: BC Decker, 1986:77–81.

DIAGNOSTIC PERITONEAL LAVAGE

Jorie Klein
Gregory G. Stanford

PURPOSE

To evaluate quickly, inexpensively, safely, and in a relatively simple surgical procedure the intra-abdominal space of patients who have sustained blunt abdominal trauma.

INDICATIONS

Patients who have a history of blunt abdominal trauma and who have an altered pain response attributable to head injury, alcohol or drug overlay, spinal cord injury, or mental retardation
Unexplained hypovolemia following multiple trauma
Suspected intra-abdominal injury associated with low rib fractures or trauma to the lower chest, flank, pelvis, or buttocks. To avoid false positive results, a supraumbilical approach may be indicated with pelvic fractures.
Patients with subsequent equivocal examinations
Carefully selected patients with penetrating stab wounds

CONTRAINDICATIONS

History of multiple abdominal operative procedures
Obvious indications for an exploratory laparotomy (free air, peritonitis)
Penetrating missile trauma
Gravid uterus in third trimester
Abdominal wall bleeding that produces a false positive result
Visceral damage
Perforating intra-abdominal injury

EQUIPMENT

Povidone-iodine solution
4 × 4 gauze sponges
Sterile gown, sterile gloves, mask, cap, goggles for two
Lidocaine 1% with epinephrine, 20 ml
Preparation tray
3-inch tape
Laboratory specimen tubes
Sedation, if indicated
Light source
Peritoneal lavage catheter (adult or pediatric as indicated)
Ringer's lactate, 500 ml or 1000 ml (pediatric patients, 10 ml/kg)
Intravenous (IV) tubing
Two 10-ml syringes
25-gauge, 1-inch needle
Two 18-gauge, 1-inch needles
Sterile towels
Peritoneal lavage tray (open or closed)
Closing suture material
Equipment to place nasogastric (NG) tube (if not placed)
Equipment to place Foley catheter (if not placed)
Restraints as indicated

PROCEDURE

1. Maintain patient's airway, breathing, and circulation; obtain baseline vital signs
2. Explain procedure to patient and family
3. Determine whether patient is allergic to povidone-iodine
4. Ensure NG tube is placed to decompress the stomach
5. Ensure Foley catheter is placed to decompress the bladder
6. Administer sedation as indicated
7. Restrain patient as indicated
8. Shave and prepare the abdomen margin to pubic area, flank to flank, and drape in a sterile manner
9. Anesthetize skin with lidocaine 1% with epinephrine
10. Direct light source

Open Procedure

11. Open lavage tray and establish sterile field
12. Open sterile lavage catheter onto sterile field
13. Open suture onto sterile field
14. Set up appropriate Ringer's lactate solution, keeping end of IV tubing sterile
15. Ensure sterile technique and universal precautions
16. Make a 3- to 4-cm infraumbilical longitudinal incision in the lower midline ring
17. Extend the incision through the subcutaneous tissue
18. Make a 1-cm vertical incision through the fascia, thereby exposing the underlying peritoneum
19. Grab the peritoneum between hemostats and open the peritoneum with a scalpel
20. Insert a standard peritoneal dialysis catheter through the peritoneum at a 45-degree angle toward the pelvis
21. Aspirate the catheter with a 10-ml syringe; if aspirate is gross blood, no further procedure is needed and the patient is prepared for a laparotomy
22. Connect the catheter tip and the Ringer's lactate infusion set
23. Infuse the appropriate amount of Ringer's lactate solution as rapidly as possible
24. Roll the patient from side to side, if possible
25. Drop the Ringer's lactate bag to the floor to facilitate the lavage fluid return by gravity siphonage
26. Remove the catheter after appropriate fluid return
27. Reapproximate the fascia with one or two sutures of O-Poly Prophylene
28. Close the skin primarily
29. Draw the appropriate laboratory specimens from the returned fluid and send to the laboratory for red blood cell count, white blood cell count with differential, amylase and other enzyme levels, and staining for bacterial and vegetable fiber
30. Apply a small band-aid dressing to the lavage site
31. Reassess the patient and obtain complete vital signs

Closed Technique

1. Steps 1–10 are the same
11. Open the peritoneal lavage kit and establish a sterile field
12. Open suture onto sterile field
13. Set up appropriate Ringer's lactate solution, keeping end of IV tubing sterile
14. Ensure sterile technique and universal precautions
15. Make a 3-mm skin nick with #11 surgical blade at the inferior ring
16. Insert the 18-gauge needle through the incision and advance into the peritoneal cavity at a 45-degree angle toward the pelvis. Two distinct "pops" should be felt as the needle penetrates the fascia and peritoneum
17. Introduce the floppy end of the guidewire through the needle and thread approximately half its length into the peritoneum. The guidewire should advance without resistance.
18. Remove the 18-gauge needle, keeping the guidewire in place
19. Advance the catheter over the guidewire with a twisting, pressing motion
20. Remove the guidewire
21. Aspirate the catheter with a 10-ml syringe; if the aspirate is gross blood, no further procedure is needed and the patient is prepared for a laparotomy
22. Connect the catheter tip and the Ringer's lactate infusion set
23. Infuse the appropriate amount of Ringer's lactate solution at a wide open rate
24. Roll the patient from side to side, if possible
25. Drop the Ringer's lactate bag to the floor to facilitate the fluid return by gravity siphonage
26. Remove the catheter after appropriate fluid return
27. Apply a small Band-Aid dressing to the skin nick
28. Draw the appropriate laboratory specimens from the returned fluid and send to the laboratory for a red blood cell count, white blood cell count and differential, amylase and other enzyme levels, and staining for bacterial and vegetable fiber
29. Reassess patient and obtain vital signs
30. Explain follow-up to patient and family

FOLLOW-UP

Positive Findings

1. Prepare patient and family for operative procedure
2. Obtain an operative and transfusion permit
3. Explain procedure and potential outcome to patient and family
4. Ensure operating room has been notified
5. Ensure patient has been admitted to the hospital
6. Continue to monitor and reassess patient
7. Ensure laboratory work is in the medical record

Negative Findings

1. Ensure patient has been admitted to the hospital
2. Explain admission to patient and family
3. Continue to monitor and re-evaluate patient

DOCUMENTATION

Procedure
Outcome
Patient's tolerance
Laboratory values
Disposition

References

American College of Surgeons. Advanced trauma life support. Chicago: American College of Surgeons, 1985:105–106.

Knezevich B. Nursing process in abdominal trauma. In: Holloway NM, ed. Emergency department nurses association. Core curriculum. Philadelphia: WB Saunders, 1985:5.

Moore E. Diagnostic peritoneal lavage. Moore E, Eiseman B, Van Way III C, eds. Critical decisions in trauma. St. Louis: CV Mosby, 1984:518–522.

Moore JB, et al. Diagnostic peritoneal lavage for abdominal trauma: superiority of the open technique at the infraumbilical ring. J Trauma 1981; 21:570.

Scott J. Peritoneal lavage. In: Mancini ME, ed. Pocket manual of emergency nursing procedures. Toronto: BC Decker, 1988:112–116.

LOCAL EXPLORATION

John D. S. Reid

PURPOSE

To distinguish patients with potentially serious penetrating injuries to the abdomen, flank, and lower back from those with superficial injuries by local exploration of the wound.

INDICATIONS

Stab wounds and lacerations to the anterior abdominal wall, flank, and lower back

CONTRAINDICATIONS

Gunshot or missile wounds
Clear indications for operative exploration
    Peritoneal signs
    Omental, visual evisceration
    Hemodynamic instability
Injuries above the costal margins (i.e., chest)
Neck injuries
Extremity injuries

POTENTIAL COMPLICATIONS

Hemorrhage from superficial vessels
Infection

EQUIPMENT

Mask, gloves, gown
Skin antiseptic
Sterile drape towels
4 × 4 gauze sponges
Syringe and needle for local anesthesia
Lidocaine (with epinephrine)
Hemostats
Scalpel
Thumb forceps
Retractors
Light source
Electrocautery (optional)
Saline for irrigation
Nonabsorbable sutures for skin

PROCEDURE

1. Expose and prepare the site of penetrating injury with skin antiseptic
2. Drape the area with sterile towels
3. Infiltrate the site with local anesthetic
4. Open and completely expose the tract of the penetrating injury
5. Assist with skin retraction and sponging of the wound as necessary
6. If the end of the tract is visualized and penetration of the abdominal cavity or vital organs has not occurred, the wound is debrided, irrigated with saline solution, and either closed or packed open as decided upon by the physician
7. If the end of the tract is not visualized or if there is penetration of the abdominal cavity, debride and close or pack the wound pending further investigations or operation

FOLLOW-UP

1. If the local exploration is negative, ensure that follow-up inspections of the wound for signs of infection and for suture removal occur
2. If the local exploration is positive, assist in arranging further investigations (i.e., peritoneal lavage, intravenous pyelogram, arteriography) or in alerting the operating room if surgery is planned
3. Ensure that tetanus immunization status is current

DOCUMENTATION

Allergies
Tetanus toxoid given, if appropriate
Type of skin preparations
Time of procedure
Complications of procedure
Sutures used
Dressing used

References

Knezevich BA, Carl L. Penetrating abdominal trauma. In: Knezevich BA, ed. Trauma nursing principles and practice. Norwalk, CT: Appleton-Century-Crofts, 1986:502–503.

Oreskovich MR, Carrico CJ. Stab wounds of the anterior abdomen. Ann Surg 1983; 198:411–419.

Thal ER. Evaluation of peritoneal lavage and local exploration in lower chest and abdominal stab wounds. J Trauma 1977; 17:642–648.

MAGNETIC RESONANCE IMAGING

Linda L. Wilson

PURPOSE

To show the relationship between vertebral bodies, disks, spinal cord, and nerve roots.

INDICATIONS

Questionable spinal cord trauma (without fracture)
Spinal cord fracture (magnetic resonance imaging secondary to computed tomography)

CONTRAINDICATIONS

Pacemaker
Metal prostheses in region of interest
Ferromagnetic aneurysm clips
Fragments of metal in eye
Nonremovable dental prosthesis
Body weight exceeding table limit

POTENTIAL COMPLICATIONS

Potential claustrophobic behavior

EQUIPMENT

Sedation, if needed
Magnetic resonance imaging compatible monitor

PROCEDURE

1. Explain procedure and the importance of remaining immobile to patient
2. Screen patient for any ferromagnetic objects (i.e., cranial aneurysm clips, foreign intraocular metal)
3. Premedicate, if necessary
4. Connect patient to monitor
5. Ensure patient/personnel have removed any ferromagnetic objects (i.e., hemostats, watches, beepers, credit cards,)
6. Transport patient to table (using backboard if necessary)
7. Position patient for type of scan ordered
8. Monitor patient's vital signs during procedure

FOLLOW-UP

Continue to monitor vital signs

DOCUMENTATION

Medication(s) administered and amount(s)
Vital signs and patient's response
Follow-up treatment and instructions

References

Bushong S. Magnetic resonance imaging: physical and biological principles. St. Louis: CV Mosby, 1988:308–335.
Shellock F. MR imaging of metallic implants and material: a complication of the literature. Am J Radiol 1988, 151:811–814.

PERICARDIOCENTESIS

Lisa B. Jones

PURPOSE

To remove fluid or blood from the pericardial sac.

INDICATIONS

Suspected cardiac tamponade with hemodynamic compromise

Appropriate treatment for a trauma patient who presents with clinical signs of a cardiac tamponade is a thoracotomy. Pericardiocentesis is helpful in establishing the diagnosis of a suspected cardiac tamponade and in alleviating hemodynamic compromise until a thoracotomy can be performed. It is not intended as a definitive treatment. A subxyphoid pericardial exploration is a better diagnostic study in suspected cardiac tamponade.

CONTRAINDICATIONS

Previous pericardial exploration

POTENTIAL COMPLICATIONS

Puncture wound to the heart
Cardiac arrhythmias
Puncture of lung, stomach, liver
Laceration of coronary artery or myocardium
Recurrence of tamponade

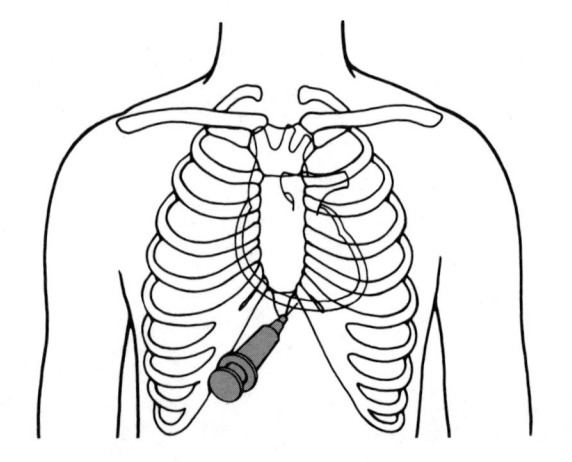

Figure 1 Needle placement for pericardiocentesis. Needle is advanced until fluid is obtained. (From Jones LB. Pericardiocentesis. In: Mancini ME, ed. Pocket manual of emergency nursing procedures. Toronto: BC Decker, 1988:70.)

EQUIPMENT

Medication for sedation
Povidone-iodine solution
Lidocaine 1%, 10 ml
Small syringe and needle for local anesthesia
Sterile drapes and gloves
2- to 3-inch 16- to 18-gauge cardiac needle with a short bevel
Stopcock
50-ml syringe
Cardiac monitor
Defibrillator
Small dressing
Hemostat
Gowns, gloves, mask, goggles

PROCEDURE

1. Explain procedure to patient if time allows
2. Sedate, if indicated
3. Ensure patient is attached to cardiac monitor
4. Ensure defibrillator equipment is at bedside and functioning
5. Prepare the skin just below the costal margin adjacent to the xyphoid and apply sterile drapes
6. Ensure sterile technique and universal precautions are followed
7. Inject lidocaine for local anesthesia as time allows
8. Attach the needle to the stopcock and 50-ml syringe
9. Insert the needle and advance slowly at a 45-degree horizontal angle under the ribs, directing it toward the midpoint of the left clavicle (Fig. 1)
10. Apply gentle suction on the barrel of the syringe
11. Stabilize the needle when fluid is returned by attaching a hemostat at the skin surface. This will prevent inadvertent penetration and injury to the ventricular wall.
12. Monitor the cardiac status throughout procedure. Elevation of the ST segment in a typical injury pattern may indicate contact with the myocardium
13. Remove all fluid from the pericardium. Substantial hemodynamic improvement will be seen with removal of 20 to 50 ml of blood.
14. Observe the blood. Pericardial blood does not clot, whereas blood obtained from inadvertent puncture of one of the heart chambers does clot
15. Prepare patient for an immediate thoracotomy if findings are positive
16. Leaving the needle secured in place with the stopcock and syringe attached may be indicated, depending on the availability of an immediate thoracotomy
17. Remove the needle upon negative findings
18. Reassess patient and obtain vital signs
19. Continue to evaluate patient
20. Document procedure and outcome
21. Document the amount of fluid removed from the pericardium

FOLLOW-UP

Positive Findings

1. Prepare patient for immediate operative intervention; notify operating suite
2. Obtain an operative and transfusion consent
3. Notify thoracic surgeon if indicated
4. Continue to monitor cardiac status and vital signs
5. Intervene with management to ensure airway, breathing, and circulation are maintained
6. Explain procedure to patient and family, if time allows

Negative Findings

1. Continue to monitor cardiac status and vital signs
2. Intervene with management to ensure airway, breathing, and circulation are maintained
3. Assess for other complications such as arrhythmias
4. Continue to re-evaluate patient

DOCUMENTATION

Visible signs of tamponade, as well as cardiac status and vital signs prior to procedure
Indication for the procedure
Allergies, and all medications used
Type of skin preparation
Time procedure initiated and completed
Physician who performed procedure
Total amount and type of fluid aspirate and whether blood clots
Any complications during or after procedure
Cardiac status and vital signs during and after procedure
Patient's disposition

References

Baxt W, ed. Trauma—the first hour. Norwalk, CT: Appleton-Century-Crofts, 1985:121.
Brunner L, Suddarth D. The Lippincott manual of nursing practice. 1st ed. Philadelphia: JB Lippincott, 1974:243.
Jones LB. Pericardiocentesis. In: Mancini ME, ed. Pocket manual of emergency nursing procedures. Toronto: BC Decker, 1988:68–71.
Sabiston D Jr, ed. Textbook of surgery. 12th ed. Philadelphia: WB Saunders, 1981:2168.

PARACENTESIS

Lisa B. Jones

PURPOSE

To remove accumulated fluid from abdominal cavity (a needle paracentesis can be done to detect intra-abdominal hemorrhage attributable to abdominal trauma).

INDICATIONS

Ascites
Suspected intra-abdominal hemorrhage attributable to abdominal trauma

CONTRAINDICATIONS

Gunshot wound to abdomen
Obstructed or distended loops of bowel

POTENTIAL COMPLICATIONS

Infection
Bleeding attributable to vessel trauma
Penetration of bowel
Shock and hypovolemia caused by fluid shifts from the general circulation to the abdomen in an attempt to replace removed fluid
Puncture of urinary bladder
Mesenteric or rectus sheath hematoma

EQUIPMENT

Skin antiseptic
Sterile drapes and gloves
Small needle and syringe for local anesthetic
Local anesthetic drug
Large bore, short beveled spinal needle
Syringe
Three-way stopcock
Sterile tubing
Sterile specimen container
Small sterile dressing

PROCEDURE

1. Inform patient of procedure
2. Have patient empty bladder or insert Foley catheter
3. Position patient in Fowler's position
4. Expose, cleanse, and drape abdomen
5. Administer local anesthetic
6. Needle paracentesis is done with patient in supine position. Needle is connected to syringe and suction is applied as needle is advanced slowly into the abdomen in four quadrants. Return of nonclotting blood is a positive result.
7. For removal of large accumulations of peritoneal fluid, a three-way stopcock is attached between needle and syringe, with sterile tubing connected to the other end of the stopcock. The tubing is connected to a sterile container.
8. Needle (intravenous catheter may be used, with needle removed after insertion, and catheter left in place) is then advanced by physician below the umbilicus, with suction applied to syringe, until fluid is obtained
9. The stopcock is then turned open to the tubing, and fluid is slowly drained into the container, which is placed below patient
10. Observe patient during procedure for pallor, cyanosis, syncope, and other signs of shock as well as pulse and respiratory status
11. Apply dressing when catheter is removed

FOLLOW-UP

1. Place patient in comfortable position
2. Record amount and kind of fluid removed
3. Monitor patient's vital signs frequently
4. Notify operating room if blood is obtained during needle paracentesis, because surgery is necessary to locate and repair injury

DOCUMENTATION

Patient and family teaching done
Type of skin preparation and anesthetic
Total amount, color, and character of fluid removed
Any complication during procedure
Vital signs following procedure
Any complications following procedure
Sterile dressings applied to site
Results of needle paracentesis

References

Brunner L, Suddarth D, eds. The Lippincott manual of nursing practice. 4th ed. Philadelphia: JB Lippincott, 1986:437.
Jones L. Paracentesis. In: Mancini ME, ed. Pocket manual of emergency nursing procedures. Toronto: BC Decker, 1988:109–111.
Luckman J, Sorenson K. Medical-surgical nursing. Philadelphia: WB Saunders, 1974:1121.
Sabiston D Jr, ed. Textbook of surgery. 12th ed. Philadelphia: WB Saunders, 1981:378.
Shires GT. Care of the trauma patient. New York: McGraw-Hill, 1979:293.

MONITORING

Arterial Line Insertion
Intracranial Pressure Monitoring
Pulse Oximetry
Pulmonary Artery Catheter Insertion

ARTERIAL LINE INSERTION

Nancy G. Brown

PURPOSE

To monitor systemic arterial pressure rapidly and to obtain direct access for analysis of arterial blood.

INDICATIONS

Diagnosis, treatment, and prevention of inadequate tissue perfusion

CONTRAINDICATIONS

Severe peripheral vascular disease
Lack of collateral circulation (ulnar)

POTENTIAL COMPLICATIONS

Hemorrhage
Air embolism
Thrombosis
Hematoma
Infection
Arterial spasm
Discomfort

EQUIPMENT

Skin preparation solution
Local anesthetic with syringe and needle
Sterile gloves and towel
Suturing material and needle holder
Systemic arterial catheter
High-pressure tubing with irrigation of 3 ml per hour or less
High-pressure bag
Transducer
Hemodynamic monitor
Heparin flush solution
Sterile occlusive dressing

PROCEDURE

1. Explain procedure to patient and/or family
2. Perform Allen's test prior to radial artery catheter insertion
3. Obtain baseline cuff blood pressure
4. Connect the equipment securely and in a sterile manner
5. Flush pressure tubing to remove all air bubbles
6. Calibrate hemodynamic monitor
7. Expose site and prepare skin with antiseptic
8. Assist physician with gloving, local anesthesia, and placement of open sterile arterial catheter
9. After catheter placement is established, connect catheter to pressure tubing, then flush tubing and display waveform on monitor
10. Identify appropriate wave form and record blood pressure
11. Assist physician with suturing of catheter if necessary and apply sterile occlusive dressing
12. Label tubing for proper line identification

FOLLOW-UP

1. Balance and calibrate the transducer every 8 hours or as indicated. Remove any identified air bubbles and keep tubing free of kinds.
2. Immobilize the extremity if necessary. Compare systemic arterial line blood pressure to cuff blood pressure every 8 hours and when required.
3. Observe monitor for appropriate waveform and troubleshoot, as required. Assess pulses, color, sensation, and temperature distal to insertion site every 2–4 hours.
4. Assess for swelling, ecchymosis, bleeding, and signs and symptoms of infection at insertion site every 2–4 hours and as required.
5. Inquire regarding any pain distal to insertion site
6. Set monitor alarm limits appropriate to patient's baseline blood pressure and current status
7. Change sterile dressing every 24 hours and pressure tubing every 24–72 hours.

DOCUMENTATION

Date, time, location, size, and who inserted catheter
Color, temperature, sensation, and pulse distal to catheter every 2–4 hours
Appropriate waveform at beginning of shift and if any changes occur
Date, time, and site condition with each dressing change
Site check at beginning of shift and every 2–4 hours.

References

Demling RH, Wilson RF. Decision making in surgical critical care. Toronto: BC Decker, 1988:53.
Halfman-Franey M. Current trends in hemodynamic monitoring of patients in shock. Crit Care Q 1988; 2:9–17.
Holloway NM. Nursing the critically ill adult. Menlo Park, CA: Addison Wesley, 1979:26–35.

INTRACRANIAL PRESSURE MONITORING

Kendra Ellis

PURPOSE

To monitor continually patients with a neurologic injury who are at risk for elevated intracranial pressure impeding an optimal cerebral functioning; to assist with an early diagnosis of elevated intracranial pressure and to calculate cerebral perfusion pressure; to evaluate medical and nursing interventions aimed at reducing intracranial pressure to maintain adequate cerebral blood flow.

INDICATIONS

Patients who have a history of head trauma and who have altered level of consciousness
Neurologic injury such as subarachnoid hemorrhage, space occupying lesion, stroke, or children with Reye's syndrome
Hydrocephalus
Encephalitis

CONTRAINDICATIONS

Existence of significant coagulopathy

POTENTIAL COMPLICATIONS

Infection, such as meningitis
Cerebral spinal fluid leak

EQUIPMENT

Portable intracranial pressure monitor
Preamp cable
Zero adjuster
Povidone-iodone scrub brushes
Lidocaine with epinephrine
Razors
Gown, gloves, masks, caps for two
Closing suture material
Sterile towels, sheets
Sedation (if needed)
Scalpel
Twist drill
Fiberoptic catheter
Sterile 4 x 4 gauze sponges
Ventriculostomy tray
Silk tape for occlusive dressing

PROCEDURE

1. Secure portable pressure monitor to bedside pole, plug in, and turn power on by moving switch to the up position
2. Connect preamp cable to extension cable
3. Press start/stop button; "888" should be displayed followed by another 3-digit number
4. Firmly connect transducer to preamp connector; display will read "—"
5. Prior to insertion of catheter, use adjustment tool to make display read "0 ± 1" by turning zero adjustment on button of transducer connector. Never adjust the zero once catheter is in vivo.
6. No leveling of transducer is necessary because the transducer is at the end of the catheter
7. If portable monitor is attached to a bedside monitor via cable, calibrate the portable monitor to the bedside monitor by pressing and holding "*" on monitor while zeroing the bedside monitor
8. Place patient in a supine position, with the head of the bed up
9. Shave the insertion site
10. Perform a 10-minute scrub with the povidone-iodine brushes
11. Assist physician with drilling a burr hole in the frontal area
12. Assist physician with assuring correct placement by performing the halo test using the aspiration or reflux of cerebral spinal fluid
13. Assist with placing a sterile, occlusive dressing around the catheter site

FOLLOW-UP

1. Document intracranial pressures
2. Calculate the cerebral perfusion pressure (mean arterial pressure minus intracranial pressure) normal 80–100 mm Hg, minial 60 mm Hg for adequate cerebral blood flow)
3. If connected to the bedside monitor, note the intracranial pressure waveform

References

Hollingsworth-Fridlund P, et al. Use of fiberoptic pressure transducer for intracranial pressure measurements: a preliminary report. Heart Lung 1988; 17(2):111–119.
Pollack-Latham C. Intracranial pressure monitoring. Part I: Physiologic principles. Crit Care Nurse 1988; 7(5):40–51.
Pollack-Latham C. Intracranial pressure monitoring. Part II: patient care. Crit Care Nurse 1988; 7(5):53–71.
Weiss M, et al. The technique of intracranial pressure monitoring. J Crit Illness 1987; 2(9):83–90.
Yano M, et al. Useful ICP monitoring with subarachnoid catheter method in severe injuries. J Trauma 1988; 28(4):476–479.

PULSE OXIMETRY

Betty M. Clark

PURPOSE

To provide noninvasive, instantaneous, and continuous measurement of arterial oxygen saturation.

INDICATIONS

Diagnostic and interventional procedures
Bronchoscopy and other endoscopic procedures
Airway management and endotracheal intubation
Central line placement
Suctioning and other routine nursing procedures
Ventilation
  Pressure-support ventilation
  Inverse-ratio ventilation
  High-frequency ventilation
  Weaning from mechanical ventilation
Patients who require a high fraction of inspired oxygen (FiO_2) because of
  Ventilation/perfusion mismatch
  Shunt
  Alveolar hypoventilation
  Impaired diffusion
Position changes may result in desaturation in patients with asymetric lung disease, refractory hypoxemia, significant ascites, or hemodynamic instability
Recovery from anesthesia in the postanesthesia recovery unit or in the intensive care unit
Titration of inotropic agents, vasopressors, and vasodilators in patients who have a low mixed venous oxygen tension and consequent arterial hypoxemia
Patients who receive muscle relaxants
Transportation of critically ill patients to and from the intensive care unit
Patients with relative or absolute contraindications to invasive oxygenation monitoring; such as impaired vascular access, coagulation disorders, or immunosuppression

CONTRAINDICATIONS

None

POTENTIAL COMPLICATIONS

Pressure sores or blisters may develop at the sensor site, particularly if circulation is compromised or edema is present. Assess skin every 2–4 hours during monitoring.

EQUIPMENT

Pulse oximeter
Sensor

PREPARATION

No calibration of the equipment is required. The diodes are precalibrated and coded during manufacturing. Calibration checks are performed internally and automatically.
No skin preparation for placement of the sensor is necessary. Skin pigmentation, nail polish, or dirty skin do not interfere with the accuracy. (Note: opaque nail coatings may decrease light transmission, rendering the oximeter inoperable. Certain blue nail polishes have strong absorption bands that may result in false low readings.)

PROCEDURE

1. Apply the sensor on an extremity without an arterial catheter or blood pressure cuff that would either continuously or intermittently reduce the arterial blood flow distally
2. Attach the sensor to the pulse oximeter
3. Adjust appropriate alarms for patient

FOLLOW-UP

None

DOCUMENTATION

Pulse oximetry data per unit standards
Sensor site every 2–4 hours
Impact of treatment modalities and interventions

References

Alexander CM. Principles of pulse oximetry: theoretical and practical considerations. Anesth Analg 1989; 68:368–78.
Daily EK, Schroeder JS. Techniques in bedside hemodynamic monitoring. St. Louis: CV Mosby, 1989:208–213.
Szalflarski NL, Cohen NH. Use of pulse oximetry in critically ill adults. Heart Lung 1989; 18:444–454.

PULMONARY ARTERY CATHETER INSERTION

Johnese Spisso

PURPOSE

To monitor hemodynamic indices, intravascular volume status, and cardiac output through continuous periodic measurements of pulmonary artery (PA) pressure, pulmonary capillary wedge pressure (PCWP), and cardiac output determinations.

INDICATIONS

Medical treatment in patients with suspected cardiopulmonary dysfunction (congestive heart failure, cardiogenic shock, myocardial infarction, myocarditis, and cardiomyopathy)

Complicated surgical procedures that require monitoring of fluid volume shifts in response to fluid administration and pharmacologic agents

Hypovolemic and/or pulmonary disorders associated with shock or trauma (septic shock, hypovolemic shock, adult respiratory distress syndrome, multisystem organ failure)

CONTRAINDICATIONS

Neonates and infants, unless insertion is performed under fluoroscopy

Patients with cardiomyopathy and/or pre-existing cardiac disease may require procedure to be performed under fluoroscopy

POTENTIAL COMPLICATIONS

Pulmonary artery infarction
Pulmonary artery rupture
Infection
Cardiac dysrhythmias
Air embolus
Systemic thrombus and/or embolus

EQUIPMENT

Povidone-iodine solution
Sterile drapes
Sterile gowns
Sterile gloves
Masks
Thermodilution pulmonary artery catheter/introducer
High-pressure tubing with fluid delivery rate of 3 ml per hour or less
High-pressure bag (300 mm Hg capacity)
Transducer
Hemodynamic monitor
500 ml bag of 0.9% normale saline or 5% dextrose in H_2O with 500–1000 units of heparin
Syringes
4 × 4 gauze sponges
Local anesthetic (2% lidocaine without epinephrine)
Emergency antiarrhythmics (lidocaine/atropine)
2–0 silk suture
Needle holder
Occlusive dressing

PROCEDURE

1. Explain procedure to patient and family
2. Ensure continuous cardiac monitoring
3. Assemble equipment
4. Prime hemodynamic pressure tubing and ascertain waveform set-up on hemodynamic monitor
5. Position patient supine
6. Assist the physician with sterile gowning, drapery, and preparation of insertion site (subclavian, internal jugular, femoral, or brachial artery)
7. Open sterile equipment (pulmonary artery catheter, introducer, suture, needle holder) onto sterile field
8. Connect hemodynamic pressure tubing to pulmonary artery catheter and flush catheter with heparinized solution prior to insertion
9. After catheter introducer has been inserted into vessel and pulmonary artery catheter is flushed with heparinized solution, prepare waveform display on monitor and zero and calibrate transducer to atmospheric pressure. Inflate/deflate balloon port with 1.5 ml of air to ensure integrity of balloon.
10. Continuously assess patient during flotation of the pulmonary artery catheter for ventricular dysrhythmias, chest pain, and shortness of breath. Have emergency medications and resuscitation equipment available at bedside.
11. Identify waveforms, then measure and record filling pressures as catheter passes through the right atrium, right ventricle, and pulmonary artery
12. Once the catheter is in the pulmonary artery, inflate balloon with 1.5 ml of air and observe and record waveform changes indicative of wedge pressure. Deflate balloon promptly and ascertain whether waveform has returned to PA pressure.
13. Assist physician with suturing of catheter and secure with sterile occlusive dressing
14. Ensure continuous fluid administration via multilumen ports to maintain patency
15. Confirm catheter placement by chest film

FOLLOW-UP

1. Re-zero and calibrate the transducer and complete a hemodynamic profile including PA pressure, PCWP, central venous pressure (CVP), cardiac output, and systemic/pulmonary vascular resistance

2. Monitor PA pressure, PCWP, and CVP every 2–4 hours or as required. Monitor cardiac index/cardiac output every 4 hours and as required.
3. Obtain mixed venous blood gas studies as indicated to determine intrapulmonary shunts, O_2 content, and O_2 consumption
4. Assess cardiac and respiratory status
5. Assess catheter insertion site for redness, edema, or exudate. Change sterile dressing every 24 hours. Change hemodynamic tubing every 24–48 hours.
6. Continuously assess pulmonary artery waveform for changes in configuration, including right ventricular migration, permanent wedge position, and dampened waveform
7. Assess catheter for cracks, open ports, patency of multilumens, and inability to wedge balloon

DOCUMENTATION

Record PA pressure, PCWP, CVP, and quality of waveform every 2–4 hours.

Record integrity/assessment of catheter insertion site and patency of catheter ports

Record response to treatment modalities and interventions

References

Shires TT. Postoperative fluid management. In: Shires GT, ed. Principles of trauma care. 3rd ed. New York: McGraw-Hill, 1985:477–483.

Valy T, Linberg S. Clinical management concepts. In: Cardona V, Hurn PP, Mason PJ, Schlipp AM, Veise-Berry SW. Trauma nursing resuscitation through rehabilitation. Philadelphia: WB Saunders, 1988:178.

THERAPEUTIC PROCEDURES

Pneumatic Pressure Device
Temporary Access for Catheter Hemodialysis
Cervical Spine Traction/Stabilization
Temperature Control Units
Wound Dressing
Steinmann Pin
Thomas/Hare Traction Splint

Closed Reduction
Cast Care
Contact Lens Removal
Eye Irrigation
Helmet Removal
Corset-Type Extrication Devices

PNEUMATIC PRESSURE DEVICE

Connie Mattice

PURPOSE

To prevent deep vein thrombosis (DVT) and pulmonary embolism. Pneumatic compression stockings are designed to support by maintaining compression of veins and capillaries. The constant compression forces blood into larger vessels, thus promoting venous return and preventing circulatory stasis. Venous stasis is the major contributing factor to thromboembolism formation. The critical time for thrombosis development in surgical patients is between anesthesia induction and the first 72 hours. The most efficient use of compression devices to promote optimal venous return is to apply them preoperatively, 8–12 hours prior to the procedure or a time that allows maximal use prior to procedure.

INDICATIONS

Prior history of varicosities, DVT, or pulmonary embolism
Over 40 years of age and especially over 60 years of age
Patients who cannot receive anticoagulants for prevention of clots
Certain types of surgical procedures, as follows:
  Orthopaedic
  Neurologic
  Extensive abdominal
  Genitourinary
  Extensive vascular
  Extensive thoracic
Procedures greater than 2 hours in length
Obese patients
Patients with suspected or apparent malignancy
Patients taking oral contraceptives

CONTRAINDICATIONS

Any local condition of existing vascular problems with which sleeves would interfere, including
  Dermatitis
  Vein ligation (immediate postoperative)
  Gangrene
  Recent skin graft
Severe arteriosclerosis or other ischemic vascular disease
Massive edema of legs or pulmonary edema from congestive heart failure
Extreme deformity of the legs
Suspected pre-existing DVT

POTENTIAL COMPLICATIONS

For optimal use, sequential compression devices should be applied on an alert patient
Evaluate for numbness, tingling, or discomfort prior to and 1 hour postfitting

EQUIPMENT

Measuring tape
Compression sleeves and unit
  Knee length (one size fits all)
  Thigh length (measure thigh)
Antiembolism stockings

PROCEDURE

1. Apply antiembolism stockings per procedure. (For optimal benefit of the sequential compression device, antiembolism stockings are recommended.)
2. Measure circumference of thigh at gluteal fold to confirm correct size of sleeves
3. Remove sleeves from plastic packaging and unfold
4. Place the patient's leg on the white side of the sleeve with the blue line centered directly behind the patient's knee (popliteal fossa) (Fig. 1A).
5. Starting at the side without the Velcro tape (Fig. 1B), wrap the sleeve snugly around the patient's leg; secure the thigh section first, then the lower leg section. Attach the Velcro tape securely to the sleeve. Note: The sleeve should fit snugly but not too tightly.
6. Plug each sleeve connector into the mating connector of the tubing assembly that leads to the control unit (Fig. 1C). Make sure that all connectors are unkinked. Align arrows on connectors and depress the latches on the sides of the connectors. Push the connectors firmly together; a click or snap sound is heard as the connection is made.
7. Turn on control unit
8. To uncouple the connectors, depress the latches and pull the connectors apart

FOLLOW-UP

1. Remove twice daily and as needed for bathing to assess skin and circulation status of lower extremities and patient comfort. Note skin condition, capillary refill, numbness, tingling of limb, plantar flexion, dorsal flexion, and pain (p).
2. Adjust pressure for compression unit to specified levels. Pressure should be highest in the ankle and decrease as it cycles to calf and thigh. High pressure alarms will activate even if the alarms are off.
3. Use compression devices until ambulation to prevent thrombosis.

DOCUMENTATION

Time and date of application
Type of sleeve used

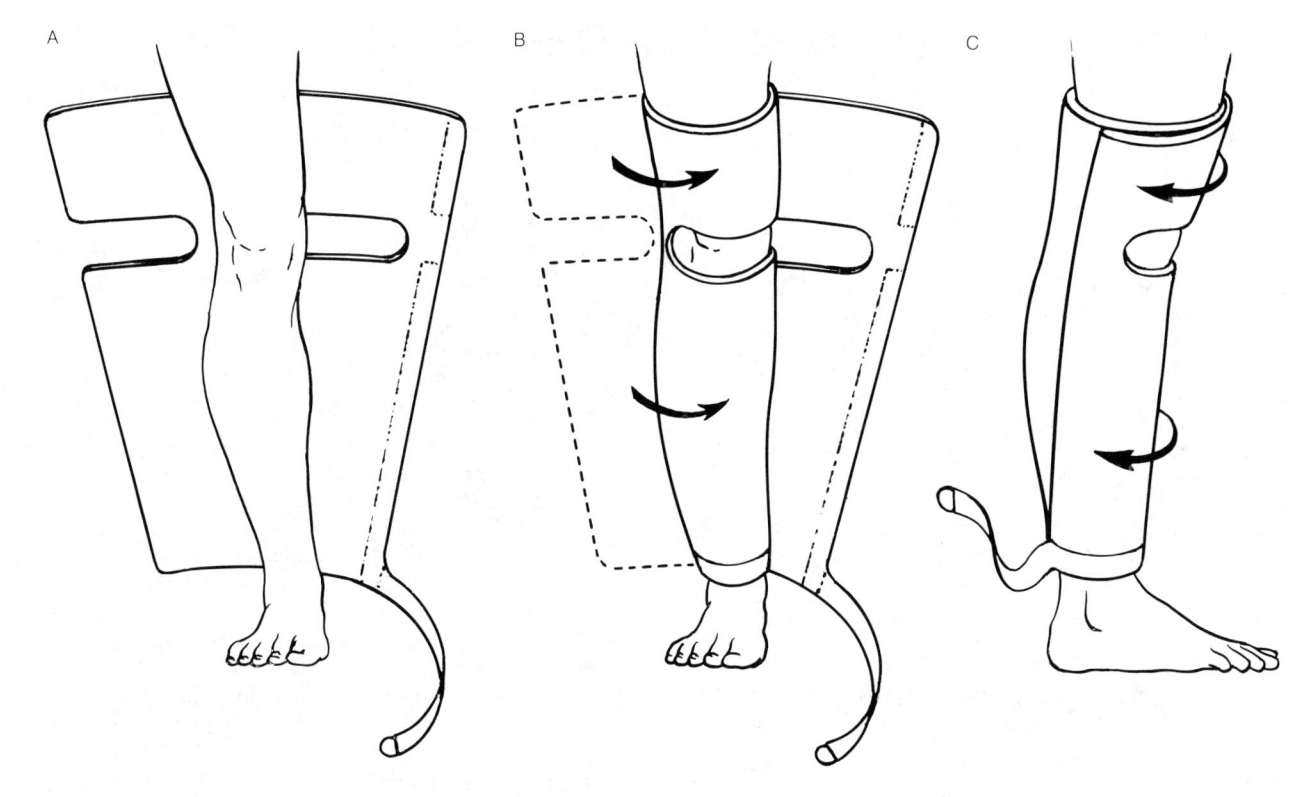

Figure 1 *A–C*, Application of antiembolism stockings. See text for detailed explanation.

To what limbs it was applied
Pressure readings
Patient's response
Time and reason for removal
Daily assessment of extremities, including removal for bathing and care

References

Barthe E. Pneumatic compression prevents deep vein thrombosis. Am J Surg 1988; 156:16B

Calditz GA, Tuden RL, Oster G. Rates of venous thrombosis after general surgery: combined results of randomized clinical trials. Lancet 1986; 19:143–146.

Inada KJ, Koike S, Shirai N. Matsumoto J, Hirose M. Effects of intermittent pneumatic leg compression for prevention of postoperative deep venous thrombosis with special reference to fibrinolytic activity. Am J Surg 1988; 155:602–605.

Nicolaides AN, Miles C, Hoare M, et al. Intermittent sequential pneumatic compression of the legs and thromboembolism-deterrent stockings in the prevention of postoperative deep venous thrombosis. Surgery 1983; 9:21–25.

Scurr JH, Coleridge-Smith PD, Hasty JH. Regimen for improved effectiveness of intermittent pneumatic compression in deep venous thrombosis prophylaxis. Surgery 1987; 105:816–820.

Tshak M, Morley K. Deep venous thrombosis after total hip arthroplasty: a prospective controlled study to determine the prophylactic effect of graded pressure stockings. Br J Surg 1981; 68:429–432.

TEMPORARY ACCESS FOR CATHETER HEMODIALYSIS

R. Bernard Rochon

PURPOSE

To allow access to the circulation for hemodialysis.

INDICATIONS

Acute renal failure or electrolyte abnormalities (i.e., hyperkalemia)
Intravascular volume overload

CONTRAINDICATIONS

Venous thrombosis at selected site of placement

POTENTIAL COMPLICATIONS

Injury to vessel
Thrombosis of vessel
Infection

EQUIPMENT

Povidone-iodine solution
4 × 4 gauze sponges
Gown, gloves, mask
Lidocaine, 1%
3 inch tape
Entry needle, 18 gauge
J guidewire
Vein dilator or introducter
Double lumen hemodialysis catheter
Fenestrated drape
Needle, 25 gauge
Needle, 22 gauge
Syringes, disposable
Suture with needle
Injection caps
Scalpel, #11

PROCEDURE

1. Explain procedure to patient and/or family
2. Prepare and drape selected site (i.e., subclavian vein, internal jugular vein, or femoral vein)
3. Anesthetize skin and subcutaneous tissue
4. Puncture vein with entry needle and establish free flow of blood
5. Pass J guidewire through needle into vessel for approximately 5 cm
6. Withdraw needle while maintaining guidewire position
7. Enlarge puncture site with #11 scalpel blade, advance dilator over guidewire, and remove dilator
8. Insert double lumen hemodialysis catheter over guide and remove guidewire
9. After catheter is positioned, venous blood should be easily aspirated. Flush with saline and establish heparin lock.
10. Secure catheter to skin with suture and place sterile dressing

References

Lally KP, Brennan LP, Sherman NJ, et al. Use of a new subclavian venous catheter for short and long term hemodialysis in children. J Ped Surg 1987; 22:603–605.

Nidus BD, Neusy A. Chronic hemodialysis by repeated femoral vein cannulation. Nephron 1981; 29:195–197.

CERVICAL SPINE TRACTION/STABILIZATION

Molly A. Seaman

PURPOSE

To provide immobilization and/or reduction of cervical spine injuries; to reduce and prevent further injuries to spine.

INDICATIONS

Known or suspected cervical injuries

CONTRAINDICATIONS

None

POTENTIAL COMPLICATIONS

Further injury from improper immobilization
Infection at site of pin insertion

EQUIPMENT

Skeletal Traction

Skull tongs (Crutchfield, Gardner-Wells)
Rope, pulley, weights
Normal saline solution
Povidone-iodine solution
4 × 4 gauze sponges
Sterile gloves
Sterile basin
Sterile scissors

Stryker Frame

Stryker frame
Sheets
Traction equipment (if applicable)

Halo-Vest Traction

Soft ware (plastic vest, sheep skin liners)
Hard ware (head pins [5], traction bars, screws)
Tools (Allen wrench, conventional wrench, torque screwdriver)
Alcohol pads
Povidone-iodine solution
Sterile gloves and drape
Lidocaine, 1% (multiple use vial)
Syringe and needles
4 × 4 gauze sponges
Tape measure

PROCEDURE

Skeletal Traction

1. Assemble equipment at bedside
2. Explain procedure to patient and family, if appropriate
3. Trim hair around pin sites
4. Cleanse area with povidone-iodine solution
5. Assist physician with tong placement
6. Attach rope and pulley

Stryker Frame

1. Explain procedure to patient; include family as appropriate
2. Apply sheets and sheepskins to posterior frame
3. With assistance of others, carefully transfer patient to posterior frame
4. Attach arm boards for patient comfort and safety
5. Care should be taken to avoid foot drop and contractures of hand (use foot board and hand rolls)
6. When turning patient, explain procedure and that patient may have a sense of floating. Reassure that frame will hold patient.
7. Remove armboards
8. Arrange anterior frame over the patient
9. Ensure the frame is locked properly
10. Ensure all tubes and lines are able to move freely as you turn patient
11. Patients with traction must be maintained in proper alignment to avoid pulling on tongs
12. Be ready to reattach patient to ventilator quickly, if appropriate
13. Turn quickly and smoothly
14. Remove posterior frame and reposition arm boards

Halo-Vest Traction

1. Assemble equipment at bedside
2. Ensure integrity of airway, breathing, and circulation prior to placement of traction
3. Maintain cervical spine immobilization with hard collar and sandbags until procedure complete
4. If patient is awake, attempt to explain procedure
5. Assist physician in measuring patient's head for halo ring
6. Prepare the selected pin sites by trimming and shaving the hair at the pin site (usually located 1 cm above both eyebrows and both ears). Cleanse sites with povidone-iodine solution and gauze.
7. Use sterile technique when opening the halo-vest unit and tools
8. Prepare anesthetic for physician to inject pin sites
9. Assist with ring placement and tightening of pins
10. Assist in measuring chest and abdomen for correct vest placement

11. Line vest with sheep skin
12. Assist in placing vest on patient while maintaining spinal immobilization
13. The vest is then secured, and the physician attaches traction bar to halo and vest

FOLLOW-UP

Skeletal Traction

1. Cleanse pin sites; watch for signs of infection
2. Provide analgesics as indicated for headaches
3. Do not add or subtract from weights unless prescribed by physician
4. Keep traction clear from dragging floor or entanglement
5. Involve family as appropriate in care of patient

Stryker Frame

1. Monitor patient's vital signs
2. Turn patient frequently
3. Perform range of motion exercises
4. Provide analgesic as ordered to promote patient comfort
5. Maintain equipment (traction, respirator, Foley catheter) to avoid dislodgment while turning
6. Involve family as appropriate in care of patient

Halo-Vest Traction

1. Cleanse pin site every 4 hours
2. Keep conventional wrench tape applied to vest for emergency removal
3. Monitor vital and neurologic signs as ordered by physician
4. Notify physician immediately regarding changes in motor function
5. Provide skin care to avoid decubitus formation under vest
6. Assist patient with ambulation during initial recovery period
7. Involve family as appropriate in care of patient

DOCUMENTATION

Patient's condition before and after procedure
Type of equipment used and location of pin site
Vital and neurologic signs
Signs of infection
Patient's turning schedule
Patient's response to treatment; provide opportunities for patient to ventilate feelings and concerns

References

Hamilton HK. Procedures. Springhouse, PA: Intermed Communication, 1983:124–128, 644–649.
Little NE. In: Case of a broken neck. Emerg Med 1989; 21:22–32.
Sumchai AP, Sternbach GL, Laufer M. Cervical spine traction and immobilization. Top Emerg Med 1988; 10:9–21.

TEMPERATURE CONTROL UNITS

Janet Neff

PURPOSE

To supplement or supplant the body's thermoregulatory ability.

INDICATIONS

When hypothermia is desired for its effect on metabolic rate and oxygen consumption (especially pertinent in head trauma)

When normothermia cannot be maintained. Trauma patients may be exposed to the elements and arrive hypothermic, or necessary interventions may induce hypothermia unless temperature controlling devices are used.

CONTRAINDICATIONS

None

POTENTIAL COMPLICATIONS

Excessive reduction or elevation of temperature
Tissue injury secondary to vascular compromise
Altered skin integrity

EQUIPMENT

Ice pack (crushed ice, waterproof container, slip cover, or ice within disposable gloves)
Grounded, engineering approved bedside fan
Cool fluids to use with lavage
Cooling/warming blanket device
  Mattress with tubes, disposable cover or light pad/sheet, hoses, machine
  Temperature probe (rectal, esophageal)
  Distilled water
Thermometer or thermistor device (within pulmonary artery catheter, Foley catheter)
Warming cabinet (temperature~40°C [(104°F]) for intravenous (IV) fluids, irrigating solutions, and blankets
Rapid warming device for IV fluid infusion and special IV tubing
Portable or overhead heat lamps

PROCEDURE

1. Assess the patient's temperature. Measurement of core temperature is most accurate, and an electronic thermometer or an infrared device (tympanic membrane) or a thermistor within a pulmonary artery catheter or Foley catheter should be used.
2. Determine the desired endpoint for thermoregulatory intervention
3. Select the appropriate means to implement plan and obtain the equipment
4. Ensure that devices are properly maintained and calibrated by biomedical engineering
5. When using any electric device to regulate temperature, be certain that there is an alarm for blanket/fluid and patient temperatures outside a safe range. Fluid warmers should not be set >40°C [104°F] for blood administration or >46°C [115°F] for crystalloid, and cooling machines should be set no lower than 15°C [60°F].
6. To use a warming/cooling mattress device, use the following procedure:
   a. Place the mattress beneath the patient with protective padding or cover. Eliminate any wrinkles.
   b. Insert the accompanying patient probe into the control jack and the patient and compare with a thermometer or thermistor reading
   c. Inspect the reservoir water level and add more distilled water if indicated. Check whether your device should have the level monitored with the unit on or off.
   d. Ensure that tubing is securely attached to mattress and unit without kinks
   e. Set the unit on automatic (temperature is monitored based on desired patient temperature) or manual (temperature is monitored based on the mattress setting)
   f. Monitor the patient's temperature periodically; frequency is dependent on the patient's initial temperature and the rapidity of temperature change
   g. The unit should be turned off prior to reaching the desired patient temperature because drift occurs. If drift is excessive, the pad, which is still cool or warm, should be removed or potentially set for the opposite direction.
   h. Skin condition should be assessed often, since sensitivity to the cooling or heating varies among patients
   i. When cooling patients, monitor for shivering and arrhythmias
7. Overhead lights are usually placed 80–100 cm (3–4 feet) away from the skin surface. Be alert to their proximity to drapes, IV lines, and monitor cords.
8. Ventilators with heated humidifiers can also elevate patient temperature

FOLLOW-UP

1. Recognize that medications are metabolized and/or detoxified at different rates dependent on body temperature
2. Be sure to explain to patient the reason for the various maneuvers undertaken (especially cooling) because these are not often perceived as pleasant

DOCUMENTATION

Patient's temperature at frequent intervals, skin care, and positioning
Complications
a. Your actions
b. Patient's outcome

References

Sollars G. Thermoregulatory emergencies. In: Kitt S, Kaiser J, eds. Emergency nursing: a physiologic and clinical perspective. Philadelphia: WB Saunders, 1990:719–753.

Review the manufacturer's literature for electrical equipment and consult with hospital biomedical engineers.

WOUND DRESSING

Janet Neff

PURPOSE

To promote healing and comfort; to reduce the chance of infection; and to support and protect the wound.

INDICATIONS

Surface trauma, such as lacerations, abrasions, or avulsions, that exposes the underlying epidermal, dermal, or subcutaneous layers or other structures

Need for continued pressure or maintenance of antibiotic therapy to wound site

Need for improved cosmetic appearance during wound healing

CONTRAINDICATIONS

Thick layers of certain types of gauze can sometimes obscure fine radiographic film findings

POTENTIAL COMPLICATIONS

Wounds that have not been fully assessed or cleansed may be ignored or assumed to be thoroughly treated on transfer to a different unit

A loose, bulky dressing may obscure significant bleeding and lead to hematoma or dead space formation

Ischemia may result from too much pressure or inappropriate application

Wound drainage and invasive devices, if not properly applied or if universal precautions are not adhered to, may contaminate other wounds or surgical incisions

Brain damage may result from excessive presure over a depressed skull fracture

EQUIPMENT

0.9% sodium chloride irrigating solution
Sterile basin or gauze "boat"
Varied sizes of gauze pads
Conformable gauze rolls
Elastic wrap
Tube gauze and applicator (or large syringe barrel)
Microporous skin tape strips (Steristrips)
Benzoin applicators
Skin preparation pads
Montgomery straps
Hypoallergenic tape

PROCEDURE

1. Ensure that the wound was properly cleansed and closed (if applicable) and that tetanus status was addressed
2. Cleanse any remaining blood from the region of the wound and planned site of dressing. Warmed normal saline is most comfortable, and a soap solution may be used to cleanse the surrounding area. Hydrogen peroxide should be avoided because it is an irritant to exposed tissue and would be hazardous if it gained entrance to a joint space; however, diluted peroxide may be necessary to remove dried blood.
3. Dressing management for an open wound is aimed toward avoiding dessication and removal of liquid wound exudate. Wet-to-dry dressings with fluffed gauze moistened with normal saline are typically used. To avoid maceration, the moist dressings should not overlay intact skin edges. A protective layer of absorbent gauze is then placed and covered with a dressing impervious to fluid. Use of Montgomery straps is often helpful with open wounds that require frequent dressing changes to maintain the surrounding skin integrity. Enterostomal supplies for skin protection are also helpful. Surgical or enzymatic debridement is necessary for any devitalized tissue.
4. Wounds with approximated skin edges rather rapidly become less susceptible to infection. Some surgeons prefer a dressing for the first 48 hours; others may require less. The same time frame is often used for allowing moisture on the site, although soaking the wound, such as in a bathtub or pool, should be avoided until healing is complete. Wounds closed with tape skin closures are least susceptible to infection. The nurse may apply these by swabbing the wound edges with an adhesive adjunct such as benzoin and attaching the tape to one wound edge (perpendicular to the wound) and pulling the other wound edge toward the taped edge for the final attachment. Snug approximation of skin edges is important. Benzoin should not contact the fresh wound edges because it is both painful and impairs the tissue's defense against infection.
5. Abraded areas of skin are usually covered with a thin layer of antibacterial cream or ointment such as silver sulfadiazine (Silvadene), neomycin sulfate–polymyxin B sulfate (Neosporin), or bacitracin. Use of water-vapor–permeable, transparent, polyurethane film dressings prevents or delays evaporation of water from the wound, thereby enhancing epithelialization. Some wounds exude too much fluid and require change of dressings or aspiration of the fluid; this raises concerns about the potential for infection within the rich medium. However, these dressings have been effective in many wounds.
6. Deep wounds or wounds at vascular sites such as the scalp or forehead should have pressure maintained to avoid formation of dead space or hematoma. This can be accomplished by folding gauze pads directly over the injured area and using conforming gauze or elasticized gauze wraps to maintain pressure over the site. When used in an extremity, pressure should be greatest over the site and distally but not as strong proximally, to promote arterial supply and venous and lymphatic return.

7. When wounds are dressed prior to cast application, either dermal continuous sutures or tape skin closure strips are usually used, unless a window will be created in the cast to allow access for removal of percutaneous sutures and close monitoring of the wound for infection.
8. Wounds over a joint require splinting to maximize healing and avoid tension on the tissues and sutures. Padded aluminum splints for digits or full extremity splints may be needed, depending on the site of injury. When securing these devices, circumferential taping must be carefully monitored. Tube gauze over a finger can be creatively applied to leave the very tip of the digit exposed for assessment of circulation and sensation.
9. Evaluate patient's level of comfort and need for analgesia. Emphasize the value of elevation of the injured part.

FOLLOW-UP

1. Teach the patient or significant other the steps involved in redressing the wound and the restrictions regarding exposure to water and return to work. It is helpful to let the patient dress the wound in the emergency department if possible and to supply the patient with similar dressings and information on where to obtain further materials.
2. Teach the patient the signs and symptoms of infection, expected changes in the wound, and how to assess for distal circulation, sensation, and motor ability. Impress upon the patient the need for follow-up evaluation of the wound and the signs and symptoms that signify an emergency.
3. Adherence to suture removal dates should be stressed to avoid epidermal track marks and prolonged irritation that might lead to infection.
4. The patient should be aware that abraded skin may develop hyperpigmentation on exposure to sunlight during the first 6 months following injury. Therefore, the area should be covered or sunblock should be applied after initial healing.

DOCUMENTATION

Neurologic, vascular, and motor status following application of dressing
Specific dressing technique employed
Teaching points covered with patient to prevent complications
Planned dates for wound recheck and suture removal
Wound care handouts sent home with patient

References

Cosgriff JH Jr, Anderson D. The practice of emergency care. 2nd ed. Philadelphia: JB Lippincott, 1984:312–315.
Simon RR, Brenner BE. Emergency procedures and techniques. 2nd ed. Baltimore: Williams & Wilkins, 1987:333–336.
Tobin GR. Wound repair and bone healing. In: Richardson JD, Polk HC Jr, Flint LM, eds. Trauma-clinical care and pathophysiology. Chicago: Year Book, 1987:253–256.
Zukin DD, Simon RR. Emergency wound care. Rockville, MD: Aspen, 1987:125–145.

STEINMANN PIN

Lisa B. Jones

PURPOSE

To reduce and immobilize a femur fracture; to decrease muscle spasm; to prevent deformity; to support and maintain alignment.

INDICATIONS

Femur fracture

CONTRAINDICATIONS

None

POTENTIAL COMPLICATIONS

Wound tract infection
Neurovascular compromise
Skin breakdown

EQUIPMENT

Steinmann pin tray
Skin antiseptic solution
4 × 4 gauze sponges
Weights and ropes
Small needle and syringe
Local anesthetic drug
Pieces of cork or other material to cover pin tips after insertion (2)

PROCEDURE

1. Explain procedure to patient
2. Cleanse area where pin is to be inserted with antiseptic solution
3. Anesthetize skin locally
4. Make a small incision at pin insertion site
5. Insert pin with manual drill device
6. Attach a U-shaped clamp to pin and connect to weights by means of a rope and pulley
7. Apply cork to pin tips to prevent injury to patients or others
8. Apply small dressings at entrance and exit sites of pin

FOLLOW-UP

1. Check for pain, swelling, discoloration, limited motion, numbness, tingling, temperature, position, pulses, and signs of infection
2. Avoid unnecessary movement of weights
3. Ensure proper alignment

DOCUMENTATION

Patient teaching
Procedure performed and extremity involved
Follow-up assessment
Complications

References

Brunner LS, Suddarth DS. The Lippincott manual of nursing practice. Philadelphia: JB Lippincott, 1982:770.
Jones L. Steinmann pin. In: Mancini ME, ed. Pocket manual of emergency nursing procedures. Toronto: BC Decker, 1988:151–155.
Schwartz S. Fractures and joint injuries. In: Schwartz S, Shires T, Spencer F, Storer E, eds. Principles of surgery. Vol. 2. 4th ed. New York: McGraw-Hill, 1984:1979–1984.

THOMAS/HARE TRACTION SPLINT

Kimberly L. Davies

PURPOSE

To immobilize fractures of the lower extremities by using traction to prevent further injury.

INDICATIONS

Suspected/obvious femur fractures
Suspected/obvious upper tibial fractures
Compound (open) or simple (closed) fractures

CONTRAINDICATIONS

Partial or complete amputation of the lower extremity

POTENTIAL COMPLICATIONS

Neurovascular compromise distal to the injury after splint application
Aggravation of vessel or nerve damage
Localized ischemia secondary to improper padding or pressure points
Infection secondary to compound (open) fractures

EQUIPMENT

Thomas/Hare traction splint
   Splint, with traction device
   Ankle hitch
   Ischial strap
   Cravats, Velcro straps
Sterile dressings (possible)
Padding material

PROCEDURE

1. Obtain history, mechanism of injury, time injury occurred, vital signs, prehospital neurovascular assessment, and interventions
2. Inform patient about the procedure
3. Remove all clothing from the injured extremity to ensure complete visual inspection. Remove shoes and boots if at all possible (Fig. 1).
4. Perform a baseline neurovascular assessment distal to the injury. Components of this assessment include palpation of distal pulses (dorsalis pedis, posterior tibial), skin temperature, color, capillary refill, and sensorimotor perception (Fig. 2).
5. Assess for possible open fractures
6. Assist with irrigation and debridement of open wounds prior to splinting. In situations in which this is not practical, simply cover with sterile, dry dressing. Do not attempt to push exposed bone ends back beneath the skin.

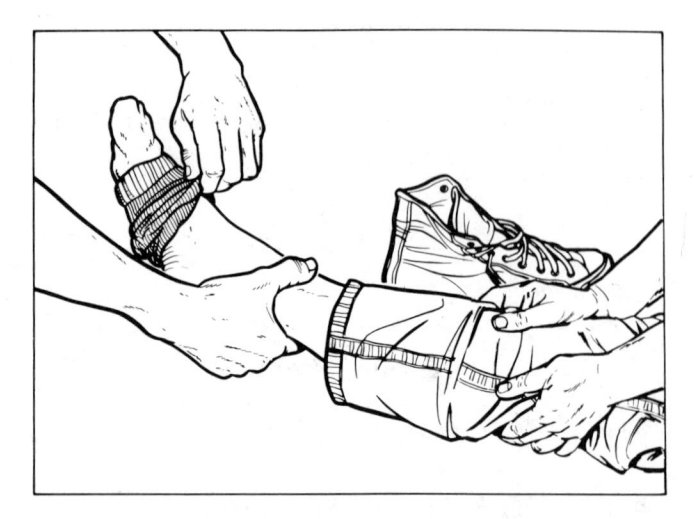

Figure 1 Visual inspection is facilitated by removal of all clothing from the injured extremity. (Figures 1 to 8 from Phillips G, Fender G, Mickelberry ME, Garbisch R. Basic life support skills manual. 2nd ed. Englewood Cliffs, NJ: Prentice Hall, 1986:170–172.)

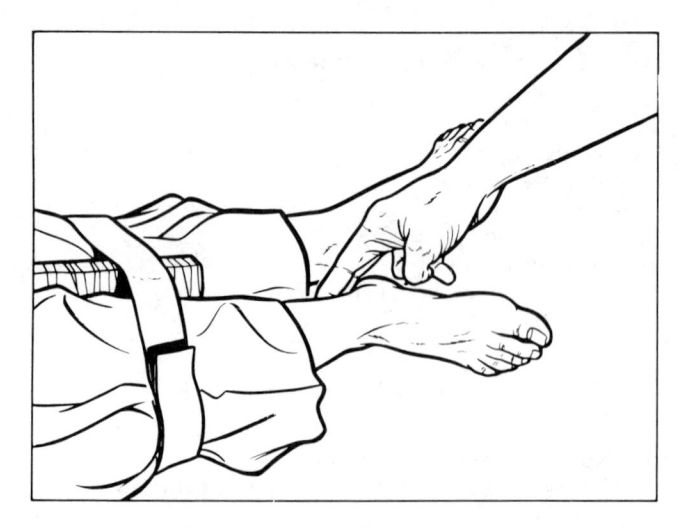

Figure 2 Perform a baseline neurovascular assessment distal to the injury, including palpation of distal pulses.

7. Obtain assistance. Proper splint application requires a minimum of two persons.
8. The assistant places one hand on the dorsum of the foot and the other underneath the calf. Manual traction is applied as the extremity is gently pulled into neutral alignment using a steady, firm force. Manual traction will be maintained until mechanical traction is engaged (Fig. 3).
9. Reassess neurovascular status
10. Apply ankle hitch (Fig. 4)
11. Adjust length of splint so that it exceeds length of the leg by approximately 6–10 inches and lock into position (Fig. 5)

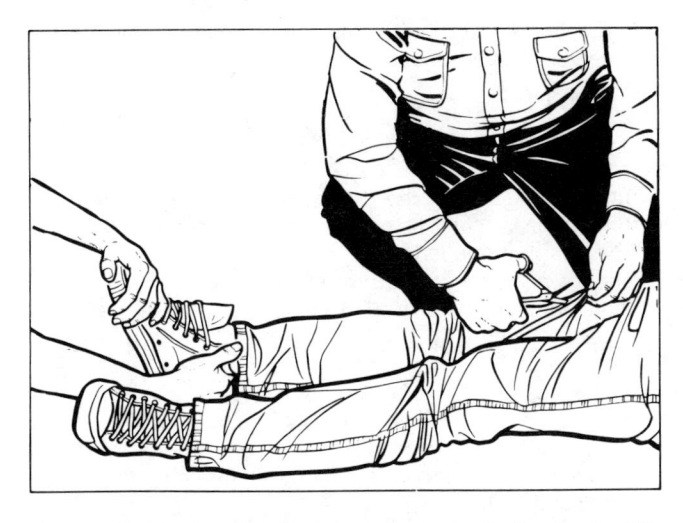

Figure 3 Maintain manual traction using a steady, firm force until mechanical traction is engaged.

12. The injured leg is gently lifted by the assistant while traction is maintained
13. As the leg is lifted, the splint is simultaneously slid under the leg until the top of the splint fits snugly at the ischium and groin
14. Pressure points and areas of contact are padded
15. Fasten ischial strap (Fig. 6)
16. Hook ankle hitch to traction mechanism (Fig. 7)
17. Mechanical traction is steadily increased while manual traction is concurrently released (Fig. 8)
18. Reassess neurovascular status
19. Secure the extremity to the splint with cravats or Velcro straps above and below the extremity. Additional placement of securing straps is recommended to provide total support of the splinted leg.
20. Gently elevate entire splint so that the foot does not rest on the stretcher

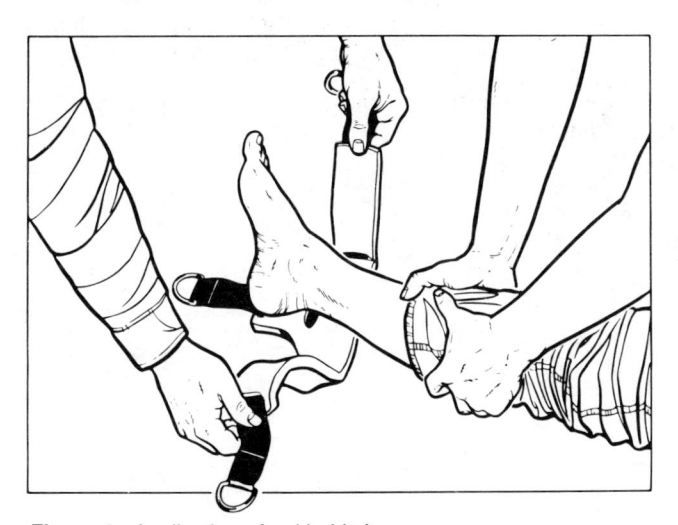

Figure 4 Application of ankle hitch.

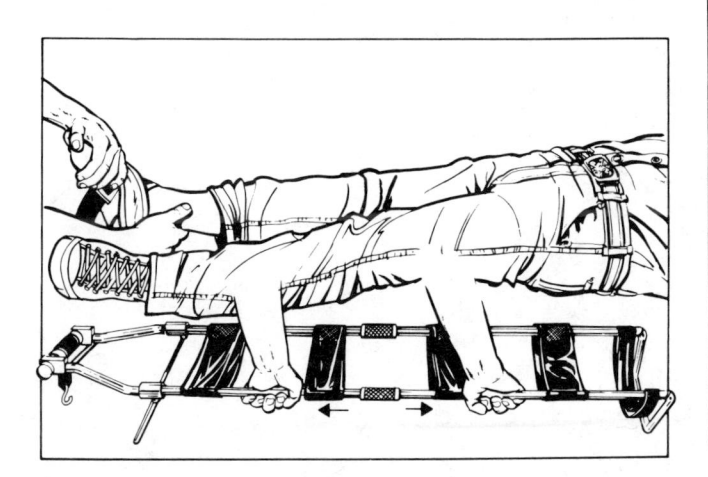

Figure 5 Lock splint into position when its length exceeds leg length by 6 to 10 inches.

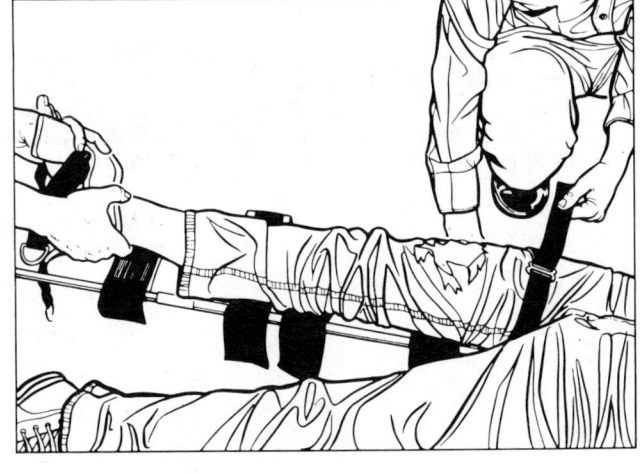

Figure 6 Fastening of ischial strap.

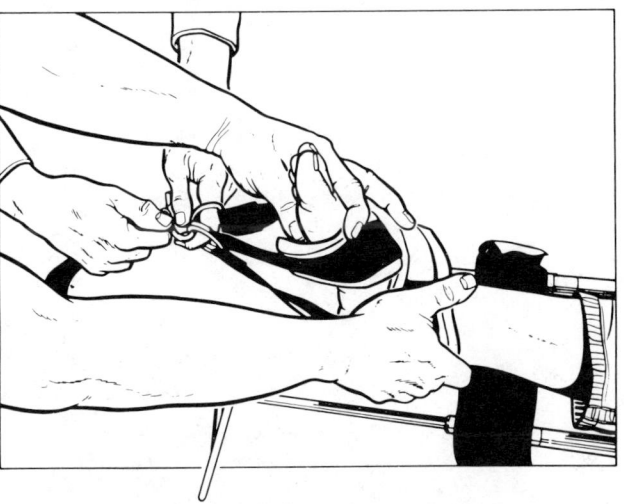

Figure 7 Ankle hitch is hooked to traction mechanism.

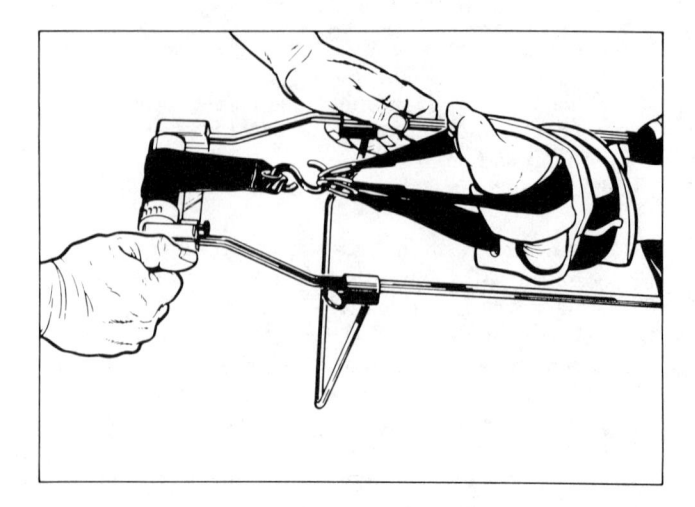

Figure 8 Steadily increase mechanical traction while releasing manual traction.

FOLLOW-UP

1. Continue to monitor neurovascular status distal to the injury with serial assessments
2. Evaluate response of the patient to splint application. Once the extremity has been adequately splinted, pain should be minimal.
3. Traction splint should remain in place until definitive interventions are made

DOCUMENTATION

Initial appearance of the extremity, description of injury
Initial neurovascular assessment of the extremity
Type of splint applied
Patient's response to the procedure
Neurovascular status post application, as well as serial assessments

References

Caroline NL. Emergency care in the streets. Boston: Little, Brown, 1983:381–395.
Knezevich BA. Trauma nursing principles and practice. Norwalk, CT: Appleton-Century-Crofts, 1986:141–152.
Lanros NE. Assessment and intervention in emergency nursing. Norwalk, CT: Appleton and Lange, 1988:326–339.
Shaw DC, Heckman JD. Principles and techniques of splinting musculocutaneous injuries. Emerg Med Clin North Am 1984; 2:391–407.
Worsing RA. Principles of prehospital care of musculoskeletal injuries. Emerg Med Clin North Am 1984; 2:205–218.

CLOSED REDUCTION

Vinette Langford

PURPOSE

To realign displaced bone ends in an effort to promote healing of a closed fracture.

INDICATIONS

Fractures of the upper or lower extremities, including
    Ulnar/radial fractures
    Humerus fractures
    Phalanges fractures
    Tibia/fibula fractures
    Foot fractures

CONTRAINDICATIONS

Where the fracture extends into the joint
Severe fractures that may require surgical fixation to provide stabilization

POTENTIAL COMPLICATIONS

Neurovascular compromise
Fat embolism syndrome
Malalignment
Compartment syndrome

EQUIPMENT

Finger traps
Counter weights
Cast padding
Cast material (plaster or fiberglass)
Ace wraps (size as needed)
Gauze rolls

PROCEDURE

1. Inform patient about procedure
2. Position patient supine with injured extremity in convenient position
3. Administer sedation if necessary
4. Place finger traps and counter weight if applicable (upper extremity fracture)
5. Administer local anesthesia
6. Ensure extremity is supported during manipulation
7. Assist with casting or splinting
8. Assess for changes in neurovascular status
9. Obtain postcasting radiographic films
10. Monitor respiratory status and level of consciousness during procedure

FOLLOW-UP

1. Continue to monitor respiratory status and level of consciousness until sedation wears off
2. Elevate extremity and apply ice-bag
3. Assess circulatory status and neurovascular status of extremity
4. Assess for other complications such as compartment syndrome

DOCUMENTATION

Initial assessment of patient including allergies
Procedure performed
Medications used
Type of cast/splint applied
Postcast radiographic film findings
Ongoing monitoring of patient's status
Patient teaching

References

Cardona VD, Hurn PD, Mason PB, Scanlon-Schilpp AM, Veise-Berry SW. Trauma nursing: from resuscitation through rehabilitation. Philadelphia: WB Saunders, 1988:525–569.

McSwain NE, Kerstein MD. Evaluation and management of trauma. Norwalk, CT: Appleton-Century-Crofts, 1987:167–193.

Sheehy SB, Marvin JA, Jimmerson CL. Manual of clinical trauma care: the first hour. St. Louis: CV Mosby, 1989:207–248.

CAST CARE

Vinette Langford

PURPOSE

To assess for neurovascular compromise in a casted extremity; to instruct patient in appropriate home care of cast.

INDICATIONS

Application of a fiberglass or plaster cast on an extremity

CONTRAINDICATIONS

None

POTENTIAL COMPLICATIONS

Neurovascular compromise
Loss of skin integrity
Compartment syndrome

EQUIPMENT

None

PROCEDURE

1. Assess extremity for neurovascular status (pain, pallor, pulses, paresthesia)
2. Assess for cast integrity (soft spots, rough edges, pressure areas)
3. Initiate appropriate interventions
4. Instruct patient in appropriate home care, as follows:
   a. Elevate extremity for 24 hours
   b. Keep the cast dry
   c. No weightbearing, if applicable
   d. Plaster cast takes approximately 24 hours to dry completely
   e. Observe for areas of skin breakdown or compromise
   f. Return for any problem

FOLLOW-UP

1. Monitor for signs of neurovascular compromise
2. Assess for cast breakdown

DOCUMENTATION

Type of cast applied
Neurovascular assessment after application
Instructions given to patient

References

Cardona VD, Hurn PD, Mason PB, Scanlon-Schilpp AM, Veise-Berry SW. Trauma nursing: from resuscitation through rehabilitation. Philadelphia: WB Saunders, 1988; 525–569.
McSwain NE, Kerstein MD. Evaluation and management of trauma. Norwalk, CT: Appleton-Century-Crofts, 1987:167–193.
Sheehy SB, Marvin JA, Jimerson CL. Manual of clinical trauma care: the first hour. St. Louis: CV Mosby, 1989:207–248.

CONTACT LENS REMOVAL

Kimberly L. Davies

PURPOSE

To remove hard or hydrophylic (soft) contact lenses from the eye.

INDICATIONS

Critically injured or unresponsive patients unable to facilitate self lens removal

CONTRAINDICATIONS

Broken, fragmented lenses
Penetrating or blunt trauma to the orbit
When initial attempts to extract the lens are difficult

POTENTIAL COMPLICATIONS

Corneal lacerations/abrasions
Aggravation of eye injuries
Damage to the lens, i.e., breakage or tears

EQUIPMENT

Penlight
Small suction bulb specially designed for removal of hard contacts (i.e., contact suction)
Two closable containers with labels
Sterile normal saline or soft lens lubricating solution
3-ml syringe

PROCEDURE

1. Timely assessment and removal are suggested to facilitate extraction, especially in the presence of associated facial injuries where edema is likely to develop. With head or facial trauma, thorough inspection is required because hard lenses may be out of position or broken.
2. If the patient is responsive, ask whether he or she wears contact lenses; if so, assist with removal and provide storage
3. For unresponsive patients, carefully inspect each eye by shining a light from side to identify the presence of a lens
4. Position patient supine
5. Mechanical removal of hard or semirigid contact lenses occurs as follows (Fig. 1):
   a. Retract upper and lower lids apart
   b. Moisten suction cup with normal saline
   c. Place small suction bulb over center of lens
   d. Gently pull lens straight off the eye
   e. Place each removed lens in separate containers with a small amount water
   f. Label containers with patient's name and differentiate between right and left lenses

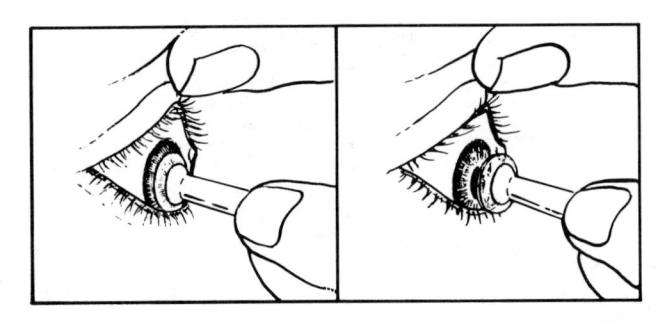

Figure 1 Technique for mechanical removal of hard and semirigid contact lenses.

6. Manual removal of hard or semirigid contact lenses occurs as follows (Fig. 2A):
   a. Retract upper and lower lids apart
   b. Gently push lids together, displacing lens off corneal surface
   c. Place lenses in separate, labeled containers
7. Manual removal of soft contact lenses occurs as follows (Fig. 2B):
   a. Soft lenses in the eye for extended periods of time can dry and adhere to the cornea. To remoisten for removal, irrigate using a 3-ml syringe (without needle) with sterile normal saline or special soft lens lubricating solution.
   b. Consult physician regarding use of topical anesthetic agent (Alcaine) if corneal reflex interferes with lens removal
   c. Retract upper lid
   d. Using index finger, slide contact downward
   e. Gently pinch lens between index finger and thumb
   f. Remove lenses, place them in separate, closable containers of normal saline or commercially prepared solution to prevent dehydration or damage
   g. Label containers with patient's name and differentiate between right and left lenses

FOLLOW-UP

1. Trauma to the orbit or eyeball may make removal difficult; if the lens cannot be removed with ease, discontinue efforts and notify physician
2. Assess each eye for particles and foreign bodies (e.g., glass, grass, metal). Note any abrasions, lacerations, or penetrating or perforating injuries.
3. A slit lamp may be used to augment visual inspection

DOCUMENTATION

Obvious eye injuries found on physical assessment
Removal, storage and location of contact lenses
Damage (i.e., breakage, tears) to the lenses

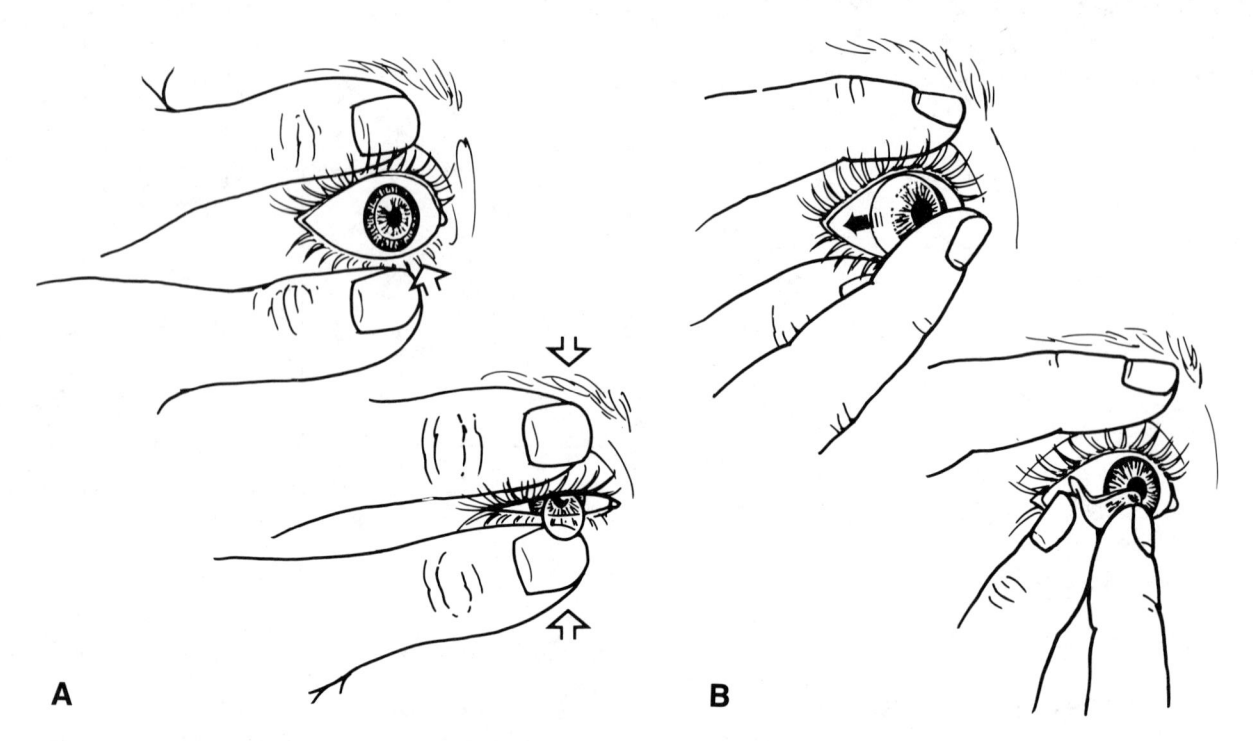

Figure 2 *A*, Manual removal of hard contact lens (right eye): Open lids wide and press down with right thumb, then slide eyelids together. *B*, Manual removal of soft contact lens (right eye): Slide lens to white of eye and pinch between thumb and index finger.

References

Budassi SS, Barber J. Emergency nursing principles and practice. St. Louis: CV Mosby, 1985:276–294.

Lanros NE. Assessment and intervention in emergency nursing. Norwalk, CT: Appleton and Lange, 1988:433–447.

Lubeck D, Greene JS. Corneal injuries. Emerg Med Clin North Am 1988; 6:73–94.

Wieck L, King E, Dyer M. Illustrated manual of nursing techniques. Philadelphia: JB Lippincott, 1986:303–309.

EYE IRRIGATION

Janet Neff

PURPOSE

To remove irritants; to prevent or reduce injury to the eye; and to preserve vision.

INDICATIONS

Foreign body sensation
Exposure of the eye to various irritants
Evidence of foreign matter in the facial region, near the eyes. Eye contamination should be assumed, especially in the unconscious patient.
    Dirt, sand, soot
    Fine glass fragments
    Chemicals (alkali, acid, gasoline, mace)
Close proximity of face to explosive forces, flame, or smoke
Patient's report of specific foreign body exposure

CONTRAINDICATIONS

Penetrating eye injury
Chemical exposure in solid form (dry powders should be brushed off or vacuumed prior to fluid irrigation)

POTENTIAL COMPLICATIONS

Injury secondary to incomplete irrigation
Abrasion induced by poor technique
Resistive movements that may jeopardize spinal precautions, if anesthesia employed is inadequate

EQUIPMENT

Absorbent, waterproof pads
Towels
2 × 2 gauze sponges
Gloves, goggles
Collection basin
Cotton tip applicators
Topical ophthalmic anesthetic drops (tetracaine hydrochloride or proparacaine hydrochloride [Ophthaine])
Bent paper clip or Desmarres lid retractor
Normal saline solution (4 1000-ml bags) at room temperature or warmed to body temperature
Wide bore, macrodrip intravenous (IV) tubing (1 or 2)
Molded scleral lens (Morgan lens) for continuous, extended irrigation
Fluorescein paper strips
Nitrazine pH paper

PROCEDURE

Preparation

1. Explain procedure to patient
2. Put on gloves and goggles
3. Assess for excessive tearing, conjunctival injection, or ciliary flush. If a penetrating object is noted, irrigation should not be done.
4. Check for presence of contact lens; remove if present
5. Evaluate degree of patient's discomfort
6. Determine visual acuity, if situation is not emergent, by the following means:
   Visual acuity for far vision with Snellen alphabet chart
   Rosenbaum or Jaeger chart for near vision held 14 inches from the eye (for nonambulatory patients)
   Gross measures such as finger counts, hand motion detection, and light perception for emergent situations or when vision is seriously impaired
7. Remove external contaminants by vacuuming, flushing, or wiping with gauze. Near the eyelids, use moistened applicators.
8. Measure conjunctival pH level in chemical exposures
9. Evert upper eyelids and expose inner lower lid to remove any obvious foreign particles. If items appear to be embedded, consult with physician for intervention. Ophthalmology consultation is often warranted. To evert upper eyelid, have the patient look down; grasp upper eyelashes with fingers; and place applicator on tarsal ridge and apply light pressure while pulling the upper lid up and outward over the applicator. A bent paperclip or retractor may be necessary to obtain full exposure.
10. Verify allergies, then anesthetize the conjunctiva by instilling 1 or 2 drops of topical anesthetic into conjunctival sac (with physician's order). This may need to be repeated during prolonged irrigation. Allow approximately 1 minute for effect.

Irrigation

1. Irrigation is an emergency procedure for chemical contamination and should begin in the prehospital setting. Alkali can cause progressive damage because it is lipid soluble and may extend through the cornea into the anterior chamber. Acid solutions cause tissue protein precipitation, thereby reducing the depth of injury; nonetheless, these are very serious.
2. Place towels, pads, and basin to absorb fluid
3. Position patient on same side as eye to be irrigated. If both eyes need rapid irrigation or if spinal precautions are being maintained, irrigation can proceed in the supine position.

4. Flush intravenous tubing with irrigating fluid
5. Begin flow of fluid slowly, then increase to full rate. The solution should flow laterally, from inner to outer canthus.
6. Be certain to irrigate beneath eyelids
7. Once major particles are removed, ask alert patient to move eyes and blink to distribute fluid
8. Swab inner canthus periodically with moist applicator
9. Irrigate each eye with 500–1,000-ml and until no further particulate matter is seen. Chemical exposures, particularly alkalis, require greater volumes of irrigant; irrigation may continue for 24–48 hours. Periodic measures of conjunctival pH level may be ordered.

Sustained Irrigation

Once gross contaminants are flushed out, sustained irrigation may be indicated. It may be helpful to insert a molded scleral irrigating lens.
1. Ensure adequate topical anesthesia
2. Flush the irrigating lens and adapter with fluid
3. While fluid is slowly flowing, have patient look down, and insert upper edge of lens under upper lid
4. Have the patient look down, retract the lower lid, and allow lid to slide back over lower border of lens
5. Maintain flow of irrigant at all times (Fig. 1). Ocular medication may also be instilled in this fashion.
6. Secure the device to prevent accidental removal. To remove, ask the patient to look up, and retract lower lid to point of lower border of lens; maintain lower lid retraction and have patient look down while retracting upper lid, and then slide lens out.
7. Remove wet linen and ensure patient's comfort and warmth

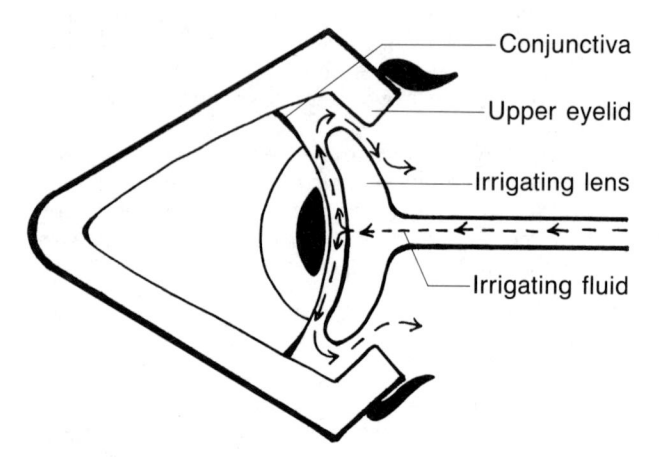

Figure 1 Method of eye irrigation using a molded scleral lens.

Fluorescein Examination

Prepare patient for fluorescein staining and slit lamp microscopy.
1. Retract lower lid and touch fluorescein strip (dry or moistened) to conjunctival sac. Ask the alert patient to blink to help distribute the dye.
2. A cobalt blue light or Wood's lamp is used to examine for areas of denuded corneal epithelium, which are evidenced by a bright green or yellowish hue
3. Generally the excess dye is flushed out following examination

FOLLOW-UP

1. Determine tetanus status and administer immunization as ordered
2. Expect administration of ophthalmic medication such as cycloplegics or antibiotics
3. Teach patient the purpose and effects of medications and techniques for their instillation as appropriate
4. Apply eye patch and teach the patient how to reapply and the hazards of a change in depth perception
5. Evaluate the patient's need for systemic analgesia
6. Facilitate ophthalmology follow-up

DOCUMENTATION

Visual ability
Level of pain
Volume and type of irrigant to each eye
Description of foreign bodies removed
Dosages and times of anesthetic drops and other ocular medications
Patient's tolerance of procedure
Patient teaching: didactic and return demonstrations

References

Burns FR, Peterson CA. Prompt irrigation of chemical eye injuries may avert severe damage. Occup Health Safety 1989; 58(4):33–36.
Deutsch TA, Feller DB. Management of ocular injuries. 2nd ed. Philadelphia: WB Saunders, 1985:61–68; 98–102; 127–131.
Lubeck D, Greene JS. Corneal injuries. Emerg Med Clin North Am 1988; 6(1):73–94.
Schaefer AJ. Ocular injuries. In: Cosgriff JH Jr, Anderson DL, eds. The practice of emergency care. 2nd ed. Philadelphia: JB Lippincott, 1984; 596–604.

HELMET REMOVAL

Bob McMullen

PURPOSE

To provide access to the airway; to expose trauma of the head, face, and neck; and to facilitate cervical spine immobilization.

INDICATIONS

Need for airway management
Need for bleeding control of facial or scalp hemorrhage

CONTRAINDICATIONS

Only one rescuer available
Rescuers inexperienced in removal technique
Patient experiences increased pain during removal attempt

POTENTIAL COMPLICATIONS

Further aggravation of spinal injury

PROCEDURE

1. Assure two rescuers trained in helmet removal technique are available
2. Inform patient of what your are going to do and stress importance that patient not attempt to help or move
3. Evaluate neurologic status
4. Rescuer 1 should be positioned at the top of the patient's head, thereby providing inline traction and stabilization
5. Rescuer 2 should untie or cut the helmet's chin strap if present
6. Rescuer 2 should then assume traction by placing one hand behind the neck, at the occipital region, and grasping the angle of the jaw with the other hand
7. Rescuer 1 removes the helmet, being careful to take the following precautions:
    a. Remove the patient's glasses first, if the helmet provides full facial coverage
    b. Spread the lower edge of the helmet so it will fit over the ears
    c. Tilt the helmet backwards slightly to clear the patient's nose, if the helmet provides full facial coverage
8. Rescuer 2 should carefully maintain inline traction and stabilize the head throughout the procedure to prevent head tilt
9. After removal of the helmet, Rescuer 1 can regain traction of the head and spine by grasping the head firmly, with the fingers of each hand positioned at the angle of the jaw and the palms positioned over the ears
10. Rescuer 1 maintains inline traction until a cervical collar is applied, and the patient is secured to a long backboard with sandbags or head immobilizer device and tape

FOLLOW-UP

1. Reassess airway, breathing, and circulation (ABCs)
2. Examine for hemorrhage
3. Assure completed spinal immobilization
4. Complete the physical examination of head
5. Re-evaluate neurologic status

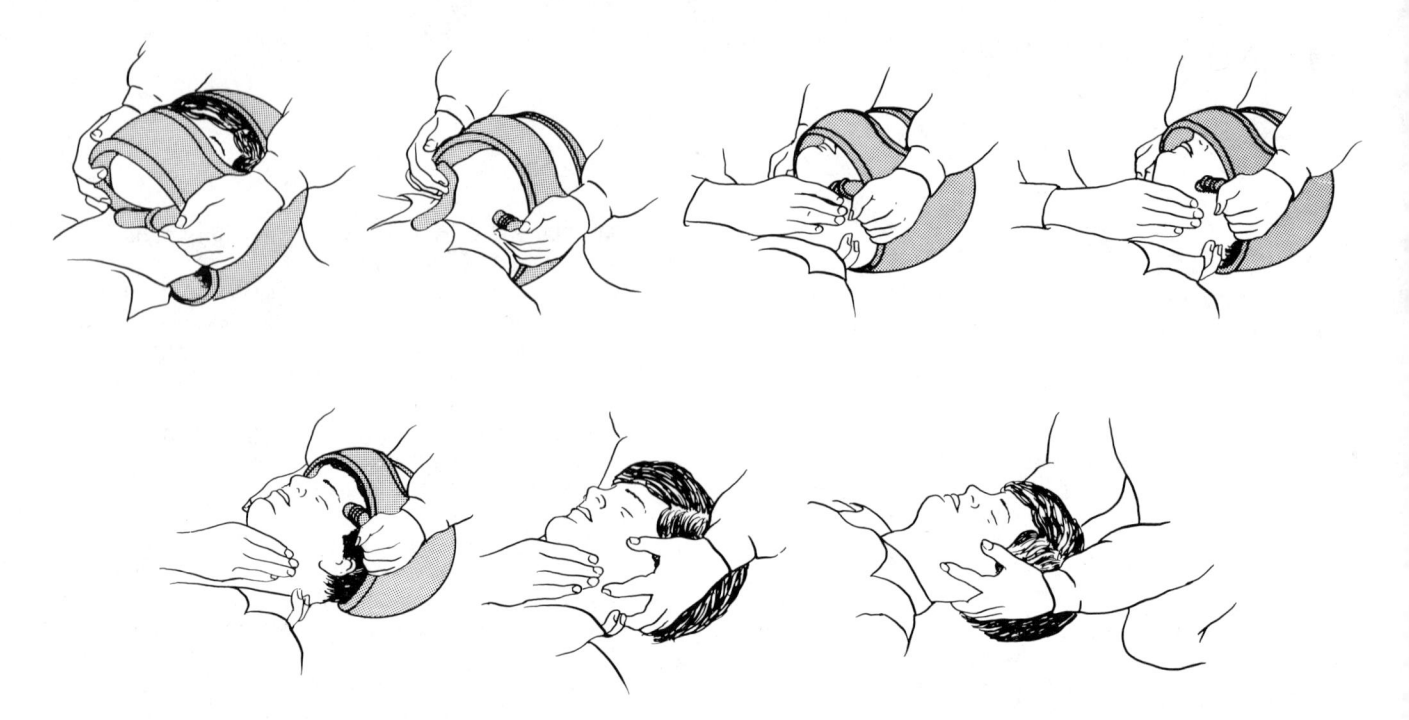

Figure 1 Removal of helmet from injured patient. (Redrawm after American College of Surgeons Committee on Trauma. Helmet removal from injured patients (wall chart). Chicago: American College of Surgeons, 1980.)

DOCUMENTATION

Initial assessment of patient with special notes pertaining to indications for helmet removal and damage to helmet (cracks, scrapes, indentations)
Procedure used and outcome
Ongoing reassessment of ABCs, vital signs, neurologic assessment and adequate spinal immobilization

References

American College of Surgeons. Helmet removal from injured patients (wall chart). Chicago: American College of Surgeons, 1980.
Caroline NL. Emergency medical treatment: a text for EMT-A's and EMT-intermediates. 2nd ed. Boston: Little, Brown, 1987:272–276.
Grant HD, Murray RH Jr, Bergeron JD. Emergency care. 4th ed. Englewood Cliffs, NJ: Prentice-Hall, 1986:270–271.
Hafen B, Karren K. Prehospital emergency care and crisis intervention. 3rd ed. Englewood, CO: Morton, 1989:255–256.
McSwain NE. Helmet removal. Curr Concepts Trauma Care 1981; 20–21.

CORSET – TYPE EXTRICATION DEVICES

Bob McMullen

PURPOSE

To provide spinal support to, and to facilitate lifting of, stable patients who need to be extricated from a sitting position or from confined spaces unsuitable for a long or short backboard. These flexible extrication devices are applied to conform closely to the patient's body.

INDICATIONS

Need for spinal immobilization during extrication of seated patient
Need for spinal immobilization during extrication of patient from confined space

CONTRAINDICATIONS

Patient's condition is unstable (e.g., cardiac or respiratory arrest, unconscious, shock); device application time is prolonged
Impaled object in chest, abdomen, or back that impedes proper application of device
Rescuers inexperienced in application of device

POTENTIAL COMPLICATIONS

Further aggravation of spinal injury, fractures, or soft tissue injury

EQUIPMENT

Cervical collar
Long backboard
Corset-type extrication device (several that are available commercially include, but are not limited to, KED, XP-1, and Greene Splint) (Fig. 1).

PROCEDURE

1. One rescuer should immediately secure manual stabilization of the cervical spine and maintain stabilization throughout the remainder of the extrication
2. Another rescuer should assess the airway, breathing, and circulation (ABCs) and apply a cervical collar. Life threatening emergencies should be ascertained and treated. If these exist, rapid extrication should follow, and the rescuer may want to reconsider use of the corset-type extrication device. In addition, oxygen should be applied at this point, if indicated, and neurologic status should be determined.
3. The corset-type extrication device should be positioned behind the sitting patient so that
   a. The smooth side (the side with no straps or fasteners) is toward the patient
   b. The patient is centered in the device
   c. The top of the device is far enough down so that it will clear the car doorway during patient removal
4. The device must next be positioned snugly up under the patient's armpits because this is where much of the weight will be borne during lifting. Failure to position the device high enough may result in excessive traction being applied to the cervical spine on lifting.
5. Fasten and make snug the straps across the abdomen and chest. If the patient is experiencing dyspnea, the top chest strap may need to be loosened slightly until ready for moving.
6. The leg straps should next be passed under each leg, attached in the fastener, and made snug and firm. Some prefer to cross the leg straps at the groin, others simply attach the right strap on the right and the left on the left; check with local protocol for clarification. In addition, prior to tightening the leg straps, it may be necessary to place some extra padding between the straps and the groin for the patient's comfort.
7. The head should next be secured to the device, either with Velcro straps or adhesive tape. It will probably be necessary to pad behind the head prior to securing it to prevent hyperextension of the neck.
8. Coexistent extremity fractures should be splinted at this point, prior to moving the patient
9. The top chest strap should be tightened, if not done previously
10. Two rescuers can now extricate the patient by lifting with the straps provided on the back of the device, and lifting the patient's legs
11. Move the patient to a long backboard, scoop stretcher, or Stokes' basket
12. Loosen the leg straps before attempting to straighten the patient's legs
13. Secure the patient to the backboard, stretcher, or basket
14. Loosen the top chest strap to relieve pressure on the chest

FOLLOW-UP

1. Reassess ABCs, vital signs, and neurologic status
2. Assure completed spinal immobilization
3. Complete secondary survey

DOCUMENTATION

Initial assessment of patient with special notes pertaining to injuries of the chest, abdomen, or back (which will be covered by the device) and initial neurologic status

Procedure used and outcome (e.g., "Patient extricated from vehicle with KED to long backboard without incident.")

Ongoing reassessment of ABC's, vital signs, neurologic status, and adequate spinal immobilization

References

Hafen B, Karren K. Prehospital emergency care and crisis intervention. 3rd ed. Englewood, CO: Morton, 1989:255–256.

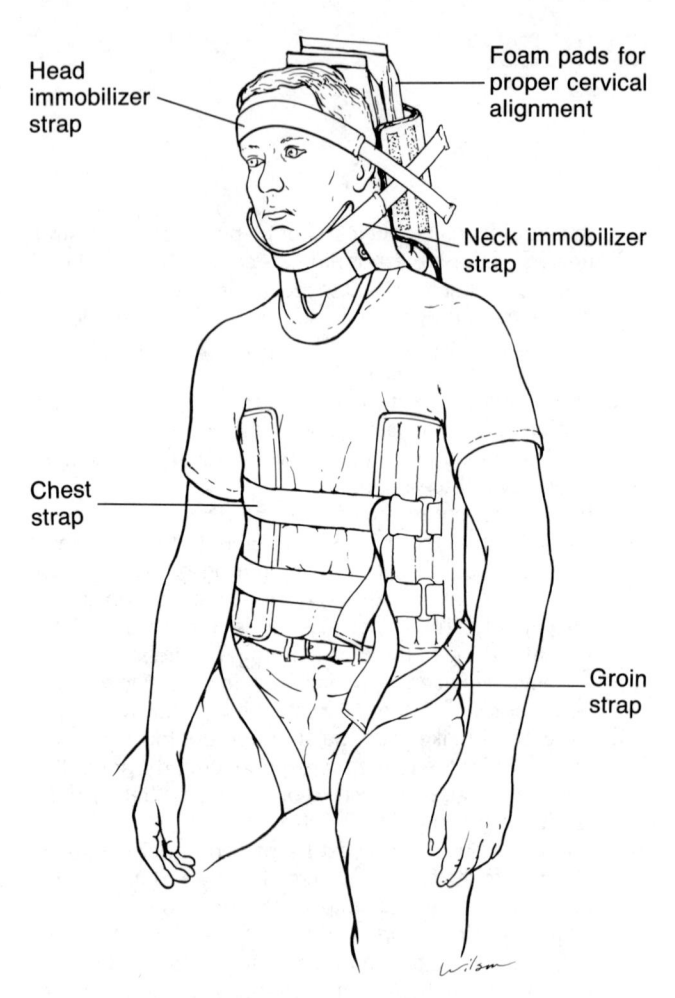

Figure 1 Corset-type extrication device.

RESUSCITATION CRITIQUE

TRAUMA RESUSCITATION VIDEOTAPING

Peggy Hollingsworth-Fridlund
David B. Hoyt

PURPOSE

To provide a valuable adjunct to education, peer review, orientation, and self critique.

INDICATIONS

Every admission that necessitates trauma team activation should be recorded on videotape

CONTRAINDICATIONS

None

POTENTIAL COMPLICATIONS

Lack of protection of tapes as confidential material

EQUIPMENT

Television monitor
Half-inch videocassette recorder with fast, slow, and pause functions
Videocamera
Wide-angle, low-light lens
Bulk eraser
Portable cart
Videotapes, half-inch size

PROCEDURE

Policy Development

1. Develop a policy and procedure for the videotape protocol
2. Specify methods for protection of patient confidentiality
3. Specify personnel responsible for tape review
4. Specify the activities for which tapes will be used
5. Specify videotaping of resuscitation in Trauma Quality Assurance Plan as a peer review and educational activity
6. Designate personnel responsible for erasing tapes on a timely basis

Staff

1. Educate all staff regarding confidentiality of peer review and educational materials
2. Educate all staff members regarding the purpose of the videotaping
3. Mount camera so that the patient's face cannot be seen on the screen
4. Label all blank tapes with sequential numbers
5. Develop audit instrument for reviewing tapes (Fig. 1)
6. Base elements of audit instrument on adherence to standards and protocols
7. Store numbered blank tapes next to videorecorder
8. Designate responsibility for operating video equipment to resuscitation nurse
9. Confirm camera position from foot of bed after turning on videorecorder and camera
10. Place blank tape in videorecorder and begin recording prior to patient admission
11. Continue taping until patient has left resuscitation bed
12. Label tape with patient's alias name and unit number
13. Record the number of the tape and patient's alias name on log
14. Place used tape in locked box
15. Remove used tapes from locked box on a regular basis for review and erasure
16. Confirm presence of all tapes by review of sequential numbers
17. Review tapes with application of audit tool
18. Initiate quality assurance process with identified issues or problem flags
19. Select tapes for review at multidisciplinary conference presentation based on team educational needs
20. Place tapes held for multidisciplinary or individual review or for nursing educational review in a secure place until used
21. Rewind all tapes and erase
22. Review problems with individual staff members or with their supervisors
23. Trend the identified problems every month and twice yearly
24. Base educational activities on identified trends
25. Add additional audit elements as trends or problems are identified

FOLLOW-UP

1. Write a periodic summary report including the entire quality assurance process from problems identified, investigation, education, remedial action, and re-evaluation plan
2. Submit summary report through quality assurance channels

DOCUMENTATION

Policy and procedure
Videotape audit tool
Meeting minutes of multidisciplinary conferences or other educational activities
Monthly, yearly trend form
Summary report for quality assurance activities

References

Hoyt DB, Shackford SR, Hollingsworth-Fridlund P, et al. Video recording trauma resuscitation: an effective teaching technique. J Trauma 1988; 28:435–440.

Patient Alias				
Unit #				
Date of arrival				
Reviewer				
Mechanism of injury				

REPORT:
Prehospital

General: _____

_____ Mechanism of injury
_____ Vital signs
_____ Rx
_____ Fluids
_____ Obvious Injuries

Team: Attending _____
Dr.1 _____
X-ray technician _____
Registered technician _____

Assessment/Management	Timely	Late	Problem	Action Taken
Airway				
Breath sounds assessment				
Circulation				
Cervical spine				
Neurologic check				
Consultants				
SECONDARY SURVEY				
Back				
Extremities				
Lavage				
Central venous pressure				
Foley catheter				
Rectal				
Inspection				
Technique				
Time art stick pressure				
Military anti-shock trousers (MAST)				
MAST removal technique				
Use of end tidal CO_2 to verify endotracheal tube (ETT)				
ETT/Ambu connect on transfer				

Problem Quality Assurance Assessment
  1.
  2.
  3.
Action
  1.
  2.
  3.
Follow-up
  1.
  2.
  3.

Nursing performance
  Vital signs, serial identity problems with intravenous lines
  Pressure bags, intravenous lines
  Warming blankets
  MAST, vital signs
  Assess level of consciousness
  Follow cervical spine status
  Early central venous pressure
  X-ray safety
  Cover gown
    Gloves
    Goggles
    Mask
    Cover hat
  Anticipate surgical airway
  Blood pressure check after ventilator
  Check intravenous rate with Dr. #1 or update fluid amounts

Figure 1 Videotape resuscitation audit form.

AMERICAN HEART ASSOCIATION THERAPEUTIC MODALITIES

Asystole
Electromechanical Dissociation
Ventricular Fibrillation
Sustained Ventricular Tachycardia

ASYSTOLE

Mary E. Mancini

A. Endotracheal intubation is the preferred method of airway management. However, if adequate ventilation can be maintained with a bag-valve-mask unit, the immediate administration of epinephrine is crucial to convert asystole to a pulse generating rhythm. Endotracheal intubation should be undertaken when possible.

B. Epinephrine (1:10,000), 0.5 to 1.0 mg, is given in an intravenous push. The drug can be administered every 5 minutes as necessary. If an intravenous line cannot be established easily and if the patient is intubated, epinephrine may be instilled into the endotracheal tube.

C. Atropine, 1 mg in an intravenous push, can be repeated in 5 minutes, if necessary, to a maximal dosage of 2 mg. If an intravenous line is not in place, consider administering atropine via the endotracheal tube, if available.

D. If still unable to convert to a life sustaining rhythm, a central line should be placed to assure delivery of drugs into the central circulation.

E. The administration of sodium bicarbonate is of questionable value and may be harmful. Consideration should be given to managing acidosis by hyperventilation. If a decision is made to give sodium bicarbonate, the dose should be 1 mEq/kg. A repeat dose of 0.5 mEq/kg may be given every 10 minutes if necessary.

F. If the cardiac rhythm is unresponsive to this therapy, consider the possibility of an alternate diagnosis. Low amplitude ventricular fibrillation may mimic asystole; therefore, defibrillation should be considered.

References

American Heart Association. Textbook of advanced cardiac life support. Dallas: American Heart Association, 1987:239.
Mancini ME. Asystole. In: Mancini ME, ed. Decision making in emergency nursing. Toronto: BC Decker, 1987:96–97.
Standards and guidelines for cardiopulmonary resuscitation (CPR) and emergency cardiac care (ECC). JAMA 1986; 21:2905–2984.

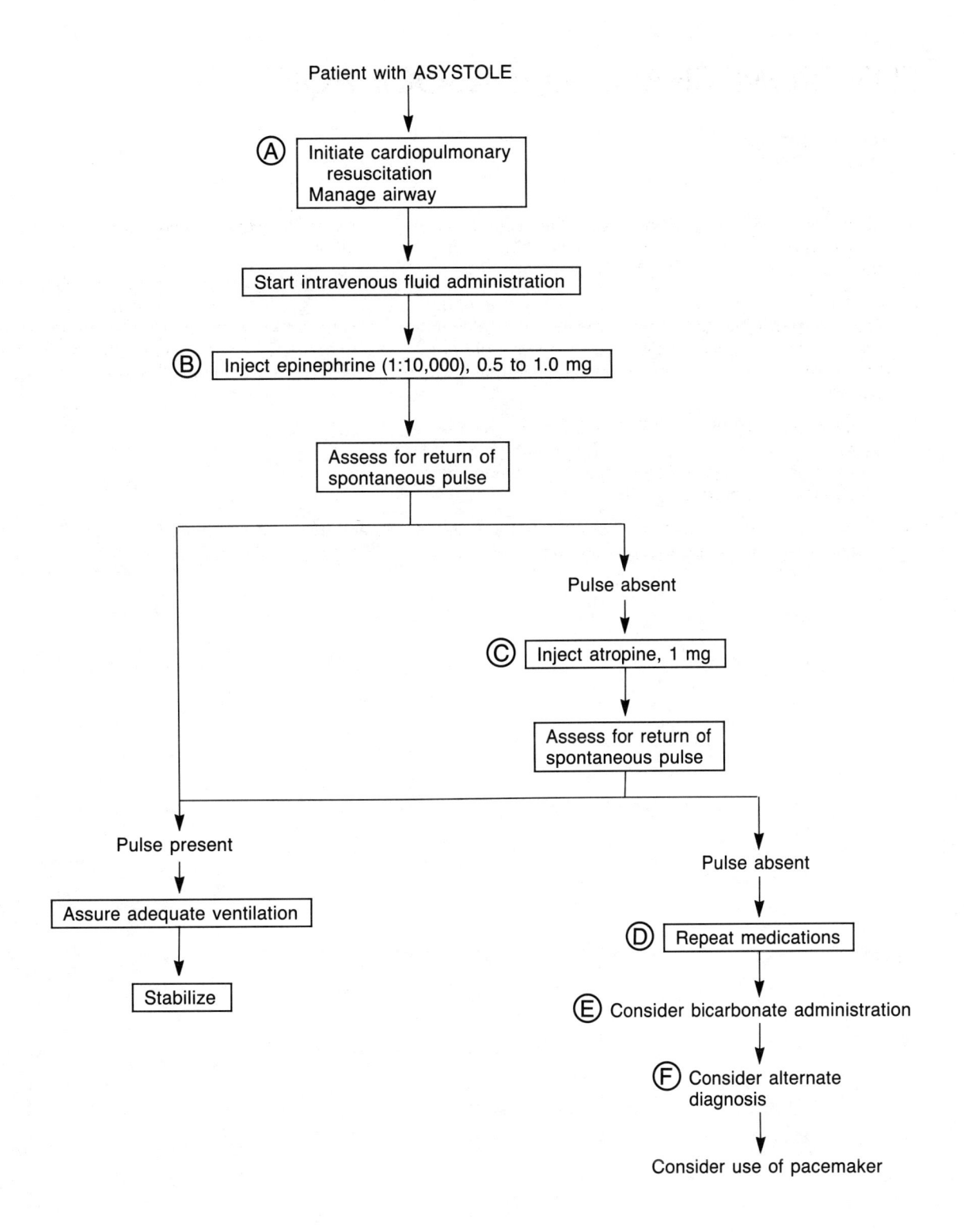

```
Patient with ASYSTOLE
          ↓
(A) Initiate cardiopulmonary
    resuscitation
    Manage airway
          ↓
    Start intravenous fluid administration
          ↓
(B) Inject epinephrine (1:10,000), 0.5 to 1.0 mg
          ↓
    Assess for return of
    spontaneous pulse
       ↙        ↘
  Pulse present   Pulse absent
                     ↓
                (C) Inject atropine, 1 mg
                     ↓
                 Assess for return of
                 spontaneous pulse
                  ↙         ↘
            Pulse present   Pulse absent
                                ↓
                          (D) Repeat medications
                                ↓
                          (E) Consider bicarbonate administration
                                ↓
                          (F) Consider alternate
                              diagnosis
                                ↓
                          Consider use of pacemaker

  Pulse present
       ↓
  Assure adequate ventilation
       ↓
  Stabilize
```

ELECTROMECHANICAL DISSOCIATION

Mary E. Mancini

A. Electromechanical dissociation is associated with a poor prognosis unless the underlying cause is rapidly identified and corrected.

B. Intubation is the preferred mechanism of airway control. However, providing epinephrine is the most critical therapy for electromechanical dissociation and should not be delayed if the patient can be ventilated without intubation.

C. Epinephrine (1:10,000), 0.5 to 1.0 mg, can be given intravenously or via the endotracheal tube if intravenous access is not established. Administration of epinephrine can be repeated every 5 minutes.

D. If resuscitation is not initially achieved with the use of a peripheral intravenous line, consider a central line to ensure delivery of medications into the central circulation.

E. Assessment of neck veins can be helpful in determining etiology. When neck vein distention is absent and there is no backflow during central line insertion, hypovolemia should be considered. When neck veins are prominent, consider pneumothorax or pericardial tamponade.

Reference

American Heart Association. Textbook of advanced cardiac life support. Dallas: American Heart Association, 1987:240.

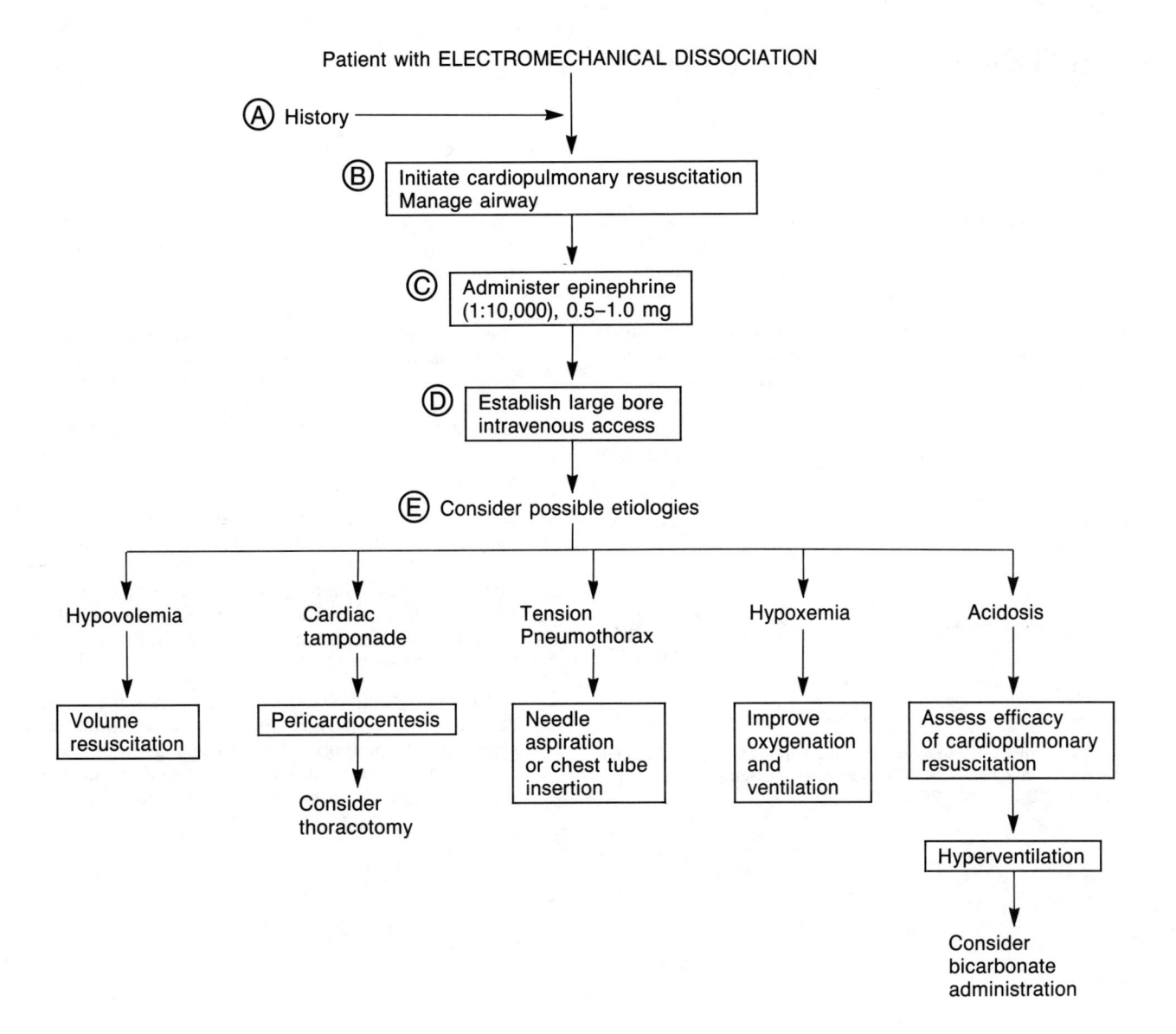

```
Patient with ELECTROMECHANICAL DISSOCIATION
                        │
Ⓐ History ──────────────▶│
                         ▼
                    Ⓑ ┌─────────────────────────────────────┐
                      │ Initiate cardiopulmonary resuscitation │
                      │ Manage airway                          │
                      └─────────────────────────────────────┘
                                    │
                                    ▼
                    Ⓒ ┌─────────────────────────┐
                      │ Administer epinephrine    │
                      │ (1:10,000), 0.5–1.0 mg    │
                      └─────────────────────────┘
                                    │
                                    ▼
                    Ⓓ ┌─────────────────────────┐
                      │ Establish large bore      │
                      │ intravenous access        │
                      └─────────────────────────┘
                                    │
                                    ▼
                    Ⓔ Consider possible etiologies
```

Hypovolemia	Cardiac tamponade	Tension Pneumothorax	Hypoxemia	Acidosis
Volume resuscitation	Pericardiocentesis	Needle aspiration or chest tube insertion	Improve oxygenation and ventilation	Assess efficacy of cardiopulmonary resuscitation
	Consider thoracotomy			Hyperventilation
				Consider bicarbonate administration

425

VENTRICULAR FIBRILLATION

Mary E. Mancini

A. When cardiac arrest is witnessed, a precordial thump may be delivered by administering one sharp blow to the lower sternum with a closed fist. This may terminate the fibrillation (Fig. 1).

B. Once a cardiac rhythm is established that generates a palpable carotid pulse, the patient's condition should be assessed and stabilized. The ventilatory status should be evaluated to determine whether endotracheal intubation is necessary. An antidysrhythmic drug infusion should be considered to prevent the recurrence of ventricular fibrillation. The reason for the episode should be determined and the disorder treated or prevented from recurring.

C. Endotracheal intubation is the preferred method of airway management. However, if adequate ventilation can be maintained with a bag-valve-mask unit, immediate defibrillation is most likely to effect conversion to a life sustaining rhythm. The effectiveness of cardiopulmonary resuscitation (CPR) should be evaluated frequently by ensuring that a pulse is being generated with each compression.

D. Electrical defibrillation should be administered as soon as possible. If a monitor is not immediately available, consideration should be given to defibrillating the patient even before a monitor is attached. As time progresses, ventricular fibrillation is likely to deteriorate to asystole. Asystole is significantly more difficult to convert to a life sustaining rhythm.

E. The patient should be evaluated for the return of a spontaneous pulse after every treatment by defibrillation or chemical therapy. If no pulse is present, a repeat defibrillation should be undertaken immediately, or cardiopulmonary resuscitation should be reinstituted rapidly.

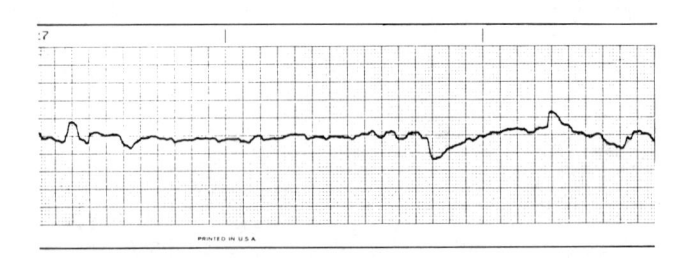

Figure 1 Ventricular fibrillation. (From Mancini ME. Ventricular fibrillation. In: Mancini ME, ed. Decision making in emergency nursing. Toronto: BC Decker, 1987:100.)

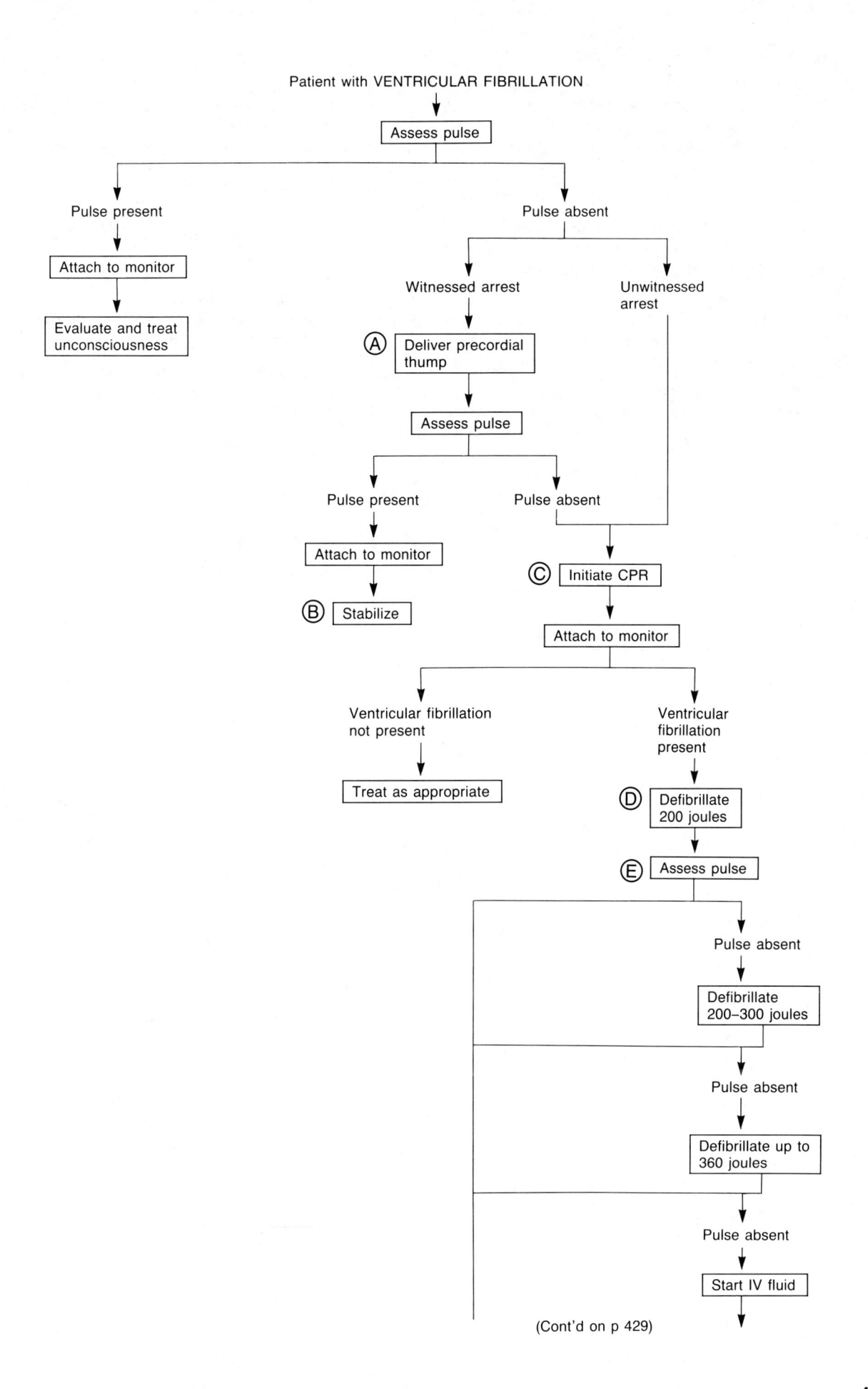

Patient with VENTRICULAR FIBRILLATION
↓
Assess pulse

Pulse present
↓
Attach to monitor
↓
Evaluate and treat unconsciousness

Pulse absent

- Witnessed arrest
  ↓
  Ⓐ Deliver precordial thump
  ↓
  Assess pulse
  - Pulse present
    ↓
    Attach to monitor
    ↓
    Ⓑ Stabilize
  - Pulse absent
- Unwitnessed arrest

↓
Ⓒ Initiate CPR
↓
Attach to monitor

- Ventricular fibrillation not present
  ↓
  Treat as appropriate
- Ventricular fibrillation present
  ↓
  Ⓓ Defibrillate 200 joules
  ↓
  Ⓔ Assess pulse
  ↓
  Pulse absent
  ↓
  Defibrillate 200–300 joules
  ↓
  Pulse absent
  ↓
  Defibrillate up to 360 joules
  ↓
  Pulse absent
  ↓
  Start IV fluid
  ↓

(Cont'd on p 429)

F. Epinephrine (1:10,000), 0.5 to 1.0 mg, is given in an intravenous push; the dose can be repeated every 5 minutes as necessary. If an intravenous line cannot be established easily and the patient has been intubated, the epinephrine may be instilled into the endotracheal tube.

G. Lidocaine, 1 mg/kg, is given in an intravenous push.

H. The initial dose of bretylium is 5 mg/kg given in an intravenous push. One may use a repeat dose of lidocaine at a level of 0.5 mg/kg instead of bretylium.

I. Lidocaine may be given in repeated doses of 0.5 mg/kg every 8 minutes until a total dosage of 3 mg/kg is reached. Bretylium may be repeated at twice the initial dose (10 mg/kg) if needed.

J. The administration of sodium bicarbonate is of questionable value and may actually be harmful. Consideration should be given to managing acidosis by hyperventilation. If a decision is made to give sodium bicarbonate, the dose should be 1 mEq/kg. A repeat dose of 0.5 mEq/kg may be given every 10 minutes if necessary. Ventilatory status should be assessed to assure the patient is adequately oxygenated.

References

American Heart Association. Textbook of advanced cardiac life support. Dallas: American Heart Association, 1987:238.

Mancini ME. Ventricular fibrillation. In: Mancini ME, ed. Decision making in emergency nursing. Toronto: BC Decker, 1987:l00–101.

Standards and guidelines for cardiopulmonary resuscitation (CPR) and emergency cardiac care (ECC). JAMA 1986; 21:2905–2984.

(Cont'd from p 427)

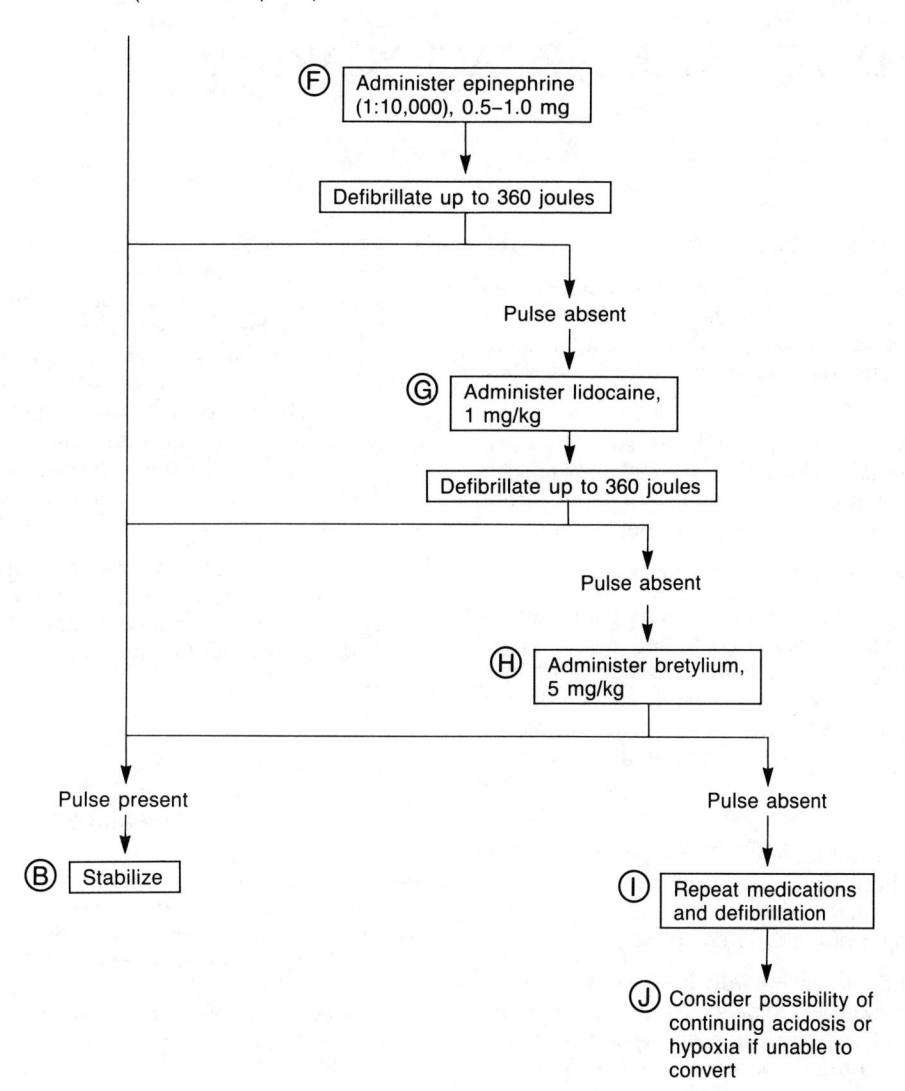

```
                    ┌─────────────────────────┐
                 Ⓕ │ Administer epinephrine  │
                   │ (1:10,000), 0.5–1.0 mg  │
                   └────────────┬────────────┘
                                ▼
                   ┌─────────────────────────┐
                   │ Defibrillate up to 360 joules │
                   └────────────┬────────────┘
                                │
                          Pulse absent
                                ▼
                   ┌─────────────────────────┐
                 Ⓖ │ Administer lidocaine,   │
                   │ 1 mg/kg                 │
                   └────────────┬────────────┘
                                ▼
                   ┌─────────────────────────┐
                   │ Defibrillate up to 360 joules │
                   └────────────┬────────────┘
                                │
                          Pulse absent
                                ▼
                   ┌─────────────────────────┐
                 Ⓗ │ Administer bretylium,   │
                   │ 5 mg/kg                 │
                   └────────────┬────────────┘
```

Pulse present → Ⓑ Stabilize

Pulse absent → Ⓘ Repeat medications and defibrillation

Ⓙ Consider possibility of continuing acidosis or hypoxia if unable to convert

429

SUSTAINED VENTRICULAR TACHYCARDIA

Mary E. Mancini

A. For a discussion of ventricular fibrillation see p 426.

B. If the patient has only minimal or no symptoms, time is available to try chemical cardioversion. If the patient starts to exhibit signs or symptoms of decompensation, the therapy for unstable patients should be initiated (Fig. 1).

C. If the patient is experiencing chest pain, dyspnea, hypotension (systolic pressure less than 90 mm Hg), congestive heart failure, or infarction, immediate action needs to be taken to prevent further deterioration.

D. The initial dose of lidocaine is 1 mg/kg.

E. Lidocaine, 0.5 mg/kg, can be given every 8 minutes until ventricular tachycardia is controlled or a maximal dosage of 3 mg/kg has been given. Be aware of the signs and symptoms of lidocaine toxicity; these include confusion, ringing in the ears, blurred vision, numbness, and seizures. Special care in administering lidocaine needs to be taken in elderly patients and those with liver disease.

F. Procainamide is administered, 20 mg per minute, until ventricular tachycardia resolves or until a total of 1 g has been administered. Be aware of the potential for hypotension or widening of the QRS complex.

G. Once the ventricular tachycardia has resolved, the patient should be evaluated to determine the reason for the episode. A continuous infusion of the antiarrhythmic drug that assisted the conversion should be initiated.

H. If the patient's condition is unstable, synchronized electrical cardioversion is the therapy of choice. A precordial thump may also be employed prior to cardioversion. The procedure and sensations that can be expected should be carefully explained to the patient. Time should be taken to answer any questions the patient may have. With each unsuccessful attempt, the energy level should be doubled until the maximal energy level of 360 joules is reached. Care should be taken to ensure that the conduction pads do not dry out with successive cardioversion attempts; otherwise, the patient may be burned.

I. If maximal energy cardioversion is not successful, an antiarrhythmic drug should be added and cardioversion tried again. The recommended order of therapy is lidocaine, procainamide, and bretylium.

References

American Heart Association. Textbook of advanced cardiac life support. Dallas: American Heart Association, 1987:241.

Mancini ME. Sustained ventricular tachycardia. In: Mancini ME, ed. Decision making in emergency nursing. Toronto: BC Decker, 1987:102–103.

Standards and guidelines for cardiopulmonary resuscitation (CPR) and emergency cardiac care (ECC). JAMA 1986; 21:2905–2984.

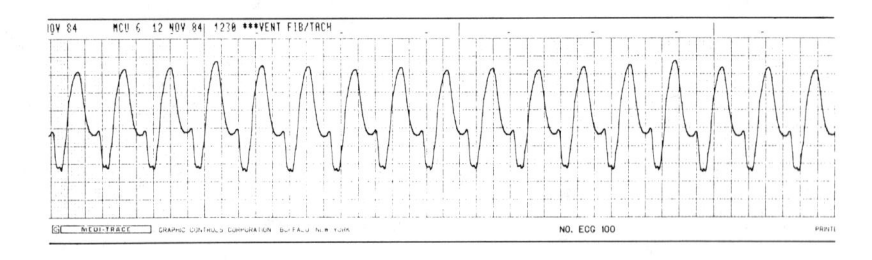

Figure 1 Sustained ventricular tachycardia. (From Mancini ME. Sustained ventricular tachycardia. In: Mancini ME, ed. Decision making in emergency nursing. Toronto: BC Decker, 1987:102.)

Patient with SUSTAINED VENTRICULAR TACHYCARDIA
↓
Assess pulse

Pulse absent → Ⓐ Follow ventricular fibrillation procedures (p 426)

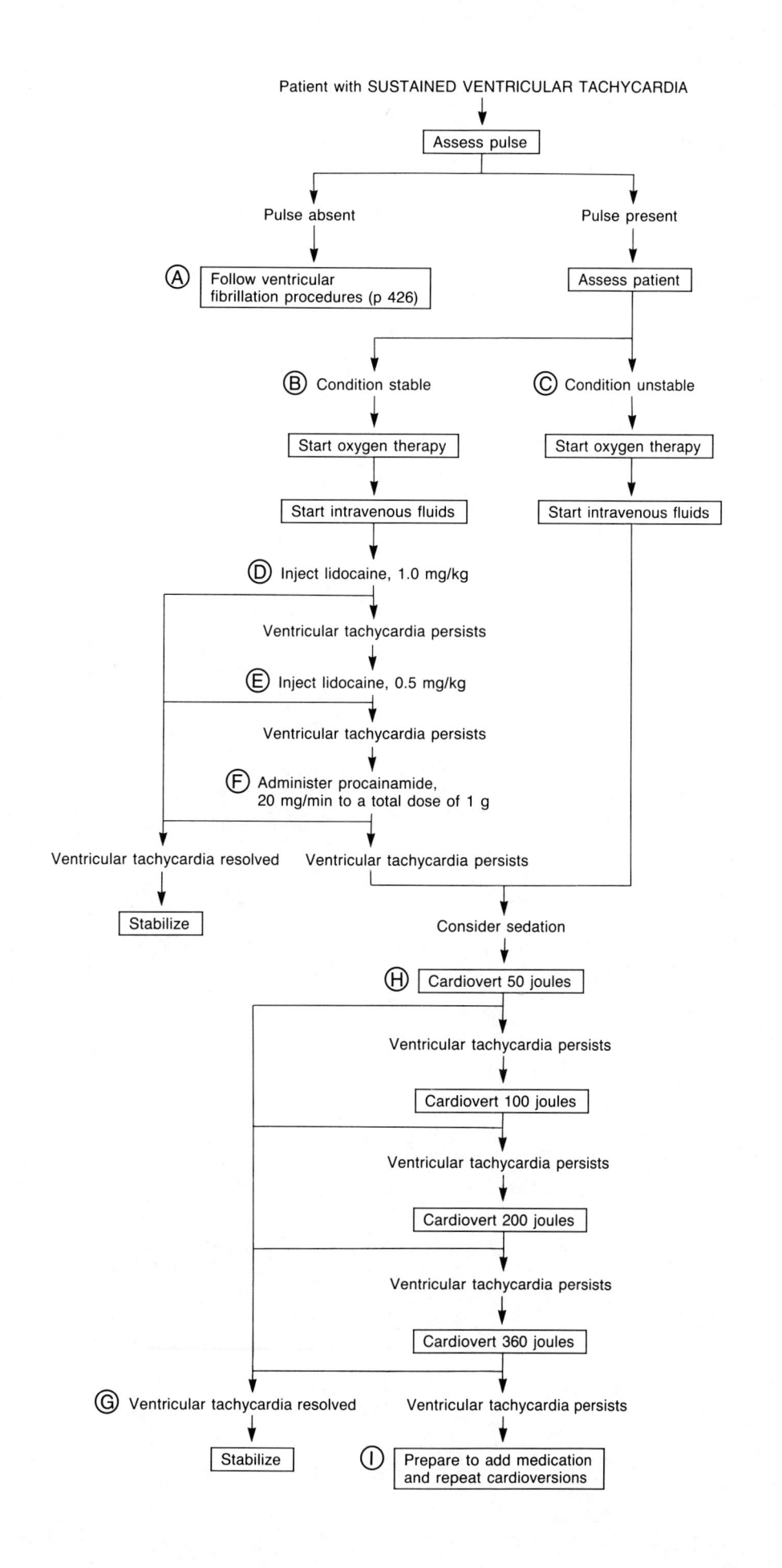

Pulse present → Assess patient

Ⓑ Condition stable
- Start oxygen therapy
- Start intravenous fluids
- Ⓓ Inject lidocaine, 1.0 mg/kg
- Ventricular tachycardia persists
- Ⓔ Inject lidocaine, 0.5 mg/kg
- Ventricular tachycardia persists
- Ⓕ Administer procainamide, 20 mg/min to a total dose of 1 g

Ⓒ Condition unstable
- Start oxygen therapy
- Start intravenous fluids

Ventricular tachycardia resolved → Stabilize

Ventricular tachycardia persists → Consider sedation

Ⓗ Cardiovert 50 joules
Ventricular tachycardia persists
↓
Cardiovert 100 joules
Ventricular tachycardia persists
↓
Cardiovert 200 joules
Ventricular tachycardia persists
↓
Cardiovert 360 joules

Ⓖ Ventricular tachycardia resolved → Stabilize

Ventricular tachycardia persists → Ⓘ Prepare to add medication and repeat cardioversions

INDEX

A

Abbreviated injury scale, 282–283
Abdominal trauma
   assessment of, 30–31, 130
   blunt, 130–333
   ileofemoral vascular injuries in, 188–889
   local exploration of, 382
   pediatric, 230–235
   penetrating, 134–135
Abruptio placentae, 258
Acetabular fracture, 164–165
Acid-base imbalance, 290–291
Acidosis
   metabolic, 290–291
   respiratory, 290–291, 294
Activities of daily living
   in head trauma rehabilitation, 338, 340
   in spinal cord injury rehabilitation, 342, 345
Acute renal failure, 304–305
Adult respiratory distress syndrome, 310–311
Air transport, 336–337
Airway disruption, in children, 228
Airway management, 26, 86–87, 358–363
   in children, 214–219
   in-hospital, 20
   in inhalation injury, 206–207
   in laryngotracheal trauma, 28, 76–77, 114–115
   in maxillofacial fractures, 68–69
   in maxillofacial soft tissue trauma, 58
   in neck trauma
     blunt, 76
     penetrating, 80–81
   pre-hospital, 12–13
   in pregnancy, 256
Alkalinization, gastric, 324–325
Alkalosis, 290–291
Amniotic fluid, in pregnancy trauma, 258
Amputation, 32, 172–175
   of auricle, 64
   rehabilitation in, 346–351
Analgesia, for rib fractures, 126
Anaphylaxis, in spider bite, 248
Anesthesia, 286–287
   local, 298
   topical, 298
Angiography
   in extremity trauma, 166, 190
   interpretation of, 186
   in knee trauma, 166
Animal bites, 58, 246–247
Ankle trauma, 166–171
Antacids, for stress gastritis, 324–325
Anti-arrhythmics
   for asystole, 422–423
   for electromechanical dissociation, 424–425
   for ventricular fibrillation, 428
Antibiotics
   prophylactic, 298
   selection of, 330
Antiembolism stockings, 394–395
Antipyretics, 302–303
Antivenom
   for snake bites, 250
   for spider bites, 248

Aortic rupture, 28, 112–113
   in children, 228
Aortography, 378
Arm. See under Extremity
Arrhythmias, 422–431
Arterial blood sampling, 368–369
   in respiratory failure, 310
Arterial injuries. See Vascular injuries and specific arteries
Arterial line, insertion of, 388
Arteriography, 378
Aseptic meningitis, 302
Asphyxia, traumatic, 28–29
Assault, 252–255
   evidence collection in, 266–269
Asystole, 422
Atropine, for asystole, 422–423
Automobile accidents
   corset-type extraction devices for, 415–416
   mechanisms of injury in, 1–2
Autonomic dysreflexia, 152, 344
Autotransfusion, 294
Avulsion, of teeth, 62–63
Axillary artery trauma, 186–187
Axonotmesis, 178

B

Bacteremia, 330–331
Bandages, 401–402
Beck's triad, in pericardial tamponade, 316
Bed-to-wheelchair transfer, in spinal cord injury, 342
Bites, 58
   animal, 246–247
   dog, 244–245
   snake, 250–251
   spider, 248–249
Black widow spider bites, 248–249
Bladder program
   in head trauma patients, 341
   in spinal cord injury, 344
Blanket, warming/cooling, 399–400
Blast injuries, 3
Bleeding
   control of, 296
     in children, 218
     initial, 20, 22
     problems in, 300–301
   in fractures, 32
   hemothorax and, 92–93
   intraperitoneal, in children, 232–233
   nasal, 60
   in penetrating neck trauma, 80–81
Blood gas sampling, 368–369
   in respiratory failure, 310
Blood pressure, systolic, in trauma score, 278–281
Blood transfusion, 22, 40–43, 294
   blood warming for, 44–45
   in children, 218
   systemic reaction to, 42
Blunt trauma. See also specific sites and types of
   mechanisms of, 1–2
Bowel program
   in head trauma rehabilitation, 340, 342
   in spinal cord injury, 342–344

Brachial artery trauma, 186–187
Brain death, criteria for, 332
Brain injury. See Head trauma
Bretylium, for ventricular fibrillation, 428
Bronchial trauma, 28
   in children, 228
Brown recluse spider bites, 248–249
Bullet wounds, 2–3. See also sites of
   debridement of, 166
   high-velocity, 164, 166
   low-velocity, 166
Burns, 3, 194–197
   chemical, 3, 200–201
   of eye, 66, 200, 411–412
   in children, 238–239
   electrical, 198–199
   of mouth, 58
   escharotomy and fasciotomy for, 204–205
   smoke inhalation and, 206–207

C

Capillary refill, in trauma score, 278–281
Cardiac arrest, defibrillation in, 426–429
Cardiac arrhythmias, 422–431
Cardiac contusion, 22, 28
Cardiac tamponade, 29, 98–101
   in children, 226
   thoracotomy for, 99, 102
Cardiac trauma, thoracotomy for, 99, 102
Cardiogenic shock, 22, 316–317
Cardioversion, electrical, for sustained ventricular tachycardia, 430
Carotid artery trauma, 48–51, 184–185
Cast care, 408
Catheter
   in hemodialysis, temporary access for, 396
   infection and, 330
   peripheral intravenous, exchange of, 374–375
   pulmonary artery, insertion of, 391–392
Central venous pressure monitoring, 294
Cervical spine injury, 146–149
   airway management in, 86–87
   assessment for
     in-hospital, 20, 26, 32
     pre-hospital, 8
   in blunt neck trauma, 76
   in children, 220–223
   traction/stabilization for, 397–398
Cesarean section, in pregnancy trauma, 258
Chain of evidence, 268
Chemical burns, 3, 200–201
   of eye, 66, 200, 411–412
Chest, flail, 28, 96–97
   in children, 224
Chest trauma
   assessment of
     initial, 20–22
     secondary, 26–28
     steps in, 124
   blunt, 28–29
   open sucking wound in, 94–95
   in children, 226
   pediatric, 224–229
   penetrating, 29
Chest tube, 366–367

433

Chest tube, (Continued)
  in children, 216, 224
  in hemothorax, 122
    massive, 92
  in open sucking chest wound, 94
  in pneumothorax, 122
  in tension pneumothorax, 88
Children
  abdominal trauma in, 230–235
  aortic rupture in, 228
  burns in, 238–239
  chest trauma in, 224–229
  extremity trauma in, 236–237
  head trauma in, 220–223
  intraosseous line in, 376
  physical and sexual abuse of, 240–241, 252
  resuscitation of, 214–219
  triage for, 210–213
Children's Trauma Tool, 210
Chin lift, for airway management, 12–13
Cimetidine, for stress gastritis, 324
Circulatory assessment
  in children, 218
  in elderly, 260
  in-hospital, 22
  pre-hospital, 12–13
  in pregnancy, 256
Clavicle trauma, 156–157
Clostridial infection, 306–307
Clothing, handling of, 266
Coagulation problems, 300–301
Cognitive rehabilitation, 338–341
Cold injuries, 3–4, 399–400
Coma
  Glasgow Coma Score for, 24, 50
  hepatic, 308
  organ donation and, 332–333
  rehabilitation in, 338–341
Communication deficits, in head trauma, 341
Compartment syndrome, 32, 170, 174
  in children, 236
  in electrical burns, 198
  fasciotomy for, 204–205
  in hip trauma, 164
Compression injuries, peripheral nerve trauma and, 178
Computed tomography, 379
  in abdominal trauma
    blunt, 131
    in children, 232–233
    penetrating, 134
  in head trauma, 48, 52
    in children, 220–223
Consciousness level, Glasgow Coma Score for, 24, 50, 278–279
Constipation. See Bowel program
Contact lens removal, 409–410
Contusion
  myocardial, 22, 28, 106–107
    in children, 228
  peripheral nerve trauma and, 178
  pulmonary, 28, 108–111
    in children, 226
Cooling devices, 399–400
Copperhead bites, 250–251
Coral snake bites, 250–251
Corset-type extraction devices, 415–416
Cottonmouth bites, 250–251
CRAMS score, 276–277
Cricothyroidotomy, 86. See also Airway management
  needle, 8, 20, 360–361
  in children, 216

surgical, 361–362
Criminal assault, 252–255
  evidence collection in, 266–269
Crisis intervention, 334–335
Crush injury, 296
Crutchfield tongs, for cervical spine traction, 397–398
Crystalloid administration, 44–45
Culture, wound, 298, 302

D

Data collection, 272–273
Debridement, 296–297
Deep vein thrombosis, 328–329
  pneumatic pressure device for, 394–395
Defecation. See Bowel program
Defibrillation, 426–429
Delayed primary closure, 298
Dental trauma, 62–63
Diagnostic peritoneal lavage, 30, 380–381
  in abdominal trauma
    blunt, 131
    penetrating, 134
  in children, 233–234
Diaphragmatic hernia, traumatic, 116–117
Diaphragmatic rupture, 28
  in children, 228
Dislocation
  of elbow, 158–159
  of femoral head, 164–165
  of hand, 160–161
  of knee, 166–167
    vascular injury in, 166, 190–191
  of shoulder, 156–157
Dispatch, emergency, 6
Diuresis, 290
Dog bites, 244–245
Dopamine, for septic shock, 320
Dressings, 401–402
Drowning, 264–265
Dysphagia, in head trauma, 340
Dysrhythmias, 422–431

E

E codes, 274–275
Ear trauma, 64–65
Elbow trauma, 158–159
Elderly, trauma in, 260–261
Electrical burns, of mouth, 58
Electrical cardioversion, for sustained ventricular tachycardia, 430
Electrical defibrillation, 426–429
Electrical injuries, 3, 198–199
  fasciotomy for, 204–205
Electrocardiography, in myocardial contusion, 106
Electrolyte imbalance, 290–291
Electromechanical dissociation, 424–425
Embolism, pulmonary, 326–329
  pneumatic pressure device for, 394–395
Emergency dispatch, 6
Emergency management. See Trauma management
Emergency medical technician–physician communication, 14
Emotional problems, 334–335
  in head truma, 341
  in spinal cord injury, 345
Emphysema, subcutaneous, 124–125
Endotracheal intubation, 20, 86–87, 358–359. See also Airway management
  in children, 214–217
Endotracheal tube, for children, 214, 216

Enteral nutrition, 288–289
Epidural anesthesia, 286–287
Epinephrine
  for asystole, 422–423
  for electromechanical dissociation, 424–425
  for ventricular fibrillation, 428
Epistaxis, 60
Escharotomy, 204–205
Esophageal trauma, 29, 75–76, 118–119, 124
  in children, 228
Evidence collection, 252, 254, 266–269
Exercise(s)
  in head trauma rehabilitation, 338, 340
  in lower extremity amputation, 351
  in spinal cord injury, 342
  in upper extremity amputation, 346
Explosion injuries, 3
Extraction devices, corset-type, 415–416
Extremity
  replantation of, 174
  rewarming of, 202
Extremity trauma. See also Fracture(s)
  assessment of, 31–32
  in children, 236–237
  deep vein thrombosis and, 328–329
  frostbite, 202–203
  in lower extremity, 164–175
  mangling/amputation, 32, 172–175
    rehabilitation for, 346–351
  open wounds in, 296–299, 401–402
  and pulmonary embolism, 328–329
  pulmonary embolism and, 326–327
  Thomas/Hare traction splint for, 408–410
  of upper extremity, 156–161
Eye
  foreign bodies in, 66, 411–412
  injuries of, 66–67
    chemical, 66, 198, 411–412
    contact lens removal in, 409–410
    fluorescein examination in, 412
  irrigation of, 66, 411–412
Eyelid, laceration of, 66

F

Facial trauma
  airway management in, 68–69
  contact lens removal in, 409–410
  evaluation of, 26
  soft tissue, 58–59
  treatment of, 70–71
Falls, mechanism of injury in, 2
Fasciotomy, 204–205
Febrile syndromes, 302–303
  temperature control units for, 399–400
Feeding, tube, 288–289
Feeding problems, in head trauma patients, 340
Femoral artery trauma, 188–189
Femoral nerve distribution, 182
Femur trauma, 164–165
  Steinmann pin for, 403
Fetal monitoring, 258
Fetal trauma, 256–259
Fibrillation, ventricular, 426–429
Field triage, 16
Finger trauma, 160–161
FiO$_2$
  measurement of, 368–369
  in mechanical ventilation, 312
Flail chest, 28, 96–97
  in children, 224
Fluid and electrolyte imbalance, 290–291
Fluid intake and output measurement, 294

434

Fluid intake and output measurement, (*Continued*)
  in comatose organ donor, 332–333
Fluid resuscitation, 290–291
  in burns, 196, 198, 238
  in children, 218, 226
    for burns, 238
  fluid warming for, 44–45, 294
  in hypovolemic shock, 22, 40–45, 184
  in multisystem trauma, 196
  Parkland formula for, 196
  in septic shock, 320–321
Fluid warming, 44–45, 294
Fluorescein examination, of eye, 412
Foot trauma, 166–171
Forearm trauma, 158–159
Foreign body
  in airway, 86
  in eye, 66, 411–412
  in wound, 298
Fracture(s)
  of acetabulum, 164–165
  assessment of, 31–32
  cast care for, 409
  of cervical vertebrae, 8, 20, 26, 76–79, 144–147, 146–149
  in children, 236–237
    in child abuse, 240–241
  of clavicle, 156–157
  closed reduction of, 407
  of femur, 164–165
    Steinmann pin for, 403
  of hand, 160–161
  of hip, 164–165
  of humerus, 158–159
  of knee, 166–167
  maxillofacial
    airway management in, 68–69
    evaluation of, 26
    treatment of, 70–71
  of nose, 60–61
  of olecranon, 158–159
  open, classification of, 168
  of orbit, 66
  of pelvis, 136–143
  of radius, 158–159
  of ribs, 28, 126–127
    in children, 228
    flail chest and, 96
  of scapula, 156–157
  of skull, 54–55, 220–223
  of sternum, 126
  of teeth, 62–63
  of thoracolumbar vertebrae, 150–153
  of ulna, 158–159
  of upper extremity, 158–159
  of wrist, 158–159
  of zygomatic arch, 66, 70–71
Frostbite, 202–203
  of ear, 64
  warming devices for, 399–400

G

Gangrene, gas, 306–307
Gardner-Wells tongs, for cervical spine traction, 397–398
Gas gangrene infection, 306–307
Gastric alkalinization, 324–325
Gastritis, stress, 324–325
Gastrostomy tube, 288
Glasgow Coma Scale, 24, 50, 278–279
Growth plate injuries, 236–237
Gunshot wounds, 2–3. *See also* sites of
  debridement of, 166
  high-velocity, 164, 166
  low-velocity, 166

H

H2 blockers, for stress gastritis, 324–325
Halo-vest traction, 397–398
Hand trauma, 160–161
Head trauma. *See also specific facial structures*
  blunt, 48–51
  in children, 220–223
  contact lens removal in, 409–410
  helmet removal in, 413–414
  initial evaluation of, 24
  neurogenic shock in, 318–319
  patient instruction sheet for, 48
  penetrating, 52–53
  rehabilitation in, 338–341
  secondary evaluation of, 26
  skull fracture in, 54–55
Heatstroke, 302
Helicopter transportation, 336–337
Helmet removal, 413–414
Hematoma
  of ear, 64
  intracranial, in children, 220
  of lung, in children, 226
  of nasal septum, 60
Hemodialysis, catheter, temporary access for, 396
Hemodynamic monitoring, pulse oximetry, 390
Hemorrhage. *See also* Bleeding
  hemothorax and, 92–93
  initial management of, 22
Hemorrhagic shock, 22
Hemostasis, 296. *See also* Bleeding; Hemorrhage
  in children, 218
  initial, 20, 22
  in penetrating neck trauma, 80–81
  problems in, 300–301
Hemothorax, 28
  massive, 92–93
    in children, 224
  simple, 122–123
    in children, 228
Heparin
  for deep vein thrombosis, 328
  for pulmonary embolism, 326, 328
Hepatic failure, 308–309
Hepatic laceration, in children, 232
Hernia, traumatic diaphragmatic, 116–117
Hip trauma, 164–165
Homeless, trauma in, 262–263
Humeral head trauma, 158–159
Hyperbaric oxygen, for gas gangrene, 306
Hypercalcemia, 290
Hypermagnesemia, 290
Hypernatremia, 290
Hypertension, intracranial. *See* Increased intracranial pressure
Hyperthermia, malignant, 302
Hypervolemia, 294
Hyphema, 66
Hypocalcemia, 290
Hypokalemia, 290
Hyponatremia, 290
Hypotension
  assessment of, 22
  in pregnancy, 256
Hypothermia, 3–4, 202–204
  in shock
    fluid warming for, 44–45
  prevention of, 44–45, 294
  temperature control units for, 399–400
Hypovolemic shock, 22, 36–39
  blood administration for, 40–43
  in children, 218
  fluid warming in, 44–45
  in multisystem trauma, 292–295
Hypoxemia, in respiratory failure, 310–311
Hypoxia, clinical definition of, 96

I

Ileofemoral vascular trauma, 190–192
Iliac vessel trauma, 188–189
Impotence, in spinal cord injury, 345
Incest, 252
Increased intracranial pressure, 24
  in blunt head trauma, 50
  in children, 220–223
  monitoring of, 389
  in skull fracture, 54
Infection, wound, 302, 330–331
  gas gangrene, 306–307
Inhalation injury, 206–207
Injuries. *See* Trauma
Injury severity score, 282–283
Intake and output measurement, 294
  in comatose organ donor, 332
Intra-abdominal infection, 330–331
Intracranial hematoma, in children, 220
Intracranial pressure, increased. *See* Increased intracranial pressure
Intraosseous line, 376
Intravenous access
  in children, 218
  temporary, for hemodialysis, 396
Intravenous pyelography, in pelvic trauma, 137
Intubation, 20, 358–359
  endotracheal, 86–87, 358–359. *See also* Airway management
  in children, 214–217
  for feeding, 288–289
  thoracic, 366–367
    in children, 216, 224
    in hemothorax, 92, 122
    in open sucking chest wound, 94
    in pneumothorax, 122
    in tension pneumothorax, 88
Irrigation
  of chemical burns, 200
  of eye, 66, 200, 411–412
  of wound, 298

J

Jaw injuries
  airway management in, 68–69
  soft tissue, 58–59
  treatment of, 70–71
Jaw thrust, for airway management, 12–13
Jejunostomy tube, 288

K

Ketamine anesthesia, 286–287
Kidney failure, acute, 304–305
Knee trauma, 166–167
  vascular injury in, 166, 190–191
Knife wounds, 3. *See also* sites of

L

Laboratory specimens, in crimes and accidents, 252, 254, 266–269

435

Laceration
  dressings for, 401–402
  of eyelid, 66
  of knee, 166
  of liver, in children, 232
  management of, 296–299
Laryngeal trauma, 28, 76–77, 114, 124
Lavage, diagnostic peritoneal, 30, 380–381
  in abdominal trauma
    blunt, 131
    penetrating, 134
  in children, 233–234
Leg. See under Extremity
Lidocaine
  for sustained ventricular tachycardia, 430
  for ventricular fibrillation, 428
Limb. See under Extremity
Liver, laceration of, in children, 232
Liver failure, 308–309
Local anesthesia, 298
Lower extremity. See under Extremity
Lung
  contusion of, 28, 108–111
    in children, 226
  hematoma of, in children, 226
  parenchymal injuries of, in children, 226

M

Magnetic resonance imaging, 383
Malignant hyperthermia, 302
Mandibular fractures
  airway management in, 68–69
  treatment of, 70–71
Mangled extremity, 172–175
Massive hemothorax, 92–93
  in children, 224
Mattress, warming/cooling, 399–400
Maxillofacial fractures
  airway management in, 68–69
  treatment of, 70–71
Maxillofacial soft tissue trauma, 58–59
Mechanical ventilation, 310, 312–315
Mechanism of injury, 1–4
Median nerve distribution, 180
Meningitis, aseptic, 302
Metabolic acidosis, 290
Metabolic alkalosis, 290
Microvascular surgery, for limb replantation, 174
Military anti-shock trousers (MAST), 32, 36, 294, 372–373
  in children, 218
  in neurogenic shock, 318
Missile injuries, 2–3. See also sites of
  debridement of, 166
  high-velocity, 164, 166
  low-velocity, 166
Motor vehicle accidents
  corset-type extraction devices for, 413–414
  mechanisms of injury in, 1–2
Motorcycle accidents
  helmet removal in, 413–414
  mechanisms of injury in, 1–2
Mouth
  dental injuries of, 62–63
  electrical burns of, 58
  soft tissue injuries of, 58
Multiple organ failure, 322–323
Multisystem trauma, 292
Muscle necrosis, in gas gangrene, 306
Myocardial contusion, 22, 28, 106–107
  in children, 228

N

Nasal trauma, 60–61
Nasogastric intubation, feeding, 288
Nasotracheal intubation, 86–87, 358–359
  in children, 214–217
Near-drowning, 264–265
Neck trauma. See also Cervical spine injury
  blunt, 76–79
  carotid artery injury in, 184
  evaluation of
    in-hospital, 20, 26
    pre-hospital, 8
  penetrating, 80–83
Needle cricothyroidotomy, 8, 20, 86, 360–361. See also Airway management
  in children, 216
Needle thoracostomy
  in children, 224
  for tension pneumothorax, 88
Nerve distribution, 180–182
Nerve trauma, peripheral, 178–182
Neurogenic bladder
  in head trauma patients, 341
  in spinal cord injury, 344
Neurogenic shock, 22, 318–319
Neurologic evaluation, 24, 32
  in children, 220–223
Neuropraxia, 176
Neuropsychological referral, in head trauma, 341
Neurotmesis, 176
Nose, injuries of, 60–61
Nosebleed, 60
Nutritional support, 288–289

O

Obturator nerve distribution, 182
Ocular irrigation, 66, 200, 411–412
Ocular trauma, 66–67
  chemical, 66, 200, 411–412
  contact lens removal in, 409–410
Olecranon fracture, 158–159
Open wounds
  dressings for, 401–402
  management of, 296–299
  sucking chest, 29, 94–95
    in children, 226
Operating room management, 292–295
Ophthalmic trauma. See Ocular trauma
Oral trauma
  dental, 62–63
  electrical, 58
  soft tissue, 58
Organ procurement, 332–333
Orotracheal intubation, 86–87, 358–359
  in children, 214–217
Oxygen, hyperbaric, for gas gangrene, 306

P

Pain, phantom limb
  in lower extremity amputation, 348
  in upper extremity amputation, 346
Pain relief, for rib fractures, 126
Paracentesis, 386
Paralysis. See also Spinal cord injury
  autonomic dysreflexia in, 152, 344
  rehabilitation in, 342–345
Paramedic-physician communication, 14
Parenteral nutrition, 288–289
Parkland formula, for fluid therapy, 196
Patient evaluation
  at emergency scene, 8–10
  in-hospital
    initial, 20–25
    secondary, 20–22
  pre-hospital, 8–17
PCO_2
  measurement of, 368–369
  in mechanical ventilation, 312, 314
Pedestrian-vehicle accidents, 2
Pediatric trauma
  abdominal, 230–234
  abuse, 240–241, 252
  burn, 238–239
  extremity, 236–237
  head, 220–223
  resuscitation in, 214–219
  thoracic, 224–229
  triage for, 210–213
Pediatric Trauma Score, 212
PEEP (positive end-expiratory pressure), 312–313
Pelvic trauma, 136–143
Penetrating trauma, 2–3. See also sites and types of
Perceptual deficits, in head trauma, 340
Pericardiocentesis, 384–385
  in cardiac tamponade, 98–101
  in children, 226
Peripheral intravenous access exchange, 374–375
Peripheral nerve trauma, 178–182
Peritoneal injuries, 30, 31
Peritoneal lavage, diagnostic, 30, 380–381
  in abdominal trauma
    blunt, 131
    penetrating, 134
  in children, 233–234
Peroneal nerve distribution, 182
Phantom limb
  in lower extremity amputation, 348
  in upper extremity amputation, 346
Phenylephrine, for neurogenic shock, 318
Physician–paramedic/EMT communication, 14
Pin, Steinmann, 403
Pit viper bites, 250–251
Placental abruption, 258
Pneumatic anti-shock garment, 32, 36, 294, 372–373
  in children, 218
  in neurogenic shock, 318
Pneumatic pressure device, 394–395
Pneumonia, 330–331
Pneumothorax, 28, 122–123
  in children, 236
  tension, 29, 88–91
    in children, 216, 224
PO_2, measurement of, 368–369
Popliteal vascular trauma, 166–167, 190–191
Positive end-expiratory pressure (PEEP), 312–313
Postural abnormalities, in head trauma, 338, 340
Pregnancy
  physiologic changes in, 256
  trauma in, 256–259
Primary closure, 298
Procainamide, for sustained ventricular tachycardia, 430
Prophylactic antibiotics, 298
Prosthesis
  lower extremity, 348, 350
  upper extremity, 346
Psychological complications, 334–335
  in head trauma, 341
  in spinal cord injury, 345

Pulmonary artery catheter insertion, 391–392
Pulmonary capillary wedge pressure, in respiratory failure, 310
Pulmonary contusion, 28, 108–111
 in children, 234
Pulmonary embolism, 326–329
 pneumatic pressure device for, 394–395
Pulmonary hematoma, in children, 226
Pulmonary parenchymal injury, in children, 226
Pulse, assessment of, pre-hospital, 12
Pulse oximetry, 392
Pyelography, intravenous, in pelvic trauma, 137

Q

Quadriplegia. See Spinal cord injury

R

Rabies prophylaxis
 for animal bites, 246–247
 for dog bites, 244–245
Radial nerve distribution, 181
Radiography
 in aortic rupture, 112
 in cervical spine injuries, 146, 147
 in diaphragmatic hernia, 116
 in hemothorax, 122
 in laryngotracheal trauma, 114
 in pneumothorax, 122
 in pulmonary contusion, 108, 109
Rancho Los Amigos Scale, for cognitive rehabilitation, 338
Ranitidine, for stress gastritis, 324
Rape, 252–255
Rattlesnake bites, 250–251
Regional anesthesia, 286–287
Rehabilitation
 in head trauma, 338–341
 in lower extremity amputation, 348–351
 in upper extremity amputation, 346–347
Renal failure, acute, 304–305
Respiratory acidosis, 290, 294
Respiratory alkalosis, 290
Respiratory complications, in spinal cord injury, 344
Respiratory effort, 278
Respiratory expansion, in trauma score, 278–281
Respiratory failure, 310–311
Respiratory rate, in trauma score, 278–281
Resuscitation. See also sites and types of
 blood transfusion in, 40–43
 in children, 214–219
 in elderly, 260
 fluid. See Fluid resuscitation
 in-hospital, 20
 pre-hospital, 12–13
 in pregnancy, 256
 in shock, 40–45
 videotaping of, 418–419
Retroperitoneal injuries, 30
Revised trauma score, 278–281
Rewarming, in hypothermia and frostbite, 202–203
Rib fractures, 28, 126–127
 in children, 228
 flail chest and, 96
Ringer's lactate. See Fluid resuscitation
Roentgenography. See Radiography
Rule of nines, for burn assessment, 194
Rupture
 aortic, 28, 112–113
  in children, 228
 diaphragmatic, 28
  in children, 228
 esophageal, 118–119
  in children, 228
 uterine, in pregnancy, 258

S

Scapular trauma, 156–157
Sciatic nerve distribution, 181
Sciatic nerve palsy, 164
Sensory evaluation, 340
Sepsis, 302, 330–331
Septal hematoma, nasal, 60
Septic shock, 320–321
Serum sickness, antivenom and, 250
Sexual assault, 252–255
Sexual dysfunction, in spinal cord injury, 345
Shear strain, 1
Shock
 cardiogenic, 22, 316–317
 in children, 214–219
 hypovolemic, 22, 36–39
  blood administration for, 40–43
  fluid warming in, 44–45
  in multisystem trauma, 292–295
 neurogenic, 22, 318–319
 septic, 320–321
 vasogenic, 22
Shotgun injuries, 3. See also sites of
Shoulder trauma, 156–157
Skull fractures, 54–55
 in children, 220–223
Smoke inhalation, 3, 206–207
Snake bites, 250–251
Sodium bicarbonate, for ventricular fibrillation, 428
Sodomy victims, male, 252–255
Spasticity, in head trauma, 338, 340
Specimens, in crimes and accidents, 252, 254, 266–269
Spider bites, 248–249
Spinal anesthesia, 286–287
Spinal cord injury
 autonomic dysreflexia in, 152, 344
 cervical, 144–149. See also Cervical spine injury
 neurogenic shock in, 318–319
 rehabilitation in, 342–345
 thoracolumbar, 152–153
Spinal trauma
 cervical. See Cervical spine injury
 thoracolumbar, 150–153
Splint, Thomas/Hare traction, 404–406
Stab wounds, 3. See also sites of
Steinmann pin, 403
Sternal fracture, 126
Stockings, antiembolism, 394–395
Strain, tissue/structure, 1
Stress gastritis, 324–325
Stryker frame, for cervical spine injury, 397–398
Subclavian artery trauma, 186–187
Subcutaneous emphysema, 124–125
Sucking chest wound, 29, 94–95
 in children, 226
Surgery, operating room management in, 292–295
Swallowing, impairment of, in head trauma, 340
Synchronized intermittent mandatory ventilation, 310
Systolic blood pressure, in trauma score, 278–281

T

Tachycardia, ventricular, sustained, 430–431
Tar burns, 200
Teeth, injuries of, 62–63
Temperature control units, 399–400
Tendon injuries, of hand, 160–161
Tensile strain, 1
Tension pneumothorax, 29, 88–91
 in children, 216, 224
Tertiary closure, 298
Tetanus prophylaxis, 298
Thermal injuries, 3–4. See also Burns
Thomas/Hare traction splint, 404–406
Thoracentesis, 364–365
Thoracic trauma. See Chest trauma
Thoracolumbar spinal trauma, 150–153
Thoracostomy
 needle, in children, 224
 tube. See Chest tube
Thoracotomy
 emergency, 102
  in children, 218
 in massive hemothorax, 92
 in subclavian artery trauma, 186
Thorax. See under Chest
Thrombosis, deep vein, 328–329
 pneumatic pressure device for, 394–395
Tibial nerve distribution, 181
Tibial vascular trauma, 190–191
Tomography. See Computed tomography
Tongs, for cervical spine traction, 397–398
Topical anesthesia, 298
Total parenteral nutrition, 288–289
Tourniquet, for snake bites, 250
Tracheal intubation, 86–87, 358–359. See also Airway management
Tracheal trauma, 28, 76–77, 114, 124
 in children, 228
Tracheostomy, 8, 20, 86–87, 362–363. See also Airway management
 in laryngotracheal trauma, 114
Traction
 for cervical spine injuries, 397–398
 for extremity injuries, 404–406
Traction injuries, peripheral nerve trauma and, 178
Traction splint, Thomas/Hare, 404–406
Transfusion, 22, 40–43, 294
 blood warming for, 44–45
 in children, 218
Transfusion reaction, 42
Transplantation, organ procurement for, 332–333
Transport, airborne, 336–337
Trauma. See also sites and types of
 mechanism of, 1–4
 multisystem, 292
 psychological aspects of, 334–335
Trauma management
 emergency dispatch in, 6
 initial assessment in, 20–24
 pre-hospital, 12–13
 scene management/patient evaluation in, 8–10
 secondary assessment in, 8–10
 triage in, 16
  pediatric, 210–213
 videotaping of, 418–419
Trauma score, 278–281
 CRAMS, 276–277
 Glasgow Coma Scale, 24, 50, 278–279

437

Trauma score, (Continued)
　injury severity, 282–283
　pediatric, 212
　revised, 278–281
Traumatic asphyxia, 28–29
Triage, 16
　pediatric, 210–213
Tube feeding, 288–289
Tube thoracostomy. See Chest tube

U

Ulnar nerve distribution, 180
Upper extremity. See under Extremity
Uremia, 304–305
Urinary output
　in comatose organ donor, 332
　measurement of, 296
Urinary tract infection, 330–331
Urologic problems, in head trauma rehabilitation, 342
Uterine trauma, in pregnancy, 258

V

Vaccine
　rabies
　　for animal bites, 246–247
　　for dog bites, 244–245
　tetanus, 298
Vascular injuries
　angiographic signs of, 186
　arterial, signs of, 188
　axillary artery, 186–187
　brachial artery, 186–187
　carotid artery, 184–185
　of knee, 166–167
　of lower leg, 168
　in neck trauma
　　blunt, 75
　　penetrating, 80–81
　signs of, 184
　subclavian artery, 186–187
　of upper extremity, 158–159
Vascular insufficiency. See also Compartment syndrome
　signs of, 204
Vasogenic shock, 22
Vehicular accidents
　corset-type extraction devices for, 413–414
　helmet removal in, 413–414
　mechanism of injury in, 1–2
Vena cava syndrome, in pregnancy, 256
Venous access
　in children, 218
　temporary, for hemodialysis, 396
Venous thrombosis, 328–329
　pneumatic pressure device for, 394–395
Ventilation, mechanical, 310, 312–315
Ventilatory assessment, 20
Ventilatory failure, 310–311
Ventricular fibrillation, 426–429
Ventricular tachycardia, sustained, 430–431
Vertebrae
　cervical, fracture of, 8, 20, 26, 76–79, 144–147, 146–149
　thoracolumbar, fracture of, 150–153

Videotaping, of trauma resuscitation, 418–419
Vision loss, 66

W

Warfarin, for pulmonary embolism/deep vein thrombosis, 328
Warming devices, 399–400
Weaning, ventilator, 312–313
Wheelchair, for spinal cord injury patients, 342
Wild animal bites, rabies prophylaxis for, 210–211
Wounds
　classification of, 166, 168
　closure of, 298
　culture of, 298, 302
　dressings for, 403–404
　infection of, 302, 330–331
　　gas gangrene, 306–307
　local exploration of, 382
　open
　　dressings for, 401–402
　　management of, 296–299
Wrist trauma, 158–159

X

X-ray films. See Radiography

Z

Zygomatic fractures, 66, 70–71